EVERYTHING YOU NEED TO KNOW ABOUT

# HEALING

RICK RENNER

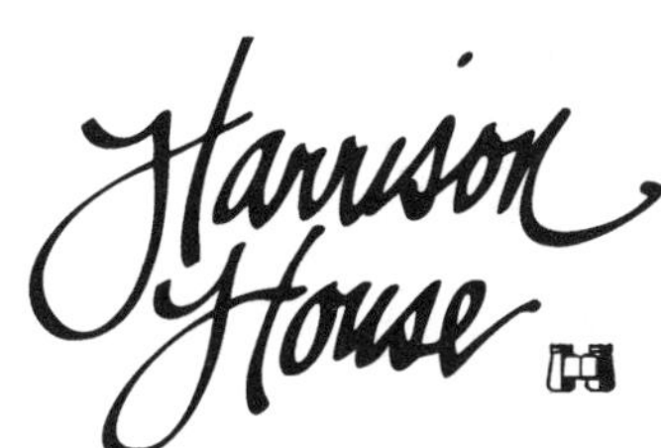

# EVERYTHING YOU NEED TO KNOW ABOUT

# HEALING

Unless otherwise indicated, all scriptural quotations are from the *King James Version* of the Bible.

Scripture quotations marked *AMP* are from *The Amplified Bible, Old Testament* © 1965, 1987 by the Zondervan Corporation. *The Amplified New Testament* © 1958, 1987 by The Lockman Foundation. Used by permission.

Scripture quotations marked *AMPC* are taken from *The Amplified Bible. Old Testament* copyright © 1965, 1987 by Zondervan Corporation, Grand Rapids, Michigan. New Testament copyright © 1958, 1987 by The Lockman Foundation, La Habra, California. All rights reserved.

Scripture quotations noted as *ESV* are taken from *The Holy Bible, English Standard Version*®, Copyright © 2016 by Crossway Bibles, a division of Good News Publishers. Used by permission. All rights reserved.

All Scriptures marked *NKJV* are taken from the *New King James Version* of the Bible © 1979, 1980, 1982 by Thomas Nelson, Inc. All rights reserved.

Scriptures quoted from the *Renner Interpretive Version*® (*RIV*) copyrighted © 2020, 2024 by Teaching You Can Trust, LLC, and published by Harrison House Publishers. Used by permission. Renner.org. Harrisonhouse.com.

*Everything You Need To Know About Healing*
Trade Paper: 978-1-6675-1239-6
Ebook: 978-1-6675-1240-2
Hardcover: 978-1-6675-1285-3
Large Print: 978-1-6675-1286-0



Published by Harrison House
Shippensburg, PA 17257-2914
www.harrisonhouse.com

1 2 3 4 5 / 30 29 28 27 26
1st printing

Editorial Consultants: Rebecca L. Gilbert and Veronica L. Bagby
Text Design: Lisa Simpson

# ENDORSEMENTS

*The following endorsements were written by those closely connected to healing ministry.*

I am deeply honored that Rick Renner would ask me to endorse his new book. As always, he has dug deeply into the truth of God's Word.

In this book, Rick shows that one of many doors we can open for sickness is worry, which is rooted in fear and comes from meditating on the lies of the devil. On the other hand, faith comes from meditating on the truth of God's WORD. The Savior's purpose, according to God's WORD, was, and still is, to destroy the works of the devil. A careful study of Scripture makes it clear that Jesus came not to only bear our sin but also our sicknesses — and to carry our diseases — so that we might walk in divine health. The moment Jesus sat down at the right hand of the Father, His blood declared that *we are healed!*

I wholeheartedly encourage you to not only read this book but to study it with your Bible in hand. I truly believe that by the time you finish, your body will be strengthened, your mind will be renewed, and your confidence in Jesus will be greater than ever before. This book is a faith-builder, and we know it is impossible to please God without faith. *Well done, Brother Rick!*

Always remember that all is well in the household of faith.

We love you, God loves you, and Jesus is Lord!

*Kenneth Copeland*
Kenneth Copeland Ministries
Fort Worth, Texas

---

The Scripture says, "God is love," so it makes perfect sense that healing is a central theme throughout the Bible. The Scripture is clear that healing is not only offered by God, it is actually His nature to heal. Still, somehow, millions of people are confused and even skeptical about whether healing is God's will. Sadly, this includes many believers.

Thank God for Rick Renner! Once again, Rick dives into the Bible, this time on the subject of healing, and lets God's Word speak for itself. In true Rick Renner style, his explanations of the original Greek words clear up any confusion about God's will for His people to be well. But then there is the haunting question everyone has asked at one time or another: "If it is God's will for me to be healed, why am I still sick?"

In *Everything You Need To Know About Healing*, Rick continues unfolding hidden treasures from the original language about the major reasons people do not receive healing. While the explanations of the Scripture are thorough, they are not complicated or difficult to understand. All are likely to find the answers to the questions they have about their own lives and others. This book is also a tremendous resource for every minister or layman who desires to help others take advantage of God's great gift of healing.

Are you in need of healing? Or do you know someone who is? Read this book. Are you a minister, a professor, or Bible teacher? You should have this book. Are you a believer who wants a solid grasp on supernatural healing and overcoming obstacles? Then get this book. With this book in one hand and Bible in the other, the answers to past failures are only a few page turns away. Again, thank God for Rick Renner!

*George and Terri Pearsons, Senior Pastors*
Eagle Mountain International Church
Newark, Texas

---

As a board-certified neurosurgeon who has practiced medicine and surgery in 10,000 patients over more than 20 years, I have treated physically and mentally disease-ridden people in all forms and presentations. This has often been a result of unhealthy habits. There were few that I've encountered who had good habits but suffered acute injury and required immediate life-saving intervention. As a result of my experiences, the Holy Spirit was clear that I was to teach on the steps leading to the tripart human's health from a faith-filled brain surgeon's perspective.

Through our ministry, The God Prescription, the Lord has facilitated collaboration with many nationally and internationally known Christian leaders to educate on the steps to living a long life. The Body Healthcare, our current work, combines member-to-member services in a national healthcare system with a goal of furthering our collective wellness. Information that reveals how to apply important wholeness principles to our global population is imperative to mitigate disease and promote health.

Dr. Rick Renner's book *Everything You Need To Know About Healing* highlights timely scriptural and medical truths to support the need for us, individually and collectively, to take ownership of our health. We must be active participants in building a healthy body and mind from good lifestyle habits of movement and diet.

Dr. Renner offers this book with a lovingly sober perspective on how our choices can lead to the need to invest "catch up" time into our spiritual, mental, and physical health later in life. We have the power to create the condition in which we would like to spend our lives now and in our latter years.

This book is chock full of "gems" that can lead us to better strategic positions for our current and future selves. He exhorts us to strive to reach that perfect peace with nothing missing or broken, literally! *Everything You Need To Know About Healing* is an accurate must-read. It will benefit you and your entire family and community for years to come!

Congratulations, Dr. Rick Renner, on a work well done!

*Avery M. Jackson III, MD*
Neurosurgeon, Trustee, Michigan Neurosurgical Institute
Great Lakes Learning
The God Prescription
The Body Healthcare
Grand Blanc, Michigan

I am honored to endorse my dear friend, Rick Renner, and this powerful, truth-filled book *Everything You Need to Know About Healing*. This is not just another book about healing — it's a life manual that shines light on God's will for wholeness in every area of our lives.

From the opening chapter, where Rick transparently shares his own story of how he came to believe in healing, to the deep biblical insights that follow, this book is both theologically rich and practically transforming. Each chapter builds with purpose — exposing seven root causes of sickness that believers often overlook, then guiding readers through the redemptive work of Jesus Christ and the many ways to walk in divine health.

I especially appreciate how Rick doesn't shy away from addressing the hard truths. He deals directly with the areas where believers sometime "self-inflict" sickness and shows how applying God's Word can bring real, lasting change. His teaching on Isaiah 53 and the meaning of redemption is outstanding, and his balance in addressing the natural aspects — diet, rest, and lifestyle — makes this book both spiritually grounded and practically wise.

Whether you're believing for your own healing, ministering to others, or simply wanting to understand God's redemptive plan in full, this book will stir your faith and renew your confidence in the healing power of Jesus Christ.

I highly recommend *Everything You Need To Know About Healing*. Read it, apply it, and watch what God will do in your life.

*Kenneth W. Hagin*
Pastor, Rhema Bible Church
President, Kenneth Hagin Ministries
Broken Arrow, Oklahoma

---

One of the greatest needs in the Body of Christ today is a clear understanding and personal experience of God's abundant provision for healing. For decades, beginning with my parents, Drs. T .L. and Daisy Osborn, our family has witnessed remarkable miracles of healing in more than 100 nations — evidence of the power of Christ's redemptive work. The remarkable results we have witnessed are the direct outcome of what we have come to know about God's plan and Christ's redemptive work.

Countless books have been written on biblical healing, but few provide the depth of practical insight found in this remarkable work by Rick Renner. *Everything You Need To Know About Healing* is more than a study — it is a life-giving guide that will open your heart and mind to the transforming truths of God's Word. You were not created to live with sickness; in these pages you will discover the keys to walking in divine health through wisdom and faith in the finished work of Jesus Christ.

*LaDonna Osborn, D.Min.*
Osborn.org
Tulsa, Oklahoma

---

God wanted someone to write a new book on healing, and the Holy Spirit chose Rick Renner to write it. In this must-read tome, God is saying, "I want to heal you, but here is what is blocking it. Here is how healing came through the Cross." Finally, here are the truths about healing and living in health, and you can learn how healing miracles are to be a normal part of our life. Read it!

*Mario Murillo*
Mario Murillo Ministries
Lafayette, Tennessee

---

This timely book *Everything You Need To Know About Healing* by Rick Renner is one of the most, if not *the* most, comprehensive study on the subject of healing that I have personally encountered. From the beginning chapter, this collection of Rick's research, personal revelation, and practical approach will be sure to unlock the reader's faith to know and expect to receive the healing flow of the Holy Spirit. Regardless of one's personal circumstances, this read will release rivers of living water to flow in you and flow through you, touching you in the deep places of your soul. This book is sure to stir both a hunger and a passion to read it over and over again. Thank you, Rick, for addressing this much-needed subject in a manner that all can both read and understand.

*Billy Burke*
Billy Burke Ministries
Tampa, Florida

---

Once again Rick Renner has produced a book that is greatly needed by the Body of Christ (and the world at large). Rick's book *Everything You Need To Know About* Healing is just that! As usual, Rick has done deep research concerning healing and covers a wide spectrum. Too often, healing (like most other Bible topics) is looked at from only one perspective. Rick covers many areas, from the spiritual to the natural. He brings out truths concerning how people get sick and how they can get well and stay well. He proves healing is definitely God's will for every person and that Jesus provided healing through His redemptive sacrifice.

This is a book that every serious Christian should have in his possession! I can assure you, all of my staff and our leaders around the world will own this book, even if I have to buy it for them myself.

*Curry R. Blake*
General Overseer
John G. Lake Ministries
JGLM.org
Plano, Texas

---

Rick Renner's books were among those I read in my formative years as a new evangelist. I was elated to learn that he now has a work available specifically devoted to the subject of divine health and healing, a ministry expression in which I am highly invested. As I read through this masterfully written work, I learned new truths and had my faith stirred to believe for and minister God's healing power.

Page after page, this book is packed with treasures, and, with precision, Renner delivers treasures that both answer the big questions and fill in the nuanced details regarding divine healing. To say I'm excited to recommend this book is an understatement. Every believer needs this book in his library. I thank God for the brilliant mind and the teaching ability of Rick Renner.

*David Diga Hernandez, Evangelist*
David Hernandez Ministries
Round Rock, Texas

---

Rick Renner writes, "My eyes had now been opened that healing and miraculous power was not just a relic of the past but still at work in the here and now!"

Every generation has the right to see healing and miraculous power at work in the here and now! God's healing and miracle power should not be just a relic of the past that we simply admire, for it is a harvesting tool, advertising God's undeniable love for mankind. But we won't just float into manifestations of His power — we must gain knowledge of the will of God and the ways of God. We must learn how to receive healing power, as well as minister it to others.

James asked, *"Is there any sick among you?"* (James 5:14). He implies that it was possible that there was no one sick among them. As the Body of Christ, we should set our faith and declare, "No more sickness in the Body of Christ!" We should not be okay with less than God's best! But to experience God's best, we have to preach it, develop our faith for it, and expect it!

That's why I so appreciate this in-depth teaching on healing that Rick Renner brings in this much-needed book that calls the Body of Christ back to living in God's best — divine healing and divine health!

*Nancy Dufresne*
Dufresne Ministries
Murrieta, California

As a physician, I've seen firsthand how connected our spiritual, emotional, and physical health truly are. Rick Renner captures this beautifully, and his insights offer a clear and hope-filled path toward real wholeness and healing.

*James Ross, MD*
Tulsa, Oklahoma

# DEDICATION

With great joy, I dedicate this book to Kenneth E. Hagin, Kathryn Kuhlman, and Oral Roberts, three ministers whom God used early in my life to open my eyes to divine healing and the miraculous power of God. God used each of them in unique ways to establish me in the biblical truth that Jesus Christ is indeed the same yesterday, today, and forever.

In the earliest part of my spiritual journey, God graciously introduced me to the ministry of Kenneth E. Hagin, and it was in one of his meetings in 1974 that I received a dramatic healing that brought resolution to a serious health issue in my life. Later I came across the radio ministry of Kathryn Kuhlman, and almost every afternoon, I waited for the moment when she would come on the air to talk about the ministry of the Holy Spirit and share testimonies of miracles that occurred in her miracle services. When it was announced that she was coming to hold one of those services in Tulsa, I attended that meeting (and others as well), and it was there that I was first visually confronted by the miracle-working power of God.

Then I attended a class at Oral Roberts University called The Holy Spirit in the Now that was taught weekly by Oral Roberts himself. As I sat on the front row each week, I hung onto every word that he spoke in that class and even recorded each lesson with the tape recorder that I always brought with me to class. Then at the conclusion of each session as others exited the auditorium, I lingered to watch as Oral faithfully laid his large hands on people who requested prayer for healing.

I am thankful that God used these three individuals to establish me in Bible truths about faith, healing, and the power of the Holy Spirit. Remarkably, as I got older and God began to use me in my own ministry, I came to either personally know or to correspond with each of these ministers before they went to Heaven. But because of their impact on my life regarding the subject of this book, I choose to dedicate my first book on healing to Kenneth E. Hagin, Kathryn Kuhlman, and Oral Roberts.

# CONTENTS

# FOREWORD
## BY RICHARD ROBERTS

Having grown up in the healing ministry, and having my own healing ministry with signs and wonders following for many years, I am deeply moved by Rick Renner's new book *Everything You Need To Know About Healing.*

As I read his personal testimony of how his search for his godly destiny led him to three individuals, Kathryn Kuhlman, Kenneth Hagin, and my father Oral Roberts, I rejoiced in the eternal truth that if you seek the Lord with all your heart, soul, and strength, you will find Him. And when you do, you'll know your true purpose and reason for being on this earth.

I've known Rick for many years. He and his wife, Denise, and my wife, Lindsay, and I are great friends. I well remember that after the Soviet Union fell, Rick was led of the Lord to build a great church in Riga, Latvia. That church was thriving and growing tremendously when all of a sudden, out of the blue, God spoke to him and told him to move to Moscow.

*Wow!* But he obeyed, and the Lord has blessed him and his ministry tremendously in Russia's capital city, and has given him favor unknown to just about anyone else.

Rick's extensive knowledge of the Greek language has given him an unusual ability to interpret Scripture and especially to shed light on the teachings of Jesus, Paul, and others concerning healing. I treasured reading the manuscript when it was first sent to me and feel quite honored that I was asked to write this brief foreword for the book.

I heartily write this foreword and believe this book will be a tremendous blessing to all who read it. Dive into it. Read every word. Submerge your spirit in it. Keep your Bible handy and refer to the many scriptures that Rick gives in confirmation.

With all my heart, I believe that as you read, you'll never be the same.

*Richard Roberts*
Chairman and CEO
Oral Roberts Evangelistic Association
Tulsa, Oklahoma

# FOREWORD
## BY ANDREW WOMMACK

I believe health and healing to be some of the most important aspects of our Christian life while we are here on Earth.

I've seen my wife and son both raised from the dead, as well as a few other people. It is such a blessing to have them still with me. My son was dead for more than four hours and was in a morgue, stripped naked with a toe tag on. When we prayed, he sat up and started talking! One year later, he gave us our granddaughter. My life would be quite different without the resurrection power of the Lord available to us today.

Kenneth Hagin used to say that healing was like a dinner bell that drew people to the Lord, and I can certainly validate that. There are countless numbers of people whom I've seen come to the Lord because of the healing videos we've produced of people who were healed of multiple sclerosis, cancer, Crohn's disease, heart problems, and many other maladies.

The good news is that healing is not just for a select few, but for everyone. It's a part of Jesus' atonement, just as much as the forgiveness of our sins. That's a radical statement, but it's backed up by Scripture. And who is better at uncovering the awesome truths of God's Word than my good friend Rick Renner!

Rick is an expositor of the Greek like no other minister I know. He can paint a word picture of biblical words that unlocks truths and makes you wonder, *How come I never saw that before?* God's truths aren't hidden *from* us, but *for* us. It takes some effort to mine the depths of God's Word, and Rick is one of the best "miners" I know. In this book, you will find treasures that are far greater than gold or silver.

God's Word is health to all our flesh and life to those who find it (Proverbs 4:22). God's Word will heal you and deliver you from all the destruction Satan is trying to bring into your life (Psalm 107:20). The faith required for healing comes from understanding the truth of God's Word (Romans 10:17), but it's only the truth you know that sets you free (John 8:32). That's where Rick is a special gift to the Body of Christ.

Rick makes God's Word come alive. I've experienced that myself and have witnessed many others have the same experience as Rick broke open the Bread of Life and shared it with us. Rick is always one of our students' favorite guest ministers at Charis Bible College, and we are not alone. Rick's ministry reaches around the world through television, teaching materials, and his phenomenal ministry in Moscow, Russia. He has more than four decades of ministry experience that has borne fruit in the lives of millions of people.

You are about to experience this for yourself as you take an in-depth study through the Scriptures with Rick on what Jesus has already provided for you. It's not a matter of getting the Lord to heal you. It's all about you just receiving what Jesus has already provided (Philemon 1:6). But as the old saying goes, "You don't know what you don't know." We are destroyed for a lack of knowledge (Hosea 4:6). But Rick is anointed by the Lord to take complex truths from God's Word and make them so simple, you would have to have somebody help you to misunderstand them!

I know the Lord wants you healed more than you want it, and I know that the Lord has gifted Rick with a supernatural ability to make God's Word come alive to those who will receive it.

Get ready to kiss your days of sickness good-bye. Actually, just kick sickness out without any good-byes. It doesn't deserve any kindness. It has never been kind to you. Treat sickness like what it really is — an attack from the devil that has come only to steal, kill, and destroy your life (John 10:10).

The Lord wishes above everything else that you prosper and be in health, just as much as He wants your soul to prosper (3 John 2). This book is a key that will unlock the truths of God's Word and open up a whole new life of health and healing to you.

I'm so glad the Lord put it on Rick's heart to write this book, and I know you'll be glad, too, as you see the truths of God's Word come alive and set you free.

*Andrew Wommack*<br>
Founder and President<br>
Andrew Wommack Ministries<br>
Charis Bible College<br>
Colorado Springs, Colorado

# ACKNOWLEDGMENTS

I have been in the ministry many decades and have written a large number of books, but this is my first book dedicated to the subjects of healing and divine health. For many years, I felt that because others had covered this topic so well, my insights would not add much to the subject. However, as I have grown older, I've begun to sense the Holy Spirit tugging on my heart that it was time for me to step into this arena to add my contributions to this important Bible topic that literally affects all of us.

As I begin to acknowledge those who helped on this project, I want to start by acknowledging the various ministers who directly or indirectly influenced my thinking about healing and divine health over the years. As a young man, I was reared in a denomination that adhered to cessationism, so not only did I not believe, I even argued against the notion that healing and miracles still occurred in our time. But upon hearing the remarkable teachings of certain ministers in my earlier years, my eyes were opened to see that healing and divine health really were purchased in Christ's redemptive work on the Cross and that they belong to anyone who will lay claim to them by faith. Among others that God notably used, I was deeply impacted by the ministries of Kenneth E. Hagin, Kathryn Kuhlman, and Oral Roberts.

But before my books are published, I always ask key individuals, whom I consider to be scripturally trustworthy and spiritually mature, to read what I have written and to alert me to anything that may need to be more accurately articulated. For this particular book on healing and divine health, I am grateful to Denise, who contemplated every word as she carefully read chapter by chapter; to Joel Renner, who has a remarkable ability to analyze spiritual truths and an interesting way of articulating them; to John Carter, Tony Cooke, and Bishop Keith Butler, dear friends who took time out of their busy schedules to read major portions of this book that I felt needed examination by a keen doctrinal eye; and to Andrell Corbin Stevens, who read portions of the manuscript and helped me communicate more accurately to my reading audience. I'm also grateful to Dr. Chip Beaulieu for the use of his meticulously researched manuscript *Our Healing Covenant* and for allowing me to use many of the translations of Bible verses on healing from his book that you'll find here in Chapter Fifteen.

I also want to acknowledge two medical doctors who reviewed every portion of this book that contained medical information or commentary. I am referring to Dr. James Ross in Tulsa, Oklahoma, who pored over every one of these sections and helped me to be correct in the way these various passages were written. I also wish to express my thanks to Dr. Avery Jackson in Grand Blanc, Michigan, a renowned neurosurgeon, who likewise read these passages to help ensure that what I had written was correct and in line with the most recent medical understanding. The contribution of these two outstanding doctors was very important, and I acknowledge them gratefully for the time they invested to help me bring you a resource you can trust.

I want to acknowledge Becky Gilbert, the chief editor at Rick Renner Ministries, who is a gifted editor with a deep commitment to Christ and who reads every word I write with spiritual eyes. I also wish to acknowledge Becky's team of proofreaders that included Roni Bagby, Pamela Page, and Beth Parker. I am likewise thankful to Pamela Page and Elizabeth Hodgson, who assisted with footnoting and compiling all the verses on healing that I've included in Chapter Fifteen of the book. I want to acknowledge Lisa Moore for her work on the front and back covers of this book — and Lisa Simpson for typesetting this manuscript in a way to make it enjoyable for readers. I also want to express my gratitude to Don Nori and the entire team at Harrison House Publishers for being the best publishing partners we have ever had in our history of writing and publishing books.

In addition, I gratefully acknowledge Maxim Myasnikov, my assistant in Moscow, who assisted me in my research of every Greek word that is used in this book — and Keith Trump, an American Bible Society scholar, awarded the highest honors for his studies in Hebrew and Greek, who examined my insights on Isaiah 53:3-5 to ensure they indeed reflect the meanings contained in the original text of the Old Testament.

Most importantly, I wish to express my heartfelt thanks to Jesus Christ my Lord, who called me and who has graciously chosen to use us and our ministry in this last-days season of the Church Age. In 1978, it was He who called me to write, promising me that if I would *"write, write, write,"* He would bless what I wrote. From that moment on, I understood my assignment was to write and that He would bless me as I did it. As I look back over the many years I've been writing, I thankfully acknowledge that He has indeed blessed what He has graciously enabled me to write.

*To Him be all the glory.*

# INTRODUCTION

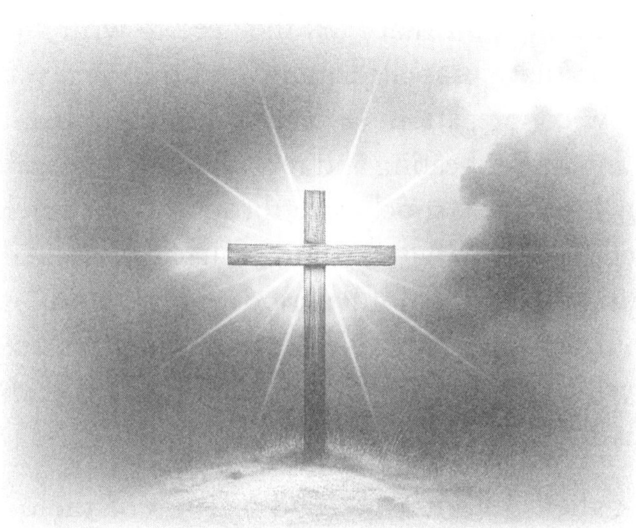

# HOPE FOR THE JOURNEY

Each year, our ministry is blessed with the opportunity to receive countless prayer requests, many of which come from individuals seeking healing for themselves or for loved ones and friends. It is a deep honor to unite our faith with theirs and steadfastly trust in the manifestation of God's healing promises in their lives. In response to our faith-filled prayers, we regularly hear from people who reach out again to let us know they (or those they know and love) received healing or grew progressively better after we prayed with them. *Oh, how we love to hear those praise reports!*

But there are also others with whom we agreed in prayer for healing who are still waiting for the answer to come, and in some cases those individuals have waited so long that it seems to them as if the answer has been endlessly delayed. Some have waited so long that hope appears to wear thin, and questions loom large: *Why does my healing remain unseen? Why does healing elude me despite my steadfast faith?* Or, *Am I doing something wrong that prevents my healing from taking place?* These instances leave people grappling with profound, and often unanswered, questions.

It is because of these people that I felt the need to write this book. However, the decisive moment that compelled me to write it *now* was a heartbreaking one. In our Moscow congregation, several faithful members fell ill, seemingly all at one time. Many found healing and recovery, but, tragically, some lost their lives. This wave of loss sent a shockwave through our church, where over the years, we have been blessed to witness numerous healings and rare instances of death due to illness. It was this painful period of illness and loss that led sincere, earnest souls within our church to ask the question: "If Jesus has indeed paid the price for our well-being, why have some of our dear friends been claimed by disease and sickness?"

It is because of their questions — and because of the questions of others who have written to me over the years with similar questions — that I decided to write this book *Everything You Need To Know About Healing*. Healing, as a subject, is vast and complex — too intricate to be entirely captured in just one volume. Yet within these pages, I've endeavored to comprehensively explore an array of topics that I believe resonate with the questions many carry in their hearts. I'm talking about topics such as:

- What are the seven main reasons why people get sick?
- What is the role of redemption in deliverance and healing?
- What exactly did Jesus' sacrifice on the Cross purchase?
- What needs to happen for a person to receive healing for the body or mind?
- When is the moment to call for the elders of the church to come anoint with oil and pray the prayer of faith?
- What is the role of diet, exercise, supplements, doctors, medicine, and a balanced life in receiving healing and maintaining health?

- What is needed for a person to stay strong and healthy as he or she grows older?
- What steps should be taken for a person to consistently live in divine health?
- What are God's scriptural promises for healing?
- *And so much more…*

## PRAYING FOR HEALING WITH ABSOLUTE CONFIDENCE

I want to emphasize once more that attempting to encapsulate every facet of the origins of disease and the mysteries of delayed healing within a single book is simply not possible. But in this book, I have chosen to concentrate on what I believe are the most crucial topics related to healing. However, as we begin this exploration, let me draw your attention to First John 5:14-15, which says, "And this is the confidence that we have in him, that, if we ask any thing according to his will, he heareth us: and if we know that he hear us, whatsoever we ask, we know that we have the petitions that we desired of him."

This passage assures us that we can possess unwavering conviction that when we petition for anything aligned with God's will, He both listens and responds affirmatively. The word "confidence" in this verse is interpreted from the Greek word *parresia*, signifying a manner of expressing oneself *boldly*, *candidly*, and with *straightforwardness.* This bold kind of speech is often translated in the New Testament as the word "confidence." Indeed, it depicts *a confident kind of speaking — a daring to speak exactly what one believes or thinks with no hesitation or intimidation.* Within this context, it means if we know our prayers are in harmony with God's will, we have the liberty to approach God with *boldness*, *honesty*, and *directness* as we present our petitions to Him.

In fact, verse 14 goes on to say that "…if we *ask* anything according to His will, he heareth us…." The word "ask" is from a form of the Greek word *aiteo*, which conveys a sense of *demanding* or *insisting.* This term paints a picture of someone who approaches prayer with authority, unafraid to present his needs and fully expects to receive what he seeks. The confidence of such a person stems from the fact that he or she is asking "according to His will." This means that individual is not just randomly asking for anything he or she wishes, but is praying "according to His will."

When you pray with the assurance that what you're praying aligns with God's scriptures, there is no need to be timid. Instead, stand firm, assert your faith, and expect God to respond!

## PRAYING ACCORDING TO THE WILL OF GOD IS THE KEY

First John 5:14 continues to say that if we are praying according to His will — or according to what God has revealed in His Word — "He heareth us." God's ear is attuned to His own promises spoken back to Him, and that is what prompts Him to take action. While our emotions and needs matter deeply to Him, it is ultimately the confident, heartfelt recitation of His promises that stirs Him to respond. Therefore, understanding what God has revealed as His will, particularly concerning healing, is of utmost importance. Indeed, First John 5:14 states that God is moved to action when He hears a believer boldly praying the promises of His Word.

But as mentioned before, God responds to prayers when they are aligned with the teachings and truths found in His Word. This is why it is crucial to align your prayers with His will. Knowing the will of God — and praying according to the will of God — is *absolutely essential* if you want to see your prayers answered. In this book, I will endeavor to show you that it is absolutely God's will for you to be healed and to live in health. You will see in the pages to come that these blessings are included in Christ's work of redemption on the Cross.

## GOD'S EXPLICIT WILL FOR YOUR LIFE

In Third John, verse 2, the apostle John expressed the will of God when he wrote, "Beloved, I wish above all things that thou mayest prosper and be in health even as thy soul prospereth."

This verse is *an unequivocal declaration of God's explicit will* for your life, and, hence, it is key for you to understand this verse. Having this verse cemented into your heart and mind will put you on a foundation so strong that you can confidently release your faith for divine healing.

The word "wish" in this verse is a translation of the Greek word *euchomai*, which expresses one's *strongest desire or will.* John was writing by inspiration of the Holy Spirit, which means this was not only John's strongest desire and will, but because the Holy Spirit was writing through him, John was expressing *God's strongest desire* for His people. This means in this verse, we discover *the explicit will of God* for every authentic believer.

Since the explicit will of God for every believer is stated in this verse, we need to really examine it to discover God's will for each of us. John wrote, "...I wish above all things that thou mayest prosper and be in health even as thy soul prospereth." The words "above all things" are an interpretation of the Greek words *peri panton*. The word *peri* pictures *a circumference* and *what surrounds you*, and the word *panton* is *all-inclusive* and pictures *everything*. As a phrase, it means *absolutely everything that encompasses you, surrounds you, and concerns you — and that means absolutely everything.*

Then John added that it was his desire (and because he was writing by the inspiration of the Holy Spirit, he was actually expressing *God's* will) that God's people "prosper." The word "prosper" is interpreted from a form of the Greek word *euodoo*, which is a compound of the words *eu* and *hodos*. The word *eu* means *good* and pictures what is *enjoyable, delightful, and pleasurable*, and the word *hodos* is the Greek word for *a road.* As the compounded word *euodoo* that

John used, it means to have *a joyful, enjoyable, delightful, and pleasurable experience on every road of life that you take.*

In the ancient world, prosperity was frequently measured by the size of one's home or the quantity of other possessions in addition to one's having enough finances so that he could freely travel abroad and take vacations.[1] For example, when Paul was ministering with such great results in Ephesus, and the idol-makers feared their "wealth" would be affected. The word "wealth" used in Acts 20:25 is translated from the Greek word *euporia*, a word similar to *euudoo* in Third John 3, because it also means *to have the ability to travel and have an enjoyable traveling experience.*

The idol-workers in Ephesus measured their *prosperity* and *wealth* by whether they had enough financial resources to travel and vacation abroad. Whether they were traveling to faraway places on expeditions to enhance their trade or their studies as explorers and hobbyists, or they were traveling and enjoying lesiure time away in a foreign land — travel was an indicator of a person's wealth and status. These idol-workers feared that Paul's preaching — and the infiltration of the Gospel into the culture, causing people to stop buying the idols they made — would affect their income to the point they would no longer be able to travel abroad and take vacations.

The way this word was used in history tells us that the word *euodoo* John used when he said it was his [and God's] will that believers "prosper" meant that God wants His people to have not only enough money to pay their basic bills, but *enough extra* to enjoy life to the point *they can travel and enjoy themselves.*

In the First Century, traveling was an outward sign of prosperity and wealth. The same might be true today in the way some measure prosperity, but, largely, people measure wealth differently in modern society — for example, by the size of people's homes or the quantity of their possessions or other resources. But the ability to travel was a pronounced mark of prosperity in the ancient world.

Maybe traveling is not your dream, but according to the verses we've seen previously, the word "prosperity" (Greek — *euodoo*) pictures *having more than enough to pay your basic bills and sufficient resources to enjoy any road of life that you will ever take.* In other words, it is not God's will for you to struggle and barely make it in life, but to have enough financially to enjoy yourself along the way.

But notice John then added that it was his strongest desire [and God's] that the people of God "be in health." The word "health" is interpreted from a form of *hugiaino*, a word that depicts one's physical health as being *healthy, in good working order, and in sound condition*, and it includes *mental soundness.* The reason it is translated as the word "whole" is, it carries the idea of *wholeness* or of *one who is complete and sound in every part of his being.*

In John 5, we discover that the word *hugiaino* is used *four times* concerning the lame man at the pool of Bethesda.

- In John 5:6, Jesus asked the lame man, "Wilt thou be made whole?" The word "whole" is from a form of *hugiaino*, which means Jesus was actually asking if he wanted *to be healthy, in good working order*, and *sound physically and mentally.*
- In John 5:9, we read that after Jesus told the man to pick up his bed and walk, he was "made *whole.*" The word "whole" is again translated from a form of *hugiaino*, which means he was immediately *made healthy, restored to good working order, and made sound physically and mentally.*
- In John 5:11, after the religious leaders asked who healed him, the healed man answered that it was Jesus who had made him "whole." The word "whole" is again translated from a form of *hugiaino*, which means he testified that it was Jesus who had made him *healthy, in good working order, and sound physically and mentally.*
- In John 5:14, after Jesus found the man, He told him, "Behold, thou art made whole." The word "whole is again translated from a form of *hugiaino*, which means Jesus jubilantly acknowledged that the man was now *healthy, in good working order, and sound physically and mentally.*

So when John wrote that it was his [and God's] strongest desire and will that God's people be in "health," it meant that God wants His people to be *healthy, physically in good working order, and sound physically and mentally.*

In Third John 2, John wrote, "Beloved, I wish above all things that thou mayest prosper and be in health...," and we covered the words "wish," "above all things," "prosper," and "health." But then John added "as thy soul prospereth." The word "soul" refers to their *emotions, mind, and will* and, herein, we find that God not only wants us to be in good physical health, but He wants His Word to transform our souls to the point that every thought — or every road the mind finds itself traveling — will be filled with the abundance of God's grace. But overall, we find that it is God's explicit will for His people *to be healthy, in good physical working order, sound physically, and abundantly blessed with good mental health.*

**The *RIV* (*Renner Interpretive Version*) of Third John 2 says:**

> **My dearly loved brothers, it is my strongest desire that you prosper in every way that concerns you — that you not only have enough money to pay your basic bills but enough extra so you can really enjoy yourselves on every road of life that you take — and that you be healthy, in good, physical working order, sound physically in every way, and that you are blessed with good mental health.**

You see, the Bible clearly states that it is God's unequivocal will for you to prosper on every road you take in life and for you to continuously enjoy the benefits of good physical and mental health. It is my heartfelt prayer that the Holy Spirit will use this book to enlighten your understanding and provide long sought-after answers that will put you on both a supernatural and commonsense path that will lead you into the healing and health that Jesus purchased at the Cross for you.

I understand the temptation of skimming through the pages of a book to find the most captivating parts. However, this book is crafted as a journey from its opening words to its closing sentence. So I encourage you to resist the urge to leap between sections. Begin with Chapter One and immerse yourself in each word until you reach the book's end. Healing and health are needed by every person — including you and those you know and love — and for this reason, I believe this book may be one of the most important books you've ever read.

As you will see, there are some sections in this book that contain health-related recommendations and medical facts. Because I am not a medical professional, I asked notable medical professionals to carefully review each of these sections to ensure they are correct.

Now that I've introduced you to where we are headed in this book and encouraged you to embark on this adventure to the very last word, the moment has finally arrived to dive into Chapter One, where I share my personal healing journey. I'm thrilled to embark on this journey with you, and I believe the pages ahead will provide answers to questions you've long sought after. May the Holy Spirit guide you through this book and use it to walk you into the healing and the healthy life God wants you to have and to enjoy!

*Rick Renner*
*July 2025*
*Moscow, Russia*

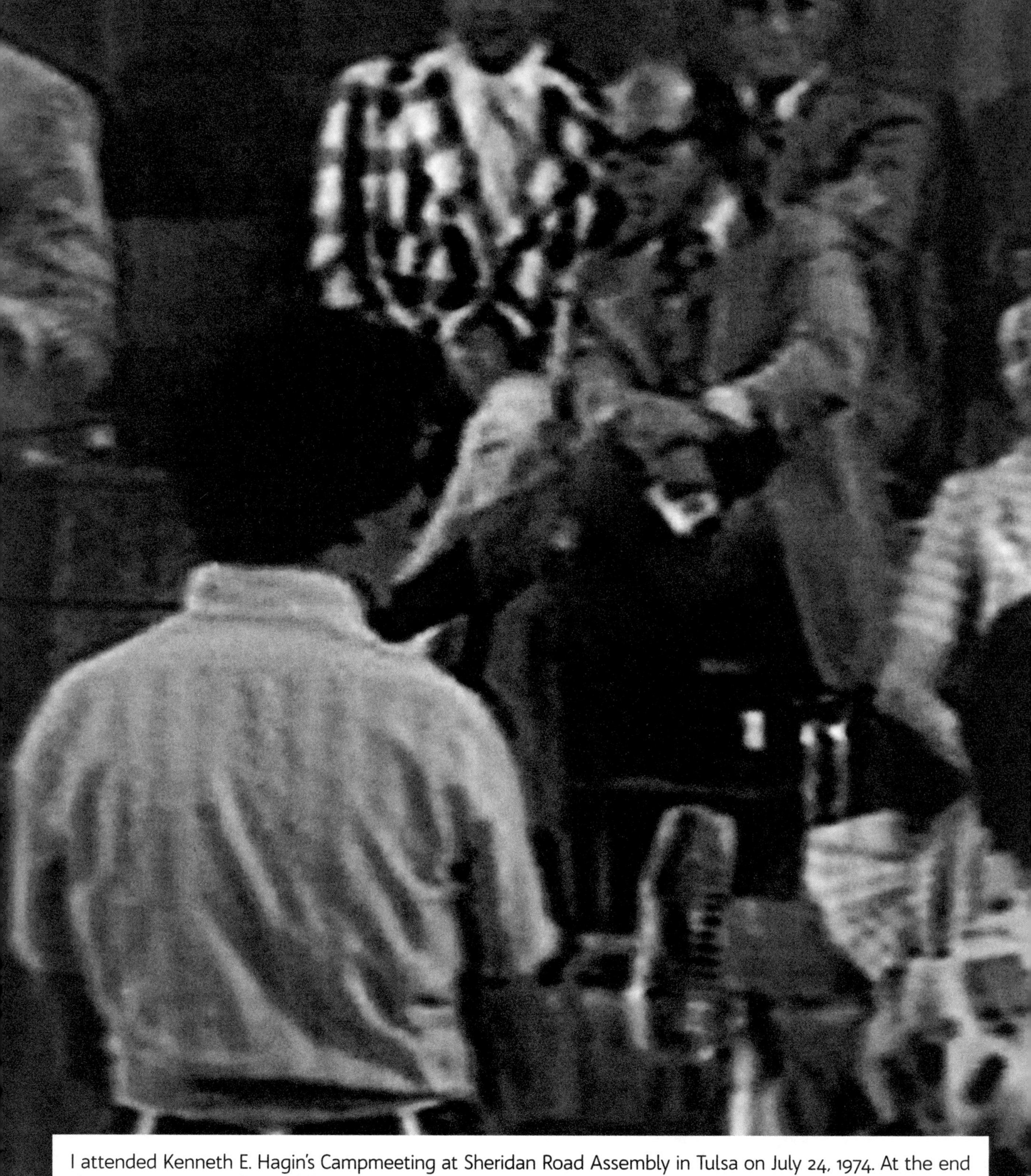

I attended Kenneth E. Hagin's Campmeeting at Sheridan Road Assembly in Tulsa on July 24, 1974. At the end that service, I went forward for prayer to commit my life to the call of God. As Brother Hagin touched my forehead, God's power flooded my whole being. Minutes later, I realized I'd been supernaturally healed of a serious kidney condition.

# ONE

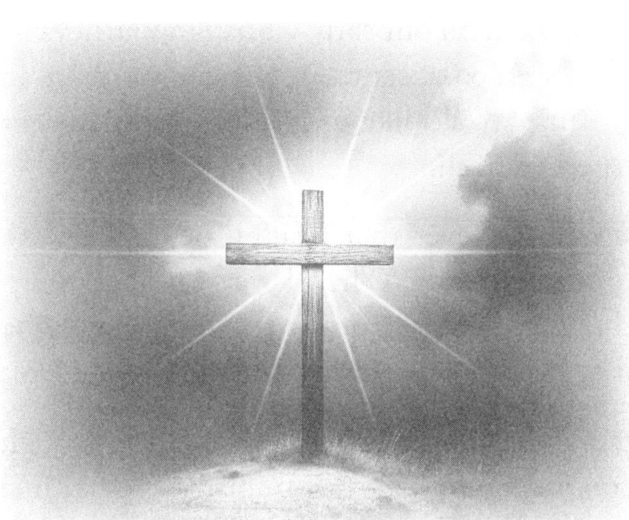

# MY PERSONAL STORY ABOUT HEALING

Our family's many decades of ministry in the former Soviet Union have been reminiscent of the vibrant days chronicled in the book of Acts. We witnessed the Gospel spreading like wildfire, saw the Church taking root, and marveled as miraculous signs and wonders manifested in the lives of countless individuals.

My wife and I and our family have seen the lame walk, deaf ears opened, blind eyes see, demons expelled, and even the dead raised. We have witnessed healings and the miracle-working power of God unleashed in the lives of those who have been saved, delivered from demon spirits, and provided for miraculously — we have seen the evil forces of hell pushed back and out of the way! In fact, we have seen so many healings and miracles, it would be impossible to list all the healings and miracles we have witnessed over the years.

But I assure you that it wasn't always this way. The following pages will reveal that Denise and I embarked on our early Christian journeys in a spiritual setting where the miraculous seemed absent. And before we delve into the wonderful subject of healing, I first would like to give you a little background about my own journey in respect to healing.

Today I am a firm believer that healing belongs to every child of God, but this was not always the case. When I was younger and growing up in my denominational church, we emphatically did not believe that God wanted to heal everyone, and in fact, anyone getting healed sounded like a far-fetched idea.

My family attended a wonderful church that God mightily used to help form the foundation for my present-day ministry — that includes the bedrock of most of my doctrinal beliefs and the basis for much of what I believe about the importance of the local church. But the big minus about our denomination and church, which I didn't even know was a minus at the time, was we did not believe in present-day healing.

The official position of our denomination was that healing (along with nearly every gift of the Holy Spirit) had been active in the Early Church in its formative years, but it and the other gifts of the Spirit had passed away with the death of the apostles. I could give you the whole doctrinal argument for why we believed this, but it would be a waste of time and beyond the scope of my purpose in this book.

Doctrinally, we were called *cessationists*, which is a theological term to describe those who believe the gifts of the Holy Spirit *ceased* at the end of the Apostolic Age. Because we sincerely did *not* believe in present-day healing (or in spiritual gifts for our age), we deemed those who practiced such things as being doctrinally off base and that whatever they were claiming to experience was merely foolish, made-up works of the flesh based on bad doctrine and a mishandling of Scripture.

Making this more interesting is the fact that I was raised in Tulsa, Oklahoma, a city that was home to notable healing ministries. Ministers like Oral Roberts, T. L. Osborn, and Kenneth E. Hagin were based in Tulsa, along with a host of other ministries noted for healing. But because we disbelieved the claims of healing ministers, we generally looked at all of them as being charlatans. It's interesting how life changes one's perspective, for after many years, Oral Robert's son, Richard Roberts, and Kenneth Hagin's son, Pastor Kenneth W. Hagin, became personal acquaintances and friends.

When I was growing up, we didn't take any of these healing giants seriously because our pastor sometimes told *healing jokes* before he proceeded to preach on Sunday mornings. I remember our congregation laughing hysterically at some of those jokes. I am telling you this to let you know that in those years, *we believed anyone who preached about, believed in, or promoted healing was a joke!*

In our church, if someone was sick — even *if* we prayed for them to be healed — we always added "*if* it is God's will." This addendum felt more like a disclaimer, a subtle contingency that hinted at uncertainty and shielded us against any failure on our part to receive the desired result.

But as a young person, it was my personal perception that no one really expected anyone to be healed. Not only that, we believed that sickness itself *could be* the will of God, so we couldn't pray with confidence for anyone to be healed. And to be honest, as I was growing up, I cannot recall *anyone* in my church community who had been healed.

While others might recall those times with a different lens, this was my impression of those days. I vividly remember our Wednesday evening prayer gatherings during which members of the congregation were invited to share the burdens on their hearts. Occasionally, someone would voice a somber prayer request, "Please pray for my relative who has stage four cancer and is dying in the hospital." But rather than praying for that relative to be healed, we usually heard a prayer that was expressed something like, "God, You know this relative is dying of cancer. We know that You are sovereign, and You could heal if You chose to heal. But since this person has not been healed yet and is so close to death, we ask You to give this relative the grace needed to embrace this cancer as Your plan for his life and give him the grace to glorify You as he dies in the hospital."

After hearing such prayers time and again, year after year as a young man, it often felt to me like these prayers for healing were more like a wish for a graceful departure than a petition for recovery. Because we didn't know of anyone who had been healed in our church, the absence of healing undergirded our incorrect belief that God was not in the healing business in our present day as He had been in the formative years of the Early Church.

## BIBLE STORIES ABOUT HEALING WERE LIKE FAIRY TALES TO ME

After our family moved to the former Soviet Union, we visited the State Hermitage Museum for the first time in St. Petersburg, Russia. On that visit, I had an experience that reminded me of my thinking when I was growing up in my church.

Inside the Hermitage's sprawling halls lies an exquisite array of religious artworks, amassed primarily during the reign of Catherine the Great. This museum, located in the former Winter Palace of the Russian czars, is fabulous beyond description and attracts millions of visitors who come to view this world-renowned art collection and to see the opulence in which the czars lived.

But on that first visit to the Hermitage, it was near the end of the Soviet Union, and communism and atheism still lingered in the lands that comprised the former USSR. It was during that first visit, as I walked past the section of paintings by a world-class master painter, that I saw a painting of Lazarus being raised from the dead by Jesus. The painting resonated with such profound emotion that I couldn't help but draw nearer, eager to drink in its every detail. As my eyes traversed the elegant frame encasing this work of art, they fell upon a small plaque nestled at the base. To my astonishment, it read, "The Fairy Tale of Jesus Christ Raising Lazarus From the Dead."

I was taken aback to find Lazarus' resurrection described as *a fairy tale*! Yet as I wandered from that painting to others that illustrated miraculous episodes from Jesus' life, it dawned on me that nearly all those paintings from the Soviet era labeled these wondrous scenes as "fairy tales of Jesus Christ."

By calling the works of Jesus "fairy tales," it put the stories of Jesus' healings and miraculous power on the same level as Cinderella, Hansel and Gretel, Jack and the Beanstock, Little Red Riding Hood, Peter Pan, and Snow White, etc. Upon encountering the description of Jesus' miraculous works as "fairy tales," my initial reaction was one of offense.

But as I began to reflect on my own experience, I realized that because we never saw anything miraculous when I was growing up, there were many aspects about Jesus' miraculous ministry that had, in reality, been a fairy tale to *me*. For me, the miracles of Jesus existed in a distant past, confined to the pages of Scripture. Our church community didn't believe in modern-day healings or the gifts of the Spirit, and we never anticipated such wonders would occur in our time. The extent of my understanding of Jesus' power was confined to what I had gleaned from our reading of Scripture, rather than from real-life experience.

Having never personally witnessed Jesus' miracle-working power, Christians try to fantasize and imagine what Jesus' healings and miracle-working power may have been like. Having never seen it, much of what they know about Jesus' healings and miracle-working power is purely imaginary or speculative — similar to the way one might view *a fairy tale* or *a legend*. To those who have never encountered such healing phenomena, something so extraordinary dwells only in the realm of the implausible.

Again, in the church and denomination I grew up in, many of us actually believed that *if* someone got sick, that sickness might have been God's will for that person. Instead of resisting ailments, we often hastened to embrace them as part of a higher purpose. It seemed we believed that our role was to navigate those trials and seek strength and solace through prayer *to cope* with them.

Countless times, I heard this sentiment, "I've visited doctor after doctor, and their treatments haven't provided relief, so I've come to the conclusion that this illness is God's plan for my life. I must seek the grace to honor Him through my suffering and to embrace this path He has chosen for me."

There were moments of desperation when individuals sought divine intervention and hoped for a healing touch. However, in most instances, when illness struck, our first instinct wasn't to rely on faith for a miraculous cure, but rather to seek the familiar remedies tucked away in our household medicine cabinet.

I personally thank God for medication and believe doctors are a blessing — God uses *numerous* avenues to counter the impacts of sickness and disease. But because we didn't know divine healing was really an option, when illness befell our household or the household of family and friends, we mostly reached for the medicine cabinet and trusted what we found there to provide relief.

Growing up, I do not recall ever having a thought about using faith to resist sickness because we hadn't really been taught about resisting the devil. If someone had told us to resist the devil or to resist sickness, we wouldn't have had a clue what that meant because the idea of "resisting" had never been introduced into our thinking.

From the pulpit of our church, the sermons echoed with themes of salvation, dedication, and surrender — marvelous cornerstones that shaped who I am today. Yet the notion of wielding faith as a shield against the devil or as a remedy for illness was unfamiliar. Plus, why would we challenge sickness when it might be seen as part of God's plan intended to teach us something? Our beliefs leaned more toward seeking grace to embrace such trials so that we might endure them with dignity and bring God glory through our suffering.

## THE BASICS OF SALVATION ARE *FOUNDATIONAL* AND *IMPORTANT*

When it came to the fundamental tenets of salvation and the dedication required for a committed life, our church was an example of excellence and unwavering faith.

Our pastor was not only a fervent lover of the Bible, but he also possessed an exceptional gift for teaching its profound truths. Looking back, I recognize how God used the teachings of that beloved pastor to instill in me a steadfast commitment to Christ and an unwavering responsibility to spread the Gospel across the globe. I am profoundly thankful to God for providing such an invaluable guide on my spiritual journey.

My family served in Sunday School and in Training Union (a Sunday night class for youth), and we sang from our hearts in various church choirs. But my family didn't just attend church services once or twice a week — *our entire lives* revolved around the activities of our church. I relate much about my spiritual journey in my autobiography called *UNLIKELY.*

Both of my parents were members of the church choir — a commitment that entailed countless hours in rehearsals at the church, always with kids in tow. We stayed late on Wednesday nights after the prayer meeting finished so my parents could attend choir practice. And because my mother taught Sunday School, I helped her set up her classroom each Saturday. With rapt enthusiasm, I'd help her decorate bulletin boards, organize chairs, and stack mimeographed lessons with pencils and pens in preparation for her teaching of God's Word the following morning.

Each Sunday, I eagerly participated in classroom activities, such as coloring, painting, and waging glitter wars with my friends in the nursery. Like all the other kids, I eventually graduated to another part of the building where the kindergarten and grade-school kids attended Sunday School. Soon I joined the children's choir and became a "Sunbeam" (for preschool through kindergarten ages) — an endearing term that anyone who grew up as a Southern Baptist will remember. These precious memories are so vivid that they will be cemented in my mind for the rest of my life.

Our family gave offerings, attended services, volunteered, and reached out to those in need. We faithfully attended revival meetings, diligently volunteered wherever there was a need, and dutifully showed up for weekly visitation, where we'd reach out both to visitors and the lost. We worked alongside our friends on special projects, befriended the surrounding community, and stood behind our pastor in support.

We gave our best, dressed our best, and did our best where the house of God and the people in it were concerned. We carried a deeply felt awe concerning our dedication and service to God — a sentiment that unfortunately seems to have dissipated in much of the Church today.

## MY OWN SALVATION EXPERIENCE

When I was just five years old, our pastor announced that our church was about to host a week-long revival meeting. Today the term "revival" conjures images of a profound spiritual awakening or a powerful divine encounter that affects masses of people.

But in those earlier days, the term "revival" was understood to mean a dedicated week of meetings that featured special sermons aimed at reaching those who were lost, rekindling the faith of those needing to rededicate their lives to Christ, and inspiring the local congregation toward greater devotion. That was the essence of what we envisioned when we spoke of a "revival."

It was a much-anticipated week of "revival" gatherings. As was the custom back then, a visiting evangelist ignited the pulpit with passionate sermons each evening. One night, the guest evangelist painted a vivid picture of Christ's Second Coming. The next evening, he delved into the dire consequences of a life steeped in sin. On the final night that week, he preached powerfully about hell — a sermon so compelling that I can still mentally see it and hear it today.

As the evangelist delivered his sermon about hell, he painted a picture of hell's infernal blaze, where flames twisted and danced with an intense, white-hot fervor. His words conjured a vision in my mind's eye, where relentless flames stretched skyward, hungrily consuming lost souls ensnared forever in their searing embrace. The minister's message was so graphic that I could visually see that fire in my mind, and I could nearly feel the heat of the flames swirling nearer and nearer. As he preached, his message reached all the way from the pulpit into my heart and grabbed hold of my soul.

I was deeply disturbed by that message in a way that would later lead me straight into the arms of a loving Savior who was and is the only way of escape from such a devastating, irrevocable eternal fate. I trembled at the evangelist's words and gripped the pew in front of me with my five-year-old fingers, lest I slip into eternity at that very moment unprepared! Oh, how I wanted to rise from my seat, step out into the aisle, and run to the altar to make my commitment to Christ, but my mother was concerned that I might not have really comprehended what I was doing due to my young age, so I held myself back and refrained.

After that week of meetings, I trembled night after night in my bed at the thought of what would happen if I died in my sleep. Every night, my precious mother looked into my eyes and spoke to my heart about what it meant to commit my life to Christ. She was attempting to comprehend the depth of my understanding at five years of age concerning Heaven and hell and choices concerning eternity. She wanted to be really sure that I understood what it meant to be unsaved, about my own need to be saved, and what it meant to repent. But even though I was five years old, I really understood, and soon everyone in my circle of family and friends would know it.

Shortly after that week of revival meetings, I found myself sitting next to my older sister Ronda in our church auditorium — strategically placed about midway between the pulpit and the back doors. As the pastor delivered the closing words of his sermon, the congregation lifted their voices to sing a heartfelt rendition of "Just as I Am."[1] My heart suddenly began to beat with urgency, stirred by an unmistakable pull, and I quietly stepped from the pew into the aisle, each movement deliberate and drawing me closer to the church's altar.

Our pastor stood ready at the altar to greet those who felt led to make a commitment to Christ. My daddy and mother in the choir loft behind him focused intently on their five-year-old son standing in front of them at the altar. My pastor reached out to take my hand and leaned down to gently ask, "Ricky, why have you come today?"

I told him that I had come to give my heart to Jesus — and on that day in 1963, I gave my heart and life to Jesus Christ, and I have served Him ever since that time. That event was the pivotal moment when I came to Christ, and as a result, the question of eternity was forever settled for me. God had used that guest evangelist and his fiery message to give me a glorious start, and from that moment forward, I had a ravenous desire for God's Word that consumed me even at a young age.

But because the church community I grew up in knew nothing about divine healing or the gifts of the Holy Spirit, we were ignorant about certain things that God wanted us to know. We focused on the sovereignty of God and generally believed most of what happened in our lives was *allowed* because it was the plan of God — and that included *sickness.*

I now understand that in many ways back then, we were uninformed. We did not believe that the devil could have been the source of sickness. Because we truly believed that God was in control, again, we thought it was our duty to accept and surrender to whatever happened as being a part of His will for our lives. We were so uninformed about the activity of the devil that if anyone said something about the devil, we surmised they needed *psychological help.* I remember a wonderful woman in our church who testified that, as believers, we had authority over the devil. She compassionately tried to open the eyes of many to the truth, but for her efforts, she was ridiculed, stigmatized, and looked upon as if she was mentally unstable.

We were so ignorant about the devil that each year on October 31, we went "all out" for Halloween by dressing up like devils and walking the neighborhood with all the other kids to collect candy. My precious mother, who led me to Christ, encouraged me each year to use my artistic flair to craft eerie depictions of demons, devils, witches, and goblins. We cut them out and proudly taped them to the front window of our house for all to see.

We were so untaught about the activities of the devil that my parents innocently bought us Renner kids a Ouija board, completely unaware of its occult connections. Back then, such things were dismissed as harmless fun and mere games not to be taken with any seriousness.

In contrast, as I mentioned, Tulsa in those years was a hub for prominent healing ministries, which meant the topic of healing occasionally surfaced in our church discussions. To combat what we viewed as egregious error, there was even a time when our pastor dedicated seven weeks to a comprehensive series aimed at challenging what he described as the misguided views of Charismatics and Pentecostals who believed that healing and spiritual gifts were still active today. We steadfastly argued and defended our doctrinal position that "those people" who believed in or who endorsed such things were off base and should be avoided like the plague.

## MY SURPRISE ENCOUNTER WITH HEALING AT A KATHRYN KUHLMAN MIRACLE SERVICE

A profound spiritual yearning took root within me in 1973 that ignited a quest for something beyond the familiar confines of my Baptist upbringing. My soul, brimming with curiosity, led me to fervently seek answers. In February 1974 at the age of 15, a transformative awakening unfolded inside me when I received the baptism in the Holy Spirit. Subsequently, I was introduced to people who *really* believed in the healing power of God and in the present-day gifts of the Holy Spirit.

With immense gratitude for my Baptist roots, which anchored me in Scripture and a life dedicated to God's service, my eyes had now been opened that healing and miraculous power was not just a relic of the past but was still at work in the here and now!

Soon I stumbled upon an extraordinary radio program that utterly captivated me. It was a daily broadcast hosted by a remarkable woman named Kathryn Kuhlman, who spoke about miracles and her relationship with the Holy Spirit. Each afternoon, I found myself eagerly tuning in to her radio program. My ears hung on her every word as she painted a vivid picture of an intimate bond with the Holy Spirit.

I had never heard anyone speak about the Holy Spirit the way I heard Kathryn Kuhlman speak. It was a whole realm of God that I had never heard about in such terms. My heart was completely captured by what I was hearing about actually experiencing a relationship with the Holy Spirit, and I wanted to experience that intimacy with Him for myself that Kathryn Kuhlman spoke about.

Every Friday on her radio broadcast, Kathryn Kuhlman played excerpts from miracle services she was holding all over the United States. When she revealed that Tulsa was next on the map for one of these extraordinary services, attending became a must for me.

The event was set to unfold at the Mabee Center auditorium, which stood on the sprawling campus of Oral Roberts University. On the Sunday the meeting was to be held, I excused myself from my church's Sunday School a little early and drove across Tulsa to ORU to attend that afternoon's miracle service at the Mabee Center auditorium.

When I arrived, a sea of people surrounded the massive auditorium. The streets and parking areas were congested with buses and carloads of determined souls who had traveled hundreds, some even more than 1,000, miles to attend this gathering. As I made my way into the building, I wondered, *Why have all these people come from so far to hear this woman preach?* It wouldn't be long before I understood.

I had volunteered to be a part of the choir, so I was allowed to enter the auditorium earlier than the crowds. I could see that the rear section of the auditorium's ground level had been transformed into an area for those battling severe and terminal illnesses. A huge crowd was standing outside, but the ushers were only allowing those who were debilitated to enter that special area so they wouldn't have to compete with the throngs of people.

From my seat, I observed a sea of individuals in wheelchairs, accompanied by oxygen tanks, IV drips, crutches, and doctors and nurses. Some were even lying on stretchers. It looked as if an entire hospital ward had been emptied and brought to the service. Some of the critically ill had been transported by family members. Others were so near to death that they had been brought to the meeting by ambulance.

One hour before the service began, the main doors to the auditorium opened and the crowd rushed in as fast as their feet could carry them. That sea of people poured into the seating area like swelling torrents through an open dam. A multitude cascaded into the seating area and swiftly filled aisles and jostled for the coveted spots nearest to the stage.

I watched as every seat was claimed and those left outside were redirected to another space where they could participate in the service via closed-circuit television. An overwhelming air of excitement and faith filled the auditorium and could be felt in the atmosphere around us.

My eyes were irresistibly drawn to the area designated for wheelchairs and stretchers. The people in that section were so sick, and I realized many had journeyed to this gathering out of deep desperation and were clinging to a glimmer of hope for a miracle. Quietly, I prayed, "Oh, Lord, please don't let them be disappointed today."

Just moments before the service began, a spokesperson approached the microphone to deliver astonishing news that miracles had already started happening among those waiting for the service to commence. I could sense my faith and the collective faith of that massive congregation rise in expectation. It was so buoyant that it seemed it could have lifted the building right off its foundation!

Then the choir director emerged, summoned everyone in the auditorium to rise, and soon the entire assembly lifted their voices in unison to sing "How Great Thou Art."[2] As we did, Kathryn Kuhlman came out on the platform to sing with us. It was my first time to see her in person. Draped in an elegant white gown, she glided across the platform with a grace that seemed almost ethereal.

Her rich, contralto voice resonated through the air as she sang, "Then sings my soul, my Savior God, to Thee: How great Thou art, how great Thou art…." As the music and instruments fell into a reverent silence, she greeted the multitude with warmth and encouraged us to sing "Alleluia." As thousands of people sang in that sacred moment, I kept thinking, "This must be a glimpse of Heaven."

After worship concluded, Kathryn Kuhlman approached the microphone to speak. One hour passed like seconds. Interrupting her own message at one point, she suddenly paused and locked her eyes onto a distant section high above in the auditorium. With an outstretched finger, she declared, "Someone right up there has just received a miracle. Stand up and claim it!" It felt as if a whirlwind of power rushed through the auditorium and suddenly miracles started taking place throughout the massive congregation.

During that gathering, I witnessed wonders unfolding in every corner as healing miracles took shape before my very eyes. In all directions around me were people experiencing miracles. Soon people were lining up near the platform to testify about what God had done in their bodies. Wheelchairs were emptied, paralyzed people got up from their stretchers and walked, blind eyes were opened, deaf ears were unstopped, and the mute began to speak.

I watched in amazement as the supernatural power of God continued on full display for hours. Everything I'd ever dreamed — everything I'd ever wanted to believe in — was happening right before my eyes. If any lingering question about God's healing and miracle-working power had tried to hide in my soul, it utterly dissolved as I watched those wheelchairs and stretchers being emptied, and people who had been unable to walk or move now walked and even ran from one end of the platform to the other. Soon the entire front of the auditorium and aisles were jammed with people who came forward to give their lives to Jesus.

That experience with the miracle-working power of God changed me and my theology forever. In truth, there is nothing like a firsthand encounter with the power of God to alter one's way of thinking and believing. After my time at that Kathryn Kuhlman service, no one could have convinced me to doubt what I had seen and experienced, for I had experienced first-hand the miracle-working power of God.

As that meeting concluded, I remember thinking, "I love my church where I grew up, but I have been told that God no longer did these things — yet I've just seen God do the impossible before my eyes!"

## MY OWN HEALING IN A KENNETH E. HAGIN MEETING IN 1974

In the spring of 1974, I was hospitalized due to a severe kidney infection. It was caused by a condition I was born with called horseshoe kidney, or renal fusion.

As a baby develops in the womb, the kidneys move into position — one on each side of the body — but sometimes the kidneys fuse together at their base and form a "U" or a horseshoe shape. In essence, they are conjoined much like Siamese twins. This condition can produce chronic kidney obstructions, kidney infections, kidney stones, kidney cancer, and even problems with the heart, blood vessels, nervous system, reproductive system, urinary system, digestive system, and bones. In those days, if the situation was serious, doctors sometimes recommended the kidneys be surgically separated.

Because I had persistent kidney obstructions, my urologist recommended a surgical procedure to separate my kidneys. But in the mid-1970s, this was considered to be a high-risk surgery, so my parents opted to explore whether medication could resolve the obstruction, hoping to sidestep the surgical risks. All of this was taking place the same summer I had become on fire for God and was in fervent pursuit of knowing more about the power of the Holy Spirit.

Through a relative, I heard that Kenneth E. Hagin was going to hold a meeting at the Sheridan Road Assembly in Tulsa. I had listened to him on his daily radio program and found comfort in listening to him because everything he taught was so solid and rooted in the Bible. He was also from a Baptist background, and knowing that he and I had a similar doctrinal foundation gave me a sense of trust when I listened to him on the radio. So I decided to attend those meetings in July 1974.

That was a historic week of services filled with the power of God — with signs and wonders and other supernatural happenings. The packed auditorium was "electric" as the anointing of God moved across the crowd. The power of God erupted, and every night more and more people packed into that space to experience a divine encounter with the supernatural anointing of God. Every evening, I sat close enough to the front of the auditorium to watch as Kenneth E. Hagin laid hands on people, and I saw so many people receiving healings and miracles.

One night during those meetings, Brother Hagin preached a message that was called, "A Man Full of Faith and Power" from the example of Stephen in Acts chapter 8. I still vividly remember that message as he described Stephen as a common man who had surrendered himself to the Lord — and as a result, he became a man of faith and power whose life was marked with mighty signs and wonders. At the end of that message, Brother Hagin asked people to come forward for the laying on of hands if they felt called to surrender to God's service.

I had always sensed a calling to the ministry, but that evening kindled a deeper yearning in my soul and spirit, and I felt urged to leave my seat to approach the altar for a divine impartation of the anointing for full-time ministry. But this whole atmosphere was unfamiliar to me, so I lingered until Brother Hagin had nearly reached the end of the line as he prayed for those who had come forward. I desperately wanted to go to the altar, but trepidation held me back. But finally, I mustered the courage to break free from my grip on the pew in front of me, and I moved to the altar to receive prayer.

By the time I got into place to receive prayer, Brother Hagin was sitting on the platform to rest before continuing. So along with a few others, I waited... and waited...and waited. Finally, Brother Hagin descended from the platform to finish laying hands on the last of us "stragglers" who had come forward.

When he passed in front of me, he murmured softly in tongues, his voice a whisper, and gently extended a lone finger toward my forehead. The moment of contact was electric as a profound surge of divine energy coursed through my being. Overwhelmed, my legs buckled, and I crumpled, finding myself on the floor — I could literally feel the power of God radiating from one end of my body to the other end.

As I lay there, it seemed like time stood still as minutes passed, or perhaps only seconds, before I rose again to my feet. When I stood, I found that I not only received a special empowerment for service, but I also received an incredible healing. I inwardly knew that God had touched my kidneys, and when I returned to see the doctor to be checked, my physician verified that I had been healed.

Now, decades later, I remain free from the ailment that once plagued me. I was healed permanently by God's mighty power on that unforgettable summer evening of 1974 in a Kenneth E. Hagin meeting. Indeed, I was supernaturally and permanently healed by the power of God on that eventful evening.

## MY EXPERIENCE WITH ORAL ROBERTS' MINISTRY

In the following months, I heard that Oral Roberts would be personally teaching a class every Tuesday night at Oral Roberts University that was called "The Holy Spirit in the Now." Oral was famous for his healing and miracle ministry, so when I heard that he would be teaching this class personally from his own experience of more than 30 years of prayer and his study of the Word, I decided to attend those classes.

In one of the classes, Oral reflected, "During my ministry, I have personally laid hands on over a million people in prayer, thousands of whom had been given up on because there was no known medical cure for their condition. I am convinced that no disease is hopeless — none is incurable — for God can heal all sickness. His power has no limits or barriers when we center our faith in Him."

Every Tuesday night, I found myself eagerly driving to Oral Roberts University, excited to participate in those remarkable classes taught by Oral Roberts. I made it a point to arrive early to ensure my coveted spot in the front row, which was directly in front of him. Each class was a spellbinding experience, and I absorbed every word he uttered. Sometimes, his proximity was such that I could almost reach out and touch him as he walked by — a living legend just within my arm's reach.

Determined to capture every nugget of wisdom that flowed from Oral's lips, I equipped myself with a trusty little tape recorder and a fresh cassette each week so I could record every word that he spoke. As Oral would begin the lesson, I'd press "play" to record what he taught in those classes, and somewhere deep in my archives, I still have a few of those old cassette tapes, and they will always be precious to me.

But while others exited the auditorium each week after class ended, I lingered at the front to watch as Oral Roberts laid his hands on people who were sick and needed healing. He carefully laid his huge hands on them and released the power of God for them to be healed, and every week, without fail, I witnessed someone who was healed at the end of those classes.

Receiving the baptism in the Holy Spirit had opened doors for me into a whole spiritual realm that earlier I had been wrongly taught no longer existed. And those multiple early experiences with the power of God changed my heart and mind and forever impacted me concerning healing and the supernatural ministry of the Holy Spirit.

## WHAT THE APOSTLE PAUL SAID ABOUT THE POWER OF GOD

We often try to appeal to people using eloquent language, yet we often miss the one definitive act that can silence skepticism, and that is *a demonstration of God's power.*

Witnessing a genuine healing or miracle can create a more profound impact than years of persuading and pleading. Indeed, there is *nothing* more compelling than a direct, personal encounter with God's power. When we allow God to "show off," that supernatural manifestation makes a far greater impact than we could ever achieve with just words.

When Paul embarked on his mission to share the Gospel with the Corinthians — people who were steeped in paganism and enveloped by profound spiritual darkness — he realized that mere words would not suffice. To truly touch their hearts, he needed to showcase God's power.

In First Corinthians 2:4, Paul wrote about the manner in which he first preached to them, when he said, "And my speech and my preaching was not with enticing words of man's wisdom, but in demonstration of the Spirit and of power." Then in the next verse, Paul told them the reason that he wanted them to see a demonstration of God's power. He said, "That your faith should not stand in the wisdom of men, but in the power of God" (1 Corinthians 2:5).

Just as I was deeply impacted by the healings and miracles that I saw in meetings with Kathryn Kuhlman, Kenneth E. Hagin, and Oral Roberts, the apostle Paul knew that miracles, healings, and other displays of God's power would have a great impact on his Corinthian listeners. Were he to rely solely on the eloquence of human rhetoric, his listeners might find room for skepticism, dissent, or intellectual debate about the message he preached.

However, a miracle unfolding before their very eyes — an irrefutable display of divine power — would strike them with such force that they could not deny the hand of God demonstrating and confirming the very words Paul spoke.

A wise man once told me, "You can't win an argument with a man who has had a supernatural experience." And it's true that when someone has had an encounter with the power of God, it puts an end to all arguments and speculation in that person about whether God is active in the affairs of men today.

Paul understood that a magnificent demonstration of God's divine power could profoundly impact his listeners. Beyond meticulously crafting a heartfelt and anointed message that would touch their hearts, he went a step further and invited God's power to work its wonders unrestrained. Confident that God's divine force would dissolve every doubt and silence every argument, Paul wisely chose to step aside and allowed God to show off, thusly confirming that the message that Paul preached was indeed the truth!

In First Corinthians 2:4, Paul said, "And my speech and my preaching was not with enticing words of man's wisdom, but in demonstration of the Spirit and of power." The word "demonstration" comes from the Greek word *apodeixis* — a word that indisputably refers to *something that is outwardly seen* or *something visible that authenticates, proves, and guarantees* the message to be true.

In the heart of ancient Corinth, where superstition held sway and demonic influences were woven throughout life, Paul knew the people needed *supernatural proof* to *authenticate* that God was behind the message being preached to them. This demonstration of power would get their attention more than anything else. Paul preached with the authority of signs and wonders to verify that he was God's man and that the message he preached was God's message. All those who saw the mighty "demonstration of the Spirit and of power" that operated through Paul knew that God was speaking to them!

Paul continued to tell the Corinthians the reason he took this approach: "that your faith should not stand in the wisdom of men, but in the power of God" (1 Corinthians 2:5). The word "stand" in this verse is the little Greek word *en*, which simply means *in*. As used here, this word describes the medium *in which* faith is *rooted.* It could be translated, "I took this approach so your faith would not be rooted in the wisdom of men...."

Then Paul continued to say he wanted their faith to be in the "power" of God. The word "power" in this verse is derived from the Greek word *dunamis*, a well-known word that denotes the mighty power of God. In First Corinthians 2:5, Paul was not merely talking about *power*, but about *tremendous power*. This word *dunamis* denotes *power that is explosive, mighty, and awe-inspiring* to those who see or experience it. Paul's words in First Corinthians 2:5 could thus be paraphrased: "I took this approach so your faith would not be rooted in the logic and wisdom of men, but so that your faith would be completely rooted in the awe-inspiring power of God."

Similarly, we also must learn to step aside to allow God to do what only He can do and to give His supernatural power an opportunity to drive truth into people's hearts. The power of God can do what you could never do by yourself — and when the Spirit of God is finished confirming the Word with supernatural demonstrations of power, all arguments will cease, the case will be closed, and the person you are trying to reach will be convinced.

## THE POWER OF GOD IS SUPPOSED TO WORK IN THE CHURCH

Just before ascending back into Heaven, Jesus instructed His disciples to stay in Jerusalem and wait for the promise of the Father, the gift of the baptism in the Holy Spirit (*see* Acts 1:4-5). He said, "But ye shall receive power, after that the Holy Ghost is come upon you: and ye shall be witnesses unto me both in Jerusalem, and in all Judaea, and in Samaria, and unto the uttermost part of the earth" (Acts 1:8).

The word "power" is again derived from the Greek word *dunamis*. As we have seen, it describes *explosive power*, but it is also notably the very word used by the Greeks to denote *a force of nature*, like *an earthquake*, *a hurricane*, or *a tornado.*

Thus, when we receive the power (*dunamis*) of the Holy Spirit, it turns into something akin to a groundbreaking earthquake that unsettles the status quo; a formidable hurricane that sweeps away all that is unholy; or a spiritual tornado that reshapes everything it encounters. Unquestionably, when God's power courses through you, you're poised to revolutionize your surroundings, and this divine power will work through you to upheave and dispel darkness.

But wait…the word *dunamis* — translated in Acts 1:8 as "power" — is also the Greek term used to denote *the full might of the advancing Roman army.* When Jesus selected this word to describe the power of the Holy Spirit, He was imparting the profound message that through the Holy Spirit's power, each of us transforms into a singular, unstoppable force that is capable of pushing back against spiritual adversaries.

In the time of the Early Church when there were no cutting-edge gadgets or complex devices that we flaunt in the modern age, believers transformed their environment like a force of nature, and like an advancing army they conquered their surroundings. Oh, let us not be so focused on what we can do that we forget what only the power of the Holy Spirit can do through us!

When the Holy Spirit is allowed to move, He shows up and shows off with all kinds of signs, wonders, and spiritual gifts — and that includes *healing* and *miracles.*

## WHY DON'T WE SEE MORE OF THESE SIGNS FOLLOWING CHRISTIANS?

As I told you, we were seriously committed Christians in the church where I grew up, but we never saw signs and wonders or healings and miracles. In Mark 16:17, Jesus said, "And these signs shall follow them that believe...." We believed in the Gospel, so why didn't we see these signs manifesting back then in our church?

A better translation of Mark 16:17 would be as follows: "These signs shall follow those who have engaged their faith and are believing...." Or to put it another way, these supernatural signs don't just automatically happen because one is a Christian. *They follow those who are believing for them.* If a believer isn't expecting these miraculous manifestations, chances are that he or she won't see them. Like anything else, signs and wonders are ignited by faith, and traditional churches seldom witness miracles or healings because they're simply not believing for them to happen.

History shows that those who frequently encounter the miraculous are those who consistently believe for it to take place. Rather than being passive, people who are aggressive about seeing the supernatural take place in their lives or ministries are the ones who see it. This means the amount of signs and wonders that "follow" you will be determined by how intensely you are *constantly believing* for them to be in manifestation.

## WHAT ARE YOU BELIEVING FOR?

So I ask, *Are you actively believing for supernatural signs to follow you everywhere you go?* Jesus didn't say, "These signs will automatically follow every Christian."

The Greek text lets us know that these signs and wonders follow those who have *engaged* their faith and are *believing*. The amount of signs and wonders you experience will be determined by how aggressively you're *continuing to believe for them to be in manifestation.*

So pray for God to increase your faith and expectancy to see sick people healed. When you confront a person who is demonized, believe that by the time you leave that person, he or she is going to be completely set free. When you find yourself in a situation that requires a miracle, rather than just passively hope something might happen, instead, engage your faith and expect to see the miraculous.

Much like anything else, signs and wonders thrive on the fuel of faith. Again, my wife and I and our family have personally observed that people who regularly experience the miraculous are those who *regularly expect* to see it.

So instead of taking a backseat approach, proactively unleash your faith and you will experience the supernatural power of God more frequently. Indeed, if you *engage* your faith, *release* your faith, and *actively believe* for these supernatural signs to accompany you, you'll see them showing up more regularly in your life.

## LEARNING THE TRUTH ABOUT HEALING AND FIGHTING THE GOOD FIGHT OF FAITH!

Regarding my own journey of healing and divine health, the transformative moment came when I witnessed firsthand the miraculous power of God in action. Yet I felt compelled to verify this for myself, so I embarked on a thorough exploration of the Bible to uncover its teachings concerning contemporary healing and the active workings of the Holy Spirit's gifts today.

Having previously been misguided by the doctrines of my denominational church, I sought help from those who not only believed in these miracles but who experienced them. I aimed to unravel biblical truths about healing and spiritual gifts — the very subjects about which I had been entirely uneducated. My yearning was to glean wisdom from those who held the Scriptures in the highest regard and who could unlock the teachings from the Hebrew and Greek.

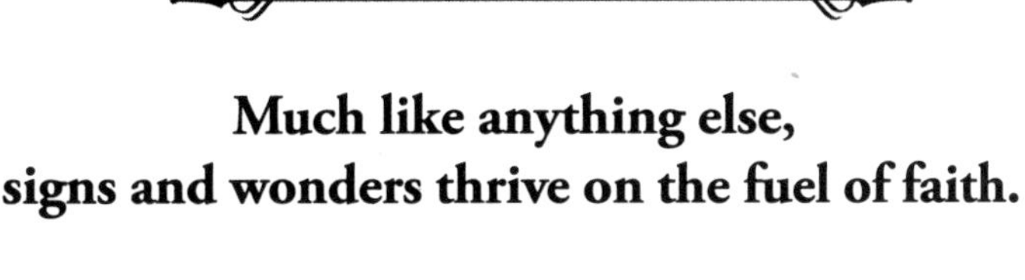

**Much like anything else,
signs and wonders thrive on the fuel of faith.**

As someone raised in a Baptist tradition, I was convinced that if something held truth, its foundation would be firmly planted in Scripture. As a part of my studies, I delved deeply into redemption with the aim of comprehending the full extent of what Jesus accomplished on the Cross.

My exploration took me to the original text of Isaiah 53:3-5 to grasp the true essence of Isaiah's prophecy regarding Jesus' suffering. I endeavored to biblically understand that His sacrificial act on the Cross encompassed not just the forgiveness of sins, freedom from guilt and shame, and peace of mind, but also liberation from physical and mental ailments.

I spent significant time investigating what it meant that we are emancipated from the curse, which encompasses Christ delivering us from the devil's dominion and ensuring freedom from sickness and pain.

I emerged from this period of exploration with the fortified belief that healing is intrinsically woven into the tapestry of our salvation. Yet despite my understanding of the Bible's teachings on this subject, I continued to see devout believers who grappled with illness, and on occasion, I myself wrestled with bouts of sickness. Most often, if sickness tried to assail me, I realized it was usually self-inflicted, like getting sick because of not taking care of my body — not resting enough, eating wrongly, or being overweight (in the past).

But even when I was doing well on all those fronts, there were still times when illness sometimes reared its head to challenge my health. In those moments, I held fast to Paul's exhortation in First Timothy 6:12 to "fight the good fight of faith."

The word "fight" in this verse is the Greek word *agonidzo*, which refers to *a struggle*, *a fight*, *great exertion*, or *effort*. It is where we get the word "agony," a word often used in the New Testament to convey the ideas of *anguish* or *conflict*. The word *agonidzo* comes from the word *agon*, which is the word that depicted the *athletic conflicts* and *athletic competitions* that were so famous in the ancient world. It pictures *wrestlers in a wrestling match*, with each wrestler struggling to overcome his opponent in an effort to hurl him to the ground in a fight to the finish.

The fact that Paul would use this word alerts us that when we step out to do anything by faith — including walking in every aspect of our redemption (which includes healing and health) — it often pushes us into a fight unlike anything we experienced before receiving this revelation. The adversary is resolute in his opposition of our journey toward healing. The conflict arises from the devil's relentless resistance to each stride we make in faith, and this might require us to battle against long-held misconceptions and doctrinal teachings that once led us to believe sickness was part of God's plan. These falsehoods must be recognized as formidable foes to be confronted and conquered. \

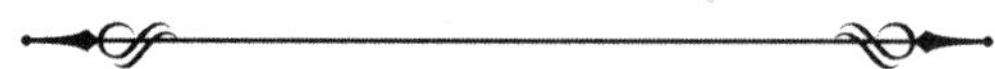

**I emerged from this period of exploration with the fortified belief that healing is intrinsically woven into the tapestry of our salvation.**

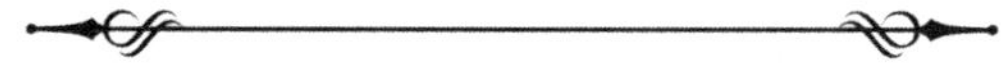

Paul recognized when we step out in faith, regardless of what it is for, we don't just effortlessly glide into what we are believing. We must fight the good fight of faith to reach a victorious position. Rather than retreat from the battle, Paul encouraged us, "Fight the good fight of faith...."

The word "good" in First Timothy 6:12 is derived from the Greek word *kalos*, which denotes *something exceptional, of the highest quality, outstanding,* or *superb*. In the context of a fight, it pictures a fighter who has given his *best effort* to the fight in which he is engaged, and, hence, he is doing a first-rate or first-class job at resisting his opponent.

But then Paul repeated the word "fight" a second time in this verse when he wrote, "*Fight* the good *fight* of faith...." This second use of the word "fight" is from the same Greek word he used at the first of the verse. It conveys the idea of *one who is giving his complete concentration to the conflict* and *who is totally focused on engaging the conflict at hand and achieving victory* — regardless of how long it takes or how much agonizing effort is required. This is far from simply gliding into victory with no hiccups or obstacles along the way.

This word "fight" reminds us that any endeavor in faith — be it walking in healing, enjoying health, or partaking in everything Christ secured through His sacrifice on the Cross — usually demands a fight. The Holy Spirit cautioned us to brace ourselves for the challenge and to pour our heart and soul into claiming the victory that Christ has won for us. Thus, if you are experiencing a fight on the path to any victory, don't feel disheartened. God is rallying you to rise, engage your faith, and give your utmost to possess what you believe is rightfully yours.

Never forget that the grandest prizes often demand the most formidable battles. Determine to overcome every hurdle and resistance in your pursuit of healing and health. Stay in the fight until you can triumphantly declare, "The fight is finished and the victory is mine!"

In my own fight to enjoy the divine health that Christ secured at the Cross, I've wielded every tool in my arsenal to combat illness. I've discovered that when sickness dares to invade my life, it is like a bandit whose aim is to steal, kill, and destroy (*see* John 10:10). Indeed, illness drains vigor, siphons finances, and consumes precious time. Anyone who has endured a bout of sickness understands its nature of *taking and taking* — like a thief intent on pilfering your life.

For me, using every means available in my arsenal to undo sickness includes standing on the Word of God, asking others to pray with me, taking vitamins or supplements, exercising, getting proper rest, going to the doctor for medical advice, and, if needed, taking medication. If sickness is an enemy that has come to steal, I will be committed to stand against it and use any method available to keep it under my feet!

## IF JESUS PAID THE PRICE FOR CHRISTIANS TO BE HEALED, WHY DO CHRISTIANS GET SICK?

In Isaiah 53:3-5, we read, "He is despised and rejected of men; a man of sorrows and acquainted with grief: and we hid as it were our faces from him; he was despised, and we esteemed him not. Surely he hath borne our griefs, and carried our sorrows: yet we did esteem him stricken, smitten of God, and afflicted. But he was wounded for our transgressions, he was bruised for our iniquities: the chastisement of our peace was upon him; and with his stripes we are healed."

In Chapters Nine and Ten, you'll discover these verses reveal the profound truth that when Christ was sacrificed on the Cross, He secured our complete redemption — and this extends beyond spiritual salvation and the forgiveness of sin. It also encompasses the payment for our grief, lack of peace, pain, shame, sorrow, transgressions, and even our physical and mental wellness.

Yet a curious question arises: "If Christ truly secured these for us through His redemptive work — if they are ours to claim as our rightful inheritance —

must we strive to possess the healing, health, or any blessings that Christ's sacrifice procured?"

Simply because an inheritance legally belongs to you does not mean you have it in your possession. In the natural realm, you might find yourself named in a will with a treasure trove of assets bequeathed by an ancestor. Yet those riches rest securely in a bank until they're rightfully claimed.

For you to lay claim to an inheritance, often you need a lawyer to explain what is written in the will to really understand what has been given to you. The journey from bequeathment to possession usually demands a meticulous process, wherein adversaries sometimes surface to dispute your rightful claim, and a battle ensues to secure what is lawfully yours.

And just as this is true in the natural realm, it is also true in the spiritual realm. Christ, at great cost, has bequeathed abundant blessings in Heaven's vaults that await your claim. But just as a person must learn of a natural inheritance and go through the process to move it into his possession, you need enlightenment and guidance to understand that certain spiritual assets are yours, and that is what I endeavor to do in this book.

Simply knowing you have a spiritual inheritance doesn't mean you'll step into it easily. The road to possession may be fraught with opposition, whether it be from the devil or skeptics who are resistant and try to coax you out of embracing the inheritance Christ secured for you.

In Chapters Nine and Ten, you will see what Christ's triumphant sacrifice on the Cross obtained for you beyond salvation, especially in regard to healing and health. My main focus with this book is to guide you to claim the healing of body and mind that is rightfully yours. But it's crucial to understand that the devil will relentlessly try to challenge Christ's highest intentions for your life and to block your access to what rightfully belongs to you by virtue of your being a child of God.

## GIVE NO PLACE TO THE DEVIL

On my personal journey of healing, I learned that in addition to knowing healing and health are in our heavenly account and belong to us, we also need to be sure that we have locked all doors, shut every window, and sealed every vulnerable crack that the devil would use to penetrate us with disease, illness, and sickness.

There are multiple "entry points" that the devil uses to enter our lives to negatively affect our health. When the devil finds one of these "entry points," or "cracks," he is able to attack us through it to take our blessing of health from us.

In Ephesians 4:27, Paul wrote, "Give no place to the devil." The word "place" is interpreted from the Greek word *topos*, which refers to *a specific, marked-off, geographical location*. It is from this word that we derive the term *topographical, as in a topographical* map. Because the word *topos* depicts *a geographical location*, it lets us know that the devil is looking for some "marked-off place" through which he can enter to steal our healing and health. For him to launch his offensive and assert dominion over these facets of our lives, he first requires an initial breach through which he can initiate his sinister scheme of devastation.

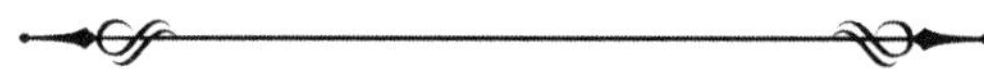

**For the enemy to launch his offensive and assert dominion over these facets of our lives, he first requires an initial breach through which he can initiate his sinister scheme of devastation.**

In Chapters Two through Eight of this book, we will see seven significant "entry points" which the devil exploits to undermine our health. There are multiple entry points, but these are the main culprits I have discovered that provide access for the ailments that plague many people. By proactively sealing these seven entry points, we can barricade ourselves against disease, illness, and sickness that seek to infiltrate our lives and effectively bar the devil from affecting our health.

Through my journey of faith, especially concerning health and healing, I've realized that when my well-being is threatened, it's crucial to introspectively assess whether I've inadvertently left any door "ajar" for the devil to access my health.

The following is a list of seven reasons why the devil continues to afflict Christians with illness despite the fact that Christ has provided healing and health for them in His redemptive work on the Cross. We'll explore each of these in the upcoming chapters, but I want you to see this summary so you'll know where we're headed. Certainly, there are additional reasons why people get sick, but these are seven primary reasons I have chosen to cover for why people fail to experience the healing and health that Jesus purchased for them on the Cross:

1. **The Biggest Culprit Is the Curse.**
2. **A Lack of Knowledge Can Open the Door to Sickness.**
3. **Disobedience Opens the Door to Sickness.**
4. **Foolishness Can Open the Door to Sickness.**
5. **Unresolved, Hidden Issues Open the Door to Sickness.**
6. **Anxiety, Fret, and Worry Open the Door to Sickness.**
7. **Devilish Attacks Can Open the Door to Sickness.**

As we continue in the next chapters, we will meticulously dissect each of these seven elements to see how they serve as "open doors" that invite disease, illness, and sickness into our bodies. For each scenario, we'll also explore strategies to securely close these open doors and ensure that sickness finds no sanctuary in our lives.

At the first of this chapter, I stated that Denise and I were reared in spiritual environments that knew little about divine healing. But once our eyes were unveiled to the biblical revelation that Christ bore the cost for our health and wholeness, we have since waged the good fight of faith to claim healing and walk in divine health. Alongside me, my wife, my family, and our ministry team have prayed in faith for multiplied thousands of people to be healed — and multiplied thousands of them have been healed!

We continue to stand with those who remain in faith for the manifestation of their healing and health. As noted at the introduction to this book, the delay feels interminable — *endless* — for some people, as if the answer will never come. It is for these precious souls that I have penned this book.

But now, it's time to turn the page to dive into the next chapter, where we will begin to explore the fundamental reasons behind disease, illness, and sickness. Together, we'll learn how to seal every entrance so that the enemy is barred from tampering with your well-being. Step by step as you read, I pray you will embrace the divine healing and health that is rightfully yours by inheritance because of Christ's sacrifice on the Cross!

Scan the QR code to watch Rick teach more on this subject.

## QUESTIONS TO PONDER AND DISCUSS

1. How does the phrase "if it be Thy will" when petitioning God nullify the effects of faith based on the passage in First John 5:14-15, which you read about in the book's Introduction?

2. What is cessationism? Can you contrast that to define continuationism and provide answers based on Scripture, not just on human experience, to defend your belief in either cessationism or continuationism?

3. Are the miracles of Jesus and the apostles, others' answers to prayers, and the moving of God's Spirit to perform miracles and do the impossible like "fairy tales" to you? If so, what did reading the scriptures in this chapter and reading about the author's experiences do to bring more understanding to your heart, strengthen your faith, and take the limits off God to move in your own life?

4. How did the Greek words in First Timothy 6:12, translated "fight the good fight," and their definitions encourage you in your own "agonizing" fight of faith for the things that are dearest to your heart? Does Rick's statement, "Never forget that the grandest prizes often demand the most formidable battles" resonate with you? If so, how? After reading this section, how will you gird yourself up afresh and anew to overcome every resistance to your faith and stand strong in your fight until you can say, *"At last — the victory is mine!"*?

5. Which of the seven main reasons for hindered or delayed healing are you the most excited to study as you continue reading this book? Least excited? Considering that it's knowing the truth that makes us free (*see* John 8:32), with what attitude or mindset will you approach these seven sections — with anticipation or dread? What healing are you expecting to receive as you read the pages of this book?

# TWO

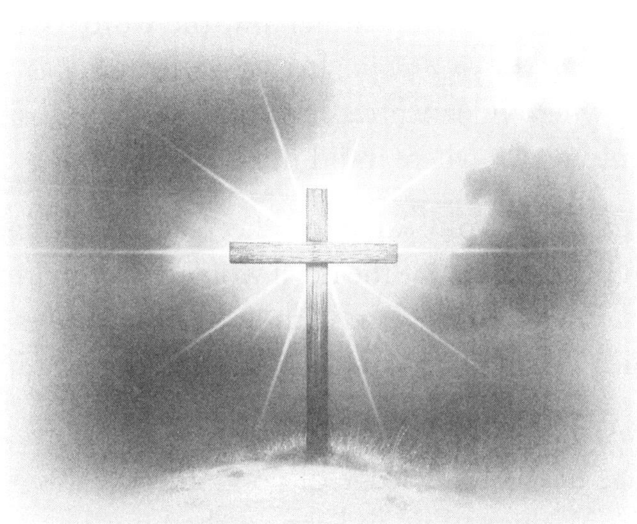

# WHY PEOPLE GET SICK – REASON NUMBER 1: THE BIGGEST CULPRIT IS THE CURSE

When illness strikes, whether it touches us personally or affects someone dear, the question of *why* inevitably follows. This search for understanding is particularly poignant for those who hold firm beliefs in healing. But when searching for answers as to *why* people get sick, we must begin by turning to the book of Genesis, where we discover the biggest culprit responsible for sickness.

After God was finished with the work of creation, He created Adam and Eve and placed them in the Garden of Eden, which was an ideal, perfect environment that was absolutely devoid of sin, sickness, strife, difficulties, and death.

Until Adam transgressed, he and Eve walked in perfect fellowship with God and experienced abundant life as God originally designed all humans to experience.

But in Genesis 2:15, we are informed that God gave Adam the responsibility to "keep" the Garden of Eden. In Hebrew, the word "keep" means *to keep, to guard, to hedge about*, or *to protect*. It is a word that was used especially to describe moments when vigilance was required to keep a sinister force from finding entrance into places where it did not belong.

The very fact that God told Adam to "keep" the Garden informs us God had warned Adam in advance that the devil would try to worm his way into the Garden, and, thus, God tasked Adam with protecting the Garden and keeping it so secure that the devil would be prohibited from penetrating it.

God had told Adam and Eve they could eat of every tree in the Garden of Eden *except* the tree of the knowledge of good and evil (*see* Genesis 2:16-17). But after the serpent seduced Eve and she reached out to eat of the forbidden fruit, it appears Adam did not want to be separated from his wife, so he willingly reached out to partake of the fruit of that tree as well — and his transgression opened a door for death, which immediately flooded, inundated, and eventually engulfed the planet.

Think of what happens when a massive concrete dam suddenly cracks and breaks under immense pressure. With a deafening roar, the dam yields as its immense structure shatters violently and releases a powerful wall of water — the torrent frothing and churning and carrying debris in a tumultuous deluge.

Like a relentless force of nature, the water spreads out across the landscape, flooding fields, roads, and buildings. Having broken free from the confines of the dam that once held it back, the water continues to spread and leaves a trail of destruction in its wake as it engulfs everything in its path, uprooting trees, obliterating manmade structures, and erasing familiar landscape.

Likewise, when the door was thrown wide open by Adam's transgression, it was as if a spiritual dam had broken, and suddenly the earth was engulfed by an evil, dark presence that quickly began to contort, pervert, and twist everything God had originally intended to be good.

With that dam broken and the door standing wide open, the very essence of evil began to consume everything in its path, and darkness unfurled its ravenous tendrils into every sphere of the planet. Evil spread and mercilessly filled the earth with its dreadful substance — a presence that carried with it death and destruction. Through the open door that Adam had unsealed by his willful transgression, death entered the world with a furious intensity.

Adam's transgression *literally* opened a door and provided an "entry point" through which death descended upon the earthly realm and enveloped it in its shadowy darkness. Adam's action was so catastrophic that in Genesis 3:17 God told him, "Because thou hast hearkened unto the voice of thy wife, and hast eaten of the tree, of which I commanded thee, saying, Thou shalt not eat of it: *cursed* is the *ground* for thy sake...."

In Hebrew, the word "cursed" is from a word that means *to bitterly and horribly curse.* God said that because of Adam's disobedience, the "ground" would be *bitterly and horribly cursed.* In Hebrew, the word "ground" depicts not only the earth itself, but everything in *the earth realm.* The words "for thy sake" mean *on account of you* or *because of what you have done.*

As a result of Adam's transgression, the earth and everything in it has become bitterly and horribly cursed. Just as God had warned them, death came rushing into the earth realm and spread into everything with its deadly presence. As a result, as God explained in Genesis 3:18, "Thorns also and thistles shall it [the earth realm] bring forth to thee; and thou shalt eat the herb of the field."

In Hebrew, the word "thorns" depicts *thorns, thornbushes,* or *dangerous, hurtful, prickly situations,* and it is figuratively used to depict *dangerous enemies.* The word for "thistles" describes *something running out of control.* It is hard to imagine, but the instant Adam sinned and threw open the door to the curse, the Garden of Eden — which means *pleasure and delight* — instantly spiraled into chaos.

**Through the open door that Adam had unsealed by his willful transgression, death entered the world with a furious intensity.**

The serene Garden once flourished with vibrant flowers, calm waters, and fragrant beauty, but after that moment, the once clear and peaceful waters became turbulent and muddied, and lush greenery twisted into tangled, thorny vines.

The Garden of Eden abruptly changed from a peaceful, well-managed haven into a chaotic, harmful, and uncontrolled environment. What was once well-tended had unraveled and transformed into an uncontrolled environment that became harmful.

God told Adam that, as a result of his transgression, he and Eve would "...eat the herb of the field" (Genesis 3:18). The Hebrew word for "herb" means *grass* or *herbs*. Such herbs and grass were different from the luscious fruit that grew in the Garden of Eden.

The words "of the field" means *country*, *ground*, *wild land*, or *battlefield.* Thus, once Adam's transgression opened the door to death, all of its death-producing consequences invaded the planet until the earth morphed from the beautiful paradise God intended it to be into a wild place and a battlefield where they would need to fight daily for survival.

When Adam's fateful choice swung open the floodgates to death, it was as if an unseen veil had been torn apart that allowed spiritual darkness to invade the world. From that moment on, a cascade of consequences swept across the earth, and the paradise that was once resplendent and with God's glory began to twist and warp under the weight of death's intrusion.

Nature, which had once thrived in its harmonious environment, now found its melody dissonant. The trees, which had formerly flourished in golden sunbeams, were suddenly overcome with strong and unpredictable winds. Rivers, once calm and purposeful, became tumultuous as their waters displayed the change. The once-clear and tranquil skies began brewing tempests that confirmed the fractured peace.

The earth quickly transformed into a wild expanse of distorted beauty and savage conflict. Animals and vegetation, which once knew abundance without end, became contenders for existence as they fought against one another for survival.

And most importantly, humanity — which was the crown of God's creation — found itself no longer in effortless communion with the world and with God. Suddenly, it was thrust into a battlefield where each dawn brought new challenges. To be clear, the moment the force of death entered the earth realm and its destructive power hit Adam and Eve, it stripped them of the glory that adorned them, and they found themselves naked and ashamed.

Being ashamed of what they had done, Adam and Eve "hid themselves from the presence of the Lord God amongst the trees of the garden" (Genesis 3:8). But Genesis 3:9-10 goes on to say, "...And the Lord God called unto Adam, and said unto him, Where art thou? And he said, I heard thy voice in the garden, and I was afraid, because I was naked; and I hid myself."

In the dawn of creation, God fashioned Adam and Eve in His own likeness and cloaked them in a radiant brilliance similar to His celestial splendor. This is the imagery Paul evoked in Romans 3:23 when he reflected on how humanity had "come [fallen] short of the glory of God."

The phrase "come short" is derived from the Greek term *hustereo*, which signifies a state of *deficiency* or *lack*. Man, who was once enveloped in brilliance, now perceived his own bare vulnerability as that glory was stripped away. Much like an unexpected wardrobe mishap that reveals and mortifies a person, Adam and Eve suddenly found themselves bereft of the luminous glory that previously adorned them. The glory of God that had once clothed them was violently stripped away by the cascading forces of death and darkness that assaulted them.

As we saw previously, when God saw what happened, He told Adam, "... Cursed is the ground *for thy sake...* "(Genesis 3:17). Many have wrongly thought that God cursed the ground, but the phrase "for thy sake" means *on account of you* or *because of what you have done.* This means it was Adam's disobedience that opened the door for the devil and death to come raging into everything in the earth realm.

The fact is that if Adam had not transgressed, these events would have never occurred, but when Adam disobeyed God's command, his disobedience literally threw open a spiritual door and provided an "entry point" for the devil and death to wreak havoc in everything in the earth realm.

Before this pivotal moment, the Garden was untouched by the jagged presence of thistles, thornbushes, or any prickly predicaments. Peace reigned over the land, unsullied by adversaries. But with the sudden descent of creation into the shadowy realm of death, a sinister transformation began.

In the blink of an eye, thorns and thistles emerged, casting a prickly pall over what was once idyllic, and death ascended the throne as the new authority. The once radiant tapestry of nature that was crafted by God's hand to be a masterpiece of beauty and good was abruptly distorted and marred by the venomous curse that contorted its once pristine essence into something completely unrecognizable.

For instance, roses, meant to embody pure beauty, found their tender branches burdened with thorns that pricked unwarily. The creatures of the earth, which had once lived side by side in blissful camaraderie, no longer lived in peace as mortality cast its long and dark shadow over them. From that moment on, the once-gentle creatures began their struggle, turning upon one another in a brutal dance of predation and survival.

In the beginning, sorrow was unknown, but with Adam's single act of defiance, the floodgates were opened, and his choice altered the fabric of earthly existence. The cascading consequences of death we see in the world today stem directly from that pivotal moment of disobedience, but they were never a part of the original divine design.

Today death's pervasive presence is still in the earth and manifests its malice in many forms — including bloodshed, disease, earthquakes, famines, hunger, murder, pestilence, perversion, sickness, strife, and war. But none of these existed before Adam's transgression. All of it was the effect of Adam's decision to disobey — it was *not* God's doing.

## 'DAMAGING' THE LORD'S REPUTATION

Today insurance companies often label earthquakes, famines, hurricanes, tornadoes, and climate change as acts of God; yet such a designation couldn't be more misleading. In reality, these devastating events are unjustly attributed to God. The truth is that God is blamed for many tragic happenings that have absolutely nothing to do with Him.

As we have seen, if Adam had safeguarded the Garden as he was instructed, such calamities would never have found a foothold. These disruptive forces are echoes of Adam's misstep. If Adam had protected the Garden as God commanded him, none of these things would have ever occurred. These troublesome natural disasters are the result of the reign of death that entered the world after Adam's transgression.

Not long after God delivered Israel from Egyptian bondage, He gave Moses the Ten Commandments, which are recorded in Exodus 20. In the Third Commandment, God said, "Thou shalt not take the name of the Lord thy God in vain; for the Lord will not hold him guiltless that taketh his name in vain" (Exodus 20:7).

Many think that taking the name of the Lord in vain means to use the Lord's name in connection with curse words. Joseph Telushkin, a respected Jewish rabbi, comments, "From Judaism's perspective, it is a *Chillul Hashem* [desecrating God's Name] to associate God with evil; that may well be why God announces that He will not forgive those who violate the Third Commandment ('the Lord will not clear one who carries His Name in vain,' Exodus 20:7). The reason would seem to be obvious: when we commit an evil act such as murdering or stealing, we discredit ourselves, but when we do evil in God's Name, we discredit God and alienate people who might otherwise have become drawn to God and religion."[1]

From Telushkin's insights, we see taking the Lord's name in vain involves wrongly associating God with actions or events that are not His doing. When individuals unjustly hold God accountable for events independent of His involvement, it tarnishes His reputation in people's minds. Reflect for a moment on how many harbor resentment toward God due to unfounded accusations linking Him to a loved one's passing, an illness, a traffic accident, or natural disasters such as hurricanes or tornadoes.

The essence of the Third Commandment crucially underscores that attributing harmful or destructive actions to God — actions He is not responsible for — constitutes "taking the Lord's name in vain."

God is profoundly displeased with those who unfairly place the blame on Him for occurrences unrelated to His will, and as the commandment states, "the Lord will not hold him guiltless that taketh His name in vain." This means that God does not wish to be erroneously implicated in events entirely disconnected from Him.

Remember, before Adam blatantly disobeyed and threw open the door for the devil and death, there was no bloodshed, disease, earthquakes, famine, hunger, murder, pestilence, perversion, sickness, strife, or war. It was Adam's disobedience that opened the door to the curse and to death in all its forms, and the effects of it have been running wild on the planet ever since. God is so against these things that, in Christ, He has given His people the authority and faith to overcome these things that are in the world (*see* 1 John 5:4).

## SCRIPTURE IS CLEAR: MAN'S SIN OPENED THE DOOR FOR DEATH TO INVADE THE WORLD

It is impossible to overstate the significance of the curse and its diabolical effects on the earth and on mankind. In Romans 5:12, Paul fully explained the tragic event that occurred when Adam disobeyed. That verse says, "Wherefore, as by one man sin entered into the world, and death by sin; and so death passed upon all men...."

The word "wherefore" is a translation of the Greek words *dia touto*, which means *on account of this*, *as a result of this*, or *consequently*. Paul herein stated that it is *on the account of* or *as a result of* what Adam did that "...sin entered into the world, and death by sin...."

The word "world" is interpreted from the Greek word *kosmos*, which refers to *everything related to the world*, including *nature* and *all human systems*. So in this verse, Paul wrote that when Adam disobeyed, sin literally entered into every system in the world, including *nature, human institutions, and all aspects of the human race and creation.*

Paul furthermore stated that with the emergence of sin came "death." The word "death" in Romans 5:12 is translated from the Greek word *thanatos*, which depicts both *physical and spiritual death.* It is also notably a word that was used to depict *a death sentence.* When Adam sinned, death entered the human race and *a death sentence* was passed onto creation.

The Greek word for "death," the word *thanatos*, is used with a definite article in Romans 5:12, and that definite article means it should be translated *the death* — it speaks of an all-pervasive death that permeated every part of the earth realm. This articulation underscores a profound, all-encompassing mortality that seeped into every corner of the earthly sphere.

Once more, we see that when Adam defied divine instruction, it unleashed a torrent of mortality upon the world as a relentless tide swept through every corner of creation and marked humanity with the indelible stain of death. Bloodshed, disease, earthquakes, famine, hunger, murder, pestilence, perversion, sickness, strife, and war, none of which marred creation before Adam's grievous choices, suddenly became grim and rampant realities.

With the proverbial gates flung wide open, Satan surged forth and plagued humankind with every conceivable torment contrary to God's original vision of goodness. It is the malevolent and twisted nature of Satan that spawned these afflictions and warped and distorted what was meant to be resplendent.

And disease, illness, and sickness, also which were previously nonexistent, became prevalent among the results of Satan's desire to afflict everything God had made to be good.

## DEATH HAS 'REIGNED' ON EARTH SINCE ADAM SINNED

In Romans 5:17, Paul wrote, "For if by one man's offence death reigned by one; much more they which receive abundance of grace and of the gift of righteousness shall reign in life by one, Jesus Christ."

The word "offense" finds its roots in the Greek word *paraptoma*, which signifies *a deliberate infraction.* When Adam extended his hand to receive the forbidden fruit — fruit explicitly prohibited by God — he did so with full awareness of his disobedience. There was no misunderstanding or confusion; God's command was unequivocal, and Adam consciously chose to defy it.

This deliberate act of rebellion — a *conscious transgression* — ushered in spiritual darkness, and humanity was consequently enveloped by the specter of death, which infiltrated every corner of existence and every part of the world's intricate designs. As captured in the original text of Romans 5:17, all of this unfolded due to one man's actions, a singular act that allowed death to gain dominion and hold sway.

The term "reigned" is derived from the Greek word *basileuo*, which conveys the notion of *ruling with kingly power.* Consequently, with Adam's disobedience, death assumed its dominion over the earth and humanity at large. Today this tyrannical rule of death manifests in myriad forms, including illnesses and diseases of every kind, bloodshed, murder, plagues, tremors of the earth, famines, hunger, pestilence, corruption, discord, war, and countless other calamities.

In Second Corinthians 4:4, Paul painted a vivid portrait of Satan when he called him the "god of this world." The term "world" comes from the Greek word *aion*, which encapsulates all that is tied to *this present earthly age and domain*. According to Paul, Satan's pervasive evil influence clouds the earthly realm, and his sinister influence leaves no stone unturned in his mission to disrupt and distress.

But regardless of the arsenal Satan may wield or the strategies he employs in the earthly realm, First John 5:4 boldly proclaims that our faith is a formidable force that transcends and triumphs over it. Satan may temporarily exercise his pervasive evil influence as the "god of this world," but our position in Christ empowers us to overcome and override his activities, and that includes moments when he dares to invade our health and well-being.

But in Romans 5:21, a mere four verses later, Paul echoed his earlier sentiment and again declared that sin has perpetually "reigned unto death." The word "reigned" is again translated from the Greek word *basileuo*, which conveys the idea of *reigning with the authority of a king.*

Paul's recurrent use of the word *basileuo* underscores his intention for God's people to grasp the gravity of the situation: When Adam consciously chose to sin, he flung wide the gates for death itself to surge forth and assert its kingly dominion over the world — its reign unleashing a cascade of grim, heinous, and dreadful consequences.

## GOD'S GRACE HAS DETHRONED THE RULE OF DEATH IN OUR LIVES

However, in Paul's writings, he also conveyed that the Cross and the resurrection of Jesus Christ empower us to overcome death and its curse. As articulated in Romans 5:17 and 21, this profound message reveals that the Cross and Resurrection grant us an abundance of grace and the gift of righteousness, and we are consequently enabled to "reign in life" through Jesus Christ.

This signifies a transformative shift where, through God's grace and the righteousness bestowed upon us in Christ, the dominion of death and its curse is vanquished. Instead of succumbing to their dark influence, we are now empowered to "reign in life by one, Jesus Christ" (Romans 5:17).

The term "reign" is once again translated from the Greek word *basileuo*, which means *to rule with royal power* or *to wield kingly authority*. Herein, we find that God's plan is for every believer to live with the sovereignty of a monarch and exert regal influence in this life. Through the triumph of Jesus on the Cross and His victorious emergence from the grave, He has shattered the dominion of death over children of God.

And consequently, even as we live in a world where death continues to hold sway over many and much of creation bears the burden of its curse, those who are in Christ are liberated from the chains of death's rule and the curse unleashed by Adam's sin.

In First Corinthians 15:55, Paul wrote, "O death, where is thy sting? O grave, where is thy victory?" Then in verse 57, Paul added, "But thanks be to God, which giveth us the victory through our Lord Jesus Christ." This of course refers to Christ's victory over death and the fact that we, as believers, not only don't feel the sting of death, but we are awaiting our own future resurrection from the dead. This element of Christ's victory over defeat belongs to every authentic believer right now!

**Satan may temporarily exercise his pervasive evil influence as the "god of this world," but our position in Christ empowers us to overcome and override his activities, and that includes moments when he dares to invade our health and well-being.**

But moving forward, in Romans 8:22, Paul gave us a perfect picture of the earth's ongoing struggle under the shadow of death, a legacy of Adam's transgression. He captures this with the words, "For we know that the whole creation groaneth and travaileth in pain together until now." This verse conjures an image of a world yearning for liberation and anticipating the day when Satan is bound and the curse of death is completely lifted.

Although believers have triumphed over death through faith, its rule persists in the world, and the planet itself longs for the promised time of renewal and restoration to God's original vision when it will be free from all the death-related effects of Satan's rule in the world. Eventually a time will come when the earthly realm will be fully restored to God's original divine plan that first existed in the Garden of Eden. At that time, all the effects of death's rule, which include disease, illness, and sickness, will vanish.

But in the same way Jesus wielded authority over the natural world during His earthly ministry, He has bequeathed to believers dominion over all things within the earthly realm, and that includes nature itself. Across two millennia, countless believers have borne witness to the power of their faith as they commanded nature's tumultuous forces — such as diverting or dissipating tornadoes and hurricanes — and saw those forces obey them. This book, however, narrows its focus to understanding how to harness our Christ-bestowed authority and our faith to transcend the impacts of disease, illness, and sickness.

By using the Almighty name of Jesus that is higher than every other name, and by embracing the promises in Scripture and wielding the regal authority bestowed upon us by Christ, every believer can transcend the burdens of the curse.

**By using the Almighty name of Jesus that is higher than every other name, and by embracing the promises in Scripture and wielding the regal authority bestowed upon us by Christ, every believer can transcend the burdens of the curse.**

If authentic Christians will embrace the truth and release their faith for it, they will rise *above* corruption, famine, hunger, epidemics, pestilence, poverty, strife, war, and innumerable other tribulations — all of which are developments God *never* intended to be a part of the human race.

## THROUGH CHRIST, YOU HAVE A FAITH THAT OVERCOMES THE WORLD

Through Jesus Christ, every believer is endowed with a faith powerful enough to conquer all the challenges this world presents — including diseases, illnesses, and sicknesses of every kind, along with every aspect of mortality unleashed by Adam's fall. As stated in First John 5:4, "For whatsoever is born of God overcometh the world: and this is the victory that overcometh the world, even our faith."

If you are born of God, this verse describes you, and it declares that if you are an authentic child of God, He has given you authority to "overcome" the "world." The word "overcome" is translated from the Greek word *nikao*, which means *to conquer, to conquest, to master, to overcome, to prevail, to subdue, and to have victory*. First John 5:4 could be interpreted, "For whatsoever is born of God conquers, conquests, masters, prevails over, subdues, and ultimately has victory over the world...."

However, in First John 5:4, the word "world" is translated from the Greek word *kosmos*, which is a metaphor for what we are divinely empowered to overcome — *the world*. In those who are joint-heirs with Christ, there resides an extraordinary authority that bestows upon each one the ability to excel and be elevated over, dominate, and ultimately conquer every opposing force, including the ancient curse set in motion by Adam's original sin.

But John continued to declare, "...This is the victory that overcometh the world, even our faith." Interestingly, the word "overcometh" is also derived from the same Greek word *nike*, which signifies *conquest*, *mastery*, or *victory*. Thus, we find that God has given to each authentic believer a faith that prevails against the world. The expression "overcometh" stems from the Greek word *nikesasa*, and given its past tense, a more fitting translation would be "having already conquered the world" or "having already overcome the world."

The word "world" again traces its roots to the Greek word *kosmos*, which refers to *everything in the earth realm*. Through faith in Christ, His Word, and His name, we gain dominion over all that the adversary attempts to manipulate within the earthly domain. This empowerment extends to triumphing over ailments, afflictions, and maladies, which were once woven into the fabric of the original curse but have since been rendered powerless for those who anchor their belief in Christ.

## JESUS RESTORED WHAT WAS LOST

So we see that through Adam's act of disobedience, a door was flung open that unleashed the rampant forces of death across the globe. In an instant, mortality seized the throne and with thorns and thistles sowed chaos and catastrophe, transforming the world into a theater of turmoil. Calamities multiplied — disease, illness, sickness, conflict, pestilence, and the fury of a rebellious climate with earthquakes, tornadoes, and hurricanes, none of which were the handiwork of the Creator. These calamities were the offspring of death and have been felt in the earth realm ever since Adam first transgressed.

But for those who embrace Jesus as their Lord, death no longer holds its former authority. Through faith in Christ's triumphant sacrifice on the Cross and His resurrection, God now intends for His children to experience a life unshackled from the curse's consequences.

Jesus reclaimed what humanity lost through the Fall, and God's ultimate plan is for His followers to "reign" with divine authority and to rule with the regal grace bestowed upon them through Christ Jesus. The authority of death has been decommissioned and dethroned, and Jesus has restored what was lost through the fall of man. In Christ, it is now God's best intention for His people "to reign" as kings and to express the kingly authority given to us in Christ Jesus!

This brings to mind what Jesus promised in Luke 10:19 when He said, "Behold, I give unto you power to tread on serpents and scorpions, and over all the power of the enemy: and nothing shall by any means hurt you."

When Jesus spoke this to His disciples, it followed His directive to venture into the world's vast fields to harvest souls in every corner (*see* Luke 10:2-11). His words were assurance that as they spread across the earth, they would be enveloped in divine safety and made immune to any sinister plot or hurdle the adversary might concoct.

The term "tread" in Luke 10:19 originates from the Greek word *pateo* and it means *to walk*. By choosing this word, Jesus promised His followers an extraordinary safeguard that would enable them to confidently step over any malevolence the adversary might unleash. He further declared, "...And nothing shall by any means hurt you." Here the word "hurt" is derived from the Greek word *adikeo*, which implies *suffering injustice* or *enduring wrongs*. Thus, Jesus assures His people that even if they encounter injustice or wrongs along the way, they will be supernaturally empowered to rise above it.

But pay heed to the terms "over," "all," "power," and "enemy" in verse 19. The word "over" is translated from the Greek word *epi*, which means *over* or *upon*, and it signifies *a superior position*. The word "all" in Greek is *all-encompassing* and refers unequivocally to *everything* the enemy might attempt. The word "power" stems from the word *dunamis*, which indicates *an immense force*, and the use of this word acknowledges that the devil indeed wields power in this earthly realm.

The word "enemy" is translated from a form of the Greek word *echtros*, which portrays *one who is not just oppositional, but fiercely hostile*, and it illustrates the devil's *malevolent disposition*. Yet Jesus proclaims that He has endowed every follower with the divine ability to tread upon and transcend all the enemy's might. Thus, irrespective of the enemy's relentless animosity and opposition, in Christ, we are granted supremacy above all adversarial power.

Significantly, the Greek construction of this phrase in Luke 10:19 includes *a triple negative*. It emphatically states in the Greek, "And nothing [first negative], no nothing [second negative], by no means [third negative], will injure or harm you."

Jesus unequivocally promised each of His followers divine protection, resolutely declaring and assuring, "And nothing, no nothing, by no means, will injure or harm you." And this is so encompassing that it would include our capacity to overcome, surpass, and triumph over disease, illness, sickness, and *any* ailment that Satan may try to send against us.

This means that by nurturing our soul and spirit with God's Word, by aligning our lives with its guidance, and by using the name of Jesus that is bestowed upon us, we have the ability to neutralize, overcome, rise above, and transcend any opposing force that comes against us. Indeed, this empowerment enables every child of God to even use Christ-given authority and faith to drive back the effects of disease, illness, and sickness so that we may enjoy health and wholeness as God originally planned.

Yet a multitude of Christians find themselves living under the effects of Adam's original transgression and unaware that the Cross confers upon them the power to counteract the schemes of Satan — *including disease, illness, and sickness* — which are results of death that flooded the earth at the time of Adam's transgression.

It is for this reason, among others, that I have crafted this book — to illuminate the path by which a faithful believer can harness faith to overcome any hindrance imposed by Satan within the earthly realm. To ascend to such a victorious stature requires instruction rooted in the redemptive work of the Cross, and it necessitates a transformation of the mind that embraces the truth that through God's grace conferred on us in Christ, we are empowered to "reign in life" across every domain.

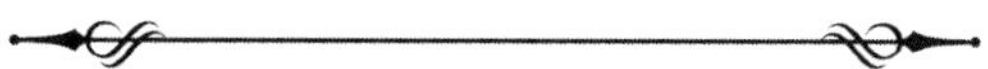

**This means that by nurturing our soul and spirit with God's Word, by aligning our lives with its guidance, and by using the name of Jesus that is bestowed upon us, we have the ability to neutralize, overcome, rise above, and transcend any opposing force that comes against us.**

Nevertheless, we see that Adam's misstep unleashed death's embrace onto humanity and wove its ominous influence across the entire human spectrum. Even when individuals strive to lead virtuous lives, eat nutritious diets, and vigorously keep fit, the shadow of death still attempts to manifest as disease, illness, and sickness. But in the chapters ahead, you will see that on the Cross, Christ wholly paid the price for our liberation from these afflictions.

In the next chapter, we'll explore another reason behind human disease, illness, and sickness. As our journey unfolds, I will shed light on fundamental reasons why believers grapple with ill health. While there may be other contributing factors, these are the primary perpetrators we will focus on that affect Christians' physical and mental well-being.

Scan the QR code to watch Rick teach more on this subject.

# QUESTIONS TO PONDER AND DISCUSS

1. In Genesis 2:15, we learned that God gave Adam the responsibility to "keep" the Garden of Eden — to keep, to guard, to hedge, and to protect it. What does this instruction to keep what God gives you tell you about the outside spiritual forces that come to steal the life and blessings God desires for every believer? What can you do as a part of your daily spiritual walk to maintain the territory and the good things God has given you? (Read Proverbs 4:23; John 10:10; and 2 Corinthians 2:11 for insight.)

2. When Adam sinned, the curse came and death flooded the Garden, leaving nothing of God's creation untouched by evil. Even worse, Adam and Eve lost their fellowship with the Lord and hid from His presence. Why is it so important to confess your wrongdoing to God and turn to Him when you've disobeyed His Word? How does shame cripple believers and prevent them from living the overcoming life in Christ that He desires for them? Read Hebrews 10:4-17 and First John 1:7 and ponder the death-defying power in the blood of Jesus that is still speaking on our behalf today!

3. Death reigned on the earth through one man's sin. But through Christ's supreme sacrifice of the shedding of His own blood, those who adhere to Him have been granted access to redemption — the abundance of grace, the gift of righteousness, and the ability to reign supreme over the tyranny of death and destruction. Besides the new birth, what demonstrations of God's power today indicate to you that others are reigning over death and destruction through Christ? Do you personally know someone who has received a supernatural healing from some physical condition or has overcome a debilitating addiction? If so, note and ponder his or her journey and testimony.

4. Why is it so important not just to read about Christ's work of redemption on your behalf — but to embrace that truth and meditate on it until it positively affects your mind, will, and emotions and your words and actions? Consider Joshua 1:8, Proverbs 4:20-22, Romans 12:2, and Hebrews 11:6

and list ways you can make your faith effectual in receiving the blessings God has to offer and has promised in His Word.

5. The words "tread," "over," "all," "power," and "enemy" in Luke 10:19 leave no room for speculation or doubt concerning God's will for you as a believer and what Jesus empowered you with in His name through His death and resurrection. Review these words as expounded on from the Greek and write down instances in which you wielded your Christ-given authority and received a positive outcome over some injustice or wrong in your life. Are you facing a challenge from the enemy right now? In what area, or areas, do you need to tread all over the enemy's might and exert your superior position in Christ over this opposition?

## THREE

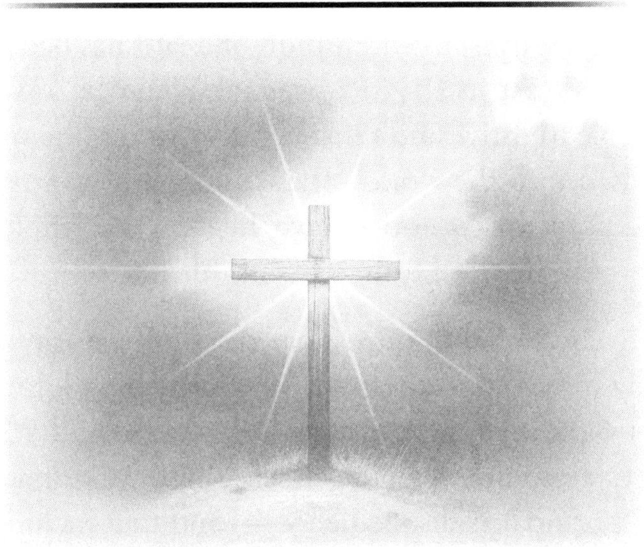

# WHY PEOPLE GET SICK — REASON NUMBER 2: LACK OF KNOWLEDGE CAN OPEN A DOOR TO SICKNESS

In the previous chapter, we saw that the main reason *why people get sick* is the curse — because death entered the earth realm due to Adam's transgression. Prior to Adam's disobedience, the earth was a haven of tranquility and protection.

However, Adam's act of defiance sowed seeds of chaos, wherein thorns and thistles sprang up and perilous circumstances took root. Death assumed a sovereign role and began to reign supreme over all living things. This malevolent shift gave rise to a plethora of afflictions, maladies, and sicknesses as side effects of the curse — all conditions that did not exist before this fateful event.

But the good news is that for those who put their faith in Jesus and crown Him as the ruler of their lives, the dominion of death has been shattered. While the curse continues to cast its shadow over the planet as a whole, God's grace empowers His people to thrive and resist bending under the weight that Adam's disobedience released into the world. Thanks to the power of Christ's sacrifice on the Cross and His victory over the grave, healing and wholeness are possible, and God's children can be freed from a life of infirmity.

Jesus' redemptive work on the Cross gave us the authority to live a life more like God originally intended. And as we have seen, First John 5:4 declares that our faith enables us to overcome and override everything that's working against us in the world's systems, including the effects of the curse that came raging into the earth as a result of Adam's disobedience — and that includes disease, illness, and sickness.

But for a Christian believer to put his faith in Christ for healing from sickness, he's going to have to *know and understand* what Christ did for him in redeeming him from the awful curse brought upon the earth and those living in it through the fall of man.

*Ignorance is not bliss!* In fact, it can be a hindrance and a blockage to the blessing of healing that God provided for every one of His children in His redemptive plan.

## WE ARE DELIVERED FROM THE POWER OF DARKNESS

When Christ rose triumphant from the grave, His resurrection unleashed an overwhelming surge of power that swept away the grip of evil for those who are in Christ. And when we embraced God's call and enthroned Christ in our hearts, God "delivered us from the power of darkness, and hath translated us into the kingdom of his dear Son" (Colossians 1:13).

The word "delivered" is interpreted from a form of the Greek word *rhuomai*, which means *deliverance*, *rescue*, or *extraction from peril.* Paul employed this term to vividly describe the transformative power of Jesus' blood and its ability to liberate every believer from the oppressive realm of darkness.

By choosing the word *rhuomai*, Paul triumphantly asserted that Christ's blood was the liberating force that extracted each child of God from the clutches of darkness. This is far from being a mere metaphorical expression, for we have been genuinely *delivered, rescued, and extracted* "from the power of darkness."

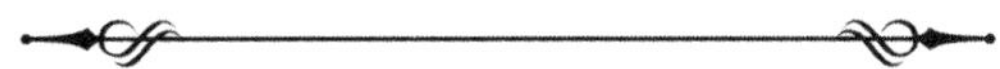

**When Christ rose triumphant from the grave, His resurrection unleashed an overwhelming surge of power that swept away the grip of evil for those who are in Christ.**

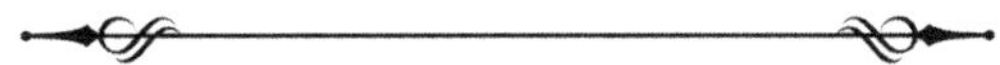

The word "from" is derived from the Greek word *ek*, which means *out* and serves as the root of our modern word "exit." The word "power" is from a form of the Greek word *exousia*, and it means *authority* and conveys the ideas of *control* or *jurisdiction*, whether over individuals or an entire domain.

The word "darkness" originates from a form of the Greek word *skotos*, which portrays *the absolute absence of light*. Paul employed *skotos* to picture the dark realm where Satan exerts control and jurisdiction over the lost, as well as in the earthly realm where he temporarily exercises his authority. Furthermore, the word "darkness" informs us that Satan's domain is so *densely dark* that it is *absolutely void of light.*

As a complete phrase, Colossians 1:13 tells us that when Christ became Lord of our lives, God literally *delivered, rescued, removed, and extracted us out from the control and jurisdiction of darkness where Satan rules.* Satan's lethal hold on us was broken, and Christ's blood became our passage out from the domain filled with death and the consequences unleashed upon the world from the time of Adam's transgression.

But Colossians 1:13 proclaims that we have not merely been extracted from the stronghold of darkness and its commanding grip — God then "translated" us into the Kingdom of His dear Son. The word "translated" is derived from a form of the word *methistema*, which is a compound of the words *meta* and *histemi*. The word *meta* signifies *a change*, while *histemi* means *to stand.* But when these words are compounded, it comes to picture *a shift in position*. While we were formerly prisoners of the oppressive reign of darkness and its tangled influence, Christ *liberated, redeemed, and extracted* us from that realm, and we were ushered into the Kingdom of God's beloved Son.

The word "kingdom" is derived from the Greek word *basileia*, which signifies *a realm governed by a sovereign*. We were formerly in the kingdom of darkness, but we now have a new standing in a realm, a Kingdom, illuminated by light, where all is to align perfectly with the redemptive work achieved by Christ on the Cross.

Romans 8:11 tells us that now the Holy Spirit dwells within you as a believer, and that divine presence carries the unparalleled force of resurrection — a divine power that is intended to unlock you from the afflictions that were associated with your former residence in the kingdom of darkness. Those old attributes of darkness are to remain back in the kingdom of darkness. But now that you have been transferred into the Kingdom of God, it is God's intention for you to experience the benefits of that realm where there are no effects of death and darkness and where God desires for you to perpetually experience everything purchased by Christ Himself for you at the Cross.

But as we have seen, despite all that Christ has achieved for His people, countless believers still find themselves ensnared in the grips of physical- and mental-health issues. This is largely due to their unawareness of the victory that Christ won at the Cross, which includes healing and health. This lack of knowledge keeps many shackled in recurring bouts of sickness because they are oblivious to the truth that it is God's will for them to live with healing and health.

## PEOPLE ARE DESTROYED FOR LACK OF KNOWLEDGE

In Hosea 4:6, God says, "My people are *destroyed* for lack of *knowledge*...."

The word "destroyed" in this verse is from a Hebrew word that means *to cease, to cut off, to obliterate, to perish, to ruin, to silence*, or even *to unravel.* The Hebrew word for "knowledge" conveys nuances of *insight, perception*, or *truth.* In the context of the phrase "lack of knowledge," the word "knowledge" refers to a person or a group of people who are *uninformed, oblivious*, or *devoid of fundamental truths.*

In Hosea 4:6, God was declaring, "My people are cut off, destroyed, perishing, brought to ruin, silenced, and undone because they are devoid of fundamental knowledge and truth."

It is interesting that in 1742, the English poet Thomas Gray coined the phrase, "Ignorance is bliss."[1] But reality shows that ignorance or a lack of knowledge wreaks havoc and ignites a chain of detrimental effects. The truth is that ignorance is the *greatest adversary* to bliss and that wherever ignorance prevails, grave outcomes are never far behind.

For example, ignorance about personal finances can pave a perilous road toward debt and a shaky financial existence. A lack of knowledge regarding one's health can lead to detrimental eating practices and invite illnesses that might have been easily sidestepped with right eating habits. Ignorance about "truth" leads to wrong beliefs, and when wrong beliefs are embraced and taught to others, they will produce adverse outcomes.

As I told you previously, my wife and I were each reared in a wonderful church environment that instilled in us a profound love for God and the Bible and taught us to be steadfast in our devotion and service to the Church. The seeds planted in us during those formative years continue to shape our lives even now. Yet when it came to matters of healing and health purchased for us by Christ at the Cross, we were devoid of this fundamental knowledge and truth.

When I say we were ignorant, I do so without any intent to offend, as my heart is filled with gratitude for the spiritual environment in which we each grew up. However, at that time we lacked knowledge about the full scope of Christ's redemptive work. We understood it to encompass the forgiveness of sins, but were unaware that it also provided healing and health.

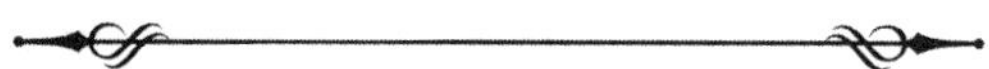

**It is interesting that in 1742, the English poet Thomas Gray coined the phrase, "Ignorance is bliss." But reality shows that ignorance or a lack of knowledge wreaks havoc and ignites a chain of detrimental effects. The truth is that ignorance is the *greatest adversary* to bliss and that wherever ignorance prevails, grave outcomes are never far behind.**

This aspect of redemption was beyond our comprehension, so we remained in the dark about this profound dimension of Christ's work on the Cross. We simply did not know that healing and health were "in the bank" and legally belonged to every child of God.

Consider again the scenario of an individual who unknowingly stands as the rightful beneficiary of a significant fortune that is securely nestled away in a bank vault. Despite being wealthy in title, if this heir remains oblivious to his inheritance, he may unknowingly trudge through life in poverty's shadow. Unseen riches lie at his fingertips, yet the veil of ignorance blinds him to what is rightfully his, compelling him to fight his way through the turbulent waters of financial struggle. Because he is uninformed about his inheritance, his wealth does nothing to elevate his status in life and he continues to live beggarly.

We actually once knew a widow who battled to make ends meet, and she prayed that God would miraculously do something to change her status and alleviate her financial stress. Then one ordinary morning was interrupted by an unexpected knock at her door. On the other side stood a lawyer who arrived to deliver news that sounded like a fairy tale. The attorney said, "A distant relative, one of immense wealth, has passed, and ever since he died, we've been searching to locate a living relative. And after much searching, we've found *you*." He continued, "It is my delight to announce that you are the rightful heir to what he left for you. A fortune is waiting for you to legally claim."

From the moment her distant relative passed away, this woman was legally the rightful owner of that fortune, yet before the moment of that surprise visit from the lawyer, she remained ignorant and unaware of her wealth. Oblivious to her inheritance, she navigated the turbulent waters of financial hardship for years. Destiny had bestowed upon her the keys to an opulent existence, but the secret treasure lay hidden for a time as she remained chained to her modest means. But when that attorney stood before her and enlightened her that she had an inheritance awaiting her, she began to live unshackled by financial stress. In fact, she directed the bulk of her wealth to support numerous ministries all the way to the end of her life.

The reality is that each of us has pockets of ignorance — but the topic of healing and health is so serious that we cannot afford to be void of knowledge on this matter. It is imperative that we grasp the teaching of the Bible that healing and health is God's will for every believer.

When Christians don't know that these blessings belong to them, it leads them health-wise to live shackled to sickness — when Christ's death and resurrection has put healing and health in the bank for them. Yet living ignorant of this fact causes them to live far below what God wants them to experience, and this is why believers can't afford to have a lack of knowledge on this matter that is so vital to their well-being.

But when my wife and I were growing up, we were not only unaware that Christ's work on the Cross encompassed provision for our healing and health, our ignorance was compounded by *mis*information. We wrongly believed that God even *intended* for us to endure disease, illness, and sickness — and clinging to this misguided belief, we actually embraced illness as a part of God's plan and believed that it was our duty to glorify God through our suffering.

However, when the truth of God's Word finally shined its brilliant light into this lack of knowledge in our lives, we discovered that the Bible promises forgiveness, peace of mind, and healing and health for the body.

## GOD'S EXPLICIT WILL FOR HIS PEOPLE TO BE HEALTHY AND WHOLE

In Chapter Nine, I will take you into some profound teaching concerning Christ's redemptive work on the Cross and all that it purchased for every child of God. In Chapter Ten, we will dive into the words of Isaiah 53:3-5, Matthew 8:17, and First Peter 2:24 to see exactly what Isaiah, Matthew, and Peter wrote about what Jesus obtained for us on the Cross.

But for now, I want to return to a quote from the Introduction, where I shared a verse that makes it clear that it is God's explicit will for His people to be healthy and whole. In Third John 2, the apostle John expressed the explicit will of God for our lives when he wrote, "Beloved, I wish above all things that thou mayest prosper and be in health even as thy soul prospereth."

I grew up reading the Bible, but never really paid attention to this verse. Because it is nestled inconspicuously in one of the New Testament's shortest books, its significance had gone unnoticed by my eyes. It wasn't until the day

I heard Oral Roberts share it that I found myself wondering, *How is it possible that I've lived my entire Christian life without noticing this verse?*

John, who was guided by the Holy Spirit as he wrote, articulated not only his own deepest desire for his readers, but also *God's* will for His people. Again, we read that John said, "I wish above all things that thou mayest prosper and be in health even as thy soul prospereth." This verse may seem very simple, but it succinctly declares God's unequivocal will for every believer.

Many translations render the word "wish" as "pray" — and, in fact, "wish" is translated from the Greek word *euchomai*, which expresses *strong desire* but can also signify *prayer* or *praying*. John begins by saying, "I wish," or "I pray." He was writing under the guidance of the Holy Spirit, which means He was desiring and praying the will of God. Thus, in John's prayer, we find that God's will "above all things" is that His people "prosper and be in health."

The words "above all things," as we've seen, are translated from the Greek words *peri panton*. The word *peri* suggests a *circumference* and symbolizes all that *encircles*, while the word *panton* is a comprehensive term representing *absolutely everything*. Together, the phrase conveys the idea of *everything that envelops, surrounds, and pertains to you* — and it truly encompasses *all aspects* of one's life.

## GOD INCLUDED FINANCIAL PROSPERITY ALONG WITH HEALING AND HEALTH IN OUR REDEMPTION

John then articulated that it was God's fervent will for His people to "prosper." The word "prosper" is translated from the Greek *euodoo*, which is a compound of the words *eu* and *hodos*. The prefix *eu* conveys a sense of whatever is *good*, and it evokes the ideas of *pleasure, joy, and delight*. The second part of this word is derived from the Greek word *hodos*, which pictures *a road*. When these words are compounded to form *euodoo*, the new word describes *encountering joy, delight, and pleasure on every road that you take in life*. It is a word in history that was particularly connected to the idea of *travel* and having *a good trip* along one's way.

In the ancient world, the benchmark of prosperity often hinged on one's financial capacity to journey to distant lands and to indulge in leisurely vacations. Take, for instance, Paul's impactful ministry in Ephesus, where local craftsmen who made idols of Artemis grew anxious about the threat to their "wealth" as a result of Paul's preaching in Ephesus.

The term "wealth" in Acts 19:25 is derived from the Greek term *euporia.* The word *euporia* is derived from the words *eu* and *poreuomai.* The prefix *eu*, again, conveys a sense of whatever is *good*, and it evokes the ideas of *pleasure, joy, and delight.* The word *poreuomai* means *to journey* or *to travel.* As a compound, it also speaks of having sufficient financial resources to journey abroad and to have enjoyable travel experiences. It is akin to the word *euodoo* that is found in Third John 2.

For the idol-makers in Ephesus, prosperity was synonymous with having the financial freedom to take holidays abroad, and these craftsmen feared that Paul's preaching, which resulted in a decline in idol sales, would endanger their revenue and, consequently, affect their ability to travel and vacation abroad.

In our world today, wealth is often gauged by the square footage of our homes, by our automobiles, or by the figures in our bank or investment accounts. Although houses and possessions also signaled wealth in the First Century, the ability to travel was a prominent indicator of affluence and prosperity.

While vacationing and traveling might not resonate as your personal dream, the Greek words used in Third John 2 tell us that true prosperity is having more than what's necessary to cover your fundamental expenses. It includes having enough financial resources to embrace any path that life presents. Simply put, it is not God's plan for His children to grapple with hardships and barely get by; rather, it is God's wish that they possess sufficient financial resources to savor the journey of life.

But then John went on to passionately express his deepest wish — and, indeed, the will of God — was that his readers, in addition to experiencing prosperity, would experience "health."

The word "health" is interpreted from a form of the Greek word *hugiaino*, which captures the ideas of *being physically fit, in optimal physical condition,* and *mentally sound.* It pictures *wholeness* and *one who is complete* and *sound* in each and every facet of his physical and mental being.

To review this critical point that I also made in the Introduction, we find the word *hugiaino* used *four times* in John 5 in connection with the lame man that Jesus healed at the pool of Bethesda.

- In John 5:6, Jesus asked the lame man, "Wilt thou be made whole?" The word "whole" is from a form of *hugiaino*, which means Jesus was actually asking if he wanted *to be healthy, in good working order*, and *sound physically and mentally.*

- In John 5:9, we read that after Jesus told the man to pick up his bed and walk, he was "made *whole.*" The word "whole" is again translated from a form of *hugiaino*, which means he was immediately *made healthy, restored to good working order, and made sound physically and mentally.*

- In John 5:11, after the religious leaders asked who healed him, the healed man answered that it was Jesus who had made him "whole." The word "whole" is again translated from a form of *hugiaino*, which means he testified that it was Jesus who'd made him *healthy, in good working order, and sound physically and mentally.*

- In John 5:14, after Jesus found the man, He told him, "Behold, thou art made whole." The word "whole" is again translated from a form of *hugiaino*, which means Jesus jubilantly acknowledged that the man was now *healthy, in good working order, and sound physically and mentally.*

When the apostle John expressed in Third John 2 his heartfelt wish, that was and is aligned with God's own will, he was clearly conveying God's explicit will for His people to be in "health"— that they would experience *physical wellness* and *be in peak condition both physically and mentally.* Indeed, it is God's will for His children *to be healthy, to be physically in good working order, and to be sound physically and mentally*!

But John continued to say "as thy *soul* prospereth." Here, the Greek word for "soul" encompasses the *emotions, mind, and will.* This speaks the truth that God's intentions stretch far beyond just our physical state. It's His divine plan for us not only to flourish bodily, but also to attain the pinnacle of emotional and mental vigor. This verse in Third John powerfully conveys that God ardently desires that His people enjoy robust health, be in excellent physical form, and be blessed with good mental health.

**The *RIV* (*Renner Interpretive Version*) of Third John 2 says:**

**My dearly loved brothers, it is my strongest desire that you prosper in every way that concerns you — that you not only have enough money to pay your basic bills but enough extra so you can really enjoy yourselves on every road of life that you take — and that you be healthy, in good physical working order, sound physically in every way, and that you are blessed with good mental health.**

This remarkable interpretation from the Greek text undeniably confirms and undergirds the truth that it is God's unwavering desire for you to flourish financially, enabling you to savor every path life lays before you, while also possessing robust physical and mental well-being.

When Third John 2 expresses God's wish for you to "prosper in all things and be in health, just as your soul prospers," it means that it is His will for you to thrive in every aspect of your life, and that includes being blessed with vibrant physical health and a sound state of mind.

In Hosea 4:6, which says people are *destroyed* because of a lack of knowledge, we are reminded of the peril of ignorance, and it shows us that God's people are destroyed when they lack understanding of His Word and His will. Often, illness grips us simply because we remain oblivious to the healing and health stored in Heaven's treasury on our behalf.

My wife and I, like many others, grew up ignorant of the truths in Third John 2 that explicitly state God's will for us concerning healing and health in our bodies and minds. Perhaps that's true of you too. It is my prayer that the Holy Spirit will use this book to enlighten your eyes and provide long sought-after answers that will put you on both a supernatural and commonsense journey into the healing and health that Jesus purchased for you. I desire that God will use this book to provide both divine insight and practical wisdom that will walk you into the healing and health that Jesus lovingly secured for you on the Cross, thus freeing you from the shackles of disease, sickness, and illness.

As you turn the page to the next chapter, you will see that another reason people get sick is *disobedience.* We will explore how disobedience throws open the door to disease, illness, and sickness, and we will also see that God's power is unleashed when disobedience is replaced with obedience.

Scan the QR code to watch Rick teach more on this subject.

# QUESTIONS TO PONDER AND DISCUSS

1. Based on what you read about in Hosea 4:6, in what ways can a person's life, including his physical or mental health, be destroyed due to ignorance of God's Word and His will?

2. Also from Hosea 4:6, what are some of the words or phrases for "destroyed" from the Hebrew text that paint the most vivid picture of someone who is cut off from the blessings of redemption? Using three or four of those words, describe the plight of someone who lacks the knowledge that healing is God's explicit will for all.

3. Based on what you read in this chapter, does the saying "ignorance is bliss" hold true concerning Scripture? How would ignorance of God's Word be a great detriment to a sick person in need of healing? To an impoverished individual in need of a financial blessing? What about the gravest detriment of all — to a sinner in need of salvation?

4. How do the words "wish," "above all things," "prosper," and "health" that were expounded on from Third John 2 give you the confidence that God supremely desires your financial, physical, and mental well-being in life?

5. What insights did you glean from the *Renner Interpretive Version* (*RIV*) of Third John 2 that undergird and solidify the truth of God's benevolence and goodness toward His people "on every road of life"?

# FOUR

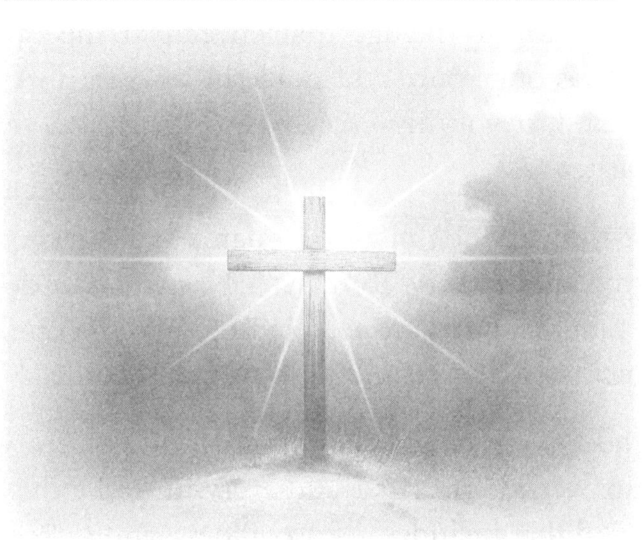

# WHY PEOPLE GET SICK — REASON NUMBER 3: DISOBEDIENCE CAN OPEN A DOOR TO SICKNESS

In the second chapter, we saw that the primary reason *why people get sick* is *the curse* that was released into the earth realm the moment that Adam transgressed. We saw on page 46 that God gave Adam the responsibility to "keep" the Garden of Eden (*see* Genesis 2:15).

As we saw previously, the Hebrew word "keep" means *to keep*, *to guard*, *to hedge about*, or *to protect*. This divine instruction meant that God had forewarned Adam of the devil's impending attempt to infiltrate the Garden, and

He commissioned Adam to act as its vigilant protector to ensure its sanctity remained unbreachable against any devilish incursion.

However, Adam knowingly violated God's instructions, and his act of defiance unleashed a deathly deluge that enveloped the earth, warping and corrupting all that was once pure and noble in its design. A malevolent force snaked across the land, devouring everything in its wake, infusing the world with its sinister spirit.

With the door thrown wide open by Adam's transgression, death stormed into existence with relentless fury. Romans 5:17 states that death surged across the world like a tyrant seizing a throne, reigning supreme until the momentous events of Jesus' crucifixion and resurrection turned the tide.

Now we have been given a faith that provides us with the upper hand, with the divine ability to override the curse and everything else this fallen world tries to throw at us — and that includes disease, illness, and sickness. Such ailments were never part of God's original design; they exist solely because of the dark reign of death instigated by Satan in the earthly realm through Adam's fall.

In the last chapter, we saw the second reason why people get sick is *a lack of knowledge.* In Hosea 4:6, God states that people are destroyed for a lack of knowledge — more specifically a lack of knowledge that Christ's redemptive work on the Cross included not only the forgiveness of sin and peace of mind, but also freedom from disease, illness, and sickness.

In this chapter, we will see that a third reason why people get sick is *disobedience.* You will discover that just as defiance against God's instructions first allowed malevolent forces to infiltrate the serene realm of the Garden of Eden, so, too, does persistent disobedience in a believer's life create vulnerabilities that enable adversarial forces to launch assaults that often manifest as ailments.

While not all forms of disease, illness, and sickness are direct assaults from dark forces, there are instances in which disobedience inadvertently leaves a door ajar for malevolence to do its work. Through this breach, malicious forces can enter, spreading disease and affliction as part of their sinister activities.

To grasp the concept of *disobedience*, let's first delve into how the New Testament characterizes *obedience*. At the heart of this understanding is the Greek word *hupakoe*, a merger of the words *hupo* and *akoe*, and the New Testament word used most commonly in connection with obedience.

The word *hupo* signifies being *beneath* or *in a subordinate role*, while the word *akoe* refers to *hearing* or *an ear*. When combined, these elements create the word *hupakoe*, which illustrates a person who is under authority (*hupo*), attentively listening with an open ear (*akoe*), and ready to receive and act upon directions. Essentially, it embodies the act of paying heed to a higher authority and executing the instructions received.

The word *hupakoe* is similar to the word *hupotasso*, which is the New Testament word signifying *submission to authority*. The word *hupotasso* is a fusion of the Greek words *hupo* and *tasso*. In this pairing, the word *hupo* signifies a position *beneath* or one who is *subservient*, while *tasso* speaks of *alignment* and *order*. The term was frequently employed in both civic and military spheres and depicted *the orderly arrangement of government* or *the strategic arrangement of troops*.

As a compound, the word *hupotasso* was used to describe *soldiers under the command of a superior officer*. In such a military setting, each soldier was acutely aware of his role, acknowledged his commanding officer, and understood how to relate to that officer. Each soldier knew his place, function, and assignment in the army, and he also understood both the rewards for obedience and the penalty for disobedience and disrespect.

In the New Testament, the concepts of *obedience* and *submission* are closely connected. In relation to our obedience to God and His instructions, both of these words tell us that we must align ourselves under God's authority and have an open heart to obey whatever He tells us to do. Like soldiers in the army, we must know our place, understand the assignment, and do whatever God instructs us to do. And as soldiers are rewarded for obedience and suffer consequences for disobedience, we must understand there are consequences for how we *do* or *do not* follow God's instructions.

## BEING 'WILLING AND OBEDIENT' OPENS THE DOOR TO GOD'S BLESSINGS

In Isaiah 1:19, God tells us, "If ye be willing and obedient, ye shall eat the good of the land." This is a powerful promise, but there is a condition in this verse that must be met for one to experience its fulfillment: we must be *willing* and *obedient.*

If we are willing and obedient to follow God's instruction, then we are promised, "...Ye shall eat the good of the land" (Isaiah 1:19). In the original language, the word "eat" implies *feasting* and symbolizes not just a mere meal, but an *abundant, celebratory banquet.* Thus, this passage assures us that an attitude of willingness and obedience unlocks the door to God's lavish generosity. In fact, we are promised that we will feast on the "good" of the land *if* we are willing and obedient.

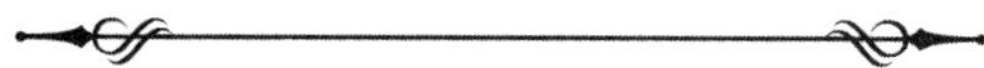

**Like soldiers in the army, we must know our place, understand the assignment, and do whatever God instructs us to do. And as soldiers are rewarded for obedience and suffer consequences for disobedience, we must understand there are consequences for how we do or do not follow God's instructions.**

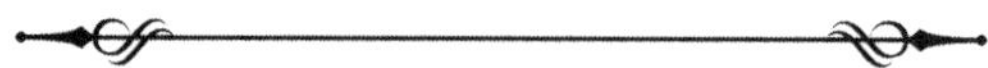

This brings us to the word "good" in this verse, which is from a Hebrew word that evokes images of abundance, blessings, prosperity, and the finest riches one can imagine. It is a term that depicts *bounty, goods, goodness, good things, and prosperity.*

Just as disobedience opened the door to a flood of death in the beginning of time, if a believer is obedient to God's instructions, it swings wide the doors to a cascade of blessings. This doesn't promise a life devoid of challenges, but when God's people are attentive to His written and personal instructions to them, they align themselves to experience a richer life in every dimension — including *vibrant health* provided by the redemptive work of Christ on the Cross, as you will see in later chapters is vividly depicted in Isaiah 53:5.

Yet in stark contrast, when God's people are disobedient to His instructions, their disobedience inadvertently invites the adversary's harmful presence, which could manifest in a myriad of ways, including illnesses and afflictions. But by embracing and adhering to God's instructions, they are divinely aligned to feast on the abundance, blessings, prosperity, and finest riches of the land, which certainly include their physical and mental health and well-being.

## THE DEVIL IS LOOKING FOR A WAY TO AFFECT YOUR LIFE

In Ephesians 4:27, Paul said, "Neither give place to the devil." The term "place" originates from the Greek word *topos*, which signifies *a distinct, defined geographical location.* It evokes the sense of *a territory*, *province*, *region*, or *zone*, and is the root of our modern term "topographical map." The implication is that the devil seeks to infiltrate every area and aspect of our lives — whether it be our finances, marriage, friendships, career, business ventures, or even *our health.*

When we disobey God's instructions to us, we unwittingly create an "entry point" — a breach that allows the devil to establish a stronghold. Therefore, Paul's message was (and still is) urgent, simple, and clear: "Neither give place to the devil." Although it may sound like a big challenge to do it, if Paul told us to give no place to the devil, that means *we are able* to close every "entry point" to prohibit the enemy's entrance into our lives.

But if you allow a door ajar in your life, even the slightest crack, the cunning devil will slip through just as he sneaked into the Garden of Eden at the dawn of time. That's the very reason God commanded Adam in Genesis 2:15 to "keep" the Garden — a directive not just to maintain it, but *to vigilantly guard, to surround with care, and to protect* it.

When God told Adam to "keep" the Garden, He was warning him to be wary, for the devil was seeking a way in, and that is why God tasked Adam to *protect* the Garden and to *keep it* secure. In the words of the New Testament, it was as though God was advising Adam, "Neither give place to the devil."

**The devil seeks to infiltrate every area and aspect of our lives — whether it be our finances, marriage, friendships, career, business ventures, or even *our health.***

The fact is, the Bible tells us we are more than conquerors through Jesus Christ (*see* Romans 8:37), so we don't have to ever let the devil run all over us. First John 4:4 declares, "...Greater is he that is in you, than he that is in the world." Yet, Paul told us, "Neither give place to the devil."

Even though the Greater One lives inside us, if we give the enemy "place" in our lives by disobeying God's instructions, the devil will find entrance into our lives through the "entry point" of disobedience, and very often, havoc is wreaked in one's health as a result.

## PETER'S AND PAUL'S ADMONISHMENT TO BE SOBER AND VIGILANT

Since the devil is looking for an "entry point" into our lives that could result in damaging circumstances, including poor health — and one of the entry points the devil uses is *disobedience* — First Peter 5:8 is important for us to understand. In this verse, Peter said, "Be sober, be vigilant; because your adversary the devil, as a roaring lion, walketh about, seeking whom he may devour."

Peter began this verse by saying, "Be *sober*." The word "sober" is interpreted from the Greek word *nepho*, which means *to be sober* and *not drunk*. It pictures *one who is free from alcoholic intoxication; free from the deliriums, delusions, and hallucinations that may accompany drunkenness; free of silly thinking and hence able to have presence of mind and clear judgment; and in control rather than being controlled by urges, impulses, whims, and fluctuating emotions.*

This word also means *to have one's wits about him*; *to be rational as opposed to irrational*; or *to be free from a drunken state in which one drops his guard and is more likely to give way to foolish behavior, unreasonable conversations, and detrimental decisions.* Simply put, the word "sober" in this verse means *to be serious-minded.*

There are six key verses in the New Testament where this word *nepho* is used.

- In First Thessalonians 5:6, the apostle Paul used it to describe *responsible living*. He said, "Therefore let us not sleep, as do others; but let us watch and be sober." Considering what "sober" means in the Greek, we could translate this verse, *"Let us watch and think clearly, not like silly drunks who drop their guard and make foolish mistakes."*
- In First Thessalonians 5:8, Paul used this word *nepho* again when he said, "But let us, who are of the day, be sober...." This could actually be translated, *"But let us, who are of the day, be clear and rational in our thinking."*

- In Second Timothy 4:5, Paul used the word *nepho* to urge Timothy to be level-headed. He said, "But watch thou in all things, endure afflictions, do the work of an evangelist, make full proof of thy ministry." That phrase "watch thou" is from the Greek word *nepho,* rendering this part of the verse, *"Keep your head on straight. Get a grip on yourself and think straight."*

- In First Peter 1:13, we find another use of *nepho* when Peter wrote, "Wherefore gird up the loins of your mind, be sober…." In early Roman times, when a runner ran, he would "gird up the loins" by grabbing the loose, dangly ends of his skirt and tucking them under his loin belt. If a runner allowed his skirt to dangle while he was running, it would get caught in his legs and hinder his race. So a good runner would tuck those loose ends under his loin belt so his legs could move freely.

  Thus, this verse means, *"Grab all the dangling ends of your life — all your loose places, your distractions, and everything that would hinder your race — and get them out of the way so you can run freely and attain your goal."*

- In First Peter 1:13, Peter again used the word *nepho* to urge his readers to be "sober" in every area of their lives. That part of the verse could be interpreted, *"Put away irresponsible and foolish thinking that leads to bad decisions."*

- In First Peter 4:7, we find the word *nepho* again when Peter called each of us to live in the light of Christ's soon return. It says, "But the end of all things is at hand. Be ye therefore sober, and watch unto prayer." That word "sober" is again interpreted from the Greek word *nepho,* making this part of the verse mean, *"Be free from the intoxications of life."* This is important, for when a person is intoxicated, naturally speaking, he drops his guard, makes bad decisions, and bad things take place as a result.

All of these multiple uses of the Greek word *nepho* bring us back to First Peter 5:8, where Peter used this word to say, "Be *sober,* be vigilant; because your adversary the devil, as a roaring lion, walketh about, seeking whom he may devour." Throughout the New Testament, the word "sober" is used as a warning to get a grip on oneself, to think straight, and to not engage in foolish thinking. But then Peter added, "Be sober, be *vigilant*...."

## THE NEED TO BE VIGILANT

The word "vigilant" tells us why we need to be sober-minded. This word is interpreted from the Greek word *gregoreo*, which means *to arouse from sleep.* It is the picture of someone who is *awake* as opposed to someone who is drowsy, sleepy, or negligent — or it portrays one who is *watchful* as opposed to someone who is careless and non-attentive. This word *gregoreo* implies *giving strict attention* to something or *being cautious and on high alert.* The best picture of the word *gregoreo* is of one putting up one's guard against a sinister force or enemy on the outside that's trying to get on the inside.

The Greek word *gregoreo* is used in 12 key verses throughout the New Testament.

- In Matthew 24:42, Jesus used it to describe the attitude we must have about His coming: "Watch therefore: for ye know not what hour your Lord doth come." The word "watch" is interpreted from the word *gregoreo* — the same word translated "vigilant" in First Peter 5:8. Its use in Matthew makes the verse better translated, *"Therefore be on your guard. Something's going to happen. And if you're not alert — if you're not on your guard — it will take you by surprise."*

- In Matthew 24:43, Jesus also said, "But know this, that if the goodman of the house had known in what watch the thief would come, he would have watched...." The word "watched" is also *gregoreo.* That part of the verse could actually be translated, *"If the goodman of the house had known in what watch the thief would come, he would have been on guard."*

- In Matthew 25:13, after Jesus had taught the Parable of the Ten Virgins, He said, "Watch therefore, for ye know neither the day nor the hour wherein the Son of man cometh." The word "watch" is again *gregoreo.* A better translation of the word "watch" here would be, *"Stay wide awake and alert, therefore, for ye know neither the day nor the hour wherein the Son of man cometh."*

- In Matthew 26:38, Jesus was in the Garden of Gethsemane when He said, "...My soul is exceedingly sorrowful, even unto death: tarry ye here, and watch with me." Again, "watch" is *gregoreo* and would be better translated in that verse as, *"Stay wide awake and alert — attentive — with Me."*

- In Mark 13:34, Jesus was commanding us to be ready for His return. He said, "For the Son of man is as a man taking a far journey, who left his house, and gave authority to his servants, and to every man his work, and commanded the porter to watch [*gregoreo*]." A better translation of the last part of this verse would be that he commanded the porter *"to stay on guard and on alert, constantly watching."*

- In Mark 13:35 and 37, we again find the word *gregoreo* translated as the word "watch." In these verses, the word *gregoreo* also implies *an attitude of watchfulness, vigilance, and of being alert and on guard.* One expositor says it means *to be on high alert.*

- In Acts 20:31, we find the word *gregoreo* in Paul's words to the Ephesian leaders. In that verse, Paul said, "Therefore watch, and remember, that by the space of three years I ceased not to warn every one night and day with tears." The word "watch" is translated from the word *gregoreo.* In this verse, it carries the idea, *"Therefore, be on your guard against outside enemy forces and be constantly vigilant and on high alert."*

- In First Corinthians 16:13, Paul said, "Watch ye, stand fast in the faith, quit you like men, be strong." The words "watch ye" are translated from the word *gregoreo,* and the verse could once again be translated, *"Be constantly on alert and on your guard."*

The Greek term *gregoreo* conveys *a persistent state of alertness and an acute awareness* that highlights the potential for unexpected events to catch us off guard. This is exactly how Peter utilized the word in First Peter 5:8 when he exhorted believers to be "vigilant." It's a divine directive that underscores our duty to remain proactive and to ensure that the adversary finds no "entry point" into our lives.

As the devil prowls and seeks to infiltrate our lives and wreak havoc, our vigilance acts as a formidable barrier that thwarts his efforts to breach our defenses and disrupt our lives.

## THE DEVIL WORKS LIKE A PROSECUTOR

In First Peter 5:8, Peter continued and said, "Be sober, be vigilant; because your *adversary* the devil, as a roaring lion, walketh about, seeking whom he may devour."

The word "adversary" is the very unique Greek word *antidikos* — and the usage of this word was well-established in the Greek culture of the First Century. It described *a lawyer who argued in a court of law* or *a prosecuting attorney who argued vehemently against the accused.* It also described *an accuser or prosecutor* who intended to bring a guilty charge against a person on the basis of information from past actions or deeds, similarly to how a legal prosecutor brings formal charges against the accused based on some legal violation.

Think about the work of a *prosecutor*; a prosecutor *prosecutes.* But to do so, he can't bring random charges against a person — instead, he has to have hard evidence against the accused. He has to have *information* of some past violation or *evidence* that some law has been broken. And with that information in hand, he can proceed to prosecute with the intention to take the violator down.

**As the devil prowls and seeks to infiltrate our lives and wreak havoc, our vigilance acts as a formidable barrier that thwarts his efforts to breach our defenses and disrupt our lives.**

But to better understand the word "adversary" — translated from the word *antidikos* — let's look at four scriptural examples of this word in the New Testament.

- In Matthew 5:25, the word *antidikos* is used twice in one verse. Jesus said, "Agree with thine adversary quickly, whiles thou art in the way with him; lest at any time the adversary deliver thee to the judge...." Although the word is translated "adversary" here, a better translation of that verse might be, *"Agree with the prosecutor quickly, whiles thou art in the way with him; lest at any time the prosecutor deliver thee to the judge...."*
- In Luke 12:58, when Jesus said, "When thou goest with thine adversary to the magistrate...," we see that same Greek word. This verse could be translated, *"When you go with your adversary, that is, the prosecutor who is bringing legal charges against you based on evidence of wrongdoing...."*
- In Luke 18:3, Jesus said, "And there was a widow in that city; and she came unto him [the judge], saying, Avenge me of mine adversary." Here, the word "adversary" (*antidikos*) describes *a ruthless prosecutor.* We could read this, *"And there was a widow in that city; and she came*

*unto him, saying, 'Avenge me from the attacks of my adversary, who is ruthlessly trying to prosecute me and take me down.'"*

- In First Peter 5:8, Peter said, "Be sober, be vigilant; because your adversary the devil...." Because the word *antidikos* is used in the Greek for the word "adversary," this verse actually tells us to be sober and vigilant *"because your adversary the devil, like a prosecuting attorney, is searching for some loophole in your life, some place of spiritual violation where you have broken a spiritual law. And like a prosecuting attorney, he will try to use that evidence to legally prosecute you and take you down."*

By using the Greek word *antidikos*, which is translated "adversary" but actually pictures *a prosecuting attorney*, Peter was informing us that the devil, like a prosecuting attorney, searches for areas of violation in your life — that is, areas where you have disobeyed or violated God's instruction. He looks for any *loophole* that he can use to prosecute you and take you down.

Even though the Greater One lives in you and you are secure in Christ, the fact is that if you have violated a spiritual law, you've created an "entry point" through which the devil can access your life. That's why it's important to judge yourself so you won't be judged (*see* 1 Corinthians 11:31) and turn from any area of disobedience in your life. Repent and close the door so the adversary has *no legal grounds* to prosecute you or attack your life.

## DISOBEDIENCE CAUSES A BREACH WHERE SICKNESS CAN ENTER

There are many violations that open a door to the devil, but in this chapter, we're focusing specifically on the underlying causes for *why people get sick.* In much the same way disobedience at the dawn of time allowed malevolence to creep into the Garden of Eden, when a Christian fails to adhere to God's instructions, it can usher in undesired influences. This breach often manifests itself in the form of *disease, illness*, and *sickness.*

Straying from God's Word invariably leads to adverse outcomes. However, beyond not adhering to the written Word of God, believers often face moments where they may overlook or neglect specific guidance imparted to them by the Holy Spirit concerning their marriage, family, business, ministry, or some step they're to take for their future. Ignoring or defying these personal instructions can push us out of sync with God's design and into vulnerable spaces where we become susceptible to attacks from Satan.

In my own journey, there were areas where the Holy Spirit gave me specific and personal instructions, which, if I had ignored or disobeyed them, could have resulted in a cascade of troubling circumstances. I'm thankful in those instances that I was spiritually sober, alert, vigilant, and obedient, not only to God's Word but to His specific instructions.

But as I write, I am also reminded of two remarkable men of faith who faced health crises after disregarding the guidance given to them by the Holy Spirit. One of these men received a clear directive to concentrate on a specific ministry area, yet he chose to veer away from this path. It wasn't until he received a cancer diagnosis that he sought answers, questioning why such a trial had befallen him.

In a moment of revelation, he felt the Lord reveal that his illness was a consequence of having strayed from the instructions he had been given and that he had inadvertently invited that affliction into his life through his disobedience. When he repented for ignoring God's instructions and realigned himself with God's purposes, the cancer disappeared. Once he got back into alignment with the Lord, the attack came to a halt.

Another nationally known minister, celebrated for his prophetic ability to discern God's will and foresee future events, unexpectedly found himself in a hospital bed with a broken arm. He was taken aback by the incident and pondered, *How could this have happened without my sensing it beforehand?*"

When he asked, "Why did this happen to me?" the Holy Spirit revealed to him that the physical mishap was a consequence of neglecting specific guidance

God had given him regarding his ministry. By turning a deaf ear to those instructions and disobeying, he had inadvertently opened a gateway for this adversity to unfold.

## MY OWN EXPERIENCE WITH DISOBEDIENCE AND SICKNESS

Allow me to recount a unique chapter from my past that intertwines disobedience and an attack on my health — a story that reaches back several decades. It was the year 1980, and I was a young man of about 22 years old, fulfilling my role as an associate pastor within a sprawling denominational congregation in Fort Smith, Arkansas.

At that time, ships carrying approximately 125,000 Cuban refugees had arrived in the United States on the shores of southern Florida. Faced with the daunting task of providing sanctuary for so many, our Presidential Administration, led by President Jimmy Carter, faced significant challenges. Overwhelmed by the cramped conditions in Florida's immigration-processing centers, federal agencies were compelled to relocate countless refugees to military bases scattered across the nation. Fort Chaffee, nestled on the outskirts of Fort Smith, became one such refuge,[1] coinciding with my pastoral journey within that bustling community.

By the time October rolled around that year, Fort Chaffee had transformed into an official resettlement hub, housing more than 19,000 Cuban refugees. But it wasn't long before news came to light that among the many displaced individuals seeking refuge at Fort Chaffee — and likely at other bases as well — were Cuban criminals whom Fidel Castro had astutely released from incarceration.

In a cunning move, Castro had emptied the island's prisons and mental institutions, dispatching both inmates and patients to American soil under the pretense of refuge. Consequently, Fort Chaffee was filled with serious Cuban offenders, and many of them grappled with both mental- and physical-health issues, including tropical illnesses.

The situation spun out of control as detainees wreaked havoc on the barracks and clashed fiercely with State Police officers. In no time, Fort Chaffee transformed into a fortress, surrounded by endless coils of razor-sharp wire and guarded by 2,000 heavily armed federal troops — it resembled a prison under siege.

Our senior pastor was a steadfast champion of the Great Commission entrusted to us by Jesus in Matthew 28:18-20. He saw the arrival of Cubans in our city as a divine opportunity to touch foreign lives without ever leaving home. Driven by this conviction, he orchestrated a robust evangelistic mission within our local church, focusing on the newcomers at Fort Chaffee. Together with church members, he organized and led church services, Bible studies, and a variety of humanitarian efforts to reach out to the Cubans, many of whom were plagued by illness, mental distress, or labeled as criminals. Our mission was to bring them the message of Christ and provide compassion to the burgeoning population of criminals, the sick, and mentally ill who were detained at the base.

Back then, I was deeply involved in volunteering at the church, stepping in wherever assistance was required, so when I learned about the need for individuals to spread the message of Christ at Fort Chaffee, I eagerly became part of a team committed to visiting the detainees there. It was astonishing to witness how Castro had deceptively camouflaged a multitude of criminals as refugees and how we, as a nation, had warmly welcomed them with open arms, not immediately grasping that we were inviting some of the world's most dangerous offenders into our midst.

One day during that period, I became *strangely ill.* Regardless of what medications I took to try to mitigate my symptoms, I couldn't seem to shake whatever it was that was afflicting me. As the sickness lingered — stretching into days — it drained my strength bit by bit. Then, on one unforgettable night, something transpired that remains vividly etched in my memory as if it had just occurred last night.

## A SUPERNATURAL ENCOUNTER IN THE MIDDLE OF THE NIGHT

I lay in bed very sick, which, in this particular case, was a sickness I became afflicted with as a direct result of my disobedience. In the middle of the night, my little dog, usually a bundle of warmth and comfort, sprang up with startling urgency. She planted herself resolutely at the foot of the bed, her growls vibrating through the darkness in a low, menacing rumble.

Suddenly, she erupted into a frenzy of barks that echoed through the room as if an unseen intruder had slunk in from the shadows. I knew no one was there except me, but despite my efforts to calm her down, she stood her ground, her growls cutting through the silence with an intensity that hinted at some invisible, malevolent presence.

When I finally, reluctantly, sat up to see what my dog was protesting, I instantly froze, my breath caught in my throat as I witnessed with my eyes wide open a dark, hooded silhouette emerge from the darkness. As I leaned forward for a closer look, I was stunned to see that sinister hooded figure step out of the darkness and stand poised at the very foot of my bed. Even now, as I recount this chilling encounter, the memory of its ghastly cloak and hood remains vivid.

As this encounter was unfolding, I'd leaned toward the foot of the bed to take a closer look. The figure responded to my movement by advancing, but instead of an anticipated gruesome, menacing face peering from beneath the hood, I saw only an unsettling void — an abyss of darkness and desolation. There was no face — the space inside the hood was filled with blackness and death, and I understood that *a spirit of death* had come for me.

I immediately began to take authority over that foul spirit in the name of Jesus and commanded it to leave. And soon, just as it had stepped out of the shadows, it retreated back into the shadows from which it had come. But when it left, *it left without me!*

When I saw that death had come to take me, I realized just how sick I really was. I woke up the next morning after a night of fitful sleep and trudged to the bathroom to begin my morning ritual. As I looked into the mirror at my reflection, I could hardly believe what I saw. My entire face looked like it had been burned, and deep wrinkles and creases covered so much of my face that I looked like a very aged, old man.

I reached for a bar of soap to wash my face, and as I did, I saw that all the skin on my hands had peeled off during the night due to the flaming-hot temperature that had afflicted my body. I was literally burned all over — and I was so sick and *still* stricken with fever that I got dressed and, as quickly as I could in my weakened condition, drove myself to the emergency room at the local hospital.

When I walked into the emergency room, the medical workers looked at me in shock. Instantly, urgency filled their steps as they whisked me away into a flurry of activity, where a sea of white coats formed a protective circle around me. I felt as though I was at the center of a human whirlwind, unable to fully comprehend the unfolding drama.

In a blink, I was registered as a patient, and soon thereafter found myself nestled into a hospital bed, tucked away in the very last room down a seemingly endless corridor. Doctors embarked on a mission to unravel the mystery behind the searing fever that gripped my body with relentless intensity and was attempting to take my life.

Eventually, the medical team inquired whether I had traveled to any exotic destinations that might have exposed me to tropical diseases. Of course, my answer was no, although I informed them that I had been frequenting Fort Chaffee, a place teeming with thousands of detainees, a good number of whom were afflicted by tropical fevers.

After thorough deliberation, the doctors determined that I had likely caught a lethal tropical fever during my time volunteering with our evangelism groups at Fort Chaffee. It was such a strange, surreal experience all around that I will never forget.

## MY DISOBEDIENCE OPENED THE DOOR TO THAT SICKNESS

Lying there in the stillness of the hospital room, I couldn't help but wonder aloud, "How on earth did I end up here? What sequence of events led to this dreadful assault on my life?" Just then, a gentle, familiar voice resonated within me — a whisper from the Holy Spirit — that said, "Rick, your disobedience has opened the door for the devil to attack you in this way. It is your own disobedience that has put you in this terrible position."

The words of the Holy Spirit left me utterly perplexed. With every fiber of my being, I had been striving to align my life with God's will. I found myself pleading, "What have I done wrong? Please reveal to me the ways in which I have strayed so far as to leave myself vulnerable to such an attack. Show me so I may truly repent!"

I want to clarify that not every illness stems from disobedience; there are countless origins and causes of sickness. However, in this particular instance, the Holy Spirit revealed to me that my own disobedience had opened the door for that attack.

The Holy Spirit gently answered my cry for help, saying, "You've turned a deaf ear in matters concerning Denise. I distinctly instructed you that she is meant to be your wife and life-long partner, yet you've disregarded my instruction and leading. I did not bring this illness on you, but it is your disobedience concerning this issue that has opened the door for these things to happen."

Deep down, I had known it was absolutely God's will for me to marry Denise and that His plan was for her to be my wife and lifelong partner in ministry.

But in my apprehension concerning the subject of marriage, I had ignored His words and His dealings. So when the Holy Spirit told me I had been disobedient in that matter, it didn't take me but *seconds* to acknowledge my disobedience and to repent. The realization stunned me into swift action to close the door to this attack.

From my hospital bed, I seized the phone, called Denise, poured out my heart to her, and set in motion a series of events that felt nothing short of miraculous. Almost immediately, my fever subsided, and I emerged from the hospital, renewed and ready to embrace our God-ordained future together. From that pivotal call, our relationship blossomed rapidly, and before long, we joyfully fulfilled God's plan by joining our lives in marriage.

## REALIGNING YOURSELF WITH GOD GIVES YOU THE POWER TO RESIST THE DEVIL

If the Holy Spirit shows you an area of disobedience in your life that may be the root of disease, illness, or sickness that you are fighting, I encourage you to ask for forgiveness immediately and make things right. James 4:7 says, "Submit yourselves therefore to God. Resist the devil, and he will flee from you." When we submit ourselves to God *first*, resisting the devil becomes doable and powerful!

The word "submit" in this verse is interpreted from a form of *hupotasso*, which is a compound of *hupo* and *tasso*. As we saw earlier on page 83, the word *hupo* means *under*, and the word *tasso* means *to arrange* or *to order*. As one word, it means *to properly arrange under*, and it was a military term that depicted *a soldier's obedience and submission to authority*. In this verse, it represents the image of someone who has thoughtfully *aligned* himself or herself beneath the authority of God and His Word. In doing so, the individual who is submitted is enveloped in the protection and oversight of God's superior power.

The word "resist" in James 4:7 is interpreted from a form of the Greek word *anthistemi*, which is a compound of *anti* and *histemi*. The prefix *anti* translates to *against*, while the word *histemi* means *to stand*. When fused together, they convey the sense of *standing against* or *holding one's ground in defiance*.

This word pictures someone who *vehemently opposes something* and *is committed to exhausting every effort to thwart it*. It embodies the ideas of *defying*, *withstanding*, or *opposing* and suggests a resistance that is both *deliberate* and *strategic*. In ancient Greek times, it was employed to illustrate the *unyielding resistance* of a foe.

In fact, James said that when resisted, the devil will "flee" from you. The word "flee" is from the Greek word *pheugo*, which translates *to flee*, *to take flight*, *to run away*, *to move one's feet as fast as possible*, or *to escape*. It paints a vivid picture of *someone's feet barely touching the ground as he flees from danger*. This term was historically used to describe a lawbreaker making *a terrified escape from a city or country where he had broken the law*.

In this context, James assured us that by aligning ourselves under God's authority, we become sufficiently fortified *to successfully repel* the devil and his attempts to afflict us. In that consecrated position of submission, the devil will "flee" from you, much like a criminal frantically evacuating a scene for fear of being convicted and prosecuted for his crime.

But James then added that the devil will flee "from" you. This seemingly simple word "from" is interpreted from the Greek word *aph*, a contracted form of the Greek word *apo*, which not only translates to *from*, but also vividly illustrates the act of deliberately *creating distance between oneself and another entity*.

In this context, it becomes clear that the devil is profoundly fearful of anyone who remains steadfastly aligned under God's authority — to the point that he wants to distance himself as much as possible from those who are submitting themselves to God, aligning themselves under the authority of God.

**The *(RIV) Renner Interpretive Version* of James 4:7 says:**

> **It is imperative that you make the decision to properly align yourselves under the authority of God — in a submitted position that actually provides you with protection. Being submitted to His authority gives you the ability to defy, oppose, stand steadfastly against, and withstand the accusing, slanderous, trap-setting behavior of the devil.**
>
> **In fact, he'll be so terrified of you that he'll move his feet as fast as he can to get away from you. Not only will he flee from you, he'll run like a criminal terrified of prosecution — so scared that he'll want to do all he can to put as much space between him and you as possible.**

The word pictures presented in this textual interpretation of James 4:7 let us know that when we repent for disobedience, God's powerful presence cleanses us and instantly gives us the ability to defy the adversary and send him fleeing.

Rather than persist in any area of disobedience that has allowed trouble to come to you, be honest with God and say:

*"Lord, I'm sorry for* [name any specific action or behavior He is convicting you of]. *Please forgive me and wash me clean with the precious blood of Jesus. Thank You for Your mercy, Your patience, and Your forgiveness — and for hearing and answering my prayer. In Jesus' name. Amen!"*

In my own case, I had ignored and disobeyed God's clear instructions to me regarding my marriage to Denise. My disobedience is what opened the door for my body to be ravaged by sickness. But as soon as I repented and obeyed, within just a short time, that tropical fever was gone and I was back to normal. By submitting to God — realigning myself under God's authority and obeying His instructions — I was empowered to resist and defy the adversary and send him fleeing.

## BE CAREFUL OF 'THE LITTLE FOXES'

People usually think that disobedience in *major matters* is what opens the door for the devil to produce troubles, but Song of Solomon 2:15 says it's the "little foxes that spoil the vine."

To fully grasp the significance of this verse, imagine these "little foxes" — standing about two feet tall, stretching a mere 25 to 27 inches in length, and weighing somewhere between 11 to 22 pounds — roughly the size of a small terrier. Although these foxes may appear innocuous, they could wreak havoc in a vineyard if left unchecked.

While they are primarily carnivorous, these mischievous creatures can cause significant damage by nibbling on plants; burrowing in vineyard soil; making paths through vines that damages leaves and fruit; gnawing on branches, causing stripped bark and exposed roots; and greedily feasting on the grapes themselves. Although seemingly insignificant, if not restrained, these tiny troublemakers can transform a flourishing vineyard into a scene of devastation.

Similarly, if we neglect to heed both the Scriptures and God's personal guidance in both the big things and the small things, we risk letting "little foxes" sneak into the gardens of our lives. These seemingly minor acts of disobedience might be the key that grants the devil entry to your life so he can sow chaos. As illustrated in the examples in the previous paragraph, ignoring God's specific directions can sometimes lead to unexpected troubles, including those that affect our health.

Disobedience is a serious issue even if in the moment it feels like something small. It might manifest as straying into sexual misconduct or dismissing God's gentle urging to take a break from an overly demanding routine. It could involve turning a deaf ear to God's Spirit telling you to join a new congregation, switch careers, avoid certain stressful relationships, or distance oneself from negative influences.

Anything along this spectrum of neglect or defiance, if left unchecked, becomes like a crafty little fox that the devil will use to exploit the "entry point" of disobedience and invade the vineyard of your life, unleashing chaos. This might include threats to your health, but once the voice of the Lord is heeded and complied with, the door to your life will remain steadfastly closed, keeping those mischievous foxes at bay and sparing your life from attack.

## BUILD A WALL OF DEFENSE TO KEEP THE DEVIL OUT

James 4:7 once again says, "Submit yourselves therefore to God. Resist the devil, and he will flee from you." Also speaking of our need to resist the enemy's attempts to access our lives, Peter similarly wrote in First Peter 5:9, "Whom resist stedfast in the faith...."

The word "resist" is from the Greek word *anthistemi*, which we saw on page 101. However, Peter enriched this notion by introducing the word "stedfast," which is drawn from the Greek word *stetereos*. This significant Greek term conveys the meaning *to bolster* or *to reinforce,* much like preparing oneself to withstand an adversary.

The inclusion of this word indicates that we must actively engage in fortifying and solidifying ourselves, ensuring the enemy's advances are rendered ineffective. But the only reason we would need to bolster and reinforce ourselves in this way is, there *is* an enemy who wants to attack us and who needs to be resisted.

**The *(RIV) Renner Interpretive Version* of First Peter 5:9 says:**

**You must intentionally and strategically make a plan by which you can resist this enemy, and you must do everything you can to bolster and reinforce yourself in faith (and in really knowing what you believe)...!**

## A REAL-LIFE EXAMPLE OF 'THE LITTLE FOX' — A BROKEN LAW AND A TRAGIC BREACH IN A WALL OF DEFENSE

Many decades ago, two sisters from one family moved to Moscow to attend our seminary. They immersed themselves in every facet of the ministry, their spirits perpetually buoyant and their faces adorned with radiant smiles. However, one night as they made their way home on foot after a long day at the seminary, they faced making a fateful choice. Instead of taking the lawful route over the bridge that spanned the railroad tracks, they opted for a more daring shortcut. With the thought of saving precious minutes, they chose to slink through a gap in the fence beneath the bridge to traverse the tracks.

The women crawled through the hole in the fence, unaware of impending peril as a train thundered along the tracks. It must have come "out of nowhere," so quickly that they had no opportunity to retreat and no way to move away from the oncoming train. The train hit them, and by the time the train roared past the scene, there was nothing left of those girls' bodies but fragments.

People questioned, "How did the devil wield the power to harm those young girls so tragically?" Yet despite my deep affection for the sisters, the explanation of this tragic loss was quite straightforward: They broke a simple but important law by venturing across the forbidden tracks, which led to their untimely demise. Had they adhered to the explicit warnings to stay off the tracks, they would be with us still, but their choice to dismiss those vital instructions unfortunately sealed their fate.

Similarly, if you examine your own life, you'll notice that the devil often strikes at the very spots where you neglected to take action or ventured into places you should have avoided. These are the tiny cracks and crevices where the devil seeks to slip through unnoticed. This is why we must bolster and reinforce ourselves spiritually because the enemy is looking for a loophole into each of our lives, and his intention once he's there is to "steal, kill, and destroy" (*see* John 10:10).

By fortifying ourselves through various means — such as immersing ourselves in Scripture, praying in the Spirit, staying in fellowship with other faith-filled believers, and walking in obedience to God's instructions — we equip ourselves to counter the subtle snares of the adversary. Engaging in these intentional practices acts as a protective barrier helps to shield us from spiritual attacks, anchoring us firmly in our faith and ensuring that we stand resilient and undeterred.

## A TRUE STORY FROM ANCIENT HISTORY TO DEMONSTRATE THE DANGER OF 'CRACKS' IN YOUR LIFE

When I contemplate the devil seeking a way to infiltrate our lives, a compelling tale[2] comes to mind, taken from history, that demonstrates the danger of "cracks" in your life. The story comes from the city of Sardis, where one of the seven churches in the book of Revelation was located (*see* Revelation 3:1-6).

Perched imminently atop forbidding precipices, the city of Sardis reigned sovereign over the landscape below, its towering fortress seemingly impervious to conquest. The inhabitants of Sardis, ensconced in their lofty domain, nurtured a haughty conviction that no invading force could breach their citadel's defenses. This mindset, however, became their Achilles' heel, a fertile breeding ground for lethargy and a dangerous complacency.

In the minds of its citizens, Sardis stood as the model of invulnerability, superior and unparalleled. Thus, entrapped in self-congratulatory delusion, they negligently overlooked the hidden flaws in the structure of their stunning metropolis, as long-formed fissures in the city's foundation had already begun their silent work of destruction. Concealed by a veil of vanity, the vulnerability of their lofty citadel remained unnoticed as nature's unsparing hand wrought havoc beneath their feet. The once-impenetrable fortifications slowly succumbed, and gaping cracks began to form at the bottom of the city's foundation. But the citizenry, prideful and smug, did not notice the massive cracks developing at the base of their trusted walls.

Initially, the fissures were minuscule, barely perceptible to the naked eye. However, as time passed, these subtle imperfections widened and deepened. Eventually, the breaches became so expansive that a person could effortlessly pass through them. But still, the inhabitants remained ignorant of their vanishing safety.

Due to the massive fractures in the walls and foundations, Sardis was losing its formidable defense, leaving an open invitation for adversaries to scale the mountain, sneak through the openings, and come directly into the heart of the city. Despite the looming threat, the residents carried on, oblivious to the precariousness of their situation.

A distant foe had been watching the city of Sardis, its eyes keen and vigilant. Yet the citizens, swathed in overconfidence, failed to perceive any threat, believing their fortress impregnable to outside forces. This misplaced pride left the city vulnerable, blind to the subtle weaknesses that had evolved into gaping breaches, which now marred its ancient walls. The enemy, ever watchful, soon discerned the gaps or "entry points" within the city's defenses.

One fateful night, under a cloak of darkness, the enemy's forces stealthily approached the towering cliffs that guarded Sardis. Like serpents, they slithered silently through the crevices, scaling upward, and slipping unnoticed into the heart of the city. With deft precision, invaders had crept through the fractures, ascending the walls and taking strategic positions over the sleeping city. Their overwhelming presence ensured that any attempt at resistance would be swiftly quashed, leaving the people of Sardis at the mercy of their newfound conquerors.

As dawn broke over the city of Sardis, its residents rubbed the sleep from their eyes, only to emerge into the streets and find themselves enveloped by a wave of shock and horror. The enemy forces had taken them. Panic gripped the people as they realized, with a sinking dread, that they were encircled and caught unaware by the looming threat that had quietly crept into their midst. They were surrounded on all sides and they were doomed. But in reality, had the city been vigilant and tended to the state of its defenses, mending any weaknesses, no adversary could have breached its formidable, impenetrable walls. Sardis fell because of *pride*.

## TAKE HEED, LEST YOU FALL

In First Corinthians 10:12, Paul said, "Wherefore let him that thinketh he standeth take heed lest he fall."

The word "thinketh" is from the Greek word *dokeo*, which can also mean *to hold an opinion, to reckon, to assume*, or simply *to think*. Within this verse, this word captures the notion of what someone *believes* about himself. Despite lacking any evidence to substantiate the individual's self-assessment, it nonetheless constitutes his steadfast self-view. Soon, the significance of grasping this concept will become crystal clear to you!

Next, Paul said, "Wherefore let him that thinketh he standeth...." The word "standeth" comes from the Greek word *histemi*, which simply means *to stand, to stand fast, to stand firm*, or *to stand upright*. But when the words *dokeo* and *histemi* are used together, as Paul uses them in this verse, it means, "Wherefore let anyone who has the *self-imposed belief* that he is *resilient, standing strong, and unshakable...*"

Paul then emphasized with grave importance the next words, "...Take heed lest he fall." The words "take heed" are derived from the Greek term *blepo*, which means *to watch, to see, to behold*, or *to be aware*. The Greek tense indicates the need not only to watch, but to be *continually watchful* or *perpetually vigilant*. In this verse, Paul passionately urged believers to maintain an unceasing vigilance over our spiritual lives and the steadfast faith we claim to possess.

He went on to say that we must be careful lest we "fall." The word "fall" is the Greek word *pipto*, which means *to fall*, but in the New Testament, it is used to depict *someone who falls into a terrible predicament* or *one who falls into a worse state than he was in before.* It can also depict *someone who falls into sin, falls into ruin, or falls into some type of failure.*

The word *pipto* emphatically describes *a downfall from a formerly presumed high and haughty position.* Therefore, it isn't just a little stumbling that Paul was referring to, but it is *a downward plummet* that causes one to sorrowfully crash!

When you put all of this together in First Corinthians 10:12, it could be understood to mean, *"If anyone has the self-imposed belief that he is resilient, standing strong, and unshakable, he is the very one that needs to be continually watchful and always on his guard, lest he trip, stumble, and fall from his overconfident position and take a nose-dive downward to a serious crash!"*

It may seem like it takes a lot of time to stay watchful and prayerful about your spiritual life, but be assured that it is less expensive and less painful to be attentive and watchful than to crash spiritually and have to repair things in your life that never had to be broken in the first place. This underscores the reason why you must pay attention to disobedience and obedience in your life, both of which bear consequential fruit.

## THE CHOICE IS YOURS

But if we are willing and obedient to God's written Word and to His instructions to us, we are divinely enabled to walk in God's blessing — and that includes *healing* and *health.* When we are disobedient to His Word and to His personal instructions to us, we move out from under His protection, and that is when the enemy finds an "entry point" to potentially produce disastrous things in our lives — and often it manifests as disease, illness, and sickness.

If you are willing to consent to what God says and to be obedient in hearing and doing His Word, obeying His instructions, He promises that "...Ye shall eat the good of the land" (Isaiah 1:19). *If* you live a life of obedience, you throw open the door to experience the blessings of God, but *if* you disobey, the door to your life will be opened for the enemy to rush in with all kinds of bad things, including attacks on your *health.*

**This underscores the reason why you must pay attention to disobedience and obedience in your life, both of which bear consequential fruit.**

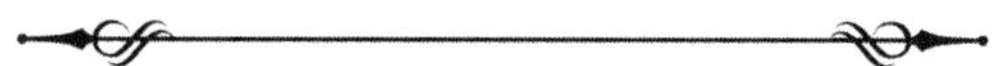

In Isaiah 1:19, God says, "If ye be willing and obedient, ye shall eat the good of the land." This powerful promise belongs to God's people, but for you to eat the good of the land, it says you must be *willing* and *obedient.* Thus, we are reminded that *it will always pay to obey.*

As we proceed to the next chapter, we will discover yet another reason *why people get sick.* Don't miss a single word of it, for what you are about to read may contain the instruction needed to bring healing and health into your life!

Scan the QR code to watch Rick teach more on this subject.

## QUESTIONS TO PONDER AND DISCUSS

1. Given the definitions of the word "keep" in God's command to Adam to *keep* the Garden of Eden, it becomes clear to see how Adam lost it all and how costly his disobedience became. Describe the ways our own failure *to guard, hedge, and protect* what God has entrusted to us can result in dire consequences, including a loss of our physical health. What steps do you plan to take to guard and keep *your* life, including guarding your heart and your spiritual walk (*see* Proverbs 4:23), after reading this chapter?

2. Why do you think James wrote about "submitting to God" before he wrote about "resisting the devil"? Refer to the Greek words and definitions for "submit" and "resist," respectively, as well as the message in Revelation 2:26, and explain in your own words why a lack of submission to the authority of God and His Word will undermine and even undo your spiritual authority against the enemy of your soul? Can you name a "little fox" in your life that you need to remove from your garden to ensure what you and the Lord are building and cultivating together remains untouched so it can flourish and thrive?

3. The adversary is portrayed by Peter in First Peter 5:8 as one who is seeking an entry point into our lives to work his destruction. But the Holy Spirit provided the answer to this hard truth when He gave Peter the words "sober" (*nepho*) and "vigilant" (*gregoreo*) as ways to stop a demonic assault before it ever gets started. Write your action steps for being sober and vigilant in your own life — both what you're already doing and what you need to begin doing.

4. Using the words "submit," "resist," "flee," "sober," "vigilant," and "adversary" from James 4:7 and First Peter 5:8, formulate a short statement of faith that you can meditate on and rehearse again and again to maintain your spiritual walls of defense against potential breaches, or openings, through which the enemy could use to intrude upon your life.

5. Since God's will is never to scare us but, rather, to prepare us, what helpful insights can you glean for your own life and well-being from the three main illustrative stories that were shared in this chapter (Rick's disobedience and deadly sickness; the two women who disobeyed the warning signs; and the retelling of the fall of "impenetrable" Sardis)? How important is it to obey both the *specific* will of God when He speaks to you or directs you — as well as the wisdom that's contained in the *general* will of God, meaning what is written in His Word?

# FIVE

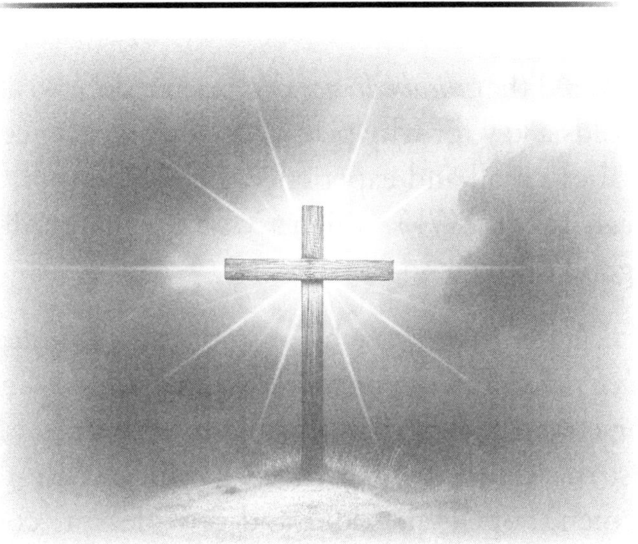

# WHY PEOPLE GET SICK— REASON NUMBER 4: FOOLISHNESS CAN OPEN A DOOR TO SICKNESS

Many people have asked the question, "If Jesus purchased our healing and health at the Cross, why do people still struggle with health issues?" Up to this point, we've uncovered three reasons *why people get sick*.

*First*, we saw the main culprit for why people get sick is *the curse* that came into the world because of Adam's transgression at the dawn of time. His act of defiance against God's command opened a spiritual door for the devil, and as a result, death and all its destructive effects came raging into the earthly realm.

*Second*, we saw that *a lack of knowledge* plays a significant role in why people get sick, for when a person lives without the knowledge that Christ paid the price for healing and health, he remains in the dark that healing and health is his by inheritance.

*Third*, we discovered that *disobedience* can open a door to all kinds of tragedy and trauma and holds a key for why people get sick. But in contrast, obedience enables us to rise above it all and experience the blessings of God. This is what is promised in Isaiah 1:19 (*NKJV*), which says, "If you are willing and obedient, you shall eat the good of the land."

Now, we will see a *fourth* reason why people get sick. Indeed, it will become clear that *foolish behavior* can fling open an "entry point" for a myriad of health problems. Of course, we know that disease, illness, and sickness are all ultimately a result of the curse that flooded the earth at the time of Adam's transgression — but just as disobedience opens the door and provides an "entry point" for the devil to tamper with our health, engaging in *foolish behavior* is another avenue through which we inadvertently open a door for the devil to affect our health.

The fact is that many times, the health challenges we face are direct reflections of our own choices. By consistently making poor decisions, we can bring about adverse effects on our health — while by consistently making wise choices, we nurture healing, vitality, and a longer and healthier life.

Earlier, we saw in Genesis 2:15, that God entrusted Adam with the duty of "keeping" the Garden of Eden. To revisit that passage briefly, the word "keeping" implies *safeguarding*, *shielding*, *encircling*, or *defending*. This word was often used to signify times when vigilance was crucial to prevent a malevolent presence from infiltrating sacred spaces.

God's command for Adam to "keep" the Garden suggests that God alerted Adam to the devil's scheming attempts to slither into their paradise uninvited. Adam was charged with the task of fortifying the Garden to ensure its defenses were so robust that the devil would find no entryway to breach.

All that God gives us requires vigilant guarding against the enemy's onslaughts. Jesus warned us of the thief's intent to steal, kill, and destroy (John 10:10). If the devil discovers a crack — an "entry point" — into our lives, he will eagerly embark on his destructive mission. And although Christ secured our healing and health through His sacrifice on the Cross, if we carelessly leave an opening for the devil, he will strive relentlessly to disrupt our health and snatch away the blessings that Christ has purchased for us in His redemptive work.

**All that God gives us requires vigilant guarding against the enemy's onslaughts. If the devil discovers a crack — an "entry point" — into our lives, he will eagerly embark on his destructive mission.**

In this chapter, we will see that *foolish behavior* is another way we open the door to all kinds of struggles, and as we proceed, I'll share my own experiences from the past when I foolishly opened a door for the devil to attack my health.

## FOOLISH BEHAVIOR OPENS THE DOOR TO STRUGGLES

I hope you'll pardon my directness, but the truth is, sadly, many individuals fall ill due to unwise decisions and reckless behavior — or to be even more blunt, they become ill because of *dumb, foolish, and stupid* actions.

Before you allow yourself to become too shocked at these three words, please know that my intention with this book is to offer assistance rather than cause offense. So please don't stop reading! Because I felt that the words "dumb, foolish, and stupid" were a bit too strong to use throughout the course of this chapter — and even politically insensitive in today's climate — I embarked on a journey to unearth an alternative expression to replace *dumb, foolish, and stupid.*

As I delved into my research, every trail I followed seemed to circle back to the words "stupid" or "stupidity." Then I ventured to explore the term "foolish," only to find its definition entangled with phrases like *a lack of good judgment, nonsense,* or *being stupid.* In my quest to find a softer and more compassionate alternative, I decided to primarily use the word "foolish" in this chapter to make the point that our wrong choices and reckless actions can indeed make us our own worst enemies.

And as you'll see, I will address my own "foolish" behaviors, sharing my unfortunate experiences and my lessons learned, to help you see how you can make adjustments in *your* life in areas where you've perhaps caused yourself problems with your physical health.

## A FEW EXAMPLES OF HOW FOOLISH BEHAVIOR CAN OPEN THE DOOR TO MANY TYPES OF ATTACKS

Admitting our own foolishness might be the last thing we want to do, yet it's often this very folly that invites a myriad of challenges into our lives, including *health problems,* which we will come to in a few moments. But before delving into how imprudence can invite health issues to come knocking on our door, let's explore a few ways that the devil attacks people through the entry point of foolishness.

For example, in the realm of finances, some people find themselves entangled in financial woes largely due to their own unwise choices. For example, using credit cards to make a quick purchase — often for things they don't really need — can feel magically easy, like the effortless wave of a wand. Yet they are usually not considering the monetary drain it will create, or they're coaxing themselves into believing it won't affect them. When the financial storm finally hits, they rightfully turn to prayer while they often lament that the devil is meddling with their finances.

While it's true that the devil may be exploiting these circumstances to unleash chaos in their bank balances and the ability to live a stress-free life, it was their series of unwise decisions that rolled out the welcome mat for disaster. Foolish decisions provided a point of entry for the devil to find his way into the middle of their finances. If they had exercised wisdom, they would have been able to keep that door closed, but repeated *foolish behavior* and *unwise decisions* threw the door open for this type of attack.

I hold no judgment against anyone who has stumbled into unwise financial choices. Denise and I, too, began our marriage decades ago with little knowledge of how to manage money and made quite a few blunders due to our lack of a budget and a long-term financial strategy. Yet thanks to God's grace and the guidance of those who generously stepped in during those formative years to teach us, we managed to steer our financial ship back on course. Today Denise and I thankfully have financial peace, and the door to monetary chaos is firmly bolted shut. It's a testament to the notion that anyone, after making financial missteps, can turn things around, learn valuable lessons, and fortify their financial world to "give no opportunity to the devil" (*see* Ephesians 4:27).

Or, also in the area of finances, how about individuals who have leaped from one job to another with such frequency that any potential employer trembles with hesitation at the sight of their resume? It's one thing to change jobs for compelling reasons — a pursuit of growth or a shift in passions — but it's quite another when the frequent transitions stem from less acceptable circumstances.

Take, for example, someone who struggles to get along with authority figures. He exits one job after another, offended over some issue each time and eager to find a new environment, only to repeat the cycle again and again. But if a person is consistently unable to get along with any employer, he or she is the common denominator, not the respective employer, who will invariably be blamed for the person's foolish lack of stability and honor of authority.

And what if a person unwisely does a mediocre job everywhere he goes to work, expecting good pay and even raises in return for his sloppy work habits? It's just a fact that people who behave unwisely in this way on the job are going to be moving on at some point, voluntarily or otherwise.

When this pattern of relentless re-employment occurs often enough, the resume, a once-proud testament to professional growth, becomes a list of weary employers and missed opportunities — a narrative that dissuades new potential employers. Potential hirers, spotting a story of instability, may hesitate, concerned that history will once again repeat itself. By consistently and *foolishly* hopping from one job to the next, this person has unwittingly marred his or her own reputation and credibility.

I think of one bright, talented individual I know of — a man whose gifts are undeniable — yet he wanders, unable to discover a true sense of belonging and keeps habitually moving from one job to another. This restless man drifts from job to job, and, unfortunately, his resume now waves like a glaring warning flag to employers, cautioning them, *"Do not hire this person because he won't stay very long."*

Although this man laments about the devil derailing his aspirations, it is the instability of his own making that has marred his reputation. The devil found an "entry point" into his life through a door he himself left ajar. But as the one who foolishly opened the door and kept it open for so long, he is the one that must shut the door to the devil and to the peril he is experiencing due to his own instability. To shut the door, he must repent, change, and learn to faithfully stay in one spot long enough for the Lord to promote him.

Certainly, I cast no stones at those who find themselves without work for various reasons — but in the scenarios I just described, it was clearly a lack of wisdom and consistent foolish behaviors that hindered God's blessings and brought destructive results that God never intended into people's lives.

Or what about the arena of mishaps and accidents that cause bodily injury or even death? Consider a man who decides to tackle an electrical issue at home. He regards precautions as mere trifles, and so, without a second thought, reaches for the tangled mass of wires. In an instant, a fierce jolt of electricity surges through them, sending him sprawling across the room, painfully reminding him of the dangers he'd so cavalierly dismissed.

If such a person claimed that the devil wanted to kill him, we would certainly agree, because John 10:10 says the devil comes to steal, to kill, and to destroy. Yet in truth, this misadventure was simply the consequence of the man's own *foolish* disregard for safety. Had he approached the task with even a little caution, he would have avoided such a shocking altercation altogether.

I am vividly reminded of a day when my father, usually a beacon of wisdom, decided to tackle some electrical work in the attic of his home. What happened that day is imprinted in my memory forever. Despite my mother's earnest pleas for caution, he dismissed her concerns with a wave of his hand. Impulsively, he reached out to grasp a bundle of electrical wires, unwittingly inviting a tempest of electricity that hurled him clear across the attic like a ragdoll in a storm.

Finally descending the ladder, his hands were blackened and burned, his hair and eyebrows singed to a crisp — evidence of his close encounter with calamity. I can still hear the tremor in his voice as he confessed, "I almost killed myself by not being careful."

Had the unthinkable happened — had he been taken from us by those unforgiving wires — it would have shattered our family, a catastrophe both devastating and absurdly preventable. Yet in that reckless moment of folly, my father opened a door for danger to strike and came perilously close to a tragic end.

Or imagine a young man who is giddy with excitement over his brand-new car, a gleaming beast of engineering and speed. Eager to share his thrill, he invites a few friends for an exhilarating spin. Determined to showcase the roaring power at his command and the thrill of his prowess behind the wheel, he pushes the accelerator with a heavy foot, flouting the boundaries of safety and speed.

Suddenly, his joyride takes a terrifying turn when the car spirals out of control, flipping repeatedly until it is a mangled wreck, its original form lost beyond recognition. Miraculously, he and his companions crawl out, shaken but unscathed, as if divine hands had shielded them from harm. They exclaim, "The devil tried to take us!" — and that would have definitely been the truth.

In that heart-stopping moment, their *foolish choices* threw wide the gates and invited the devil to take their lives. With hearts pounding, they thank God for their improbable deliverance, but it was a stark reminder that *foolish actions* open a door and provide an "entry point" for the devil to create disaster.

What I just described to you was a hypothetical scenario. But this actually happened years ago when our son Paul experienced an unforgettable "adventure" after purchasing his first car, a spirited little red vehicle. He was so thrilled to show off his car that he invited his brother Philip and a friend to join him for a whirlwind drive through the serpentine streets of downtown Moscow.

Eager to showcase the car's power, Paul floored the accelerator, while there was ice on the road, and it sent them racing toward an abrupt bend along the Moscow river's canal. Suddenly, the car jumped the curb and collided with a formidable concrete barrier, then hit a concrete electrical pole, and the car was sandwiched between the canal railing and the light pole, which fortuitously stopped them from landing in the canal.

Astonishingly, all three young men emerged unscathed from the mangled wreckage. It was a miracle that they hit no pedestrians and that the car did not plunge into the water of the canal. When my wife and I laid eyes on the crushed remains of the car, we were at a loss for words, unable to fathom how anyone survived the harrowing ordeal.

We are thankful that God miraculously protected all three of those men that day, but it was *foolish* behavior that triggered that attack, which God's grace and angelic forces circumvented. The accident was so severe that the city of Moscow constructed a permanent barrier where the accident occurred to prevent it from ever happening to anyone else.

We're talking about ways poor judgment and foolishness can trigger destructive outcomes in multiple areas of our lives. Now imagine with me a husband and wife locked in endless discord with never-ending arguments and unresolved tension that persist in their marriage. Their once vibrant home now echoes with the sounds of constant conflict, leaving no room for peace. Slowly, this persistent turmoil seeps into the lives of their children and begins to affect their schoolwork and cloud their emotional well-being.

Day turns to night, weeks blur into months, and years pass by as the family is drawn deeper into a web of strife — each tug at the now-fragile threads of the marriage threatening to unravel it completely. What might have begun as minor disagreements snowball into overwhelming emotional turmoil, financial strain, and the looming threat of separation and dissolution.

More often than not, this type of destructive cycle in a marriage can be traced back to the activity of the devil, who stealthily slipped through a cracked door left ajar, spread seeds of contention, and exploited the vulnerability of the situation, creating chaos within the home. During heated and contentious moments, thoughtless and foolish remarks, reckless threats, and impassioned ultimatums often arise and pour fuel on the fire, intensifying the turmoil.

But by recognizing the enemy's attack and slamming the door shut to this insidious intruder, peace can reign again, and the family can find its way back to unity. The devil is the master of strife, and he uses it to "steal, kill, and destroy" marriages and families. Just as we read in First Peter 5:8 in the last chapter, the enemy is always looking for an "entry point" into people's lives, especially families, so that he may devour them.

Throughout our many years of ministry and walking alongside countless individuals who were suffering in this area, my wife and I have witnessed the unfolding of similar stories in marriages and families time and time again. Every marriage and home has challenges, but when both marriage partners are willing to work together, to submit to the authority of the Word of God, and, if needed, to seek professional help, the door to the enemy can be shut tight and he can be pushed out. We have seen countless remarkable stories of couples who have taken ownership of their vulnerabilities and sin — whether it be neglect of a spouse, betrayal, bitterness and resentment, or a myriad of other challenges — and they've turned their situations around to the glory of God.

By addressing these issues head-on and barricading their home against future intrusions, many have experienced profound healing and restoration. Of course, this process requires mutual effort, and there are times when one partner's endeavor to secure their home is thwarted by the other's indifference, leaving the entrance to turmoil still unguarded.

The devil is perpetually seeking a breach through which to unleash chaos within a family. It is through these openings, these "entry points," that he creeps in — and this is why the Bible passionately urges us to remain vigilant and to "give no place to the devil" (Ephesians 4:27).

These examples offer just a glimpse into the many types of assaults that arise from foolish behavior. While countless instances exist, this chapter will now narrow its focus to explore how foolish behavior acts as an entry point for the devil to undermine one's health and overall well-being. Let's delve deeper into these illustrations of how one's physical health can be affected by sickness and disease.

## FOOLISHNESS THAT RESULTS IN DISEASE, ILLNESS, AND SICKNESS

Remember that in the opening of this book, I asked you to journey with me to the very last word of this book. Now, I kindly implore you once more not to skip this section, even if the truths within it may make you uneasy. Let every sentence unfold before you in its entirety and remember that I am addressing reasons *why people get sick* to help those who are sick to receive healing and to step into the life of health that God wants them to experience.

In addition to the previously mentioned issues, which often stem from the open doors and "entry points" we leave ajar for the devil, we must acknowledge that many health issues also arise from unwise decisions and imprudent behavior. I don't wish to offend or upset anyone, but we must frankly admit that some of the physical and mental issues that people experience are *self-inflicted.*

Beyond simply unleashing their faith to achieve the healing and health they seek, they must acknowledge where they have left a door open and take action to seal any lingering cracks and to close all "entry points" to ensure that health concerns are once-and-for-all overcome and remain a thing of the past.

## IN SPITE OF OUR FOOLISH BEHAVIOR, GOD REMAINS OUR HELPER!

In Hosea 13:9, God says, "O Israel, thou hast destroyed thyself; but in me is thine help."

At the time Hosea penned this striking verse, Israel was teetering on the edge of ruin, mostly by its own hand, having been ensnared by reckless decisions and careless oversight. Yet amidst the chaos and the mess of their self-sabotage, in His infinite compassion, God offered a lifeline when He said, "O Israel, thou hast destroyed thyself; but in me is thine help."

As we proceed through this chapter and see numerous types of self-inflicted health challenges that arise from misguided actions and poor behavioral choices, we can still hear God saying to each of us, "Despite the fact that some of your troubles are of your own making, you'll find help in Me!"

And let us also never forget that Psalm 23:1 says the Lord is our Shepherd. Picture the tireless role of a shepherd, who, time and time again, retrieves wayward sheep that have blundered into ditches and ravines. These sheep, not the wisest of creatures, repeatedly find themselves entangled in the same snares despite previous rescues.

Similarly, Jesus our Great Shepherd (*see* Hebrews 13:20), vigilantly guards His flock. When we falter and sink into the pits of our own making, He is ever ready to lift us out. His boundless compassion reaches us even when our physical ailments or mental burdens stem from our own heedlessness, which may have inadvertently left a door ajar for the adversary's mischief to ensue.

Satan frequently seizes the opportunity to exploit the circumstances we've created through our own carelessness. And in the midst of them, he whispers accusations and tries to convince us that divine aid is out of reach because we are suffering due to our own foolish behavior. Yet like a tenderhearted Shepherd, Jesus stands ready to help, offering His guiding hand even when we've wandered into messes of our own creation.

As we journey forward, we will explore a few specific ways we may have inadvertently invited the devil to burden us with disease, illness, and sickness. While this isn't an exhaustive list, my aim is to illustrate scenarios that many can relate to easily. To set the stage, I'll start by sharing a personal story from years back, when I unknowingly gave the devil an "entry point" that threatened my well-being and tried to cut my life short.

## BEING OVERWEIGHT OPENS A DOOR TO SICKNESS

In this section, I wish to share an experience from my own life that was very unpleasant. Although I didn't enjoy it when it happened, God used it to produce a significant, necessary change in my life.

Years ago my family gathered courage to address an "elephant in the room" that had taken the form of my expanded waistline. Over a number of years,

I had *foolishly* allowed myself to grow larger and larger. But this intervention, driven by my family's genuine concern for my well-being, set in motion a journey toward a much healthier version of myself.

Like many who carry extra weight, I had spent countless hours gazing into the mirror, eventually becoming so familiar with my size that I failed to notice what others saw — the reality of my obesity. Clad in black for years to try to visually mitigate my burgeoning size, I believed I'd effectively tucked away my dilemma, shrouding it at least partially from view. Yet my family, with their keen eyes and abundant love, recognized my unhealthy state, and they cared enough to confront me and guide me toward the path of weight loss. For their courage and support, I will always be profoundly thankful.

Embarking on my weight-loss journey, I made an appointment with a doctor for a thorough check-up. As he meticulously documented the details on my medical chart, his eyes lingered on the scale's glaring revelation that revealed I weighed nearly 320 pounds. While jotting down the figure, he muttered under his breath the phrase "morbidly obese."

The words struck me like a lightning bolt. Stunned, I turned to him and asked, "Could you repeat that, please?"

He answered, "Sir, you are morbidly obese."

"I'm what?" I asked him again.

He answered, "You are morbidly obese."

Being labeled "morbidly obese" felt like both a sucker punch and a slap in the face. Little could have been more shocking to my ears, so I asked him again, "Morbidly obese?"

The doctor's words, though hard to swallow, were another catalyst for an immediate and transformative decision to turn my life around. I share this with you because I have profound empathy and understanding for those grappling with weight challenges. I want you to know that every word you read from me is steeped in genuine compassion, devoid of condemnation. If you or someone dear to you is battling with excess weight, you're well aware that it feels like an inescapable prison. Yet I assure you, the keys to freedom are within reach!

Personally, I found that I had to face the truth head-on, both seeing and hearing it, and I know I'm not alone in this. Often, it's when we're forced to confront the truth that it sparks the necessary change we need, even if it's uncomfortable to take in and process.

That's precisely what happened to me, and I couldn't be more grateful for it. But for me, it also meant that I needed to work with a physical trainer and go to a special gym that specializes in helping people to regain *mobility*, which I did, and I continue to go there to this day.

While that I suffered with excess weight — and with it, high blood pressure, back and feet pain, and regularly losing my balance and falling — I made multiple prayer requests for healing. But one day, I heard the Lord speak plain and clear, "Quit asking people to agree with you for healing. You do not need healing. You need to lose weight. If you do that, these problems will disappear."

I recognize some individuals face thyroid complications that contribute to their larger size. However, medical experts confirm that the prevalence of such issues is often overstated by those grappling with their weight. For most, the root of excessive weight can be traced to unhealthy eating habits that trigger metabolic dysfunction and hormone imbalances, a lack of physical activity, emotional struggles, and other factors.

In numerous instances — and indeed, *numerous* is the right term — people find themselves battling weight-related ailments because they permitted their weight to spiral out of hand. It's as if the devil had exploited a weak spot — an "entry point" — in their lives, and through it, he created a stronghold to both ravage and shorten their lives. Yet no matter the origins behind the accumulation of extra pounds, the keys to freedom are available.

To show the devastating effects of being overweight and obese, I refer to material from my book *Last-Days Survival Guide*, where I document how being overweight presents a risk of a number of health conditions. The website of the CDC (Center for Disease Control) states that people who are overweight and obese are at increased risk for many serious diseases and health conditions, including:[1]

- High blood pressure (hypertension)
- High LDL cholesterol, low HDL cholesterol, or high levels of tri-glycerides (dyslipidemia)
- Type 2 diabetes
- Coronary heart disease
- Stroke
- Gallbladder disease
- Osteoarthritis (a breakdown of cartilage and bone within joints)
- Sleep apnea and breathing problems
- Some cancers (endometrial, breast, colon, kidney, gallbladder, and liver)
- Mental illness, such as clinical depression, anxiety, and other mental disorders
- Body pain and difficulty with physical functioning
- Bone problems
- Low quality of life
- Many causes of death (mortality)

Individuals carrying excess weight face numerous challenges, frequently experiencing health issues, increased absenteeism from work, and reduced physical mobility that interferes with daily life. In many cases, the physical pain they suffer due to obesity triggers the need for painkillers, which often cause chemical imbalances in the brain and more weight gain — and the cycle feels hopelessly endless and hard to stop, like a merry-go-round ride that never ends.

The prevalence of excess weight and obesity is skyrocketing, wreaking havoc in personal lives and creating alarming consequences on a national level. This burgeoning statistic has actually turned the issue of obesity into a pressing concern for national security as healthcare costs push the system toward the brink of economic disaster.

The list of potential ailments connected to being overweight and obese highlights some issues that can largely be alleviated with weight loss. But shedding pounds after a significant gain demands unwavering dedication. I speak from experience, as I personally faced this challenge years ago. But with the power of God, the unwavering support of my family, guidance from a fitness trainer, and my own determination, I managed to drop more than 100 pounds. Before achieving this, I battled fiercely with my weight, and I *really* struggled as I carried what amounted to the weight of a small human being around on my body!

In addition to grappling with the embarrassment of my expanding physique and the constant need to upsize my wardrobe, as I already shared, I was also wrestling with high blood pressure and a recurring tendency to take unexpected tumbles. I was becoming immobile simply due to the difficulty of moving my large physical size.

If I hadn't gotten a grip on where I was headed, it was inevitable that other issues would have developed. But having just recently undergone the most intense physical checkup in my life, I am thankful to God that the medical report shows I am in top-notch condition. My bloodwork is so spectacular that my doctor said, "Oh, how I wish that my bloodwork was as good as yours!"

But before I overcame this battle with obesity, the Lord had instructed me to stop asking for healing prayers — and, rather, to lose weight and my problems would go away. So instead of repeatedly seeking prayers for my blood pressure and frequent falls, it was time to take responsibility for the situation I had allowed in my life and to firmly close the "door" that I had left ajar for the devil to slip through.

This pivotal choice marked the beginning of a transformative chapter in my life, and I can declare with assurance that anyone wrestling with weight issues can triumph over it by using the right tools and by receiving the strength that faith provides.

If you find yourself in a similar condition, I want to encourage you that by losing weight, it is likely your blood pressure will normalize, the pain in your joints will disappear, back and feet pain will also subside, and you'll find that many symptoms of diabetes or insulin resistance will leave — *and you'll feel so much better about yourself.*

If you've inadvertently allowed excess weight and obesity to creep into your life and overtake you, it's time to take a stand. Repent, seek support, turn a fresh page, and journey toward the version of yourself that reflects the vibrant, healthy being you are meant to be. Embrace the healing and health that await you, stepping boldly into the life you deserve and the overall health that is your birthright as a child of God.

People overeat for various reasons ranging from nervousness and stress to depression to simply an inordinate love of food. Pertaining to overindulgence, the words "gluttony" and "lasciviousness" often come to mind.

Focusing on the word "lasciviousness," I must point out that this word in the New Testament is derived from a Greek word that captures the idea of excess both in the areas of food and sex, and it means *overindulgence in food* or *an unrestrained lifestyle that is particularly characterized by rampant sexual indulgence.*

The word "lasciviousness" is listed as the principal sin among the transgressions of Sodom and Gomorrah, and it played a significant role in God's decision to obliterate those cities. But from a linguistic point of view, in God's mind, lasciviousness includes *an overindulgence in food*, and it is just as wrong and perverse as unrestrained sexual activity outside of marriage.

I believe that when we honestly assess the damaging effects of excessive eating and what it does to a person — or to a nation systemically, where healthcare is the number-one industry and obesity-related morbidity rates are skyrocketing — we can better understand why God would view this as a "perverting" act that destroys one's health and life. To keep eating excessively, while at the same time requesting healing prayers for physical ailments that are connected to being overweight, is futile. But God is so good that He will heal us time and again in spite of ourselves.

As God said through Hosea, "O Israel, thou hast destroyed thyself; but in me is thine help" (Hosea 13:9). Although we may be reaping self-inflicted health challenges arising from our own misguided actions and poor behavioral choices, God is still saying to each of us, "Despite the fact that some of your troubles are of your own making, you'll find help in Me!"

God delivered me from the bondage of this stronghold, so I speak on this topic with an empathetic heart and the insight of someone who understands just how deeply it can wreak havoc across various facets of life. Many are so confined and inhibited that they find themselves building their entire lives around their physical size.

For example, they can only ride in the front seat of certain automobiles; they avoid certain shopping malls and vacation destinations due to the required amount of walking to visit those places; they can't use a bus, a van, or some types of SUV transportation because of a lack of strength in their leg muscles to make the upward step into the vehicle; and some must even purchase more than one seat when using public transportation.

If you or anyone you care about is wrestling with the challenge of being overweight or obese, take heart — it is not a permanent fate. Breaking free requires patience and persistence, but I stand as proof that liberation is within reach. Once the door to obesity is closed, the result will be healing and health springing forth in your life — and new mental freedom that is exhilarating!

**If you've inadvertently allowed excess weight and obesity to creep into your life and overtake you, it's time to take a stand. Repent, seek support, turn a fresh page, and journey toward the version of yourself that reflects the vibrant, healthy being you are meant to be. Embrace the healing and health that await you, stepping boldly into the life you deserve and the overall health that is your birthright as a child of God.**

## BEING IMMOBILE OPENS A DOOR TO SICKNESS

Another serious factor that provides an "entry point" to disease, illness, and sickness is *immobility*, regardless of one's size. Getting up and physically moving eliminates many problems related to immobility, but by foolishly allowing oneself to become sedentary, a person can provide an entry point for the devil to assail him or her with all types of health issues. This isn't just a concern for individuals grappling with excess weight, for many who are slender also find themselves hindered by a lack of movement.

It seems society today is even designed for immobility. For instance, does your neighborhood have sidewalks? If not, you're not alone, as a shrinking number of new communities include them, reflecting a shift in lifestyle where strolling has become nearly extinct. Nowadays, the average household owns multiple cars, turning walking in most places, especially suburbia, into a nostalgic memory from the past.

In today's fast-paced world, strolling for leisure or necessity seems like an archaic tradition, unless you lace up your sneakers with the explicit intention of clocking exercise steps. Outside major cities, spotting someone on foot is now a rarity, and when you do, you can almost bet they're purposefully marching toward their fitness goals. Daily foot traffic consists mostly of short jaunts from the living room chair to the kitchen, a quick shuffle to the bathroom, or a tired trudge to the bedroom. Otherwise, it's a brisk walk to the car to embark to a destination.

Such is our aversion to walking that even at destinations like shopping centers, malls, or places of worship, we perform "vehicular ballet" through parking lots, twirling around and around in search of the elusive closest spot — all this effort just to trim a few steps off our route! Instead of simply parking farther out, many contently idle in their cars, eyes peeled for a prime space near the entrance to minimize the distance they must travel on foot.

Motionless living, characterized by the absence of consistent, physical activity, plays a significant role in the rise of weight gain, obesity, insulin resistance, diabetes, and debilitating immobility, alongside numerous other health issues that could largely be resolved if individuals embraced a more active lifestyle. This crisis of a sedentary existence has escalated to such an extent that shopping malls and grocery stores now provide motorized carts to aid individuals who are unable to navigate aisles unaided, allowing them to glide through their shopping journeys with assistance.

In various parts of the world where automobiles are scarce and walking is woven into the fabric of daily life, the number of physically inactive individuals is remarkably lower. Do you remember when spotting someone using a motorized cart was a rarity? Nowadays, it feels like these carts are omnipresent. Just recently, I found myself weaving between them as I navigated the aisles of an American grocery store.

While we are grateful for the technology that aids those with genuine mobility challenges, it's important to recognize that much of the immobility epidemic is self-imposed. By consciously choosing to incorporate physical activity into our daily routines, we could significantly alter the landscape of this issue.

The workplace environment has also undergone a transformation and has morphed into a reality where individuals are tethered to their computer screens, often remaining stationary for extended periods. This persistent gaze into the computer is not only a drain on one's mental well-being but is also a culprit in the creeping tides of weight gain and the erosion of physical agility.

As someone who writes multiple books annually, I frequently find myself ensconced in my chair and drawn into the creative process. Without a conscious nudge to break this sedentary cycle, hours can slip by in immobility, and when I do eventually rise, my body protests with discomfort. However, by setting a mindful rhythm of movement every couple of hours, I discover a remarkable improvement in my physical ease and agility.

Years ago, when I grappled with obesity, it was a condition that nearly rendered me immobile. As I mentioned, my back and feet seemed to always hurt, so I avoided walking, which contributed to my being even more inactive. Time slipped by as I remained ensnared in a cycle of endless sitting. Finally, I resolved to slam the door shut on this "entry point" for the devil and reclaim my vitality.

Facing my enduring habit of immobility, I began to make deliberate choices. Rather than seeking the nearest parking spot or riding an elevator, I embraced the walk from a distant parking space and saw staircases as opportunities to revive my strength and mobility. My journey back to physical health was also greatly supported by my visits to the gym and the aid of an inexpensive trainer, an important ally who guided me in safely shedding the chains of a sedentary lifestyle and reigniting the spark of movement in my life.

Instead of engaging in activity, many find themselves ensnared in the comforts of a couch or the embrace of a favorite chair, eyes glued to the flickering TV screen or endlessly scrolling through their phones. A person can't live like that and expect to be healthy.

**Time slipped by as I remained ensnared in a cycle of endless sitting. Finally, I resolved to slam the door shut on this "entry point" for the devil and reclaim my vitality.**

If you don't move physically, you will lose the ability to move. You can request prayer, go to the doctor, and throw medication at your symptoms, but if you don't take care of your physical body, you're not going to have the kind of health God wants you to have.

This sedentary lifestyle is no path to well-being. Our bodies are like finely-tuned instruments that thrive on movement; neglecting them leads to inevitable decline. You may seek prayer, consult with doctors, or rely on medication to mask symptoms, but without physically moving, the state of health you desire will remain elusive. So I encourage you to embrace activity and honor the gift of movement — it's essential for a life of vitality.

If you've found yourself trapped in the web of a sedentary lifestyle, breaking free requires a determined leap into action. Instead of daunting yourself with the prospect of running a marathon right away — an endeavor likely to lead to frustration and defeat — begin with small, achievable steps. Commit to moving in ways you can manage, make it a habit, and gradually increase your efforts.

This steady progression will help you rebuild your strength and agility. Remember, inactivity can be a door or entry point for the devil to come flooding in to undermine your health and well-being. However, by nurturing a habit of regular movement, you effectively bar the door to many issues associated with inactivity and keep unwelcome forces at bay.

## NEVER TAKING TIME TO REST OPENS A DOOR TO SICKNESS

Another reason people get sick is because they *foolishly* do not take time to rest, and this wrong decision opens a point of entry for the devil to affect their heart, mind, and body. Once again, I will use an example from my own life to make the point.

Many years ago, I saw myself as invincible and never in need of rest or a vacation. In the end, I learned a valuable lesson that altered the rest of my life for the better. At the time, Denise and I were practically living in two different cities — in two countries — simultaneously because we were leading two large churches in two different nations at one time.

Our cross-border existence was a whirlwind of bleary-eyed drives through tangled traffic leading to the airports, marathon sessions standing in immigration lines, and the relentless hauling of cumbersome baggage from one land to another. Upon reaching our destinations, we would plunge headfirst into meetings with our teams, barely catching our breath. I assured myself this juggling act was doable, and we did it week after week over the course of several very intense years.

As time passed, my mind became clouded, and I began to make unwise decisions. In the middle of the night, we often found ourselves awakening in perplexity, unable to recall where we were. We became so physically and spiritually weary that we would fall asleep if we sat still just for a few minutes. Then a moment came when many issues came crashing down all at once. With urgency, I called those with spiritual authority in our lives, and they quickly came to our side. At their insistence, we took time to recuperate and to design a new lifestyle where the rhythm of productivity danced gracefully with the melody of rest.

Seizing this unfortunate but opportune moment, the devil had attempted to unleash chaos into our lives that would have been destructive. But by heeding the wisdom of our overseers and embracing a new way of living, Denise and I found strength to shut the door to the devil and close his "entry point" into our lives.

Truth be told, what I faced was rooted in pride. I believed I was immune to the need for rest that other people seemed to require. I fancied myself as unstoppable and thought that I could charge ahead tirelessly without consequences. I disregarded the wisdom embedded in the Fourth Commandment, which says, "Remember the sabbath day, to keep it holy" (Exodus 20:8). To make matters more complex, I didn't know *how* to rest, and I perceived periods of downtime as nothing more than squandered moments when I could be doing something productive.

Looking at our present schedule might not strike you as traditional "rest." Yet Denise and I have discovered a harmony between labor and leisure that suits us perfectly. This balance has unlocked a new level of productivity in our lives. While rest might mean different things to different people — some see it as a few hours of downtime each day, others as regular days off, or occasional vacations — what truly matters is finding your own rhythm. This unique dance keeps you revitalized and shields you from the pitfalls of physical, mental, and spiritual exhaustion.

This is an area where I find myself perpetually seeking help from the Holy Spirit, for I am a hard worker who thrives on productivity. Take, for instance, our infrequent visits to the United States to speak and minister at various kinds of events all over the nation. When we do come to America, we aim to make every moment count, and we therefore cast our net as wide as possible to touch countless lives.

On a recent visit, Denise and I embarked on an ambitious 31-day journey during which we were scheduled at a staggering 57 events. Our determination to maximize our impact was admirable, yet by the journey's end, I was physically sick, and it took nearly two months for me to regain my vitality. The issue wasn't a lack of healing; rather, it was my unrealistic scheduling — cramming in the impossible without a single pause for rest — and it opened the door for physical sickness.

The reality is, finding the delicate equilibrium between work and rest is like locking the door to the devil and preventing him from infiltrating one's health and relationships. Conversely, by recklessly charging ahead without pausing to breathe, we inadvertently fling open a door and invite him to assail our spirit, soul, and body.

While this can be difficult, making prudent choices is beneficial in thwarting numerous health challenges. Should you find yourself having taken a misstep or two, seek God's forgiveness and embark on a path of wiser decisions. In doing so, you will close the door the devil has been using to access you, and you'll pave the way toward the life that Christ purchased for you at the Cross and is yours by inheritance!

## WHAT YOU SOW IS EXACTLY WHAT YOU WILL REAP

As we further discuss how *foolish behavior* and *unwise choices* can open the door to sickness, I would be remiss not to highlight a fundamental principle that governs us all. This is the age-old truth known as the "law of sowing and reaping."

Even those who aren't particularly spiritually inclined communicate this sentiment when they echo the saying, "What goes around comes around." Much like gravity's inescapable pull, the law of sowing and reaping influences every facet of our existence and stands as an undeniable law that is unchallenged.

And as you will see in the next pages, the law of sowing and reaping also has great application to healing and health. The actual law of sowing and reaping is found in Galatians 6:7 where the apostle Paul wrote, "Be not deceived; God is not mocked: for whatsoever a man soweth, that shall he also reap." What

Paul was saying in this verse is so emphatically true that he began by telling us not to question its validity. That is why he said, "Be not deceived; God is not mocked...."

The word "deceived" has its roots in the Greek word *planao*, a word that conveys the idea of *being swayed by an external influence* or *causing one to stray from the right path, to be misled, or to wander aimlessly.* When Paul penned this verse, he did so with a forceful directive and a stern prohibition. His emphatic tone could be accurately interpreted as an admonition to "put an end to being deceived."

It appears some individuals had been "misled" about the efficacy of the law of sowing and reaping. This is not surprising, for this eternal principle still encounters doubt from those who are unwilling to acknowledge its truth. But Paul boldly proclaimed with conviction that "...God is not mocked...."

The word "mocked" finds its roots in the Greek word *mukteridzo*, which conveys the image of *someone disdainfully turning up their nose at another, exuding an air of ridicule*, or *derision.* It paints a picture of an individual insolently proclaiming, "Really? You can't possibly buy into that silly notion of sowing and reaping. How naïve must one be to think that what you plant is what you will harvest!"

But Paul unabashedly proclaimed, "...Whatsoever a man soweth, that shall he also reap." The word "soweth" comes from the Greek word *speiro,* a word that denotes *any* seed that is planted. The emphasis on *any* seed highlights that this principle extends to every aspect of life. It pertains to love, labor, time, patience, kindness, forgiveness, bitterness, finances, selfishness, and even seeds that one sows concerning *health.*

Expanding the meaning of "soweth" is the Greek word *ean,* translated as "whatsoever." This little word signifies *whatever, whatever thing*, or *no matter what a person sows.* Through this linguistic choice, Paul revealed that this is a divine principle echoing throughout all aspects of existence without exception.

Like the inevitability of a sunrise, whatever seed you plant, in any realm of life, will eventually sprout into its corresponding harvest.

The Greek tense envisions sowing not as a singular act, but as an ongoing, habitual practice. Thus, it might be rendered as, "...Whatever a person plants again and again and again — constantly planting, planting, and planting...."

In other words, this describes *a constant, steady, perpetual sowing of seed.* The law of sowing and reaping declares that for any seed you sow constantly, this divine law will kick into action and you will gather a bounty from what you have planted. The word for "reap" is in the same Greek tense, meaning it could be translated, "You will reap, reap, reap, reap, and keep on reaping and reaping."

As a whole, Galatians 6:7 could be interpreted, "Don't let anyone pull the wool over your eyes! You might scoff at this divine law, but it is absolutely fixed and unchangeable. The law is that whatever you continuously plant in the garden of your life — regardless of what sort it is — that is inevitably what will be your harvest." This law is so fixed that it means if you constantly:

- Sow *love*, you will certainly reap a harvest of *love.*
- Sow *patience*, you will certainly reap a harvest of *patience.*
- Sow *kindness*, you will certainly reap a harvest of *kindness.*
- Sow *forgiveness*, you will certainly reap a harvest of *forgiveness.*
- Sow *bitterness*, you will certainly reap a harvest of *bitterness.*
- Sow *strife*, you will certainly reap a harvest of *strife.*
- Sow *money*, you will certainly reap a harvest of *money.*
- Sow poor *health habits*, and you will certainly reap a harvest of *poor health.*
- Whatever you sow — regardless of what it is — is *exactly* what you will reap.

Hence, if you're going to reap what you sow, maybe you ought to figure out what you want to reap and then start planting those kinds of seeds to assure you'll get the harvest you wish for your life. Plant seeds today that will grow into the life you envision for tomorrow.

Remember that the law of sowing and reaping is a timeless truth and a divine principle that touches every aspect of existence and is never denied. You are currently living in a harvest of what you have sown in your past. *Never forget that sowing and reaping is a universal law that applies to everyone and to everything.*

But immediately after Paul wrote about the law of sowing and reaping, he added, "For he that soweth to his flesh shall of the flesh reap corruption; but he that soweth to the Spirit shall of the Spirit reap life everlasting" (Galatians 6:8).

Here again, we see the word "soweth" — the Greek word *speiro* — which means *to scatter* or *to sow*, as in *sowing seed*, and the verb tense used here indicates *continuously sowing*. It means the opening part of the verse could be rendered, "For he that soweth, soweth, soweth, and soweth to his flesh...." The Greek word for "to" is *eis*, a word that means *into* and, hence, pictures one who habitually sows *into* his flesh or *into* the flesh realm.

This portrayal paints a vivid picture of someone who panders to the flesh. Instead of pausing to evaluate the long-term consequences of his actions, he gives in to impulse and momentary pleasure. This picture portrays the flesh like an insatiable beast — always wanting more, no matter how much it is fed. Gratifying the flesh can yield temporary satisfaction, but it often results in a cycle of destruction.

In this state, the person prioritizes short-term satisfaction over long-term well-being. Rather than resist the voice of the flesh, he instead gratifies it, indulges it, and makes provision for it. Essentially, he satisfies its demands and bows to its commands because the appetite of the flesh knows no bounds — its desires are insatiable, ever hungry to consume every aspect of a person until it holds complete sway over his life.

The flesh will urge you to rest beyond what is necessary or to be driven to the point of getting very little rest. The flesh will coax you to linger in a state of laziness or push you with overactivity to the detriment of your physical and emotional well-being. The flesh will impassion you to indulge far more than you should until your life is steered by these cravings and becomes a turbulent, chaos-strewn path marred by idleness, self-degradation, neglect of responsibilities, or unnecessarily broken health — all due to a lack of stewardship and care.

In fact, following the flesh's whims can become the most arduous trail one can tread. It clamors to dominate you, yelling for control, insisting on being the ruler. Unless you bring these urges to the Cross and subdue them through the power of the Spirit, they will persist and eventually coax you to succumb, unleashing their detrimental consequences upon your life.

If you don't mortify the flesh by the power of God's Spirit, you'll find yourself serving your own self-consumed lifestyle, and you'll find yourself pandering to the hankerings of the flesh. As a result, Paul said you will "reap corruption." The word "reap" is translated from the Greek word *theridzo* which means *to harvest* or *to reap.*

The word "corruption" is the Greek word *phthora,* which evokes images of *decay, degradation,* or *putrefaction.* Consequently, investing in the desires of the flesh will culminate in harvesting unpleasant and repulsive outcomes in your life. If you sow into your flesh, you will end up reaping really putrid and stinking situations in your life.

Imagine your health as a flourishing garden. If you neglect its care and simply go along with cravings to overeat, oversleep or succumb to the siren call of the couch, or if you allow ambition to drive you to work nonstop without pause, these seemingly innocuous choices will eventually bear the fruit of various health woes.

Think about the person who keeps his lifestyle revved like a car engine with the gas pedal pressed to the floor continually, allowing little to no reprieve.

What appears to be minor indulgences or weaknesses are actually seeds that can sprout into a tangled mess of significant health challenges. What seem like small actions, repeated habitually, will produce a cascade of serious health issues.

But in Galatians 6:8, Paul continued to say, "...He that soweth to the Spirit shall of the Spirit reap life everlasting."

Once more, we encounter the term "soweth," derived from the Greek word *speiro*, meaning *to scatter* or *to sow*, as one who *plants seeds*. Here it signifies an ongoing act of sowing, and we could render this segment of the verse as, "He who constantly sows and sows and sows to the Spirit shall, from the Spirit, reap a harvest of eternal life."

This paints the image of someone who turns away from indulging the flesh, choosing instead to invest in the Spirit. Consequently, this person "reaps" eternal life. The word "reap" translates from the Greek word *theridzo*, which, as we've seen, conveys the idea of *harvesting* or *reaping*. What this person reaps is called "life everlasting." In Greek, it depicts a life so wondrous that it defies measure.

Hence, if you make the decision to stop foolishly repeating actions that produce negative and putrid results — and you determine instead to surrender to the Spirit — the scripture promises you will harvest a life overflowing with immeasurable, abundant joy and blessings.

## YOUR BODY BELONGS TO JESUS CHRIST

We need to understand that once we gave our lives to God, our physical bodies became the property of Jesus Christ. In First Corinthians 6:19, the apostle Paul wrote to the Corinthian believers because they were living way below God's holy standards.

Out of shock over the reports that had reached his ears, Paul said, "What? know ye not that your body is the temple of the Holy Ghost which is in you, which ye have of God, and ye are not your own?"

Notice the first word of this verse begins with the word "what." In Greek, it's more than just a simple word — it's an exclamation that mirrors Paul's astonishment. It's as if he was so baffled that he asked, "What? Have you not yet comprehended…?" He followed with the words "know ye not," which are translated from the Greek words *ouk oidate.* Here, the word *ouk* conveys an emphatic *no*, and *oidate* stems from *oida*, meaning *to comprehend* or *to grasp something fully*. Piecing these elements together, we see that Paul was essentially expressing, "What? Do you not yet understand? Do you really not get it? Have you not realized that…?"

Even the seemingly simple word "that" carries profound significance. In Greek, it is the word *hoti*, and it underscores a pivotal truth Paul was eager to convey: "What? Know ye not *that* your body is the temple of the Holy Ghost?" (1 Corinthians 6:19).

Paul's use of the word "that" points the Corinthians to the truth that our bodies are indeed God's temple. The Greek word for "body" is *soma*, and it refers to *the physical body*. The moment we surrender our life to Jesus, God swoops in and transforms our physical body into a divine container of the Holy Spirit and we become His temple.

The word "temple" in this verse is the Greek word *naos*, and it describes *a grand sanctuary* or *a richly adorned shrine*. Picture vaulted ceilings, lustrous marble, granite, and glimmers of gold and silver, all embellished with intricate decorations. This word not only conveys the opulence of sacred architecture, but also speaks to the most revered, concealed section of a temple. It's the very term employed in the Old Testament Septuagint to refer to the *Holy of Holies*, where God's presence dwelled.

If Jesus is your Lord and Savior, the Holy Spirit has moved inside you and has become a permanent resident in your life. You are now a walking, breathing sanctuary. That's what Paul was communicating to the Corinthians and to us when He said, "…Your body is the temple of the Holy Ghost which is in you…" (1 Corinthians 6:19).

The word "in" here is the Greek word *en*, and it specifically identifies the location where the Holy Spirit is — *inside us*. Paul further elaborated, saying, "...Which ye have of God...." Here, the words "ye have" are translated from the Greek word *echo*, which means to *contain*, *hold*, or *possess*. Essentially, Paul was saying, "We are the holders, the possessors, or the containers of this remarkable gift which we have *of* God."

The word "of" in this context comes from the Greek word *apo*, and it means directly *from* God. The profound change we underwent the day we were saved is not a result of personal rehabilitation or reform. It is something we received as a gift *directly from God*.

Paul went on to say, "...Ye are not your own. For ye are bought with a price..." (1 Corinthians 6:19-20). The words "not your own" in Greek mean *emphatically not your own* and underscore the absolute relinquishment of personal ownership. The word "bought" is a translation of the Greek word *agoradzo*, a word that refers to *the liberation of a slave from the bustling marketplace* — a metaphor for the ultimate act of redemption.

This freedom given to us came at a "price." The word "price" is translated from the Greek word *time*, which signifies *a cost that is substantial and priceless*. The indescribable cost for our redemption was the blood of Jesus. Because of the marvelous work of His grace in our lives, we are not our own anymore. Our body, soul, and spirit belong to Him who loved us and gave Himself for us.

## 'GLORIFY' GOD IN YOUR BODY

Knowing we were purchased by the blood of Jesus, Paul continued, saying, "...Therefore glorify God in your body, and in your spirit, which are God's" (1 Corinthians 6:20). Basically, Paul said, "As a result of and in response to what Jesus did, glorify God in your body and in your spirit."

The word "glorify" is translated from the Greek word *doxadzo*, a form of *dokeo*, which means *to access*, *to estimate*, *to think*, or *to ponder*. The use of this word lets us know that in order to glorify God we need to value the weight and the worth of how we can best bring God glory in our "body" — which again is the Greek word *soma*, the term for *the physical body*.

Most believers focus solely on glorifying God in their spirit, and while that is certainly included in First Corinthians 6:20, we are also instructed to glorify Him in our body. When Jesus died, He redeemed both our spirit and our body. Therefore, it is no longer ours but His, and He wants us to make a well-thought-out decision of how we can best glorify Him with it — it is His temple, after all.

This principle of taking good care of what God has entrusted to us was established back at the beginning of creation. The Bible says, "And the Lord God took the man, and put him into the garden of Eden to dress it and to keep it" (Genesis 2:15). Even though Eden was a perfect paradise, God still placed Adam in charge of it and told him to dress it and keep it. And as we have seen, the word "keep" means *to guard* and *to protect* something.

Similarly, God has entrusted each of us with the stewardship of our physical bodies. It is God's will for us to develop our bodies and to guard and protect them as the dwelling place of God, and in doing so, we "glorify God with our body."

## LEARN TO MANAGE YOUR BODY IN 'SANCTIFICATION AND HONOR'

Consider what Paul says in First Thessalonians 4:4: "That every one of you should know how to possess his vessel in sanctification and honour." What's interesting about this verse is that in the original Greek, there are two words that don't appear in the *King James Version*. It actually says, "That every one of you should know *of himself* how to possess his vessel in sanctification and honour" (1 Thessalonians 4:4).

This means each of us has to become familiar with our own self and know how to "possess his vessel." The word "possess" in this verse is the Greek word *ktaomai*, which means *to control, manage, or win the mastery over.* It clearly depicts personal mastery and implies that you should master your body and not allow your body to master you.

Here Paul called the physical body a "vessel" — using the Greek word *skeuos* — which is the word for *a utensil* in the kitchen or *a tool* in the toolbox. Specifically, it is used here to depict the human body as *an instrument in God's hands.*

Paul even told us how we are to manage and master our body when he said, "...In sanctification and honour" (1 Thessalonians 4:4). The word "sanctification" is the Greek word *hagiasmos*, which means to treat something as *holy, consecrated*, or *sacred.* It's taken from the word *hagios*, the word for *holy.* We are also to treat our body in "honor," which is the Greek word *time*, describing *price*, *value*, or *worth.*

Here time refers to something of immense cost and extraordinary value. Again, we have been redeemed out of Satan's control by the precious blood of Jesus, which makes us holy and priceless in God's eyes. Therefore, what He calls holy and priceless, we also need to call holy and priceless and treat it as such.

Although God's Spirit dwells inside us, if we don't take care of and maintain our physical bodies, they will end up broken, in pain, or out of commission. And that condition is not indicative of your body being the precious dwelling place of the Spirit that was purchased by Christ's blood.

But to master your body — to truly steward your physical being — it's essential to nourish it with the right foods, engage in regular physical activity, and practice good hygiene. Simply lounging around in front of the TV, aimlessly browsing the Internet, or playing online games for hours every day, for example, will put you on a fast track to health issues. A conscious choice to take charge and keep your body active and agile is crucial to maintaining your body's vitality. As the old saying goes, "If you don't use it, you'll lose it."

## HOW ARE YOUR EATING HABITS?

I encourage you to ask yourself, *What kinds of foods am I putting into my body?* Are they healthy and full of life, or are they processed and empty of nutrition? This is not meant to condemn you, as all of us could probably come up higher in this area of our lives.

Again, if you're not eating healthy, please don't feel condemned. This was an area that I personally struggled with for years. I have candidly shared how I had gained so much weight that it resulted in physical ailments and hindered mobility. But it's a fact that to a great degree, what you eat will determine how you feel and what you're able to do.

The apostle Paul gave us a practical yardstick regarding what we eat, what we drink, and everything else we do. In First Corinthians 10:31, he wrote, "Whether therefore ye eat, or drink, or whatsoever ye do, do all to the glory of God."

In my own journey to experiencing the healing and health that Christ intended for me to have, I had to come to a place where I asked myself some hard questions — and these are questions you may want to ask yourself:

- *Am I eating in such a way that brings God glory?*
- *Does my weight glorify God?*
- *Am I just eating out of boredom or am I actually hungry and in need of nutrition?*
- *Are the things I'm putting into my mouth good for my body?*
- *Can I eat unhealthy foods and enormous portions to the glory of God?*

For me, the clear answer to all these questions was a resounding no! When God reminded me of First Corinthians 10:31, I knew that I had to repent for not taking care of my body. With God's help and the encouragement of others,

I made the decision to master my body and to learn how to have healthy discipline and boundaries regarding the food I ate.

I was the only one who had the power to change what I was doing. I alone could make the decision to break bad habits and learn to master new ones — and the same is true for you. I prayed for God's strength every day and committed to one deliberate choice after another that I was going to align my eating and drinking habits with a higher purpose and learn how to eat and drink "to the glory of God." Again, God's Word says, "Whether therefore ye eat, or drink, or whatsoever ye do, do all to the glory of God" (1 Corinthians 10:31).

Eating to the glory of God is about submitting your diet and your relationship with food to the lordship of Jesus. Regardless of your weight or size or how out of shape you are, you can turn it around by praying and developing a godly, practical plan and following it.

One day at a time — one decision at a time — you can get started and become more fit and mobile than you thought you could be. You'll feel better physically and feel better about yourself emotionally. You may even be able to get off many of the medications you've been on once your doctor gives you the go-ahead to do so.

## ANOTHER WORD ABOUT MOBILITY

Another area that I really had to come to grips with was exercise. It seems that for many, exercise is a matter of either passionate commitment or outright aversion. Before I made the big change in my life, exercise was virtually nonexistent in my life. Nevertheless, as God got my attention about my dietary choices, He also got my attention that my workout regimen needed a significant overhaul. My workout regimen up to that time was walking from one room to another in the house or walking from a parking lot to wherever I needed to be, and that was about it. If I needed to go upstairs in a building, rather than use the stairs, I would search for an elevator or escalator to avoid walking up a flight of stairs. As noted earlier, a sedentary life leads to immobility!

But God used key scriptures to help me make positive changes in my eating and exercising. The first verse was First Corinthians 9:27, where Paul said, "But I keep under my body, and bring it into subjection…."

The words "keep under" are a translation of the Greek word *hupopiadzo*, which describes *the area of the face below the eyes.* The one thing located in this region that can often get us in a lot of trouble is our *mouth*. In order to truly bring our body into submission, we have to learn to take authority over our mouth — and that includes *our appetite.*

The second verse the Holy Spirit used to help me, which is often misinterpreted, is First Timothy 4:8, which says, "For bodily exercise profiteth little…." Although it appears this verse is downplaying the value of exercise, a closer look at the original meaning shows that it actually encourages exercise!

Take, for example, the words "bodily exercise," which are the Greek phrase *somatike gumnasia*. This phrase is a compound of the word *soma* — which is the same word for the *physical body* that we saw in First Corinthians 6:19 — and the word *gumnasia*, which means *exercise* and is where we get the word "gymnasium." The word *gumnasia* is derived from the Greek word *gumnadzo*, which was used to portray *naked athletes* who exercised, trained, and prepared for competition in the athletic games of the ancient world. Hence the phrase "bodily exercise" carries the idea of *exercising with all of one's might in order to develop oneself.*

In the ancient world, the seemingly odd practice of shedding one's garments was deemed necessary in order to eliminate all hindrances that otherwise could have impeded an athlete's movements. Therefore, the use of the word *gumnasia* — translated here as "exercise" — carries the idea of removing laziness, sluggishness, all excuses, and anything else that would hinder physical movement. Furthermore, people in the ancient world believed discipline of the body was one of life's chief concerns and that it was essential for physical, mental, and even spiritual advancement.

What was Paul really getting at when he claimed that physical exercise "profiteth little"? To grasp his point, we must look at the word "profits," which comes from the Greek word *ophelimos*. This word means to be *indebted* or *obligated* to do something. Originally rooted as a legal term, it conveyed the necessity of upholding one's legal and moral responsibilities. In this passage, it means we have an undeniable duty to engage in physical exercise.

This brings us to the word "little," which is the Greek word *oligos*, and it describes something that is *short-lived*. The use of this word tells us that the effects of physical exercise are *temporary*. Yet according to First Timothy 4:8, the Holy Spirit is telling us through Paul that we have a moral obligation and an undeniable duty to physically exercise — even though it is only profitable in this temporal life.

When we make a decision to discipline ourselves, strip off laziness and excuses, and develop our physical body, it contributes to developing ourselves mentally and spiritually as well. In fact, we are called to steward and develop our *whole* man — spirit, soul, *and* body — which are inseparably one. And one part will invariably affect the other parts, positively or negatively, depending on the care and attention we give to these matters.

If you find yourself constantly saying, "Exercise is just too tough for me. I'm too big, and I get winded after just a few steps," start by surrendering to the lordship of Jesus in this area of your life — and then start doing something. Begin with the smallest of steps, for even a few small steps and some movement is better than endlessly sitting or standing still.

*Some movement is better than no movement.* If you can only walk three minutes, walk three minutes. If you get in a pool and just move your arms and legs in the water, do that. Rather than search for the parking space closest to a door, park farther away and take the opportunity to walk. Rather than search for an escalator or elevator, use the stairs as an opportunity to lift your legs and strengthen your muscles.

The point is, *begin to move*. Make a plan and begin to work that plan. Where you start is not where you'll stay. You will improve with time because God's blessing is on your efforts, and He wants to help you experience better health than you ever thought possible.

## THE DECISION IS YOURS: WHAT KIND OF HARVEST DO YOU WANT TO REAP?

In this chapter, we've uncovered how reckless actions can serve as an invitation to illness, much like leaving a gate ajar for unwelcome guests. Picture the devil as a stealthy lion on the prowl, seeking those whom he can devour. When he encounters someone heedlessly treading down a path of foolishness — and that includes someone who treats his body or mind foolishly — he seizes the chance to sneak in and wreak havoc by stealing, killing, and destroying.

If you've been crossing the line concerning the care of your physical body and health, are you going to continue doing what is foolish and leave an "entry point" for the devil to ravage your health, or will you change your behavior and thereby seal every entrance for the enemy?

**The point is, *begin to move*.
Make a plan and begin to work that plan.**

By indulging in unwise, flesh-driven decisions, you plant seeds that are bound to yield bitter and harmful fruit, and that includes unwanted health issues. The good news is, if illness strikes as a consequence of imprudent actions, God will enable you to close the door to that ailment when you make the choice to change.

If you are currently suffering from sickness due to the misguided choices you've made in the past, it's time to take an honest inventory with God and with yourself. Acknowledge the missteps that have led you here. To halt the ongoing cycle of illness and sickness in your life, be genuinely repentant and seek God's help so those detrimental seeds cease to bear fruit. If needed, ask others whom you trust to help you.

Through these actions, you can shut the door to what the enemy is trying to do to your health. The harmful seeds you planted can be uprooted, and you can begin to plant positive seeds that produce boundless blessings, goodness, and better health.

The law we saw in Galatians 6:7 states that everything we do in life is a seed that eventually produces a harvest. If you carry on foolishly in respect to your flesh, you're going to reap a disastrous harvest. This principle is never violated, so don't deceive yourself into thinking that somehow you will be an exception. This divine law applies to every one of us, so make sure you're planting the right seeds so you can reap a good harvest in your health!

But now…let's move to the next chapter where we will delve into another reason why people get sick. Prepare to be astonished by what you're about to discover. The upcoming pages will open your eyes to another significant reason why many fall ill despite the fact that Jesus secured healing and health for every child of God.

Scan the QR code to watch Rick teach more on this subject.

# QUESTIONS TO PONDER AND DISCUSS

1. In this chapter were both real and hypothetical examples of the ways foolish decisions and actions can open the door of destruction in people's lives — financial mismanagement, a poor work ethic, disregarding laws of safety, allowing strife in relationships, overeating, eating poorly, sleeping too much or too little, obesity, a sedentary lifestyle, and over-activity without giving the body time for recovery and recuperation. Did you see yourself in any of these categories? Which one(s) applies to you? If you're overweight, you can't simply lose the weight you desire to lose overnight — but what steps can you take *right now* toward righting some of your unwise life choices and begin setting you on a new course of healing and health?

2. Hosea 13:9 says, "O Israel, thou hast destroyed thyself; but in me is thine help." Just as it was true then, it is true today that so much of the trouble we face is trouble we have brought on ourselves through poor judgment. How does this verse encourage you to turn *toward* God, not *away from* Him, when you miss it in some area of your life? Find three more scriptures that talk about God's mercy and His desire to forgive you and help you, and write them out for further meditation.

3. Do you have someone who can speak into your life when you're making consistent decisions in the wrong direction, such as persisting in not getting enough rest — or eating so poorly that your health is being affected? If so, who is that person? If not, think about someone you'd like to ask to help keep you accountable in stewarding or *keeping* that which God has given you, including your health. Reach out and ask that person to pray for you and encourage you in areas where you need to improve, whether it's the care of your health, your finances, your relationships, etc. List those areas you'd most like help with. Most importantly, make the Lord your Partner in your endeavors to glorify Him with your life. Perhaps journaling will help you draw near and pour out your heart to Him in areas where you struggle.

4. Were you shocked to learn of some of the serious physical conditions that can occur because of obesity and a sedentary lifestyle? List three conditions you were surprised to see on the list in this chapter. Do you know someone who is suffering needlessly because of a failure to take measures to lose weight or to exercise more to strengthen himself or herself? Are you comfortable sharing this information with him or her from a heart of care and concern? Will you commit to praying for this person for the strength to act on the truth that will eventually bring freedom to his or her life? If so, consider Philippians 2:13 as you do.

5. Prior to reading this chapter, did you understand that you belonged to God not just in your spirit, but also in your spirit, soul, *and* body? (*See* 1 Corinthians 6:19.) Using Romans 12:1, write out a statement of consecration that will help you daily *yield* the ownership of your entire being— spirit, soul, and body — to the Lord.

## SIX

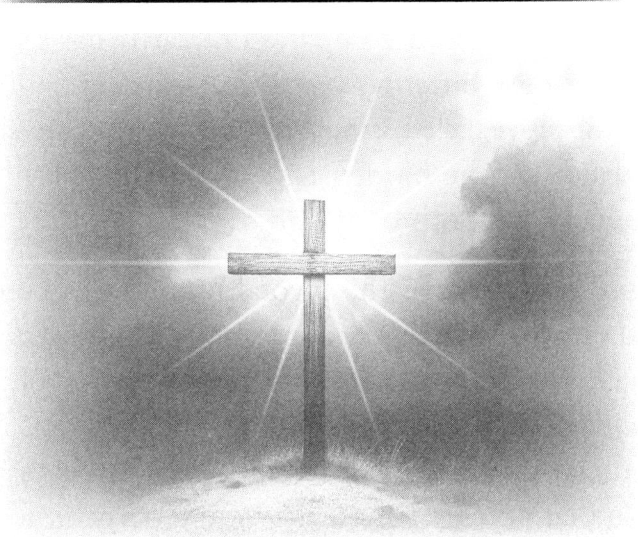

# WHY PEOPLE GET SICK — REASON NUMBER 5: UNRESOLVED, HIDDEN ISSUES CAN OPEN A DOOR TO SICKNESS

In the preceding chapter, we explored another reason *why people get sick* — and that is repeated *foolish behavior*, which creates entry points for the devil to produce a myriad of health problems in one's life. Now, as we delve deeper in our journey, we will shift our focus to *unresolved, hidden issues* that can also provide a point of entry for a wide array of ailments, diseases, and sicknesses that undermine our health.

I am grateful to the pharmaceutical pioneers who have meticulously engineered a vast spectrum of medications, addressing an infinite number of physical and mental ailments. Thanks to groundbreaking scientific advancements in medicine, there now exists a remedy for almost every conceivable disease, illness, and affliction imaginable.

However, no pharmaceutical company on Earth has ever conjured a pill potent enough to dissolve bitterness, offense, strife, and unforgiveness. And now scientific findings reveal that these emotional states are significant culprits in deteriorating health — the hidden entry points the devil uses to infiltrate one's life to wreak havoc on both body and mind.

In earlier chapters, we've seen the pivotal moment in Genesis 2:15, where God entrusted Adam with the sacred duty of *safeguarding, shielding, encircling, and defending* the Garden of Eden. This divine directive implied that Adam was forewarned of the devil's sly intentions to infiltrate paradise. Thus, God tasked Adam with the crucial mission of fortifying the Garden, ensuring its defenses were so formidable that no crack or crevice would permit the devil's entry.

We've seen — and we will see it more fully in Chapters Nine and Ten — that Jesus' redemptive work on the Cross not only paid for the forgiveness of sin, but it also included peace of mind and healing and health for the body and mind. But many believers still become sick and wonder why, and one reason is because they have unresolved, hidden issues that serve as entry points for havoc to be wrought in their body and mind. It is of paramount importance that we know how to identify these vulnerable areas, and then learn how to close the door to the potential of their negative effects on the body and mind.

To be clear, an unresolved, hidden issue in a person's life has to do with his or her mind or emotions — I'm talking about *the soul* or the unseen part of man that lies beneath the surface of his or her physical being.

For example, wounds in the form of disappointment, pain, or grief often lie in the soul, unseen and untended to beneath the surface — but these things can cause serious problems in a person's physical and mental health and well-being if they continue to be hidden and unresolved.

People have valid reasons to feel wounded — whether from past traumas or recent troubling events — and as a result, they may find themselves entangled in a web of bitterness, resentment, conflict, and seeming inability to forgive. But if these emotional states really are culprits that the devil uses to attack and deteriorate one's health, it is essential for us to find a path to freedom from these negative attitudes and emotions so that we are not physically and mentally affected by them long-term.

## KEEP YOUR HEART WITH ALL DILIGENCE

While science has only recently affirmed the long-term detrimental affects of bitterness, offense, strife, and unforgiveness, Proverbs 4:23 has always told us, "Keep thy heart with all diligence; for out of it are the issues of life."

The word "heart" paints an image of the core from which all life's actions spring forth. It serves as the fountain of one's being, and thus, whatever blossoms within this innermost realm, whether good or bad, will inevitably shape the entirety of one's external existence.

- If a person is inwardly filled with peace, peace will dominate his outward life.
- If, however, resentment takes root in his soul, the world he encounters will be tinted with its harsh brushstrokes.
- If his inner being harbors grievances against others, the harvest he reaps will be laden with fruits of discord.
- If strife and unforgiveness lurk beneath the surface of one's thoughts and emotions, like a hidden compass, they will steer the journey of his existence along a difficult path.

People are acutely conscious of the physical discomforts that visit their bodies, yet they remain remarkably unaware of the turmoil and discord simmering within their souls — an upheaval that invariably impacts their physical and mental well-being. While we have blood pressure cuffs for monitoring cardiovascular strain and thermometers for temperature readings, no tangible instrument exists to diagnose a heart entangled in bitterness, resentment, conflict, and unforgiveness.

Assessing the state of one's heart demands a willingness to be open, truthful, and attuned to the voice of the Holy Spirit. The heart holds such paramount importance in the state of our whole life, including our physical health, that Proverbs 4:23 advises us to "keep" it with all diligence.

**If strife and unforgiveness lurk beneath the surface of one's thoughts and emotions, like a hidden compass, they will steer the journey of his existence along a difficult path.**

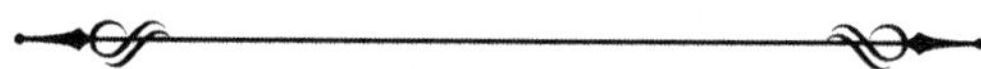

In the original text, the phrase "keep thy heart with all diligence" carries the meaning of *above all guarding*, and it emphasizes the critical importance of conducting a thorough examination of our inner self to ensure it is devoid of bitter seeds that could yield disastrous results in our life.

We are reminded of Matthew 15:19, where Jesus teaches that all evil originates from the heart. This further highlights the necessity of being vigilant about our inner condition. Above all, we must safeguard our heart, meticulously defending the inner sanctum of our being, for whatever festers at the core inevitably influences every aspect of our existence.

One way to gauge if bitterness, resentment, conflict, and unforgiveness are taking root within you is to pay attention to your speech. Whatever resides in a person's heart eventually finds its way through his words. As Jesus observed, "For out of the abundance of the heart the mouth speaketh" (Matthew 12:34).

The mouth serves as a conduit for what is stored in the heart — thus, if one's heart is filled with bitterness, the corrosive influence of offense will permeate his attitudes and reveal itself through his spoken words and reactions in various situations. No gravitational force is potent enough to keep what is in the heart from spilling out through speech, and ultimately, it will betray its own presence. *Never forget that the mouth is the great revealer of the heart.*

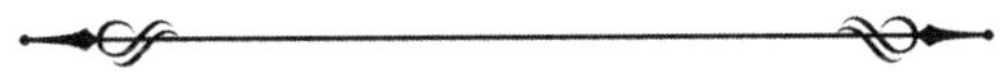

**One way to gauge if bitterness, resentment, conflict, and unforgiveness are taking root within you is to pay attention to your speech.**

## THE LONG-TERM BENEFITS OF A SOUND HEART, AND THE LONG-TERM EFFECTS OF UNRESOLVED, INNER ISSUES

But Proverbs 14:30 tells us, "A sound heart is the life of the flesh: but envy the rottenness of the bones."

In the original text, the words "sound heart" actually mean a "heart of health" and paint a vivid picture of one's heart — and by extension, one's emotions — being in harmonious balance. Recognize that the "heart" symbolizes the deepest essence of a life, and its condition profoundly shapes and impacts one's body, mind, and, ultimately, the surrounding world.

But Proverbs 14:30 also states that when a person's core is in healthy balance, it manifests as vitality and health in his physical life. Essentially, inner turmoil invariably reveals itself in one's body or mind. However, when the internal state is nurtured and flourishing, it generously radiates its positive influence throughout the entire body and into all aspects of life.

Conversely, when the inner essence of a person is unbalanced, it inevitably leads to chaos in their external demeanor. This is echoed in the last part of Proverbs 14:30, which states, "...But envy [is] the rottenness of the bones." Here the word "envy" symbolizes a toxic internal state that gnaws away at a person's very being, like a pervasive illness eroding the bones and marrow of their existence.

Proverbs 17:22 likewise says, "A merry heart doeth good like a medicine: but a broken spirit drieth the bones." We will look at this verse piece by piece, but here we once more encounter the pivotal role of the "heart" and its impact on an individual's existence. A heart that thrives in wellness and harmony fosters a vibrant synergy between body and mind. However, when it is burdened with fractures and frailties, the cracks inevitably extend outward and mirror turmoil in both the physical and mental realms of that person's life.

When Proverbs 17:22 refers to a "merry heart," it pictures someone whose inner being is in prime condition. This verse assures us that such a state of being has a profound impact on the physical body, so much so that it enhances its vitality and well-being.

Indeed, experts in the field of psychoneuroimmunology have observed that maintaining a good inward condition equips one to fend off onslaughts of illness and mental strain.[1] Again, we see that the heart wields an extraordinary influence over both the body and the mind.

That is why Proverbs 17:22 goes on to say that a merry heart "doeth good like a medicine." The original wording actually says it "works a good healing." In essence, when one's inner core is at peace, it plays a pivotal role in rejuvenating and sustaining both a person's physical and mental well-being. However, the verse continues by stating that a "broken spirit drieth the bones."

This implies that a heart in the grip of bitterness can have a profound impact on the body, robbing it of vitality and strength. Modern medical and psychological research validate that such adverse influences debilitate the body and undermine the immune defenses,[2] just as all negative emotions do.

## WHEN ENVY AND STRIFE ARE ALLOWED TO FESTER, THEY RESULT IN EVERY EVIL WORK

In James 3:16 we read, "For where envying and strife is, there is confusion and every evil work." This passage holds immense significance, as it reveals that when jealousy and discord, along with all their offspring, take root in a person's inner being, they catastrophically unlock a door for every evil work, and that includes a lack of healing and poor health.

In this verse, the word "envying" finds its origins in the Greek word *zelos*, and it paints a portrait of *an individual fiercely absorbed in ensuring their own goals take the spotlight*. It illustrates *a person driven by competition, seething with discontent when others surpass them in accomplishments or accolades*. This mindset festers *with jealousy*, *envy*, and *bitterness* toward those who possess what they covet. It embodies the disposition of someone who *smolders with irritation — consumed by a jealous ire, incensed and provoked by another's success*.

The word "strife" in James 3:16 stems from the Greek word *eritheia*, which originally described *a political faction*, often leading to its translation as *a party spirit* due to its ties to political realms. This term depicts scenes of individuals or collectives aggressively championing their agendas. But in this context, it predominantly embodies *a self-centered ambition*, focused more on personal desires and the fulfillment of individual whims than on attending to the needs of others. It paints a picture of *someone so intent on achieving personal goals that he is willing to compromise on principles, bend the truth, and even sever relationships to get what he wants*.

This self-serving, introspective attitude is so preoccupied with personal aspirations that it becomes oblivious to other people's aims and dreams. If unchecked, it can insidiously morph into *a divisive party spirit*, driving wedges and fueling *discord* among people.

The word "confusion" in this verse is interpreted from the Greek word *akatastasia*, which is the prefix *a* with the words *kata* and *stasia* (from *stasis*) attached. The word *kata* carries a sense of what is *dominating,* while the word *stasia* means *to stand.* It could picture *that which is done according to order or that which is dominated by order.* Yet when an *a* is added to its beginning, it serves to negate the meaning and shifts the word's essence to picture *anarchy*, *chaos*, or *rebellion,* carrying images of *instability, discord, and turmoil.*

Then James said where these exist, there is "every evil work." The word "every" is a translation of *pan*, an *all-inclusive word* that means *all* and leaves nothing out. The word "evil" is translated from *phaulos*, a Greek word that denotes that which is *rotten* or *stinking*, such as *maggot-infested meat.*

Through his choice of words, James vividly illustrated that when a person becomes internally entangled with emotions like bitterness, offense, conflict, and unforgiveness — along with their troublesome companions — it acts as an open invitation for every kind of evil. As we have seen from other verses in this chapter, this evil includes the onset of disease, illness, and sickness.

**The *RIV* (*Renner Interpretive Version*) of James 3:16 says:**

> **For it is a fact that whenever one is driven to see his view or agenda adopted at the expense of others, and he is irritated, irate, annoyed, provoked, fuming, or incensed at those who have other views — so filled with strife in his heart that he is blinded to the desires or needs of others — and jockeys for advantage or position even at the expense of others — there is anarchy, chaos, confusion, and insubordination. And that leads to instability, upheaval, unrest, and absolutely every kind of dead, decaying, foul, and stinking activity and business.**

James 3:16 indisputably shows that if bitterness, offense, strife, and unforgiveness rage in the heart, it invariably throws open a door to disaster of every type, and this would certainly include attacks on healing and health.

## WHAT MEDICAL AND PSYCHOLOGICAL SCIENCE TELL US ABOUT THE LONG-TERM EFFECTS OF BITTERNESS, OFFENSE, STRIFE, AND UNFORGIVENESS

Today there are many scientific studies that show if unresolved, hidden issues are left unchecked, they can rapidly surface and spread in one's life like wild weeds that suffocate a garden. Because this possibility exists, it is imperative that we do all we can to seal every entry point that the devil would want to use in this way to poison us and make us unhealthy in our body and mind.

In life, nearly everyone has felt the sting of another's words or deeds. Maybe it was a parent's relentless criticism that marred your childhood, or a colleague's betrayal that undermined your work. Or maybe you discovered infidelity in your marriage, or perhaps you endured the trauma of physical or emotional abuse at the hands of someone you trusted. These are very difficult experiences that can etch deep scars and kindle lingering anger, bitterness, and resentment, causing far-reaching effects on one's physical and mental health.

In fact, if such unresolved, hidden issues are not dealt with, they can ripple through the body and mind and wreak havoc. The fact is that Jesus' redemptive work on the Cross included paying the price for the healing and health of our body and mind, but if we allow such negative feelings to simmer without closure, they can open the door for both psychological and physiological disorders. This underscores the intricate bond between our emotional landscape and our physical well-being.

Due to modern studies in the realms of psychology and medicine, we know that the physiological and emotional effects of harboring such inner turmoil includes the following:

### Heart Disease

Recent research reveals that harboring bitterness, nursing offense, cultivating strife, and clinging to unforgiveness can ramp up stress hormones like cortisol and adrenaline. This biochemical surge elevates blood pressure and accelerates heart rate. Left unchecked, this toxic combination will gradually wreak havoc on the cardiovascular system, leading to an increased risk of heart disease. We live in a day when medicine is readily used to deal with these issues. But in many cases, although medications can address the manifestation of disease, they cannot heal the underlying issues of bitterness, offense, strife, and unforgiveness that are at the root of these physical issues.

### Digestive Problems

According to medical experts, harboring unaddressed and concealed emotions like bitterness, resentment, conflict, and unforgiveness might take a toll on one's digestive system. These negative emotions can worsen gastrointestinal conditions by intensifying the body's stress responses. Research shows they can aggravate symptoms of acid reflux and irritable bowel syndrome. And while ulcers are primarily caused by infection or medications, stress and unresolved emotions can magnify their severity and slow their healing. Thankfully there is medication to help with all of these symptoms, but many of these ailments would disappear if a different state of mental and emotional well-being existed in the core of a person's life.

### Immune Dysfunction

Lingering bitterness, grudges, conflict, and a heart unwilling to forgive can produce long-lasting stress and emotional chaos in a person's life. These undermine the immune system and leave it less capable of warding off illnesses and infections. As a result, the body's defenses falter, leaving it vulnerable to various ailments and extending the time it takes to heal from them. Thankfully, there is medication to help with such problems, but many of these would not be needed if peace replaced the other unresolved, hidden issues.

### Sleep Apnea and Insomnia

The unresolved issues of bitterness, offense, strife, and unforgiveness contribute to inner turmoil and stress that disrupt sleep. Scientific evidence suggests that the persistent absence of restful sleep increases the risk of an array of health complications such as diabetes, heart problems, obesity, and a deterioration of mental well-being. Again, we are thankful there is medication to help with such problems, but many of these would cease to hold sway if genuine peace replaced unresolved, hidden issues.

### Mental-Health Disorders

When a tangled web of unresolved issues — like bitterness, grudges, conflict, and an unwillingness to forgive — lie beneath the surface in a person's life, it stirs a silent storm within. These covert battles can fuel mood disorders such as anxiety and depression, and the perpetual stress of clinging to such negative emotions can even disturb the delicate balance of one's brain chemistry.

It's this hidden turbulence that often gives rise to shifts in mood and behavior. Although these and other related disorders can be medically treated, they can often be permanently eradicated when the unresolved, hidden issues of a person's soul are dealt with and resolved.

### Dysfunctional Relationships

Unresolved bitterness, festering offenses, simmering strife, and unspoken unforgiveness can quietly undermine one's capacity to thrive in relationships. These concealed remnants from past connections can weave a web of confusion and cloud a person's judgment, hindering his ability to welcome those he truly needs in his life.

Consequently, this invisible baggage not only casts a pall over his personal journey, but also ripples outward to create waves of discord for those within his circle. The weight of negative emotions like these can affect those near us, fray the threads that weave our relationships, and erect barriers that prevent us from forging profound and meaningful connections with others. Such dysfunction can also result in the loss of important relationships in our lives, resulting in unhealthy isolation.

## Increased Anger

When people harbor deep-rooted bitterness and grudges and allow strife to brew, it is like they are planting seeds that often blossom into a tangled mess of conflicted emotions, frequently producing anger as a result. The emotional tempest this creates can dramatically alter the journey we share with our loved ones and all our connections — family, friends, and colleagues. When anger is left unchecked, it can build invisible barriers between us and others, cause our friendships to crumble over trivial matters, and fuel our own disproportionate reactions to events in our lives.

As a result, our relationships may begin to drift apart, propelling these cycles of resentment and anger to continue. Ultimately, this can lead to rash decisions, a cloud of pessimism looming over us, and a torrent of hurtful remarks tinged with sarcasm being said at the wrong time. This emotional turbulence will likely result in withdrawal, isolation, and spirals of depression and anxiety, leaving us trapped in an emotional storm of our own making.

## Decreased Self-Esteem

Recent research reveals that clinging to emotions like bitterness, offense, strife, and unforgiveness often undermines one's self-image, and this erosion of self-esteem frequently exacerbates a spectrum of mental-health issues, such as depression and even Post-Traumatic Stress Disorder (PTSD). Scientific studies indicate that when one's inner being is disrupted, this internal dissonance tends to foster the absorption of negative thoughts and feelings, making individuals more susceptible to anxiety, fear, and discouragement.

To summarize, research shows that unresolved, hidden issues can contribute to *heart disease, digestive problems, immunity dysfunction, insomnia, mental health disorders, increased anger, and decreased self-esteem.* But in addition to the points I just briefly described, there are many other additional negative psychological or social consequences that can affect the quality of a person's life when he or she has unresolved, hidden issues, including dysfunctional relationships.

I urge you to recognize that the effects of clinging to the toxic feelings of bitterness, offense, conflict, and unforgiveness extend far beyond mere physical consequences — the results delve deep into the realms of our emotions and our mental well-being. When these negative forces are left to simmer, they can stealthily lay the foundation for profound challenges both in our bodies and in our hearts and minds — and indeed in the circumstances of our lives.

Holding on to unresolved attitudes exacts a steep emotional toll that burdens both heart and mind like a relentless storm. These emotions fuel toxic fires in the soul and gradually erode our peace and joy. And harboring unforgiveness doesn't stop at wreaking emotional chaos, for it can seep into the body and ignite a cycle of pain and distress in our health. Such a heavy load is unforgiving and leaves echoes of its impact on mental, emotional, and physical health that linger far beyond the initial problem.

## JESUS DESCRIBED THE EFFECTS OF UNRESOLVED, HIDDEN ISSUES OF BITTERNESS, OFFENSE, STRIFE, AND UNFORGIVENESS

The enduring impact of internal turmoil is so significant that Jesus addressed it in Luke 17. In this crucial chapter, He painted a vivid illustration of the corrosive consequences of harboring resentment, taking offense, nurturing conflict, and clinging to unforgiveness. These emotions, if left unchecked, can pollute the spirit and seep into the circumstances of our lives in an insidious pool of spiritual sludge. Moreover, Jesus imparted wisdom to His disciples on how to cleanse their hearts of such destructive sentiments.

Luke 17:1 begins this important passage by saying, "Then said he [Jesus] unto the disciples, It is impossible but that offences will come...."

First, I want you to notice that Jesus indisputably said it is "*impossible* but that offences will come" in this life. The word "impossible" in the original Greek text literally means *impossible*. The *New International Version* translates it, "Things that cause people to stumble are bound to come, but woe to anyone through whom they come." The *Amplified Bible* interprets it, "Stumbling blocks [temptations and traps set to lure one to sin] are sure to come, but woe (judgment is coming) to him through whom they come!" These agree with the intent of the Greek text, which depicts offense as an event that *will surely happen* at one point or another in every person's life.

The word "offenses" finds its roots in the Greek word *skandalon*, which also forms the basis of our English word "scandal." This tells us that when an offense takes place, it ignites a tempest of scandal within the emotional and mental landscape of a person. It's similar to an unexpected snare that causes one *to trip, to fall*, or *to stumble.*

Often translated as *a stumbling block* or *a stumbling stone*, offense can describe the jarring ordeal of encountering behavior that is so far removed from our expectations that it makes the soul *falter, totter*, or *wobble* and leaves us reeling inwardly.

This event catches you so off guard that you almost *lose your footing* — and your once-esteemed opinion of a person takes a dramatic plunge. At the heart of every offense lies either *something someone did or said* or *something someone neglected to do or say.* In one way or another, he or she failed to meet the spoken or unspoken expectation you held, and it left you stumbling in your emotions.

At some junction in our journey, we've all brushed against the sting of offense, and it is a wound that can cut deep. Yet in Luke 17:1, Jesus assured us that as long as we live and breathe, there will be the potential for offense, so we must combat it and refuse to allow it to have a place in our hearts and minds.

The fact is that human beings are enigmas who are wrapped in layers of unpredictability. Just when you believe you've got them figured out, they surprise you with actions that leave you dumbstruck, sometimes doing or failing to do things you wouldn't have imagined in your wildest dreams.

**Often translated as *a stumbling block* or *a stumbling stone*, offense can describe the jarring ordeal of encountering behavior so far removed from our expectations that it makes the soul *falter*, *totter*, or *wobble* and leaves us reeling inwardly.**

Even the most devout Christians, those who immerse themselves in hours of prayer, study the Scriptures diligently, and strive to live a holy life, occasionally find themselves acting in ways they'd rather not. This is simply part of the human condition. So if you let yourself get ruffled every time someone falls short of your expectations, you'll find yourself living in an up-and-down, roller-coaster existence in your heart and mind!

## A REAL-LIFE EXAMPLE OF A PERSON WHO WAS SHACKLED TO BITTERNESS, OFFENSE, STRIFE, AND UNFORGIVENESS

If we fail to rein in feelings of bitterness, offense, conflict, or unforgiveness, they can brew within us and create an entry point for malevolent forces to seep into our lives. In this chapter, we've witnessed how these corrosive emotions can manifest in physical ailments and that those ailments will continue to persist if the deeper emotional issues are not dealt with.

But let me illustrate this with a true story that paints a powerful picture of how such emotions can wreak havoc on the well-being of a believer, depriving that person of the healing and health that Jesus secured for him through His Cross and resurrection.

Decades ago, Denise and I knew a precious woman, who is now in Heaven, but although she was free to walk the streets of our city in the former Soviet

Union, she was inwardly as bound as any person I've ever ministered to in a real prison filled with inmates. Her early life had been filled with pain and mistreatment that left indelible emotional scars, and she was shackled to horrible memories that kept her bound.

Others we'd known and ministered to had similar experiences in life to this woman, but they had learned to move forward with life. This woman remained emotionally frozen, and like a ghost, her past haunted her present and tortured her soul. Enveloped in a cocoon of old grievances, she had retreated inward to a world of isolation.

We counseled her again and again, but then we watched every Sunday at church as she sat there in the congregation, surrounded by others yet untouched by their warmth because she had an impenetrable barrier that separated her from those who had friendship or kindness to offer.

Resentment and unforgiveness from events from long ago, which in her case were inflicted by people who no longer were living, caused this dear woman to cast harsh, unwarranted judgments on all who endeavored to approach her. It was as if she was playing a mental and emotional game of "get before you're gotten" with ghosts from her past. Her present company of sincere believers were simply innocent bystanders of the grief she'd failed to shed.

Eventually her hurts morphed into a shield that barred the gates of trust and cast unfounded aspersions on the very community of faith that she needed. Her entire facade was marked by the harshness that festered within her, and her body became ensnared by a crippling disease that seemed to mirror the bitterness she harbored deep in her soul — an outward testament to her unresolved pain.

I'm sorry to report that she died in this miserable, wounded condition, although real, supernatural help from Jesus was available and had been presented to her on many occasions just in our experience with her. The hurts this woman once experienced — and no doubt they were real — had been meditated on, nurtured, and held fast for so long by this woman that no one could get through to her. And she passed from this world, though saved, with that offense clasped tightly in an unyielding grip in the recesses of her soul.

This may seem like an extraordinary example — something I wish were merely an exaggeration — but it is, in fact, a stark reality for a large swath of people who ought to be experiencing the healing and health Jesus provided for them by His redemptive work on the Cross. The sad truth is that the Body of Christ is home to many who bear wounds from the past that continue to cast shadows over their current lives and affect their relationships and their bodies and minds.

In this chapter, I don't want to simply diagnose the root of the problem for my readers. I want to assure you that if you are among those who have been abused, betrayed, deserted, hurt, let down, wounded, stabbed in the back, or rejected by your parents, family, or friends — healing is possible, and a brighter future awaits you where the ghosts of yesterday no longer haunt your present.

The echoes of past torment are being orchestrated by dark forces to try to dictate the course of your life today. Left unchecked, those offenses and the backlash of torment they caused will completely derail you. And such inner turmoil can fester and eventually manifest in physical ailments or even mental struggles. *But you don't have to live today with the residual effect of what the devil did to you yesterday.*

Remember that Luke 17:1 says as long as we live in this world, we will bump up against the potential for offense. This means sidestepping every potential offense in life would be like trying to dance through raindrops without getting wet.

Hence, learning how to handle such issues is essential if you want to keep your heart free from bitterness, offense, strife, and unforgiveness, along with its accompanying fruit of *heart disease, digestive problems, immunity dysfunction, sleep apnea and insomnia, mental-health disorders, dysfunctional relationships, increased anger, and decreased self-esteem.*

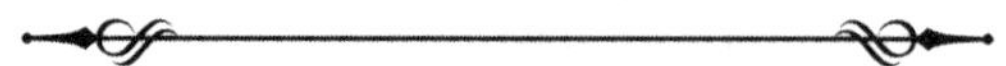

**You don't have to live today with the residual effect of what the devil did to you yesterday.**

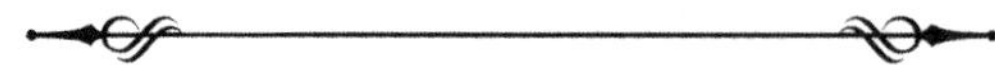

## TAKE HEED TO YOURSELF

When Jesus addressed the ever-present potential for bitterness, offense, strife, and unforgiveness in Luke 17:3, He told the disciples, "Take heed to yourselves: if thy brother trespass against thee, rebuke him; and if he repent, forgive him."

Notice that Jesus said, "Take heed to yourselves...." This counsel is crucial, for when one is hurt and offended, the instinct is to fixate on the one who wronged us, rather than to introspect. It's tempting to recount the person's misdeeds and — to anyone within earshot — to seek empathy and, knowingly or not, spread the negativity to others.

Bitterness is a tangled web that can impede your spiritual journey, and God's presence cannot thrive in the midst of such toxic thoughts. That's the reason why it's of utmost importance that you obey Jesus' command to "take heed to yourself." The fact is that when one is offended, he often wants to get a grip on his offender. But Jesus says, "Get a grip on *yourself*."

Even though a person may have really done wrong — or you perceived he failed you in some way — rather than focus on his misdeeds and allow your inner attitudes to poison you, instead you must get a grip on your own emotions so that you are not poisoned by the scandal of offense.

But Jesus went on in Luke 17:3 to say, "...If thy brother trespass against thee, rebuke him; and if he repent, forgive him." The word "trespass" is translated from the Greek word *hamartano,* which denotes *breaking rules*, *committing a wrong*, *crossing boundaries*, or *committing some type of violation.*

Hence, it means if your brother *violates* you, you are to rebuke him — and the word "rebuke" comes from the Greek word *epitimao*, which means *to forthrightly and directly admonish*. Then if he repents, you are to *forgive* him.

At times, facing a disagreement head-on can prove beneficial, leading to the resolution of the problem at hand. However, there are instances when people find themselves trapped in an endless loop of discussions, revisiting every minute detail, yet reaching no fruitful conclusions.

Sometimes bringing a third person to the table to hear the conversation proves helpful. But eventually, one must weigh whether revisiting the issue repeatedly is a worthy endeavor or if it merely exacerbates the hurt. When a solution remains elusive, sometimes the wisest course is to step back and entrust the matter to God.

Whether or not a direct conversation yields the response we desire, it remains vital to embrace forgiveness, even if the one who caused the pain fails to comprehend the impact of his actions or refuses to acknowledge his wrong. Luke 17:3 says if a brother or sister repents, we should forgive that person, implying that it is for his or her sake that we do so. But if no such repentance is made, forgiveness is nevertheless in order for all the previously mentioned reasons — so that the inner storm of chaos caused by unforgiveness will not work its destructive aftermath in the body and mind *and life* of the person who clings to it.

Jesus said we are to "forgive," which is translated from the powerful Greek word *aphiemi*, which means *to permanently dismiss*, *to liberate completely*, *to discharge*, *to send away*, or *to release*. The best modern-day translation of this word "forgive" is *let it go*. Thus, Luke 17:3 could read this way: "If your brother *violates* you, *be straightforward* and *deal with it*, and if he repents, *let it go*."

The reality is that you might have endured a significant wound or genuine wrongdoing in the past that caused you great pain. It could have even taken something from you that can never be given back. However, if you hold on tightly to these negative emotions — choosing not to forgive and clinging to anger, bitterness, offense, and strife — these emotions will slowly dismantle your life. Sadly, *a past-tense problem* will become *a present-tense issue* when you refuse *to forgive* and *let it go.*

**Even though a person may have really done wrong — or you perceived he failed you in some way — rather than focus on his misdeeds and allow your inner attitudes to poison you, instead you must get a grip on your own emotions so that you are not poisoned by the scandal of offense**

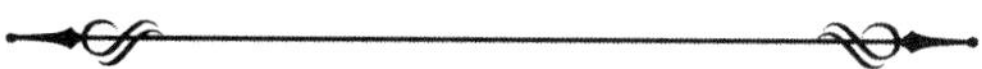

"Letting it go" does not mean you deny what was done to you or that you are to remain in close proximity to the person who caused you harm. Indeed, if a person has continually been caustic, you need to put space between that person and yourself. Staying near where others continue to hurt you will only make it more difficult for you to forgive them, to be healed, and to move on.

The book of Ecclesiastes reminds us in chapter 3 that there is a time and place for everything under the sun. Verse 5 affirms that there is "a time to embrace, and a time to refrain from embracing" — and this shows us the delicate balance between connection and detachment and highlights that there are moments to hold others close and times when it is imperative to step back. Then in verse 7, we are reminded that silence and speech each have their seasons as well and that silence often serves as a balm for healing. Indeed, there are times when we must back off and provide distance and silence in order to be healed after being injured.

But often, even though people manage to physically and temporarily distance themselves from someone who has caused them pain, those past painful memories cling stubbornly and end up steering the course of their lives long after the events have passed. To change this negative trajectory, it is crucial for our own well-being to heed Jesus' instruction to forgive that person and to let the sin or offense go.

**If you hold on tightly to these negative emotions — choosing not to forgive and clinging to anger, bitterness, offense, and strife — these emotions will slowly dismantle your life. Sadly, *a past-tense problem* will become *a present-tense issue* when you refuse *to forgive* and *let it go.***

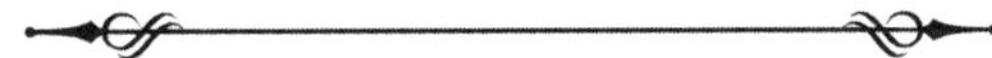

Someone once compared the act of clinging to past grievances to sipping a vial of poison, foolishly expecting it to harm the one who wronged you. Yet, ironically, it is *you* who bears the brunt of the venom. As already evidenced, such festering resentment can ripple through your physical health, emotional state, and mental clarity, leaving you affected on all fronts.

There comes a time when you must release the grip of past grievances and get over the offense for your own benefit. Whatever hurt lingers from bygone days or whatever offense weighs heavy on your heart, know that freedom is within your grasp. Someone may have really committed an offense against you by speaking or acting inappropriately — or even cruelly — toward you, but at some point you have to release it and get over the offense for your own benefit.

If you struggle with horrific realities of infidelity, rape, murder, or other terrible events that have occurred to you or someone you know, these are serious and very painful offenses that often and correctly require legal action. In this passage, Jesus never told us to deny what others have done, but urged us that regardless of what they have done, for our own sakes — even if a legal action is required — we are to forgive them.

Jesus commands each of us to forgive our offenders, but the tough part comes when someone commits the same offense over and over. In the framework of ancient Jewish law, individuals were obliged to forgive their neighbors three times in a single day. However, Jesus elevated this benchmark and set the bar at seven times a day — effectively doubling the expectation — and then he added one.

Forgiving someone once or twice for repeating the same misdeed within a day is a formidable challenge, but to offer forgiveness seven times in such a short span seemed so daunting that the disciples could only respond by imploring, "Lord, increase our faith" (*see* Luke 17:5). This was the equivalent of saying, "Oh Lord, this is a tough challenge, and we're not sure we're up to doing what You have told us. Please strengthen our faith and help us!"

In Hebrews 4:12, the Word of God is likened to a sharp, two-edged sword. This metaphor serves as a powerful reminder that God's Word can pierce through our facade and touch the core of our being as it delivers uncomfortable truths that are tough to embrace. Yet this divine scalpel has the unique ability to excise the ailments within us if we choose to heed its instruction.

Choosing to let go of an offense can be very difficult to do, but Jesus gave the clear directive that if someone has wronged you even multiple times in a single day and seeks your forgiveness with genuine repentance, we are bound to forgive them each and every time. And as we submit to this divine instruction, it releases the Holy Spirit to wield His mighty sword to slice away at the bitterness and resentment that has tried to root itself inside us. I want you to understand that Jesus' unequivocal message in this passage is that we must *get a grip on ourselves and choose to let it go.*

So regardless of whether the wrongdoing was born of purpose or thoughtlessness, the reins are in our hands, and we alone must choose whether to remain chained by this hurt or to liberate ourselves by releasing it.

As I said earlier, nurturing grudges and clinging to toxic feelings is like drinking poison and expecting someone else to suffer. And this, my friend, is one reason why people get sick. Eventually the poison inside begins to harmfully take its toll on the body, heart, and mind.

**There comes a time when you must release the grip of past grievances and get over the offense for your own benefit. Whatever hurt lingers from bygone days or whatever offense weighs heavy on your heart, know that freedom is within your grasp.**

## THE EMOTIONAL AND PHYSIOLOGICAL EFFECTS OF FORGIVENESS

Having looked at the ramifications of unforgiveness and its toll on our well-being, let's now turn to see what science says regarding the emotional and physiological advantages of embracing forgiveness and seeking peace. You'll soon uncover how heeding the teachings of Jesus creates a protective barrier and how it shuts the point of entry that the enemy has used to access you and your health.

Earlier, I listed the physiological and emotional ramifications of bitterness, offense, strife, and unforgiveness — but now I want you to see what medical science reports happens as a result of letting go of these negative emotions.[3]

### Improved Heart Health

Recent scientific studies suggest that embracing forgiveness can be a boost for your health, significantly improving cardiovascular markers (blood pressure, heart rate, and stress recovery). Moreover, forgiveness combats stress, transforming stress into peace and a soothing balm for your heart, much like a gentle salve for the soul, which resultantly fosters a heartier and healthier life.

### Lower Blood Pressure

Studies reveal that holding on to grudges can act like a silent agitator that sends one's blood pressure and heart rate on an upward journey while burdening arteries with undue stress. This internal turmoil can damage one's cardiovascular health by contributing to inflammation, endothelial dysfunction, and arterial stiffening. All these negative processes raise the risk of atherosclerosis and heart disease. In short, chronic stress and hostility can lead to reduced arterial flexibility, which increases cardiovascular risks.

In contrast, individuals who embrace forgiveness tend to enjoy notably lower blood pressure levels compared to their grudging counterparts. Furthermore, studies reveal a strong connection between the act of forgiving and reduced heart rates, as well as a decrease in heart-related symptoms, when compared to those who cling to past grievances.

### Stronger Immune System

Research indicates that holding onto grudges can affect our immune system by diminishing it's resilience, whereas embracing forgiveness enhances immune efficiency by reducing stress and inflammation.

### Improved Mental Health

Research indicates that embracing forgiveness can lead to a significant reduction in depression, anxiety, and hostility. Evidence supports that forgiveness may enhance parasympathetic activity (slower heart rate and calmer physiology.) Those who practice forgiveness often experience enhanced psychological well-being and improved social connections, processes that are linked with serotonin and oxytocin regulation. Furthermore, as forgiveness grows, levels of stress and mental-health challenges tend to diminish. Some experts suggest that it is a reciprocal relationship in which mental stress and forgiveness significantly influence each other.

### Fewer Symptoms of Depression

Research suggests that harboring resentment toward others can worsen symptoms of depression. Furthermore, individuals with unforgiving mindsets frequently exhibit increased muscle tension, elevated heart rates, and higher blood pressure. In contrast, forgiveness seems to buffer physiological stress responses and improve mood-regulating neurochemistry. It can also ease the symptoms of PTSD. Thus, those who embrace forgiveness tend to navigate life with less depression and greater contentment and find themselves more at peace with their circumstances.

### Improved Self-Esteem

Research indicates that releasing grudges bolsters emotional resilience and fortifies the ties that connect individuals, which leads to enriched relationships. Further findings reveal a close partnership between forgiveness and self-esteem and illustrate that those who practice forgiveness tend to possess a more robust emotional resilience and an enhanced self-image that fuels their confidence. A growing body of research suggests that individuals who practice forgiveness are better equipped to confront challenges, thus amplifying their confidence and sense of self-worth.

To summarize, we see that it is a medical and scientific fact that practicing forgiveness contributes to *improved heart health, lower blood pressure, a stronger immune system, improved mental health, fewer symptoms of depression, and improved self-esteem.*

While it's undeniable that modern medicine offers a vast arsenal to tackle numerous health challenges, the insights I just described cause me to ponder whether many of these issues could be alleviated through something as simple as forgiveness. The power of forgiveness on one's well-being is so profound it prompts me to consider its healing potential — not just for those who seek forgiveness, but equally for those who offer it. Instead of allowing grudges to fester and inadvertently compromise our health, why not take a preventative measure against illness by embracing forgiveness as a regular practice in our lives?

## WHY JESUS LIKENED BITTERNESS, OFFENSE, STRIFE, AND UNFORGIVENESS TO A SYCAMINE TREE

In Luke 17:6, we read, "And the Lord said, If ye had faith as a grain of mustard seed, ye might say unto this sycamine tree, Be thou plucked up by the root, and be thou planted in the sea; and it should obey you."

In this passage, Jesus drew an analogy between these internal toxins and the sycamine tree, instructing His followers, including *us*, on how to eliminate such negativity from our lives. It's no mere chance that He chose the sycamine tree for this metaphor. Why not a plum, apple, or orange tree? Was there a specific reason Jesus selected the sycamine to represent bitterness, offense, strife, and unforgiveness?

In my own quest to unravel the mystery of this question, I delved into the archives of botanical science, eager to unearth the attributes of the sycamine tree. What I uncovered was nothing short of illuminating and astounding. By considering the following fascinating details about the sycamine tree, I believe you'll grasp precisely why Jesus chose this particular tree to symbolize the toxic emotions of bitterness, offense, strife, and unforgiveness.

### FACT NUMBER 1:<br>IN EGYPT AND THE MIDDLE EAST, THE WOOD OF THE SYCAMINE TREE WAS THE PREFERRED WOOD FOR BUILDING CASKETS.[4]

*Caskets!* Just think of it — the tree that was most commonly used to make caskets is the example Jesus used to depict bitterness, offense, strife, and unforgiveness! The sycamine tree was the preferred wood for building coffins because it possessed these characteristics:

- It grew quickly, which was beneficial because large amounts of this particular wood was needed for making coffins.
- It grew in many different kinds of environments, which made it easily accessible.
- It grew best, however, in dry conditions.
- Its wood was very durable, which was a desired quality for coffins.

Taking a look at this, I can understand why Jesus likened the sycamine tree to unforgiveness, because, just like the sycamine tree:

*Bitterness, offense, strife, and unforgiveness grow very quickly.* These inner toxins, like a plant, sprout with alarming speed, and in no time, they take root, spiral wildly, and expand until they engulf everything in their path. This unruly plant of bitterness finds its fertile ground in the heart, where it seeks to dominate and overshadow any space it inhabits.

*Bitterness, offense, strife, and unforgiveness grow in every environment.* These inner toxins know no boundaries, and they flourish in every corner of the world. Regardless of one's origins, residence, cultural background, or social standing, unforgiveness sprouts within human hearts universally. It pervades all walks of life and is experienced globally.

*Bitterness, offense, strife, and unforgiveness grow best in dry conditions.* These inner toxins find their strongest roots in arid spiritual landscapes. They flourish in places untouched by repentance, devoid of joy, and barren of the Spirit's fruits. In these parched environments, unforgiveness spreads and prospers.

*Bitterness, offense, strife, and unforgiveness will bury you.* These inner toxins, like the sycamine tree, are the materials the devil uses to craft a coffin from which escape becomes ever more elusive. It's a stark reminder that these negative emotions can be our most efficient gravediggers and hasten us toward being put six feet under.

### Fact Number 2:
### The sycamine tree had a very large and deep root structure.[5]

In the arid landscapes of the Middle East, the sycamine tree boasts some of the most intricate and profound root systems in the region. This formidable tree can soar to impressive heights of more than 30 feet, yet its true strength lies beneath the earth. There, its roots delve deep into the ground and form an extensive underground network. This subterranean fortress renders the sycamine almost indestructible, and even if chopped down to the stump, it defiantly resurrects itself. Time and time again, the roots relentlessly surge upward to breathe new life into the world above.

It's no surprise that Jesus chose the sycamine tree to illustrate the nature of bitterness, offense, strife, and unforgiveness. Just like this resilient tree, unforgiveness needs to be uprooted completely, or it will continuously resurface. Its roots burrow deep within the human soul, and only through sincere repentance, empowered by the Holy Spirit, can these roots be fully extracted to prevent their persistent return.

### Fact Number 3:
### The sycamine tree produced fruit that was bitter to eat.[6]

The sycamine tree and the fig tree bear a striking resemblance to one another. Their respective fruits seem to look nearly the same. Although the sycamine mirrors the fig tree's inviting exterior, in a cruel twist of nature's deception, the sycamine's fruit is bitter. The moment this fruit touches the tongue, its true nature is revealed — an overwhelming bitterness turns anticipation into disappointment and leaves a bitter and sour aftertaste.

In the days of the New Testament, figs were prized treasures and too costly for poorer people. Those with less to spend turned instead to the fruit of the sycamine tree, a humble stand-in for the luxurious fig. Yet the sycamine's fruit was notoriously sharp and acrid.

To endure its bitterness, one had to nibble cautiously, before setting it aside for a reprieve, only to return later for another tentative bite. Rarely would one muster the resolve to consume an entire piece in a single sitting. Its intense tartness demanded patience and persistence in nibbling it over a long period of time.

Jesus compared the astringent fruit of the sycamine tree to the corrosive nature of bitterness, offense, strife, and unforgiveness. For example, much like one would sample the sharp fruit of the sycamine tree — tasting it reluctantly, contemplating its harshness, yet ultimately reaching for another bite — so do people indulge in the bitterness of their grievances.

They ruminate over their resentments, putting them aside momentarily, only to revisit the seething cauldron of their discontent. They dwell over their grudges, let them stew in the depths of their hearts, and step away briefly, only to return to the sour recollection repeatedly. It becomes a relentless cycle of chewing on the bitterness and inevitably returning for more.

When people marinate in the sour brine of bitterness and resentment, fixated on injustices, real or perceived, they internalize these corrosive emotions toward those who have harmed them or those whom they deem their enemy. Eventually, their unyielding unforgiveness transforms them into something equally bitter. Curiously, much like those who are unlucky enough to have once tasted the sycamine fruit, individuals who perpetually brood over bygone grievances find themselves ensnared in a cycle of spiritual poverty as they chew on the fruit of their own discontentment.

### Fact Number 4:
### The sycamine tree was pollinated by the sting of a wasp.[7]

Remarkably, the sycamine tree owes its pollination to a wasp that punctures the very core of its fruit with its stinger. The pollination of the sycamine tree hinges on this intimate interaction, and thus, a sting is required for the sycamine tree to be pollinated.

Think of all the people you know who have uttered words like, "I've felt the sting of that person before, and I refuse to endure it a second time. The pain they caused cut so deep that I'd be foolish to let them near enough to inflict such hurt again!" Is it possible that these people were "stung" by a situation specially designed by the devil to pollinate their hearts and souls with bitterness, offense, strife, or unforgiveness? *Is it possible that Satan's "wasp" got to them?*

The truth is that when you shield your heart from bitterness, offense, strife, or unforgiveness, *you disarm the devil* and leave him powerless to plant these toxic seeds within you. The most effective strategy to shield yourself from the corrosive impact of these emotions is to resolve to never let offense take root. Perhaps you've already been "bitten," but by avoiding the stinging effects of that venomous wasp, you will prevent unresolved, hidden issues from ever taking hold, and it will spare you the arduous task of uprooting it later.

All of this information makes it crystal clear why Jesus chose the sycamine tree to illustrate the perils of harboring bitterness, offense, strife, or unforgiveness. Harboring these emotions is like opening a door that invites the enemy and his destructive power into your life. They are the materials of "coffins" that the devil wants to use to put you six feet under.

And as we have seen, bitterness, offense, strife, or unforgiveness rapidly develop roots that grow deep into your mind and emotions and eventually control every facet of your existence. Their bitter fruit is used by the devil to tempt you to chew on it repeatedly, and clinging to these negative emotions will put you into a cycle of poverty that robs you of the richness of a fulfilled spiritual life.

## HOW TO UPROOT AND REMOVE THAT TREE!

Now with this clarity about why Jesus chose the sycamine tree for His illustration and the weight of its significance apparent, let's delve into Jesus' instructions about how to uproot bitterness, offense, conflict, and unforgiveness from the depths of our lives.

In Luke chapter 17, Jesus provides a profound lesson on uprooting the deeply ingrained feelings of bitterness, offense, conflict, or unforgiveness from our hearts. He guides us on how to cast these persistent emotions into a barren realm where they can never take root in us again.

**And as we have seen, bitterness, offense, strife, or unforgiveness rapidly develop roots that grow deep into your mind and emotions and eventually control every facet of your existence.**

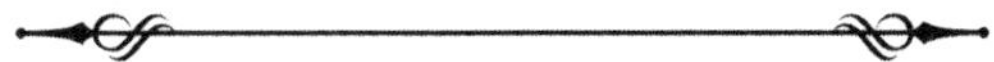

In Luke 17:6, Jesus said, "...If ye had faith as a grain of mustard seed, ye might say unto this sycamine tree, Be thou plucked up by the root, and be thou planted in the sea; and it should obey you." Notice that Jesus said, "...Ye might say unto this sycamine tree...."

When someone comes to terms with the fact that he's wrestling with feelings of bitterness, offense, conflict, and an inability to forgive, he needs to do more than just pray and seek forgiveness; he needs to address these negative forces head-on.

In this passage Jesus highlighted the power of the verbal command by saying, "...Ye might say unto this sycamine tree...." This suggests that instead of letting your thoughts rule over you, the time has come for you to speak directly to your thoughts and command them to follow your lead!

If you wait until the mood strikes, you might never get around to it. Relying on your feelings alone is like trying to swim in a pool of quicksand. You see, emotions are impulsive and unpredictable and will craftily convince you that you're justified in holding on to bitterness, offense, strife, and unforgiveness. But instead of being a puppet to these wayward feelings, seize control and command them into submission.

In short, it's time to stop pointing fingers outward and start taking responsibility for your own liberation. It's time for you to become the conductor of your own emotional orchestra. Or as Jesus said, it's time to face that "sycamine tree," uproot it entirely, and pave the way for new freedom!

- If you don't speak to your emotions, they *will* speak to you.
- If you don't take authority over your emotions, they *will* take authority over you.
- If you don't rise up and conquer those feelings of bitterness and unforgiveness, they *will* rise up and conquer you.
- If you don't take authority over your emotions and tell them what to think, what to do, and how to react, they *will* tell you what to think, what to do, and how to react.
- It's time for you to do the talking and take command of your thought life!

You have to speak to bitterness, offense, strife, and unforgiveness as the enemies they are. These toxic agents are not mere emotions, they are invaders that aim to infiltrate the depths of your being, unravel your life, and affect your healing and health. You must stand as a steadfast guardian of your heart and resolutely refuse to harbor them for even a moment.

This might require verbally confronting these forces repeatedly, like a gardener who tirelessly pulls out weeds, until their grip is loosened and they're banished permanently from your inner life. Freedom demands a relentless spirit that declares, "I will seize the roots of this toxic growth and uproot it from the depths of my soul — relentless in my pursuit until liberation is my reality!"

**You have to speak to bitterness, offense, strife, and unforgiveness as the enemies they are. These toxic agents are not mere emotions, they are invaders that aim to infiltrate the depths of your being, unravel your life, and affect your healing and health. You must stand as a steadfast guardian of your heart and resolutely refuse to harbor them for even a moment.**

## COMMAND THOSE ATTITUDES TO BE PLANTED IN THE SEA!

But in Luke 17:6, Jesus further said, "...If ye had faith as a grain of mustard seed, ye might say unto this sycamine tree, Be thou plucked up by the root, *and be thou planted in the sea*; and it should obey you."

Jesus didn't suggest merely cutting issues down to their roots or setting them aside. He understood well that doing so might only allow them to take root and grow anew. Instead, He instructed they be "planted in the sea."

In the harsh, salty embrace of the sea, life cannot flourish, and a plant is doomed — its hope of revival drowned in brine. It becomes, quite literally, *a dead thing*. The sea's salt utterly erases its potential for life, and no effort or time can coax it to sprout again.

In this metaphor, Jesus provided the powerful lesson that when confronting unresolved, hidden issues that produce bitterness, offense, strife, or unforgiveness in life, it is not enough to simply trim them back. These must be fully uprooted and cast away to a realm where they cannot regenerate — into waters that ensure their demise. Thus, they become dead issues, forever severed from the soil of your life and incapable of returning to haunt or hinder your journey.

And notice what Jesus said next, "...And it should *obey* you." The word "obey" is the Greek word *hupakouo*, which means *to obey* or *to submit.* It is the exact Greek word that would be used to describe children who are commanded to obey their parents. And here, we find that out-of-control emotions behave just like an out-of-control child. They rant, rave, and carry on all day long — *until* you finally stand up and tell them to straighten up and act right. Indeed, your flesh will pout, throw a temper tantrum, and carry on to a ridiculous extent until you decide that enough is enough.

If you don't take control over your emotions, they will take control over you. But once you rise with resolute authority, address your emotions, and wield the power vested in you through Jesus Christ, you'll find that your emotions and thoughts will fall in line with your directives!

- If you don't take authority over your emotions and flesh, they *will* continue to dominate and hound you.
- If you'll stand up to your destructive emotions and plant them in the sea forever, they *will* obey you, and you will be free!

## A RESULT OF NOT DISCERNING THE BODY OF CHRIST

An example of the consequences of unaddressed internal issues among believers becomes clear in Paul's correspondence with the Corinthians. The church in Corinth was overflowing with spiritual gifts — including the gifts of healing and the working of miracles — yet despite the vast number of these gifts in the church, many of the congregation were plagued by illness and were even succumbing to premature, untimely deaths. As Paul wrote to them, he made it clear that they were sick and dying because of unresolved inner issues.

After Paul shared what many have come to know as the Communion verses, he wrote this sobering warning about receiving Communion: "Wherefore whosoever shall eat this bread, and drink this cup of the Lord, unworthily, shall be guilty of the body and blood of the Lord" (1 Corinthians 11:27).

The word "unworthily" in this verse is the Greek word *anaxios*, which means *unworthily*, *unfit*, or *not equal to the task*. The fact that the Holy Spirit moved Paul to write this warning tells us that some people who come to the Lord's Table are unfit to take Communion because their behavior and inner attitude does not correspond to what Communion represents. Furthermore, Paul stated that some who took Communion "unworthily" had inadvertently opened a door for sickness and even death to enter their lives.

The clearest example of a person taking Communion "unworthily" is Judas Iscariot during the Last Supper. Although he sat at the table with the rest of the disciples and pretended to be in covenant with them and with Jesus, he had already cut a deal with the Jewish leaders to hand Jesus over to them. Satan had entered Judas' heart and sown seeds of betrayal, yet in that embittered state, he ate the bread and drank of the cup as if everything was all right.

Despite this inner turmoil and deceit, he reached out to partake of the bread and wine and feigned that he was in covenant with the rest of them, but, covertly, he had already made a deal to betray Jesus. His actions were unworthy, and he became "guilty" of the body and blood of the Lord.

The word "guilty" is interpreted from a form of the Greek word *enochos*, which describes someone *charged*, *indicted*, or *liable*. This is a person who is held responsible for a wrong action, behavior, or motive. Here we see that God views Communion with profound seriousness, and it is incumbent upon us to do likewise. Our focus must extend beyond the mere elements of the ritual; we must grasp the profound significance of the sacred covenant that Communion embodies, which is covenant with Jesus Christ and with His Body, the Body of Christ. By receiving the bread and wine (or juice), we declare that we are in covenant with God and with one another.

Paul penned this cautionary message to the Corinthians because they were filled with unresolved, inner issues, and their behavior had devolved into discord and litigation. The congregation had splintered into factions: some pledging allegiance to Paul, others pledging to Apollos, and still others proclaiming their loyalty to Christ.

Amidst the strife and venomous gossip, the Corinthian church had become a raging, relational mess. Despite the turmoil in them, these church members were shamelessly partaking in Communion — the sacred act of partaking in the body and blood of Jesus — as though all was harmonious, when, in reality, it was not.

In verse 29, Paul went on to say, "For he that eateth and drinketh unworthily, eateth and drinketh damnation to himself, not discerning the Lord's body" (1 Corinthians 11:29). The word "damnation" here is the Greek word *krima*, which describes *a decree, a judgment*, or *a verdict with an adverse consequence*. Just as immutable laws govern the physical world, there are spiritual laws that we are bound to obey. Violating these spiritual laws — such as breaking a covenant — inevitably triggers negative consequences that cannot be avoided.

Hence, if you partake of "the bread and the cup" of Christ with an insincere heart that is not honoring the Lord and upholding His covenant, you open a door for negative consequences to come upon yourself for "not discerning the Lord's body" (*see* 1 Corinthians 11:29).

The words "not discerning" in Greek depict one's inability *to discern, to judge, to appreciate*, or *to be truthful concerning something*. In this verse, it describes one who lacks discernment and does not rightly value Christ's sacrificial covenant for all His people, nor His command that we be "one."

## SICKNESS CAN BE A CONSEQUENCE OF NOT DISCERNING THE BODY OF CHRIST

Paul then added, "For this cause many are weak and sickly among you, and many sleep" (1 Corinthians 11:30). The opening phrase, "for this cause," is a translation of the Greek words *dia touto*, which means *for this explicit reason*. Many believers were weak and sick in Corinth because they had taken Communion unworthily. That is, they were in broken relationship with each other, yet they continued to partake of Communion as if all was well among them.

The word "many" is the Greek word *polloi*, which indicates *great numbers.* The word "weak" is *asthenes*, which describes *a wide range of infirmities*. It is an all-encompassing term that embraces all forms of *disease, illness, sickness, and weaknesses.* This word also conveys the idea of someone who is fragile and must be treated with supreme care due to ill health. Thus, Paul in essence said great numbers of people were "weak and sickly" in the Corinthian church because they had taken Communion unworthily.

This brings us to the word "sickly." This word is translated from the Greek word *arrostos*, and it describes *a state of poor or fragile health* and depicts a person with such a weak and broken condition that he or she is *critically unwell.* This word depicts one who is devastated by sickness, perhaps invalid, bedridden, or comatose.

Ironically, Paul was addressing a congregation that was overflowing with the gifts of the Holy Spirit — gifts that included healing and miracles. In fact, there were so many manifestations of these gifts that they couldn't be counted. Yet despite healings and miracles occurring all around them, numerous believers there still found themselves "weak and sickly."

In First Corinthians 11:30, Paul also said "many sleep." The word "many" here is the word *hikanos*, which describes *a sizeable or significant number*. And the word "sleep" is the Greek word *koimaomai*, which refers to *death*, and it is where we get the word *coma.* Why were so many Corinthian believers experiencing disease, illness, sickness, weakness, and even untimely deaths? The answer lies in the fact that they inwardly held issues toward one another, which fractured their physical and mental well-being.

Paul continued to urge them — *and us* — to make an inward examination to see if their hearts were in alignment with the commitment represented in the act of Communion. If yes, then we can freely partake of it. But if we, like Judas Iscariot, have inward issues that are unresolved and we are inwardly conflicted with others, we should not partake of Communion until those issues are resolved.

In fact, Paul said, "For if we would judge ourselves, we should not be judged" (1 Corinthians 11:31). The word "judge" is translated from a form of the Greek word *diakrino*, which depicts one's ability *to discern, judge, be truthful*, or *come under scrutiny*. Hence, if we will be truthful and take a scrutinizing look at our attitudes, inward thoughts, and actions and be willing to confront the truth that we need to change and submit to the Lord's correction — thus laying aside those hidden, unresolved issues — it will keep the door closed to negative consequences.

So before any sincere believer partakes of the elements of Communion, he should take time to soberly examine himself to see if he is really walking out his covenant with God and His Church — His own Body — or if there is anything he is allowing to keep him from being in sync with others.

## STEPS TO REMOVE BITTERNESS, OFFENSE, STRIFE, AND UNFORGIVENESS

In this chapter, we have seen that unresolved, hidden issues have great consequences that affect one's health. We have also seen in Luke 17:1 that Jesus said it's simply a reality of life that from time to time, situations will arise that entice and tempt us to become bitter, offended, upset, and unforgiving.

But in Ephesians 4:31, Paul instructed us, "Let all bitterness, and wrath, and anger, and clamour, and evil speaking, be put away from you, with all malice." This verse is God's directive to us, and if God tells us that we are to remove these toxins from our lives, it means we *can* remove them.

Since we all encounter this conundrum sooner or later, I've crafted eight simple steps based on Scripture and my personal experiences to help you maintain emotional equilibrium and ward off bitterness, offense, strife, and unforgiveness. These eight steps may not seem deep or profound, but if they can help keep your heart free of strife and offense, they are mighty and powerful!

1. **Ask God to reveal the root of bitterness in your life.**

   I recommend you read Hebrews 12:14-15, where the root of bitterness is addressed very clearly. Ask the Holy Spirit to empower you to remove it and to ensure that it never takes root again. Once a root of bitterness is addressed and uprooted, it can shut that door forever and it will become a dead issue in your life.

2. **Don't allow yourself to become a judge of another person's inward motivation. God is the only One who sees the heart.**

   You may think another person's actions reveal a heart that isn't right with the Lord. But you really don't know what is in that person's heart, so leave it alone. It's best to steer clear of playing the role of judge. Jesus cautioned us, "Judge not, that ye be not judged" (Matthew 7:1). Keep in mind, judgment is a boomerang; throw it out, and it's bound to boomerang back to you with greater force!

   After giving your all to gently and thoughtfully addressing an issue with another person, and you still find dissatisfaction with the outcome, perhaps it's time to let the Lord deal with the deeper matters of someone else's heart that you can neither see, nor correct. Instead of getting upset with that other person, take a look in the mirror and ask yourself if you are the one who needs to change and grow up this time. Take time to let the Holy Spirit help you reassess what you're seeing, hearing, and feeling. Go to the Word of God and let its light shine into the deepest recesses of your heart so it can expose any inward wrong attitudes or unresolved issues from your past.

3. **Give others the benefit of the doubt.**

   Individuals frequently behave in manners that are misconstrued by those around them. Perhaps they are unaware of how their actions are being interpreted, inadvertently conveying attitudes or intentions that starkly contrast with their true desires. Have you ever found yourself on the receiving end of a misunderstanding? Has anyone ever doubted the purity of your motives? Were you stunned by how far from reality others' perceptions of you strayed, even though you were confident that your intentions were genuine and well-meaning?

   This happens to everyone from time to time, so just as you want others to believe the best about you, it's important for you to reverse that grace and believe the best about others. Jesus gave us this principle in Luke 6:31 when He said, "...As ye would that men should do to you, do ye also to them likewise."

4. **Be forgiving when others act ugly.**

   When someone irks you and you're on the verge of taking offense or feeling upset over their imperfections, pause for a moment to consider the countless times others have shown grace toward your own missteps and shortcomings. Before rushing to judge, ask yourself, "Have I ever behaved poorly or spoken harshly?" It's likely that you've found yourself guilty of the same actions that have you riled up in the current situation.

   Reflect on the importance of embracing others in the same way that Jesus Christ has warmly and generously embraced you. Romans 15:7 says,

"Wherefore receive ye one another, as Christ also received us to the glory of God." Consider how Jesus welcomed you and me. Did He demand perfection before extending His love, or did He embrace us in the midst of our imperfections? Gratefully, He welcomed us in our entirety — flaws, faults, quirks, and all!

Since the time you became a child of God, have there ever been moments when you've stumbled and felt that you've fallen short in the eyes of the Lord? Surely we've all been there. Yet Jesus has never turned His back on you or was so disheartened as to sever the bond between Himself and you. In Romans 15:7, we are urged to receive each other just as Christ has received us, and that means we need to do a lot of forgiving and overlooking in life!

I encourage you to quit focusing on the faults and flaws of others and start concentrating on how to be more forgiving and merciful. If you give mercy, you'll receive a harvest of mercy in your own life. Take the route of mercy, and you'll never be sorry.

You might be surprised to find that sometimes it's best to turn a blind eye to another's missteps and simply let it go. If you'll take this approach to life, you'll have a lot less emotional disappointments and problems with your nerves and even your physical well-being. Offer the forgiveness and kindness you hope to receive from others and watch how it transforms your world.

5. **Ask yourself, "What would Jesus do in this situation?" and, "What instruction has the Holy Spirit given me?"**

Jesus went to the Cross and died for those who hung Him! He could have released enough power to defend Himself, instead He "...committed himself to him that judgeth righteously" (1 Peter 2:23).

Is it possible that this time, you need to be quiet and follow in the steps of Jesus (*see* 1 Peter 2:21)? Very often, it is best to let God be your Defender.

Of course, you must deal with problems when they arise, especially if they are of a severe nature, but never forget that God is a God of justice, and you can entrust yourself, along with your situation, to Him.

6. **Let God's Word, like a mighty sword, slice its way into the deepest recesses of your being to extricate the toxins that have been growing there.**

   Hebrews 4:12 says that God's Word is a sword and that it pierces to the deepest parts of our being. If you will allow the Holy Spirit to insert that mighty blade into your life, He will use it like a surgeon's scalpel to remove the areas where bitterness, offense, strife, and unforgiveness have grown inside you and to heal all your diseases.

   As noted before, God's Word has the divine ability to pierce through our facade and touch the very core of our being. If you allow this divine scalpel to do its work, it has the unique ability to excise whatever is foul within us. If we heed its instruction, even if it's hard to do, it will eventually lead to the freedom that God longs for you to experience in life.

7. **Regardless of why you think your offender(s) did what he (or they) did, make a decision to forgive and to let it go.**

   In Luke 17:3 and 4, Jesus commanded us to "let it go" and to release our offenders for what they have done to us. This doesn't mean they didn't do wrong; it simply means that rather than live shackled to them and their trespasses, as well as your grievances against them, for your own sake, you have chosen to release it, let it go, and move on with your life in Christ.

   Remember this is precisely what God did for you when He forgave you. Psalm 103:3 says, "Who forgiveth all thine iniquities; who healeth all thy diseases." Isn't it interesting that *forgiveness* and *healing* are linked in this verse. Psalm 103:12 says, "As far as the east is from the west, so far hath he removed our transgressions from us."

As you forgive, healing will come to you. But as you release your offenders from their offense, make sure you plant that issue in the sea where it never produces again. As God did for you, ask Him to help you to remove it "as far as the east is from the west."

8. **Make a decision to start speaking to yourself every time your thoughts try to hound you with pain from the past.**

The pain from the past may be real, but remember, you hold the reins of your destiny. Instead of letting your emotions run you in every direction, it's time to stand firm and unleash your commanding voice to tell bitterness, offense, strife, and unforgiveness that their rule in your life is over!

It is possible that in addition to these eight steps, the Holy Spirit will show you other ways to shut the door to bitterness, offense, strife, and unforgiveness. But by heeding His guidance, He will show you how to navigate around the enemy's attempts to stir turmoil in your spirit against loved ones, colleagues, and friends.

However, ignoring the Holy Spirit may cause the door to your life to be opened for accumulating grudges, resentments, hostilities, animosities, and anger, and with each conflict left undealt with and every wound unhealed, this could affect your healing and health and prohibit you from experiencing what Jesus purchased for you on the Cross. Forgiving may seem incredibly hard to do, but I assure you that this difficulty pales in comparison to the agony of living with bitterness, offense, strife, unforgiveness, and poor physical and mental health.

## IN SUMMARY

We've seen that although Jesus' redemptive work on the Cross paid for the forgiveness of sin, peace of mind, and healing and health for the body and mind, the troubling reality persists that many believers still struggle with illness.

A significant factor contributing to this paradox may be the presence of unresolved and concealed problems. These underlying issues serve as entry points for havoc to be wrought in the body and mind.

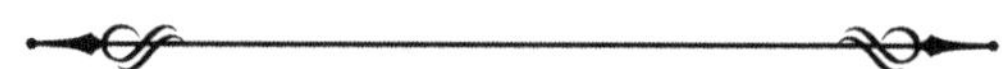

**Ignoring the Holy Spirit may cause the door to your life to be opened for accumulating grudges, resentments, hostilities, animosities, and anger, and with each conflict left undealt with and every wound unhealed, this could affect your healing and health and prohibit you from experiencing what Jesus purchased for you on the Cross.**

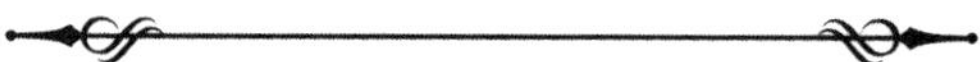

If the issue of bitterness, offense, strife, and unforgiveness is not put to rest, these attitudes and emotions can hinder you from experiencing the healing and health that belong to you as a child of God. In fact, when these things are tolerated and begin to fester within, they can increase the risk of *heart disease, digestive problems, immunity dysfunction, insomnia, mental health disorders, dysfunctional relationships, increased anger, and decreased self-esteem.*

But we have also seen that even medical research shows us that when forgiveness is practiced, it contributes to *improved heart health, lower blood pressure, healthier immune functioning, improved mental health, fewer symptoms of depression, and improved self-esteem.*

God wants each of His children to prosper and be in health (*see* 3 John 2), but if we cling to bitterness, offense, strife, or unforgiveness, these will act as barriers to stop us from experiencing God's best plan for us. Therefore, we must commit wholeheartedly to the practice of forgiveness and thus clear away obstacles that could otherwise impede us from experiencing the healing and health that Jesus secured for us through His redemptive work on the Cross.

But there are more compelling reasons for why believers endure disease, illness, and sickness, despite the fact that Jesus paid the ultimate price for their healing and health. In the upcoming chapter, we will explore the next crucial factor that contributes to why so many find themselves battling ailments in both body and mind.

Scan the QR code to watch Rick teach more on this subject.

# QUESTIONS TO PONDER AND DISCUSS

1. Throughout the ages, science "catches up" with God at various intervals and sneaks glimpses into spiritual truths that aid mankind in every sphere of life — including the fields of medicine and psychology. While science has only recently affirmed the long-term detrimental effects of bitterness, offense, strife, and unforgiveness, Proverbs 4:23 has always told us, "Keep thy heart with all diligence; for out of it are the issues of life." Look up that verse in various translations and write why there's such a connection between one's internal posture and health and the success he will enjoy outwardly as he navigates life.

2. From the study of Proverbs 17:22 in this chapter, make the distinction between a "merry heart" and a "broken spirit" — and between "medicine" and "dry bones." The contrasts are no accident — they're scriptural confirmation that what we allow to work within us consistently, whether good or bad, will work on the outside of us, also whether good or bad.

3. In James 3:16 we read, "For where envying and strife is, there is confusion and every evil work." How does the *RIV* of this verse expand your understanding of how envy and strife manifest and what the ramifications are of these sinful forces when they're allowed to operate in us against others?

4. From the verses you read on forgiveness in this chapter, formulate a statement about why forgiveness benefits *you* when you've been wronged — and why it's a detriment to your life and health when you withhold forgiveness. The future can be bright in spite of the most hurtful experiences in life — but unforgiveness and bitterness will dull the path, slow the steps, and present constant obstacles and challenges to future dreams of happiness. How would you articulate to someone who's struggling a scriptural case for forgiving and completely releasing those who have wronged him or her?

5. Review the four attributes of the sycamine tree and ponder their stark parallels to the power of offense if one doesn't deal with it *intentionally* and *immediately*. Also review the eight steps to ridding oneself of bitterness, offense, strife, and unforgiveness. Which one(s) stood out to you as something you need to have a conversation with the Lord about? Which one(s) were new to you and revealed something about the power of offense to *make* and *keep* you sick in body and mind — and about the power of forgiveness to liberate you?

# SEVEN

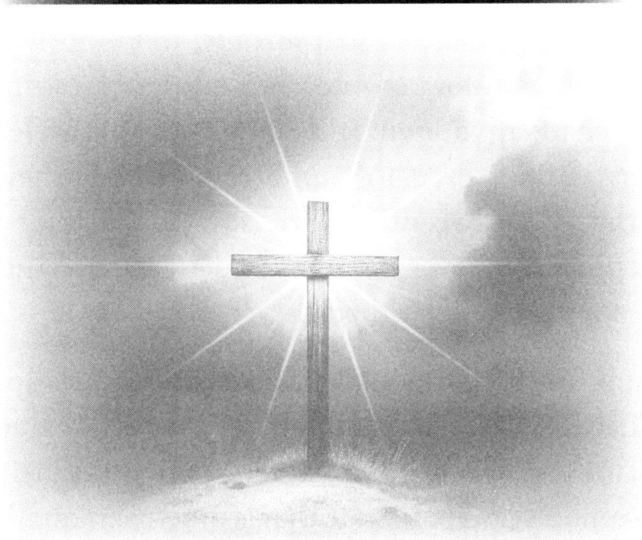

# WHY PEOPLE GET SICK — REASON NUMBER 6: ANXIETY, FRET, AND WORRY CAN OPEN A DOOR TO SICKNESS

By way of review, the reasons *why people get sick* that we've covered so far are as follows: 1) the curse; 2) ignorance, or a lack of knowledge; 3) disobedience; 4) foolishness (foolish actions and behaviors); and 5) unresolved, hidden issues. All these reasons can provide entry points for the devil to find his way in and produce a myriad of health problems in a person's life.

You might be thinking, *What about old age? Doesn't old age produce health issues for people?* I have deliberately not mentioned age and the complications that may come with it because I cover that in detail in Chapter Fourteen.

But in this chapter, we will see that anxiety, fret, and worry are also *entry points* that the devil uses to affect one's healing and health. By the time we are done with this chapter, you will *really* understand why Jesus said, "take no thought" for your life, not even for tomorrow (*see* Matthew 6:25) and why He reminded us that "the fowls of the air…sow not, neither do they reap, nor gather into barns; yet your heavenly Father feedeth them." Then Jesus posed the question, "Are ye not much better than they?" (*see* v. 26).

Despite the unwavering care of a benevolent Heavenly Father, a sea of countless individuals find themselves engulfed in anxiety, fret, and worry over the cares of today, tomorrow, and even matters far beyond their control. Anxiety disorders have become a silent epidemic that is quietly entangling approximately 50 million adults (nearly 1 in 5) in the United States in their invisible chains. These emotions respect no boundaries and affect people indiscriminately across all ages, genders, and races. The truth is, anxiety, fret, and worry are temptations that nearly every person confront at some point in life. But let's be clear about what we mean by *anxiety*, *fret*, and *worry*.

- *Anxiety* is *feeling uncomfortable, fearful, nervous, tense, or worried* about a real, imaginary, or perceived threat that might or might not happen in the present or future.

- *Fret* is being *nervous* or *worried*, and it comes from an Old English word that means *to consume, devour, eat, or gnaw* and pictures an inner issue that *eats* or *gnaws away* at a person.

- *Worry* is *overthinking a problem*, and it results in *distraction*, *depression*, and *a lack of peace*.

- *Anxiety*, *fret*, and *worry* are interconnected, tangled emotions and thoughts that lead to a mental wrestling match with unpredictability.

And while all three of them have distinct characteristics, they each have an inseparable connection with *fear*, as we will see in the next section.

- *Fear* is a disconcerting emotion that emerges when one is confronted with perceived dangers or looming threats. It produces physiological and psychological reactions, and it is linked to anxiety disorders.

## ANXIETY, FRET, AND WORRY ARE ROOTED IN FEAR

In Second Timothy 1:7 we find that "fear" is described as *a spirit* — an adversary sent to paralyze us. In examining Timothy's experience, it's clear from this passage that he was grappling with this "spirit of fear," which crept into his life and was sapping his strength and clouding his judgment.

Timothy was at the helm of a persecuted congregation during a turbulent era, and he was acutely aware that his leadership role put him at risk of severe persecution. Although no tangible threat against him is known to have materialized, the mere possibility loomed large in Timothy's mind and unsettled his mental equilibrium. As he witnessed unrest and decline around him, it seems that fear tightened its grip, and that is what prompted Paul to tell him, "For God hath not given us the spirit of fear...."

The word "fear" in Second Timothy 1:7 is rooted in the Greek word *deilia*, which signifies *a fear* or *apprehension* that compels one *to recoil* or *to act with timidity*. This type of dread drains one's capacity to confront challenges directly and makes him or her withdraw and succumb to cowardice. Because of the situation occurring toward believers in that day, Timothy found himself ensnared in an incapacitating fear, and that is why Paul reminded him that God had not given him a spirit of fear.

You must understand that fear is a spiritual force that hauntingly emerges when we sense looming threats or dangers. This emotional upheaval can give rise to a surge of aggression, a protective huddle, or a desperate sprint away, which is commonly referred to as the fight-or-flight response. Many believers in Timothy's church had taken the flight approach and had abandoned the faith to save their skin. But in Second Timothy 1:7, Paul exhorted Timothy to hold his ground, reminding him, "For God hath not given us the spirit of fear...."

## 'FEAR HATH TORMENT'

In First John 4:18, we are told that "fear hath torment." The word "fear" is interpreted from the Greek word *phobos*, which simply means *fear*, and it is where we derive the word "phobia." A phobia can be described as *an intense and often irrational fear or aversion to certain objects or situations where the perceived danger far outweighs reality*.

Currently, *millions* of people in the United States grapple with one or more phobias — some estimate up to ten percent of the population *or more* suffer with such conditions, which vary from minor inconveniences to severe disturbances. Those affected by phobias are often painfully aware of the disproportionate nature of their fear, but they find themselves unable to conquer them. If left unchecked, these phobias can spiral into an anxiety disorder that is characterized by an unwavering and disproportionate terror induced by specific triggers.

First John 4:18 tells us that those who live in the grip of "fear" are subject to "torment." The word "torment" is derived from the Greek verb *koladzo*, a word that describes whatever is *torturous* and pictures the act of *torture* itself. By definition, torture is the action or practice of inflicting severe pain or suffering on someone as a punishment or forcing him to do or say something. Throughout history, torture has been used to shatter a victim's spirit — to dismantle him emotionally, mentally, and physically as a method of punishment or as a means of bending the will of the tormented to the will of the tormentor.

In history, there have been many forms of physical torture that Christians and non-Christians alike have suffered, some of which are discussed in my book

*No Room for Compromise.*[1] As noted in that book, Romans were savage in their methods of torture. Within the vast stretches of the Roman Empire, diverse and terrifying torture techniques served to suppress criminals, dissenters, and adversaries of the state. Among these was the ghastly *rack* — a sinister device that embodied the very essence of agony. Although the precise origin of this monstrosity remains veiled in mystery, ancient texts point toward its debut in the hands of the Greeks.

The first known mention of *the rack* was in 356 BC when its twisted gears were used to coax a confession from an arsonist who was believed to be responsible for burning the Temple of Artemis in Ephesus. Then in 328 BC, this notorious contraption took center stage again as Alexander the Great employed it to extract a confession from the lips of a conspirator who plotted his assassination. The Roman historian Tacitus also tells us that this infamous device was employed in a grim bid to unravel the identities of plotters who dared try to assassinate Nero. We are also informed by Early Church fathers Tertullian and Jerome that this instrument of torture also played a dark role in the persecution of Early Christians, including St. Vincent who endured its horror in 304 AD.

The "rack" was a gruesome apparatus that was crafted from a sturdy rectangular wooden frame that was slightly elevated above the ground and each end of it boasted a sinister roller. The unfortunate soul subjected to its cruelty would find his ankles shackled to one roller while his wrists were bound to the other. As the malevolent operator went about his sinister task, he would turn a handle connected to a top roller and methodically tighten the chains. This slow, deliberate tension would relentlessly pull the victim's limbs, wreaking havoc on his shoulders, hips, knees, and elbows.

The oppressor slowly manipulated an array of pulleys and levers, and with chilling exactitude, he turned the roller, subjecting the victim to a crescendo of pain. Joints would audibly surrender, one by one, until the final tear severed the victim's resilience and agony was fully attained. Picture the terror as a tormentor deftly maneuvered the gears of the rack, with its relentless wheels inexorably stretching a soul to the brink, all in the pursuit of extracting a confession or administering a grim chastisement.

Keep this in mind as you read the words of First John 4:18 that say "fear hath torment." Fear, like a perpetrator, is a spiritual force that puts you on the rack, and from there the devil begins his demented and sick business of twisting your emotions and mind into a mess as he attempts to pull you apart. This insidious power seeks to fracture the human spirit, unravel the emotional and mental fabric of the mind, and bend the victim's will to mirror that of the tormentor's dark intent.

Those who are ensnared in perpetual states of anxiety, fret, and worry find themselves tugged mercilessly in every direction, teetering on the brink of what they can endure. Their stomach churns with uneasiness, their heart races like a runaway train, their imagination blazes tirelessly, and their sleep becomes elusive. This relentless assault becomes so decimating that it eventually negatively affects both their physical and mental health.

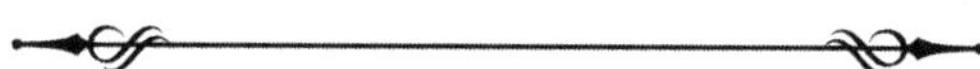

**Fear, like a perpetrator, is a spiritual force that puts you on the rack, and from there the devil begins his demented and sick business of twisting your emotions and mind into a mess as he attempts to pull you apart. This insidious power seeks to fracture the human spirit, unravel the emotional and mental fabric of the mind, and bend the victim's will to mirror that of the tormentor's dark intent.**

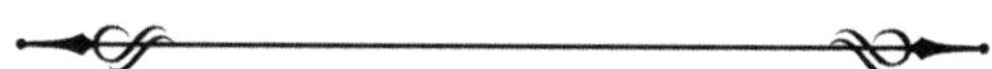

Those ensnared by anxiety, plagued by constant fretting and worrying, find themselves caught in the fierce grip of fear. Some might even express, "I feel so torn by this situation." It's as though an evil force has stretched them upon a rack and is pulling them apart. On one side, they're yanked toward the edge by relentless worries about their children — a tension so overwhelming it takes a toll on their body and mind. On another side, they're dragged toward distress over financial woes. And yet, in another twist, they're being wrenched apart by anxieties about the future. Each turn of the rack's mechanisms further unravels their emotions, mind, and physical health.

## GOD'S LOVE CASTS OUT FEAR ALONG WITH ANXIETY, FRET, AND WORRY

Feelings of anxiety, worry, and fretfulness are fear-induced, and their manifestation often reveals a person's struggle to fully trust in the boundless love of God. First John 4:18 declares, "There is no fear in love; but *perfect* love casteth out fear...."

The word "perfect" might seem distant and unattainable, yet it is a translation of the Greek word *teleios*, and it denotes *completeness, maturity, and perfection.* It tells us that when a person fully embraces the love of God, that divine love begins the process of *completing*, *maturing*, and bringing that believer into *perfection.* But this same Greek word is also used to illustrate the progression of a student who advances from one educational level to the next; it thereby symbolizes a continuous upward journey or an upward trajectory in life.

On one hand, when fear takes hold, it conjures a storm of "what if" scenarios that haunt the mind, but on the other hand, if believers allow themselves to be enveloped in the embrace of God's love, it calms this inner turmoil. Where fear torments the mind, unsettles the inner man, and fills a person with anxiety and distress, if the profound love of God is truly embraced, its divine touch liberates the mind from the clutches of fear.

In fact, First John 4:18 states very clearly that perfect love actually *expels* the presence of fear. The words "casteth out" originate from the Greek words *exo ballei.* The Greek word *exo* means *out* and illustrates the idea of *something existing beyond a boundary rather than within it.* Meanwhile, the word *ballei*, a form of the word *ballo*, means *to throw* or *to toss.* When these words are used together, as they are in First John 4:18, they convey the message that when God's love is firmly rooted in one's life, it not only completes, matures, perfects, and sets the individual on a higher path, but its powerful presence seizes any lingering fears within the person and hurls them out!

Thus we find that God's love and fear are not meant to coexist. When God's love is increased in a person's life, its transformative power goes to work to eradicate the essence of fear from one's inner being — and as fear is cast out, so are its agitating companions of anxiety, fret, and worry.

## A MAJOR REASON WHY CHRISTIANS DON'T EXPERIENCE HEALING AND HEALTH

Jesus' redemptive work on the Cross *emphatically* included the full payment for forgiveness of sin, freedom from guilt and shame, peace of mind, and healing and health for the body. We saw in Chapter One that the words of Isaiah 53:3-5 confirm that Jesus secured all these blessings on our behalf. As we journey further into this book, in Chapter Ten we'll explore these verses in even greater depth and clarity along with others related to the subject of healing and health. Yet in spite of the fact that Christ purchased healing and health for His people, there are vast numbers of faith-filled believers that continue to grapple with illness despite their faith in, and affirmation of, these promises.

But we have seen repeatedly that just as God tasked Adam with the sacred duty of tending the Garden of Eden and preventing any trace of evil from infiltrating its bounds, so, too, are we charged with safeguarding our lives. We must vigilantly seal every potential breach against the adversary. Should he discover even the slightest crack, he will seize the opportunity — much like the devastating entry of the curse and death that dawned upon the world through Adam's misstep — and try to unleash chaos and destruction of every kind. This havoc extends to relentless attacks on the health and healing promised to God's children, secured by divine covenant and Christ's sacrifice on the Cross.

When relentless anxiety, fret, and worry find a place in us, it's like opening a door for the enemy to invade our mind and emotions and create turmoil that can be paralyzing. These negative forces are notorious for their detrimental effects on health, and at a moment's notice, they can spark a host of severe physical complications in a person's body.

While medications can provide a temporary shield by dulling symptoms, if anxiety, fret, and worry are the underlying culprits, the remedy will only offer a fleeting respite. As grateful as we are for the help of medication and every available resource to foster healing, health, and repair, it is crucial that we address the root cause, which could be a deep-seated spirit of fear that is fueling the anxiety, fret, and worry.

To get a sense of how destructive long-term anxiety, fret, and worry are to one's health, let me shed light on some health issues intricately linked to these feelings. If you find yourself battling any of the following symptoms, following your doctor's advice and medical recommendations is crucial. However, it's equally important to pause and ask, *Am I inadvertently inviting these issues into my life by allowing anxiety, fret, and worry to take center stage?* While medication can be beneficial, relying solely on it might just be covering up the underlying problem. Without addressing the core issues, there's a chance these challenges will resurface because the true root remains untouched.

Medical science affirms that the following are sometimes a result of long-term anxiety, fret, and worry — or the risk factors associated with these conditions are increased when anxiety, fret, and worry are present.[2] While the redemptive sacrifice of Christ on the Cross has already secured your liberation from these burdens, let's take a moment to recognize the destructive effect these harmful emotions can have on the body. Consider this a brief overview, and we will return to a few of these in greater detail later.

- Brain fog (difficulty with focus and memory)
- Coronary artery disease (increased risk)
- Depression
- Difficulty sleeping
- Difficulty swallowing
- Digestive disorders
- Dizziness
- Dry mouth
- Easily tired
- Fast heartbeat
- Fatigue
- Feeling tense
- Headaches
- Heart attack (increased risk)
- Inability to concentrate
- Irritability
- Muscle aches
- Muscle tension
- Nausea
- Nervous energy
- Rapid breathing
- Shaking
- Shortness of breath
- Suppression of the immune system
- Sweating
- Suicidal thoughts
- Trembling
- Twitching
- Vomiting

This list, although not exhaustive, outlines the diverse ways anxiety, fret, and worry can manifest their impact in our lives. Beyond these general bullet points on how the body responds to anxiety and worry, let's delve deeper into how these culprits serve as an *entry point* for the devil and his darkness to wreak havoc on vital human systems.

## A DEEPER LOOK AT THE EFFECTS OF ANXIETY, FRET, AND WORRY ON THE BODY AND MIND

Medical studies indicate that when anxiety, fret, and worry storm within someone, adrenaline is released to course throughout the body, and as a result, the heartbeat quickens, blood pressure rises, and that hormonal release sets off a chain of physiological responses.

For those who are trapped in chronic anxiety, fear can manifest as persistent chest pain (that may or may not be heart-related, but it is a serious symptom that requires medical evaluation), nagging back pain, throbbing headaches, and the unsettling flutter of heart palpitations. The immune system may falter, and because muscles remain in a perpetual state of tension, more severe physical responses can be triggered along with aches and pains. Psychologically, the mind may become a breeding ground for dread, irritability, and tension with the potential to spiral into panic attacks or to pave a path toward depression.

Stress, which can come as a result of these emotions, can also increase muscle tension and pain perception, as well as exacerbate fibromyalgia symptoms and other symptoms related to inflammation in the body.

I listed many diverse ways anxiety, fret, and worry can manifest in the human body, but now let's look more specifically at how they can negatively impact our most vital systems. Remember that the word "fret" means to *consume*, *devour*, *eat*, or *gnaw away at*. In each of the following instances, you will see how anxiety, fret, and worry literally gnaw away at one's health. We'll look at the impact of these nuances on the *cardiovascular system*, *central nervous system*, *respiratory system*, *excretory and digestive systems*, and *immune system*. Let's begin with the long-term impact on the cardiovascular system.

### Cardiovascular System

Science shows that living in a whirlwind of anxiety and incessant worry for an extended duration can spell trouble for the heart and the circulatory system. The relentless drumbeat of an elevated heart rate, coupled with the surge of stress hormones and heightened blood pressure, exacts a formidable toll on the body. Amplified anxiety levels unleash stress hormones that compel the heart to race at a brisker, more forceful tempo that impairs blood-vessel function and promotes arterial stiffness, known as atherosclerosis.

If this cycle repeats itself consistently, it contributes to arterial stiffening and higher cardiovascular risk. It also indirectly heightens the threat of hypertension, heart attacks, and strokes. Additionally, anxiety and worry flood the system with stress hormones that can spike blood sugar, which ordinarily serves as an energy boost — but for individuals grappling with excess weight, this sugar rush causes glucose to be stored as fat and can pave a path toward heart disease and stroke as well as present increased factors for kidney disease through hypertension.

*Think of it... much of this is unleashed by anxiety, fret, and worry!*

**Central Nervous System**

The central nervous system serves as the command center of your body. Heightened levels of anxiety, fret, and worry unleash a torrent of stress hormones that speed up your heartbeat and breathing, elevate your blood-sugar levels, and rush blood to your limbs. Over time, this can take a toll on your heart, blood vessels, muscles, and various other systems.

As the nervous system conducts its relentless symphony of physical responses, the body's resilience gradually wears thin. And when anxiety, fret, and incessant worry take center stage, they can trigger panic attacks, prompting the brain to unleash a flood of stress hormones.

This hormonal deluge can spiral into a storm of increased sympathetic activation and a release of cortisol and adrenaline, causing headaches, dizziness, and even depression. When the floodgates of stress hormones are left wide open for too long, the risk rises for potential metabolic issues, weight gain, and a cascade of other health complications.

*Again... much of this is unleashed by anxiety, fret, and worry!*

## Respiratory System

Anxiety, fret, and worry can also stir a swelling storm in the chest or thoracic region of our body that often manifests as troublesome respiratory symptoms, such as rapid, shallow breathing. For those without pre-existing respiratory conditions, this is a fleeting inconvenience, but for individuals already grappling with respiratory challenges, such as asthma and chronic obstructive pulmonary disease (COPD), anxiety, fret, and worry can intensify breathing troubles. Research additionally shows that a sudden surge of anxiety, fret, and worry can trigger or worsen asthma symptoms. Moreover, when anxiety tightens its grip, it can accelerate breathing to an alarming pace and culminate in hyperventilation and sometimes even spiral into full-blown panic attacks.

*Think of it...much of this is unleashed by anxiety, fret, and worry!*

## Excretory and Digestive Systems

Likewise, anxiety, fret, and worry can escalate to incite inward queasiness and even unexpected and unwanted vomiting. Over time, anxiety, fret, and worry can signal their presence through stomach pain and the worsening of symptoms associated with ulcers. As if these conditions weren't already enough, if a person experiencing these symptoms then chows down on fatty and sugary foods, it can send the stomach into overdrive and lead to an intensified condition of acidity. This excess acid then makes its unwelcome journey upward, resulting in the burning discomfort of acid reflux.

Yet the chaos does not end there, because anxiety, fret, and worry also unleash their destructive influence upon the intricate workings of digestion. Those who are plagued with constant anxiety, fret, and worry frequently find themselves bouncing between the extremes of diarrhea and constipation. This relentless cycle ushers them into an ordeal of pain, bloating, and discomfort, provoking agonizing muscle spasms within the intestines. It's as if the bowels begin to mirror the anxiety, fret, and worry harbored in the mind. It becomes evident that these symptoms will worsen conditions like irritable-bowel syndrome (IBS) and aggravate inflammatory-bowel disease (IBD) flare-ups like Crohn's disease and ulcerative colitis. Thus we see that anxiety, fret, and worry set the stage for many digestive woes.

*Think of it...all of this is unleashed by anxiety, fret, and worry!*

**Immune System**

Long-term anxiety, fret, and worry additionally unleash chemicals and hormones that quicken the pulse and breath. When anxiety, fret, and worry persist, they cause the body to remain stuck in high gear, and it never receives the message to relax and return to its normal rhythm.

This continuous state of unrest chips away at immune defenses and leaves one more susceptible to infections and illnesses. Thus, an excess of anxiety, fret, and worry can chip away at the body's natural armor against colds and viruses by weakening immune defenses.

And when relentless anxiety, fret, and worry continue, the body responds by kicking into overdrive and signaling the endocrine system to flood the body with "emergency" hormones. Among these is cortisol, which is associated with suppressing the immune system — and chronic immune suppression may impair cancer surveillance as well as infection resistance in the body.

Chronic anxiety, fret, and worry are also associated with exacerbating the symptoms of Graves' disease and may contribute to the onset of other autoimmune diseases, such as inflammatory-bowel disease, multiple sclerosis, certain types of arthritis, *and more* in vulnerable individuals.

Thus, it is clear that anxiety, fret, and worry don't just steal one's peace of mind — these factors impact every corner of the body, rob people of their health, and make them vulnerable to a host of health challenges.

*Think of it...much of this is unleashed by anxiety, fret, and worry!*

## 'TAKE NO THOUGHT' FOR TOMORROW!

The words of Jesus in Matthew 6 carry profound weight, but when they are paired with these modern medical insights, they reveal an even deeper meaning behind His guidance to "take no thought" for our lives, not even what will happen tomorrow. It was in verse 25 that Jesus spoke to the disciples about the futility of worry. He said, "Therefore I say unto you, Take no thought for your life, what ye shall eat, or what ye shall drink; nor yet for your body, what ye shall put on. Is not the life more than meat, and the body than raiment?"

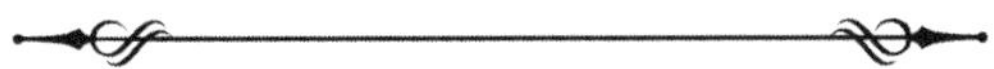

**It is clear that anxiety, fret, and worry don't just steal one's peace of mind — these factors impact every corner of the body, rob people of their health, and make them vulnerable to a host of health challenges.**

The words "take no thought" are translated from the Greek words *me merimnate.* The particle *me* signifies *no* and serves as *a negating force.* The word *merimnate* is derived from the word *merimnao*, and it pictures one in a state of being *anxious*, *fretful*, or *worried.* It pictures a mind overwhelmed by the necessities of life or the unpredictable nature of the future. Essentially, this phrase can be interpreted as "do not worry" or "cease your worrying."

For many years, I did not like this verse and tried to avoid it. The notion of living without a shred of worry seemed too impossible to me. In fact, I sidestepped almost every New Testament passage urging me to cast aside my worries. I was anxious, fretful, and worried about many things, but Denise, with gentle persistence, would echo the words of Jesus and remind me of the uselessness of anxiety. She would particularly remind me of Jesus' words about the "fowls of the air." We are told in Matthew 6:26 that Jesus said, "Behold the fowls of the air: for they sow not, neither do they reap, nor gather into barns; yet your heavenly Father feedeth them. Are ye not much better than they?"

To illustrate the unwavering faithfulness of God and the pointlessness of anxiety, Jesus drew His disciples' gaze upward to the birds in the sky. While the term "fowls" might be more classically used, the word "birds" captures the essence more vividly. Imagine finches, seagulls, sparrows, and pigeons soaring overhead — all familiar birds that grace the skies over Israel. Jesus remarked that these creatures "sow not, neither do they reap, nor gather into barns; yet your heavenly Father feedeth them."

When Denise and I are in Israel, we particularly enjoy watching the birds on the patio at a certain restaurant, which we always notice are quite plump. The sparrows are so big, in fact, we even wonder how they manage to fly. Unlike most humans who must plant and harvest for their food, these birds seem blissfully unbothered by concerns of sustenance. With no thought spared toward their next meal, they fill the skies with melodies and welcome each new dawn with joyful songs. Despite their carefree existence, they rarely die from hunger, for they are consistently nourished by God's generous hand, as He meets their needs with care.

Then Jesus asked the thought-provoking question, "Are ye not much better than they?" This was the equivalent of saying, "If God faithfully feeds and provides for creatures such as the birds of the air, aren't you better than birds, and don't you see that this means God will also provide for you?"

As I mentioned, when Denise and I are in Israel, we delight in watching the rather well-rounded birds that inhabit the area. Their rotund appearances often tickle our sense of humor and leave us marveling at their ability to take flight despite their size. Denise frequently remarks with amusement, "Rick, just look at these birds. They live without fretting about today, tomorrow, or the days to come. They don't worry about where their next meal will come from or how their needs will be met." She usually follows by saying, "Rick, we should aspire to be like birds, who trust in the assurance that God will faithfully provide for their well-being."

This is absolutely true, yet people spin themselves into a tizzy with anxiety, fret, and worry about these very things. Despite Jesus' assurance that God will tend to their needs, they tenaciously hold on to their habit of anxiety, fret, and worry, and in doing so, they inadvertently open a door for darker influences to wreak havoc on their physical and mental well-being.

We have seen that even modern medicine acknowledges an association between these emotional states and a range of health challenges, such as the *autoimmune disorders* we just saw, including *Graves' disease* and *multiple sclerosis*, among others. Chronic stress and unresolved psychological distress can trigger flare-ups and worsen symptoms, and they may contribute to the onset of disease in genetically predisposed individuals.[3]

We have seen the principle in Genesis 2:15 that just as God charged Adam with keeping the Garden, God has charged you to "keep" your life and to make sure the adversary never finds an *entry point* to access your world. But when anxiety, fret, and worry are active, they don't just rob one of peace of mind, they throw the door wide open for the enemy to attack every corner of the body and make him or her vulnerable to a host of health challenges.

## MY PERSONAL EXAMPLE OF ANXIETY, FRET, AND WORRY

I was prone very early in life to anxiety, fret, and worry. As I was growing up, I often heard people say, "I'm just worried to death" about this or that. Such expressions echoed through my church and home so often that they sculpted my perception to the point that I thought anxiety, fret, and worry were essential components of a person's existence. In my eyes, if someone wasn't consumed with anxiety, fret, or worry about something, it meant something was wrong with him. To me, the hallmark of being a responsible adult was having anxiety, fret, or worry over matters, big or small — and, conversely, to my way of thinking at the time, living a life devoid of these was the height of irresponsibility!

Even after I was filled with the Holy Spirit, I had to deal with anxiety, fret, and worry. There were rare occasions when I sailed through a day unburdened by concern, but then I'd find myself pondering the anomaly of my lightheartedness and would question what defect in my heart allowed for a day free of worry. I'd diligently dig to unearth some elusive source of distress, and once I successfully conjured a worry to hold on to, a sense of relief would wash over me, as for me, it meant my ship had finally righted its course back to responsible living!

But in the early years of our marriage, God opened the door for Denise and me to serve as assistants to a wonderful pastor in a very large denominational church. This precious man, whom I really needed in my life at that time, was a scholar and theologian of the highest order, and he was a strict disciplinarian. Not only did he demand the best and highest of himself, but he demanded the best and highest of every person who served alongside him in the ministry. He was anointed, brilliant, exacting, demanding, and absolutely unbending in his expectations of those who served in his inner circle. There were times when he could be austere and harsh with those who worked closest to him, and that included *me.*

Oh, how fervently I yearned to win the approval of that pastor and to be a shining example in the church where we found ourselves in those early years. The pastor's expectations were ceaseless, and at times, it felt as if I was stretched upon a metaphorical rack, as he urged me relentlessly to achieve *"more, more, more."* Yet I rose to the challenge and did my best to meet his demands with resilience and excellence. A diamond must endure immense pressure to truly sparkle, and I believed that God was using the unyielding pressure of our pastor to polish me and to make me shine. However, not many were able to weather the stringent path that our pastor set before those aspiring to be earnest disciples. But I resolved to be among the few who would endure, survive, and emerge, brilliantly radiant, for withstanding the journey.

There were times when our pastor could be quite stern, and often I felt like an anvil that was being constantly pounded by a hammer. In fact, there were times when his words fell very heavy, but I embraced his rigorous guidance and believed God was using him to teach me to have order in my life and to be disciplined. Despite the intensity of his reproofs, challenges, or scrutiny that he gave me — and there were *many* instances when that happened — I was thankful for the shaping of my character that resulted from his mentorship.

I was driven by a deep desire to be at his side, so I volunteered to assist him in any way he needed. I found joy in vacuuming his car and cleaning it until it gleamed, polishing his shoes to perfection, tidying his yard by raking leaves, and accompanying him with his books where he needed them. Whenever he offered, I gladly traveled with him to meetings, and I was thankful for each opportunity. My heart leaped at the chance to be near him, and I cherished every second of that remarkable season. During those times, he poured wisdom from the Word of God into my life and helped ground me in sound doctrine.

When I initially joined his team, I felt it to be a special honor and a coveted opportunity to be part of something so big and important. But soon, it morphed into *a grueling ordeal.* Every week he would *demand* a report from each of us on the pastoral team *in advance* on how many anticipated converts we would each be responsible to see come forward to receive Christ in the upcoming Sunday service. He wanted to know *exact* numbers — which he meticulously wrote down on his pad — and the following Sunday, he expected the numeric results to match our predicted answers! He would ask, "Exactly how many souls will you personally be responsible to talk to and see walk the aisle this Sunday? How many in-home visits and phone calls will you personally make before the weekend's services?"

Because of his relentless pressure, I found myself becoming ensnared in anxiety, fret, and worry. The old habits of worry that I had grown up with were stirred up again, and I soon found that I was "worried to death" that I would disappoint him in some way. I woke up worrying, I went to bed worrying, and worry about failing him haunted me throughout each day. Denise would plead with me to relax, but I didn't know how to relax. I literally lived in a continual state of anxiety, fret, and worry about failing to meet his expectations. The thought of facing him with inferior results left me living in a state of dread and feeling cornered and overwhelmed.

The truth is that I was sold out to the Lord, and because I was committed to following any directive from the pastor, every week I spent several nights visiting people in their homes. I also set a personal challenge that I wouldn't let a week go by without calling *at least* 200 individuals to invite them to Sunday school. In addition, I was working feverishly to see how many people would walk the aisle on Sunday morning to either give their lives to Christ or to join the church so that I could reach the criteria expected of me. I lived at this pace week after week, month after month. As the weekend services approached, a storm of anxiety, fret, and worry brewed within me, as I worried intensely about whether I would meet my altar quota. The thought of falling short by even *one* person sent shivers down my spine, as it meant facing his verbal criticism at the pastoral staff meeting the next morning.

After several years of living like I was trapped in a pressure cooker — and being eaten up with anxiety, fret, and worry — the situation escalated so severely that I found myself hospitalized because I was suffering from multiple bleeding ulcers. The bleeding was so profuse that the doctor was taken aback by my alarmingly low blood count. As I lay in my hospital bed and watched blood flow into me from bags suspended on racks, my doctor perched on the edge of my bed and gravely warned, "Rick, it's not normal for someone your age to be suffering like this. You have to rein in this worrying habit, or it will invite further health complications. I know you don't wish for an early death, but the way you are headed is not good. It's imperative that you find a way to stop this worry that is dictating your life."

I wish I could tell you I found a solution for anxiety, fret, and worry back in those days, but it continued nearly unchecked for many years. Instead of being set free from it, I merely learned how to cope with it, but coping with it wouldn't prove to be a long-term solution. This *entry point* for the devil was wide open, and I fought with anxiety, fret, and worry for many years.

## ANXIETY, FRET, AND WORRY CONTINUED TO *HOUND* ME

A year later when Denise and I began our teaching and traveling ministry with our young boys at our sides, I was still plagued by anxiety, fret, and worry. I was *worried* about taking care of Denise, I was *worried* about feeding and raising our sons, I was *worried* about whether or not anyone would want to have us minister in their churches, I was *worried* about if we were well-liked, I was *worried* about whether others saw us with approval, and I was *worried* about our traveling schedule.

But most persistently, I was *worried* about finances, as we were starting our own ministry and felt a financial strain as we were trying to get things established in those early years. In those days, my mind was a factory ceaselessly producing an overrun conveyor belt of *worry*, with each new worry piling onto the next.

Despite my constant battle with anxiety, worry, and stress, which were thieves of my peace and barriers to my connection with Denise and our sons, God's unwavering faithfulness shone bright and showered our ministry with abundant blessings. Invitations from churches flooded our calendar and people were eager for us to speak and conduct extended meetings. I found myself teaching at seminars and conferences, and, remarkably, my books began to capture the attention of a vast audience. Somehow, the finances always arrived just in time to settle our obligations.

Yet even in the midst of these successes, I remained ensnared in a habitual cycle of anxiety, fret, and worry, and I was unable to enjoy the blessings that enveloped us. God's gracious hand was evident, but just as quickly as I'd catch a glimpse of His benevolence, a wave of worry would invariably crash over me and drag me back into the depths of fretting over what lay ahead.

This habit of anxiety, fret, and worry even persisted as Denise, our young sons, and I embarked on our most daring adventure to relocate to what was once the Soviet Union. Guided by the Holy Spirit, we set out to establish the first Christian TV network in the USSR and felt the Lord's call to physically build the first church building in more than 50 years in the city where we lived. The financial demands of these assignments weighed heavily on my mind, and during the long season of those days and nights, I found worry was my frequent companion.

Anxiety, fret, and worry not only disturbed my peace, they also took a toll on my physical well-being. I had constant heart palpitations, I couldn't sleep, I experienced horrible acid reflux, my stomach was always upset, and despite having no significant changes in my eating habits, I began to gain more and more weight, which added to my anxiety, fret, and worry. Although I didn't realize it back then, *one symptom of anxiety, fret, and worry* is *weight gain!*

Soon the architectural plans for the church were approved and massive bulldozers moved onto our church land to prepare the ground for pouring the foundation of the new building. However, just as the process started, I was informed that the land we purchased was of such a swampy nature that it would be impossible to build on it. And although this was surprising, we knew this was the plot of land on which we were to build the church, so we refused to quit.

Relentlessly, bulldozers dug into the supple peat moss in a tireless search for the elusive bedrock we needed to begin building the foundation of our building. Gnawing into the earth and carving their way through the ebony soil, the bulldozers roared over the property, the sound of their engines producing an incessant clamour.

Our persistence was rewarded when, at last, we reached a resolute bed of sand, which we uncovered at 12 feet deep, stretching down to 15 feet in some places. Yet this triumph was quickly overshadowed by the next daunting challenge:

Our structure, which was destined to span roughly the size of a football field, demanded that all the unstable peat moss from the same abysmal depth be completely removed *and then moved off the property* so we could replace it with expensive, denser dirt that could hold the piers and support the foundation!

Once the bulldozers had finished their monumental excavation, I descended into that newly unearthed abyss and traversed nearly the expanse of a football field. The air carried the earthy aroma of mold and decay that was fed by the moisture that clung to each clump of soil, which disintegrated beneath my touch as I brushed my fingers against the damp walls of the massive hole. My feet slipped in particularly damp places, breaking my stride so that I had to regain my balance to resume my small journey.

We were now the owners of the biggest hole in the nation. This gargantuan abyss had not come cheap in terms of time, effort, or resources. The endeavor was bigger than anticipated — it had been fraught with difficulties, it had been exhausting, and it had drained our coffers. We relied as a ministry on the giving of our partners, so our ability to keep making progress depended on what people had given.

Every penny we'd stewarded on that project up to that point had been meticulously allocated to carving out this monumental pit, and now our finances echoed emptily back at us. Adding fuel to the fire, the city had imposed a near impossible, exacting deadline and demanded the project's completion within a mere 22 months — if we failed to meet this timeline, they had the legal authority to seize the land, along with every ounce of investment we'd poured into it.

I explored every possibility to trim our budget and even contemplated whether I should scale back the TV network that the Holy Spirit inspired us to launch. Yet it became clear to me that this wasn't the path He intended. Diminishing the network would deprive countless individuals across the former Soviet Union of their initial exposure to the teaching of the Bible. Our mission felt formidable: to construct the church building without incurring debt, while simultaneously maintaining and growing the TV network. Accomplishing both at once seemed like an insurmountable challenge. Still, it was the charge that had been entrusted to us.

We had exhausted our funds, and it left us with no option but to hit pause on the building's construction and await a fresh influx of resources. Meanwhile, the looming 22-month deadline for the entire project weighed heavily on me and sparked anxious thoughts, like, *What will people think of us now, abruptly pausing our progress like this?*

The thoughts of judgment from others nipped at my heels — it was a relentless chorus of my own doubts that truly hounded me and haunted my every step like a bloodhound on the scent of a trail, and mine was the scent of failure. I'd walk around that huge hole in the ground, and a sinister voice that cunningly used Scripture as a weapon taunted me: *You're no better than the fool who laid the first stone of a tower without measuring the cost, doomed to never see it reach the sky. You're incapable of completing what you set in motion. You've failed your family, your team, and your partners.* My mind went into overdrive, and I could imagine people saying, "All you have to show for all your efforts is a big hole."

Remarkably, winter swept in with relentless force and unleashed a blizzard that blanketed the landscape with mountains of snow. The fierce and enduring snowfall rendered nil any hope of continuing construction, forcing all activity to come to a halt. This unexpected pause in the project was a blessing because it arrived just as we had depleted every cent allocated for its progress. I had cried out for deliverance, and God answered me with snow!

In those winter months when construction came to a standstill, we hoped for a financial miracle to reignite our building efforts. By day, anxiety gnawed at my spirit and rendered me incapable of focusing on other pressing matters. My temperament grew fragile, quick to anger, and prone to irritation. By night, sleep eluded me, as I tossed and turned in a storm of anxiety, fret, and worry. I would slip into bed, wrestle with my thoughts, rise in frustration, and repeat the cycle until morning's light crept in — an unhealthy routine that haunted me for months.

Each evening, Denise would reach over to me in bed and gently remind me, "Rick, entrust these worries to the Lord. Jesus said that He cares for the sparrows and nourishes them with what they need. If His love extends to sparrows, it surely embraces us, too, and we will have what is needed for His plans."

Denise constantly reminded me to think of the "sparrows" until the verses about the sparrows begin to grate on me. I found myself filled with frustration and thinking, *It's simple enough for you to tell me to recall the sparrows and dismiss worry when you're not the one fielding calls for the funds needed to push this project forward. You blissfully drift into dreamland each night, unburdened by responsibility, so spare me the bird talk when what I truly need is cash!*

As time passed, my digestion began to reel with issues that had my stomach in turmoil and me making frequent trips to the bathroom. Furthermore, nausea visited me frequently and led to bouts of vomiting. My heart raced regularly, as if trying to outrun a storm, and it sent my blood pressure soaring. No doubt, I was dealing with a classic presentation of IBS and high cortisol levels. This uneasy mix of symptoms, accompanied by excruciatingly sleepless nights, formed a miserable existence for me.

Yet in all honesty, although the situation was indeed dire, I had *allowed myself* to be ensnared and pulled into anxiety, fear, and worry. Throughout my life, these turbulent emotions had hounded me off and on, but under the financial pressure of that monumental project and the deadline imposed on us, they'd reached their crescendo and plunged me into a living nightmare as I became consumed by my own dilemma and concerns.

Then one night, at about 2:00 a.m., I found myself restless, twisting and turning in bed like the tide of the sea. Denise, from her side of the bed, pleaded for me to sleep and to quit moving the bed. Realizing the injustice of my inner storm robbing her of rest, I slipped out of the bed and wandered to my office that was sequestered on the far side of our apartment. Overwhelmed by my thoughts, I pressed my forehead onto the hard surface of my desk as tears ran down my cheeks. Between sobs, I muttered, "Oh Lord, I feel like I'm standing on the edge of failure. I know that You are faithful, but I just don't see where the kind of money we need is going to come from, and I am so afraid."

Out of nowhere, I felt a gentle nudge on my left shoulder. Startled, I glanced up to find our little Joel, who was quite young then, standing by my side. I asked him what brought him out of bed, and he replied, "Daddy, something woke me up and told me to find you. Why are you crying?" I whispered back, "Joel, I'm just anxious about the money we need to finish the building." With the innocence of a child and a wisdom beyond his years, he planted his hands firmly on his hips, gazed directly at me, and said, "Aw, Dad, hasn't God shown you His faithfulness yet?" Then, as if understanding that his assignment was finished, he turned, walked back down the hallway, and went back to bed.

That experience jolted my cluttered thinking back to reality. Just as a drunk person's thinking is clouded because he is intoxicated, I'd found myself engulfed in an intoxicating overdose of anxiety, fret, and worry — a potent brew I couldn't seem to stop sipping. Then, just as a steaming cup of coffee can rouse a drunk from his stupor, the wisdom in Joel's words immediately cleared my mind and brought clarity to my senses.

That evening after Joel went back to bed, I found myself drawn to my Bible, and flipped it open to Philippians 4:6. In that moment, God revealed to me six steps to *banish* anxiety, fret, and worry from one's life permanently. The insights I gathered from that verse liberated my thinking, and I know they'll bring freedom to you too.

## SIX STEPS TO FREEDOM

We have seen that prolonged episodes of anxiety, fret, and worry can be associated with increased risk of physical and mental problems, including flare-ups of *autoimmune disorders*, such as *Graves' disease*, *inflammatory-bowel disease*, *multiple sclerosis*, *rheumatoid arthritis*, and *systemic lupus erythematosus*, to name a few. It is clear that when these troublesome emotions are allowed to persist, they provide an *entry point* for the devil to rob you of the healing and health that was purchased by Christ in His redemptive work on the Cross.

In this chapter, I've identified a possible culprit behind why some individuals fall ill. More importantly, I aim to offer a remedy to help you shut this entry point that the adversary is perhaps exploiting in your life to infringe upon your physical and mental well-being. I found a way to close the door in my own life, and that is what I want to share with you next. If you'll embrace the instruction found in Philippians 4:6, I believe peace will flood your being and begin to usher in a resurgence of healing and health both in your mind and body.

The big breakthrough came in my life on that night when I reached for my Bible and opened it to Philippians 4:6. That verse says, "Be careful for nothing; but in every thing by prayer and supplication with thanksgiving let your requests be made known unto God."

I needed to cast aside the swirling storm of anxiety, fret, and worry that was clouding my mind so I could focus on life and ministry and the plan of God for my life in the freedom that Christ purchased for me as a believer. And there in Philippians 4:6, I discovered a beautiful, methodical guide that showed me exactly how to release my anxious thoughts and find peace. As I embraced each step of this divine guidance, my inner turmoil melted away, and in its place, peace enveloped my heart and filled it with calmness and clarity. Since that time, I have applied these simple steps to my life again and again, and I have lived without anxiety, fret, and worry. Sure, those emotions have occasionally come calling, but I have mastered the art of leaving them unanswered on the doorstep.

The magnitude and multitude of challenges that my wife, our sons, our ministry, and I have encountered on our journey defy embellishment. Sometimes, these hurdles have felt colossal and insurmountable. When negative emotions threaten to envelop me with their relentless grip, I find refuge in Philippians 4:6, and time and again, this guiding verse stands as a guard, prohibiting the entrance of anxiety, fret, and worry and restoring peace to my heart.

## STEP 1: 'BE *CAREFUL* FOR *NOTHING*'

In Philippians 4:6, Paul said, "Be careful for nothing; but in every thing by prayer and supplication with thanksgiving let your requests be made known unto God." The *first step* we find in Philippians 4:6 is "be careful for nothing." The Greek text exactly says *meden merimnate* and conveys this command with precision. The word *meden* means *in no way*, *none*, *nothing*, or *not at all*. It pictures what should be nonexistent in the life of a believer.

The word *merimnate* is derived from the word *merimnao*, and it means *to be anxious*, *preoccupied*, or *fretful*. This is the same word Jesus used in Matthew 6:25 when He told His disciples, "...Take no thought for your life...." In the context of most of the New Testament, *merimnao* portrays a mental state fraught with anxiety over life's essentials or over uncertainties of the future — a fragmentation of one's focus caused by spiraling thoughts of concern. These words "be careful for nothing" could be correctly rendered, "Don't worry about anything — and that means nothing at all!"

In this initial stage of sorting through the tangled cords of anxiety, fret, and worry, it's crucial to embrace absolute honesty with both God and ourselves. Instead of resigning ourselves to this inner chaos as a normal part of our existence, we need to recognize that God deems it unacceptable and believes it should have no place in our lives. True liberation always begins with confessing our sins, and we must reach a point where we understand that living in stress and worry is not aligned with God's plan for us. It's essential to acknowledge the toll it's taking on our body and mind and be ready to turn away from it and step boldly toward a life free from turmoil.

## STEP 2: 'IN EVERY THING BY *PRAYER*'

The *second step* we discover in Philippians 4:6 is found in the word "prayer," which in this verse is translated from a form of the Greek word *proseuche* and is the most commonly used word for prayer in the New Testament. This particular word and its various forms are used approximately 127 times in the New Testament. It is a compound of the words *pros* and *euche*. The preposition *pros* conveys the idea of moving *toward* and suggests *nearness*. Throughout the New Testament, the word *pros* consistently paints a picture of an intimate connection or symbolizes an up-close and personal engagement with another entity.

The second part of the word *proseuche* is taken from the word *euche*. The word *euche* is an old Greek word that describes *a wish, desire, prayer*, or *vow*. In its original usage, this word encapsulated the act of a person making a solemn promise to God that was driven by a pressing need or heartfelt desire. This person would commit to offering something precious to God in exchange for receiving a positive response to his or her prayer in return. Therefore, embedded within this word is the concept of *a sacred exchange* wherein one offers up something of value to receive something deeply wished for or yearned after in the deepest way.

This tells us that instead of carrying anxiety, fret, and worry about anything, we are to come near to the Lord in order to give Him whatever is concerning us and then ask Him to give us something back in exchange for the worries we have given Him. So give Him your anxiety, fret, and worry, and ask Him in exchange to give you His peace. This verse emphatically means that when you give God your problems, in return, He gives you His peace.

Maybe there's been a moment in your past when you've encountered such an extraordinary exchange. Picture a time when your thoughts were tangled in chaos, and upon entrusting your troubles to God, a miraculous peace washed over you and dissolved your anxieties. This "exchange" is the step that Paul encouraged us to take when anxiety, fret, and worry attempt to seize your mind or emotions.

## STEP 3: '...AND *SUPPLICATION*'

The *third step* Paul wrote about is found in the word "supplication." The word "supplication" in Greek is *deisis*, a word that vividly illustrates *an individual facing some form of deficiency in his life that prompts him to fervently advocate for these needs to be met.* The *King James Version* translates *deisis* as "supplications," which means *to beg, beseech,* or *earnestly appeal.* It paints a portrait of someone in such dire need that the person is driven to cast aside his or her pride and summon the courage to passionately, forcefully, and desperately implore others for assistance or relief.

One of the most striking illustrations of the Greek word *deisis* is found in James 5:16, a renowned passage that declares, "...The effectual fervent prayer of a righteous man availeth much." In this verse, the word *deisis* is rendered as "fervent prayer." Here we find *deisis* embodies *a deeply passionate, earnest, honest plea and a sincere prayer that is offered with gravity.* It approaches God with utmost seriousness and fervently implores Him to act and address a pressing need that the praying person is confronting in his life.

In times of distress, when anxiety and worry weigh heavily upon your heart, you are encouraged to turn to the Lord with a sincere and earnest plea for His assistance. Paul's choice of words implies that you can approach God with great confidence and ask Him to act on your behalf — and you need not be shy or hesitant in your prayers. Speak to God openly, sharing your innermost feelings, the challenges you encounter, and the desires you wish for Him to fulfill.

## STEP 4: '...WITH *THANKSGIVING*'

Following this, Paul unveiled the *fourth step* to overcoming anxiety, fret, and worry. He urged us to, first, "be careful for nothing," and then to do the last two steps — pray and make supplication — with "thanksgiving." He said to share our petitions with God and to do it with a heart brimming with gratitude.

The word "thanksgiving" in this verse is the Greek word *eucharistia*, which is a compound of the words *eu* and *charis*. The word *eu* means *good* or *swell,* and it denotes *a general good disposition* or *an overwhelmingly good feeling about something.* The word *charis* is the Greek word for *grace.* But when these two words are compounded to form the word *eucharistia,* it describes *an outpouring of wonderful feelings that freely flow like grace from the heart in response to someone or something.*

By choosing this word, Paul emphasized that when we sincerely ask God for something, it should be accompanied by a genuine expression of gratitude from the heart. Even though our request has just been made and its fulfillment isn't visible yet, it's fitting to thank God ahead of time for granting what we've asked.

This act of preemptive gratitude is a testament to our faith, and it's vital to pair our heartfelt requests with equally fervent thanksgiving. In other words, let your gratitude be as fervent and impassioned as your initial request!

## STEP 5: 'LET YOUR *REQUESTS* BE MADE KNOWN UNTO GOD'

Paul then gave us the *fifth step* toward liberation from anxiety, stress, and worry when he wrote, in effect, "Make your requests known to God." The word "requests" originates from the Greek word *aitema,* which is derived from the word *aiteo.* This word "ask" dismantles any notion that you are merely a lowly worm that is undeserving of boldly entering God's presence.

Within the New Testament, the word *aiteo* depicts a person who confidently insists or demands that a particular need be fulfilled, all while approaching and addressing his superior with deep respect and honor. Moreover, this word conveys a strong sense of anticipation, as one fully expects to obtain the requested outcome.

Thus, this word *aiteo* paints the portrait of an individual who prays with authority and a firm expectation that their request will be granted. This means when you pray about a need that is concerning you, as long as your prayer is based on the Word of God, you can do so with a sense of authority and fully anticipate that God will fulfill His promises and respond to your petitions.

## STEP 6: '...BE MADE *KNOWN* UNTO GOD'

As a *sixth step*, Paul encouraged us to "...let your requests *be made known* unto God." The word "known" is derived from the Greek word *gnoridzo*, a word that means *to broadcast*, *declare*, or *make something known very clearly*. Essentially, this means when you approach God with your requests, you should do so with great boldness. Articulate precisely what you need and express it with such clarity and confidence that all of Heaven takes notice. You see, when you stand before God to share your requests and do it with Scripture backing you up, it gives you the right to be remarkably bold and forthright!

**The *RIV* (*Renner Interpretive Version*) of Philippians 4:6 says:**

> **Don't worry about anything — and that means nothing at all! Instead, come before God and give Him the things that concern you so He can in exchange give you what you need or desire. Be bold to strongly, passionately, and fervently make your request known to God, making certain that an equal measure of thanksgiving goes along with your strong asking. You have every right to ask boldly, so go ahead and insist that God meet your need. When you pray, be so bold that there is no doubt your prayer was heard. Broadcast it! Declare it! Pray boldly until you have the assurance that God has heard your request!**

In those moments when anxiety, dread, and fear came knocking and their tendrils threatened to entwine me in their grip, I discovered a path to freedom by embracing the six steps outlined in Philippians 4:6. I realized that I no longer had to be consumed by these crippling emotions for the rest of my days. Before I discovered these straightforward steps, I regularly battled inner turmoil and unsettling health issues that were related to ongoing anxiety, fret, and worry. But by diligently applying the principles in Philippians 4:6, I was able to firmly close the entry point that allowed the enemy to infiltrate my life. If you find anxiety, fret, and worry sneaking into your world, know that you, too, can firmly close that door by embracing these six simple steps.

## IN CONCLUSION

Thus far in this book, we've explored the various causes of illness, including how individuals can inadvertently offer the devil an *entry point* to compromise their well-being. We've also uncovered actionable measures to fortify ourselves against such intrusions.

Beyond what we've already discussed, it's undeniable that there are moments when, despite doing everything right, a person finds himself besieged physically and mentally, and as a result, he endures attacks in his body and mind.

As we turn the page to the next chapter, we'll discover that even when all seems to be in order, malicious forces can strike to bring about disease, illness, and sickness. Together, we'll explore how Jesus dealt with the demonic realm and its connection to disease, illness, and sickness, and we'll see how to take necessary measures to fend off these sinister assaults!

Scan the QR code to watch Rick teach more on this subject.

# QUESTIONS TO PONDER AND DISCUSS

1. Because human beings are in a higher class of creation than animals, including birds, read the following in Matthew 6:26 for consideration: "Behold the fowls of the air: for they sow not, neither do they reap, nor gather into barns; yet your heavenly Father feedeth them. Are ye not much better than they?" In what way does this truth bring comfort to your mind? Do you believe this in your heart — do you possess the assurance that even in times of dire need, your Heavenly Father will take care of *you*? Why or why not?

2. Review the descriptions of *anxiety*, *fret*, and *worry* in this chapter and describe in your own words how these emotions are rooted in *fear*. How does knowing and believing the love of your Heavenly Father alleviate these oppressive conditions? (*See* 1 John 4:16-18.) Write out one or more of the following verses — Psalm 34:4; Luke 12:32; Philippians 4:6-7; and Second Timothy 1:7 — to meditate on. Keep them in your personal journal or somewhere you can refer to them to use for further study.

3. Were you surprised to learn that it has been scientifically and medically proven that anxiety, fret, and worry can negatively affect your physical health? Scripture bears this out as well: "A calm and peaceful and tranquil heart is life and health to the body..." (Proverbs 14:30 *AMP*). Can you name a time when anxiety and worry affected *your* physical health? Are you experiencing the physical effects of worry right now? If so, what can you do to regain a calm, peaceful, and tranquil heart? Consider Isaiah 26:3 and Hebrews 12:2 in framing your answer.

4. Jesus commanded us to "take no thought" for our lives, not even for tomorrow (*see* Matthew 6:25,34) by worrying, fretting, and having anxiety about what the next day will bring. Using First Peter 5:7 as your guide, write down the things that are troubling you in your mind right now and imagine yourself casting every one of those things, one by one, over onto the Lord. Since the Scripture says to cast them on the Lord "once and for all," practice

reminding yourself throughout the day that He has your cares and you no longer have to carry them.

5. Have you begun taking the "six steps to freedom" as enumerated on pages 228-234? Which of these six steps have you mastered in your spiritual walk — and which one do you struggle with the most? Ask the Lord to walk you through these steps and help you transform your thinking so that even the things that greatly bothered you in the past have no effect on your peace-filled heart and mind in the future.

# EIGHT

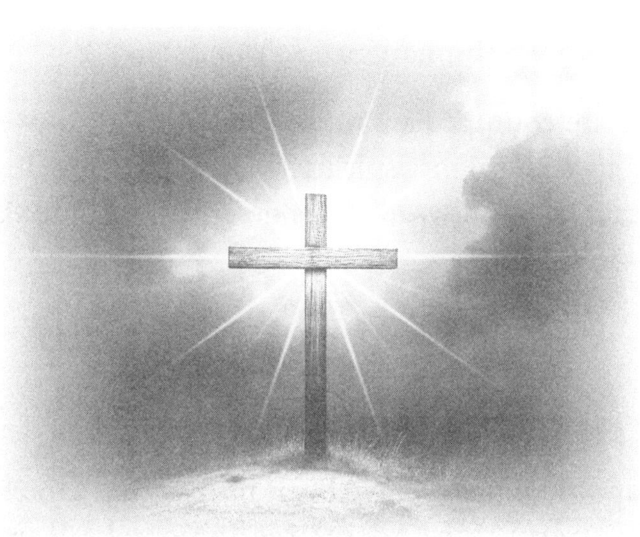

# WHY PEOPLE GET SICK — REASON NUMBER 7: DEVILISH ATTACKS CAN OPEN A DOOR TO SICKNESS

In addition to the reasons *why people get sick* that we have covered so far, it is also possible that unsolicited devilish attacks can open a door to sickness. We must remember that the Bible says, "For we wrestle not against flesh and blood, but against principalities, against powers, against the rulers of the darkness of this world, against spiritual wickedness in high places" (Ephesians 6:12).

If Adam had never transgressed, the scourge of death and its harrowing companions — disease, illness, and sickness — never would have entered the earth's domain. However, as revealed in Romans 5:12, Adam's ill-fated decision to transgress God's command flung wide the gates for Satan to storm into the earthly realm. Now the adversary's presence is undeniable, and he and his hordes have been unleashing attacks upon humanity ever since Adam's monumental fall that left its mark on the human race.

Thankfully, we are equipped with the tools needed to overcome the devil. God has endowed us with mighty spiritual weapons that include His Word, the blood of Jesus, other spiritual weapons as described in Ephesians 6:14-18, and the power of the Holy Spirit.

**The adversary's presence is undeniable, and he and his hordes have been unleashing attacks upon humanity ever since Adam's monumental fall that left its mark on the human race.**

But it is a fact that, at times, the attacks we encounter have nothing to do with our mistakes. The devil and his cohorts conspire to place obstacles in front of us that are aimed at thwarting God's purpose for our lives. But by aligning ourselves with God's divine authority, we are given all the strength and command we need to repel every attack of the devil and to ensure his retreat.

If you have addressed all the issues in the first six reasons why people get sick, you are already on your way to experiencing healing and better health. To review, those six reasons are as follows:

- Reason Number 1: The Biggest Culprit Is the Curse
- Reason Number 2: A Lack of Knowledge Can Open a Door to Sickness

- Reason Number 3: Disobedience Can Open a Door to Sickness
- Reason Number 4: Foolishness Can Open a Door to Sickness
- Reason Number 5: Unresolved, Hidden Issues Can Open a Door to Sickness
- Reason Number 6: Anxiety, Fret, and Worry Can Open a Door to Sickness

But beyond the six reasons discussed previously, another often overlooked factor is the direct attack of devilish forces. It may surprise some to consider that disease, illness, and sickness can be a direct assault from the devil himself. The problem began with Adam's transgression, which flung open the floodgates for evil and death to sweep across the world. In that pivotal instant, the authority bestowed upon Adam was seized by the devil, and the devil and the rule of death twisted everything that had been made pure and good by the Creator, turning it into something distorted and malevolent.

However, through the cross of Christ and what He accomplished by His death, burial, and resurrection, those of us who have received Jesus have been given authority over the enemy and a faith that overcomes the world (*see* 1 John 5:4). If we will embrace what He did for us and learn how to walk in faith and operate in common sense, we can override most of the effects of the curse and the rule of Satan in the earth. I warn you that this is a large chapter that contains insights you have not likely ever read in such detail.

## SATAN IS A MASTER AT CREATING HINDRANCES

First, we need to understand that the devil is a master at creating hindrances of all types. In the pages before you, I want to give you two compelling instances from the New Testament in which Satan sought to attack and thwart the advancement of the Kingdom of God.

We will begin with an episode from Paul's life and then look at an encounter that occurred in the ministry of Jesus. In these narratives, we will discover two prime examples of how the devil and his cohorts launch seemingly arbitrary assaults for a myriad of reasons. While these examples are not about an attack of disease, illness, or sickness, they do demonstrate the fact that Satan often attacks to stop one's progress.

**Through the cross of Christ and what He accomplished by His death, burial, and resurrection, those of us who have received Jesus have been given authority over the enemy and a faith that overcomes the world.**

In First Thessalonians 2:17-18, Paul wrote, "But we, brethren, being taken from you for a short time in presence, not in heart, endeavoured the more abundantly to see your face with great desire. Wherefore we would have come unto you, even I Paul, once and again; but Satan hindered us."

In verse 17, Paul wrote about how he and his companions were filled with an overwhelming desire to reunite with the Thessalonians, exerting themselves tirelessly to fulfill that wish. They yearned so intensely for this encounter that verse 18 notes their persistent efforts to make it happen "once and again." However, their endeavors were met with constant obstacles, as Paul acknowledged that "Satan hindered us."

In this passage, Paul used the term "Satan" — derived from the Greek word *satanas*, which pictures *an adversary who despises, accuses, slanders, or plots against*. Embedded in this very name is the idea of *one who conspires against*. It's astonishing how Satan orchestrates chaotic circumstances to obstruct and thwart our progress, and this is the essence of what Paul was stating in this verse. In essence,

Paul remarked, "We were en route to visit you, with every intention of reaching our destination. However, unimaginable events began to unfold. We exerted every effort to be with you. Indeed, I, Paul, made repeated attempts. Yet Satan, the master at creating conspiracies and chaos, worked to impede our attempts multiple times."

The word "hindered" is translated from a form of the Greek word *egkopto*, which means *to cut in on* or *to elbow out of the way*. Imagine a race in which a runner is making good progress until a rival suddenly barges in, using his elbow to shove the other runner off track, attempting to knock him out of the race. This is the imagery Paul used to communicate the truth that Satan did everything possible to elbow Paul and his team away from their intended destination.

But beyond the athletic metaphor, the Greek word *egkopto* also paints a picture of *an obstructed road*. Frequently, travelers in the ancient world encountered a road broken up so badly that it created an impasse. Such an obstacle would force them to retrace their steps and find another route to reach their destination, as their originally intended path lay thoroughly blocked.

Considering these nuances of the word "hindered," Paul was conveying to the Thessalonian believers: "We set out with every intention to visit you, but Satan relentlessly tried to shove us off track and thwart our journey. Time and again, he erected obstacles so insurmountable that we found no way around them. Our attempts to find alternate paths were met with constant disruptions, as the devil spun wild and conspiratorial plots to derail our plans and prevent our arrival."

While I am certainly not magnifying the devil or suggesting that he has the power to ultimately stop us, these scriptures show us that, like Paul, we must persevere when our path is blocked, and if needed, we must even blaze another trail. If our resolve is unshakable, we can rise above any assault.

Yet Scripture makes it crystal clear that ambushes exist — challenges that strike when we're on the right path. These unexpected hurdles frequently target those steadfast in faith who are walking in obedience, and they are designed to halt them from making progress.

## EVEN JESUS DEALT WITH SATAN'S ATTEMPTS TO BLOCK HIM

Jesus came under such an attack when He was preparing to cast a legion of demons out of the demoniac of Gadara. Violent and destructive winds seemed to come *out of nowhere* to capsize Jesus' boat and drown Him and His disciples in the middle of the Sea of Galilee. Mark 4:37 says, "And there arose a great storm of wind, and the waves beat into the ship, so that it was now full."

Notice it says, "And there arose...." The words "there arose" are translated from a form of the Greek word *ginomai*, a word that is used more than 200 times in the New Testament, so its meaning is well documented. The word *ginomai* can describe *something that happens unexpectedly* or *something that catches one off guard.*

For instance, the word *ginomai* is used in Acts 10:9-10 to describe how Peter received his vision, which revealed that salvation had become available for Gentiles. Those verses say, "On the morrow, as they went on their journey, and drew nigh unto the city, Peter went up upon the housetop to pray about the sixth hour: and he became very hungry, and would have eaten: but while they made ready, he *fell into* a trance."

Especially notice the words "fell into." This phrase is derived from the Greek word *ginomai*, and because the writer Luke used a form of the word *ginomai*, we know that Peter didn't expect this visitation to occur that afternoon. He was waiting on dinner when *suddenly* — *unexpectedly* — he "slipped into" a trance. This was an encounter with God that caught Peter off guard.

Also, when John told us how he received the book of Revelation in Revelation 1:10, he used the word *ginomai,* saying, "I was in the Spirit on the Lord's day...." The words "I was" are taken from the word *ginomai.* Therefore, we know from the use of this word that John was not expecting to have a visitation that day. The vision came *unexpectedly*, taking him *completely off guard* as he looked up and found himself standing in the realm of the spirit.

Again, this same word, which contains an element of *surprise*, is used in Mark 4:37 to tell us that Jesus and His disciples didn't expect bad weather on the water that night. Many of Jesus' disciples were fishermen before they were called into the ministry, so they knew the weather of the sea. If a natural storm had been brewing, these men never would have taken their little boat out. Therefore, you can be sure that when they began their journey that night, it was a perfect night for sailing.

But the Bible says, *suddenly and unexpectedly*, "there arose" a great storm of wind. Notice Mark said it was "a great storm of wind." The word "great" is taken from the Greek word *mega*, which denotes *something of magnificent proportions.* It is where we get the idea of "megabills," "megawork," "megatired,"and "megaphone." By using this word, Mark let us know that this was a megastorm!

Also notice that Mark doesn't say it was a thunderstorm or a rainstorm; he told us it was "a great storm of wind." The word "wind" is taken from the word *lailaps*, and it describes *turbulence* or *a terribly violent wind.* Therefore, the storm that came against Jesus that night was an unseen storm. A person couldn't see this storm, but he could feel the effects of it. This was an attempt of the enemy to destroy Jesus and His crew before they reached their destination.

On the other side of the sea, in the country of the Gadarenes, Satan had a prized possession: the demoniac of Gadara. The devil knew that if Jesus' ship reached the other side, he would lose his grip on that man and Jesus would perform one of the greatest miracles of His ministry.

It was when Jesus was on the edge of a breakthrough that this unexpected attack of violent and destructive turbulence came down upon Him and His disciples to try to kill and destroy them. The devil didn't want Jesus to arrive at the country of the Gadarenes. This was a preemptive strike of the devil to prevent or undo the work of God. This was also a great opportunity for the disciples to learn that Jesus Christ is Lord of the wind and the waves. After He exercised authority over this unseen turbulence and spoke to the waves of the sea, the Word says that "…the wind ceased, and there was a great calm" (Mark 4:39).

The fact that this attack came just as Jesus was on the brink of a major miracle is not uncommon, for this is often the moment when Satan chooses to attack. If such attacks came against Jesus, we can be sure that the enemy will attempt to do this to us as well. Therefore, we must mentally and spiritually prepare ourselves to deal with demonic attacks. We are to "put on the whole armor of God" (*see* Ephesians 6:13) and take authority over the wind and the waves that come against our lives — our families, our businesses, or our bodies — just as Jesus took authority over the wind and the waves that came against Him.

But Mark 4:39 tells us that when the wind and the waves ceased that night, "…there was a great calm." Verse 37 previously told us that this storm had been a *great storm*, but when everything was said and done, Jesus had matched a great storm with a *great calm*. If the adversary has created a great sickness in your body, Jesus Christ wants to match it with a *great healing*. Whatever the devil does, Jesus Christ wants to match that attack with an even greater blessing in your life!

**It was when Jesus was on the edge of a breakthrough that this unexpected attack of violent and destructive turbulence came down upon Him and His disciples to try to kill and destroy them.**

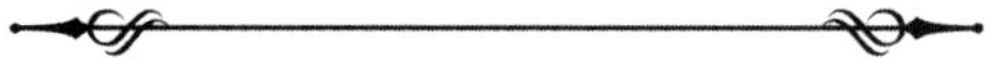

## PAUL'S THORN IN THE FLESH

In my book *Apostles and Prophets*, I comment on Second Corinthians 12:7, where Paul wrote about how the devil launched yet another attack to thwart his progress. Paul was bursting into new realms of revelation, and it was so threatening to the domain of darkness that it provoked the devil into mounting assaults against him with the aim of diverting his focus and distracting him. In this greatly misunderstood verse, Paul wrote, "And lest I should be exalted above measure through the abundance of the revelations, there was given to me a thorn in the flesh, the messenger of Satan to buffet me, lest I should be exalted above measure."

The words "exalted above measure" are a translation of the Greek word *huperairo*, a compound of the words *huper* and *airo*. The word *huper* means *over, above, and beyond.* It depicts *something that is way beyond measure* and conveys the idea of *something that is greater, superior, higher, better, more than a match for, utmost, paramount, or foremost.* It could also describe *something that is first-rate, first-class, top-notch, unsurpassed, unequaled, and unrivaled* by any person or thing. The second part of the word *huperairo* means *to lift up, to raise*, or *to be exalted.*

When these two Greek words are compounded to form the word *huperairo*, it speaks of *a person who has been supremely exalted.* This is a person who has been *magnified, increased, and lifted up to a place of great prestige and influence.* Although *huperairo* could be used to express the idea of a person who haughtily exalts himself, this is categorically not the idea Paul had in mind when he wrote this verse. Rather, Paul used the word *huperairo* to depict one who has been greatly honored and recognized due to something he has written, done, or otherwise achieved.

Because Paul was an apostle, we know that God had graced him with supernatural insight and revelation. In Second Corinthians 12:7, Paul indeed referred to the "abundance of the revelations" God had given him. And all New

Testament ears who heard the word *apostolos* — the Greek word for "apostle" used to describe Paul's ministry office and calling — knew this depicted a spiritual leader who possessed supernatural insights and who had the potential to lead others from one spiritual dimension into the next spiritual dimension or level.

Paul said he had received an "abundance" of such revelations. The word "abundance" is from the Greek word *huperballo,* a compound of the word *huper* and the word *ballo,* meaning *to cast* or *to throw.* When these two words are compounded to form the word *huperballo*, they describe *something that is phenomenal, extraordinary, unparalleled, or unmatched.* It is like an archer who aims for the bull's-eye, but when he releases the string and shoots his arrow, his arrow flies way *over the top* of and even *beyond* the target.

Paul used this word *huperballo* — here translated as the word "abundance" — to explain that the revelations he had received were not only unparalleled in quality, but the vast number of them were far beyond what anyone else had ever received. As an apostle, he was enabled to go into new geographical regions, but he was also able to journey into spiritual realms and dimensions and to receive spiritual truths in a greater way than others.

Paul preached these "abundant revelations" as he traversed the regions surrounding Asia and the Mediterranean Sea. Everywhere he went, he preached what had been divinely revealed to him, and as he preached, his power, authority, and fame grew greater and greater. Those who heard Paul were enabled to journey with him into spiritual truths they probably would have never accessed if they had not been in his apostolic presence and heard his apostolic voice.

Due to these revelations and his boldness to preach them, Paul became one of the most influential apostles in history. In Second Corinthians 12:7 Paul wrote, in effect, that Satan was so alarmed by the progress he was making with the Gospel that the enemy launched a full-scale attack to impede his progress. Satan didn't want Paul to be recognized or magnified to a greater extent, so the devil attempted to ruin him, to destroy him, and to discredit the message he preached. How? Paul said he was afflicted with a "thorn in the flesh."

The word "thorn" is the Greek word *skolops*, a word used to describe *a dangerously sharp, spiked instrument or tool.* However, this word was also used to describe *the stake on which an enemy's head was stuck after being decapitated.* Some have suggested that the words "in the flesh" refer to a physical sickness, but this cannot be confirmed by any scripture in the New Testament and should be taken as unsubstantiated conjecture.

People have even gone so far in their imaginations as to assert that Paul suffered from malaria, epilepsy, eye disease, club feet, or a hunched back. Paul may have dealt with physical symptoms of sickness from time to time, as most of us have. But all these speculations are ridiculous. If he had suffered these physical infirmities as his "thorn" that beleagured him time and again, it would have been physically impossible for him to travel the vast distances he did to do his ministry.

However, what is clear is that Satan wanted Paul's head on a stake! He wanted to eliminate this man of God and put him completely out of the picture. The words "in the flesh" most likely describe a type of event that was a constant source of irritation to the apostle Paul that caused him personal distress, and it kept occurring over and over again. This is why he referred to it as a "thorn in the flesh."

Some allege that God sent the thorn to keep Paul from being prideful about his many revelations. But Paul plainly wrote it was a "...messenger of Satan to buffet me..." (2 Corinthians 12:7). It was not a messenger from God, but rather a messenger of Satan sent to attack and distract him. The word "messenger" is the Greek word *angelos*, a word that can describe *an angel*, *one who is sent on a special mission*, or *a messenger who is dispatched to perform a specific assignment*. This was a "messenger of Satan" — perhaps a demonic entity — that was sent directly from Satan himself to buffet Paul and to restrict the progress of his ministry.

This thorn in the flesh categorically did not come from God; otherwise, Paul would have called it a "messenger of God." But Paul plainly stated this thorn in the flesh was a "messenger of Satan" — a special force that had been dispatched to keep Paul from gaining additional status and prestige and to prevent him from taking the Gospel further and higher into the world scene.

Paul was preaching to kings, governors, and world leaders. He was establishing churches, writing New Testament Scripture, and pushing back the forces of hell. His personal influence was growing and his impact was increasing day by day. The revelations that God had given him were about to change the course of human history. So fearing that Paul's influence would grow too great, Satan strategically sent forces that had been instructed to create disturbances to "buffet" the apostle.

The word "buffet" is the Greek word *kolaphidzo*, a Greek word that comes from the word *kolaphos*, a word that describes the *fist* or *knuckles*. When it becomes the word *kolaphidzo*, as Paul used it in Second Corinthians 12:7, it refers to *beatings with the fist*. The Greek tense describes *unending, unrelenting, continuous, repetitious beatings*. This means Paul was not telling us of a single event, but of a series of many events. The word *kolaphidzo* ("buffet") gives us our greatest insight into the "thorn in the flesh" Paul was writing about in this verse.

Paul endured many afflictions during his ministry, but some of the greatest afflictions he faced were due to religious leaders who so fiercely opposed him. These religious leaders included Jewish leaders who hated him and his message, and they also included false brethren who were constantly trying to displace him in his position of authority and usurp his apostleship in the local churches. Paul was resisted outside the church by leaders of the Jewish faith who hated him, and he was opposed from within by those who wanted him out of the picture so they could take his place of prominence inside the church.

Thus, the biggest "thorn" in Paul's life was the fact that he had to deal with these different groups of people who covertly planned the problems and hassles he frequently faced in the ministry. A special messenger from Satan, perhaps even a demonic angel, had been sent to incite and stir up these people against Paul.

In light of these Greek words, consider this fresh *RIV* (*Renner Interpretive Version*) of Paul's words in Second Corinthians 12:7:

> **Because of the phenomenal revelations I have received and on account of the vast number of these revelations that God has entrusted to me — and to hinder the highly visible progress I am making in the Lord's cause — a special messenger has been sent from Satan to harass me with constant distractions and headaches. There's no doubt about it! Those whom Satan has stirred up against me want my head on a stake! Satan is using these people to constantly buffet and distract me in an attempt to keep me from reaching a higher level of visibility and recognition and to sidetrack me from preaching my revelations.**

Paul's thorn in the flesh was his way of saying the devil was using people (and other attacks) again and again to try to keep him distracted solving those "people problems" that hindered him from making significant Gospel advancements. But despite the fact that Satan wanted to thwart Paul's progress, he was unable to do so because Paul forged ahead with the power of God.

## A POSITION OF SUBMISSION TO GOD EMPOWERS US TO RESIST THE DEVIL

In James 4:7 we find that when we are living in submission to God, it gives us the power to resist the devil and he will flee from us. That verse says, "Submit yourselves therefore to God. Resist the devil, and he will flee from you."

The word "submit" is the Greek word *hupotasso*, a compound of the words *hupo* and *tasso*. The preposition *hupo* means *under*, and the word *tasso* means *to arrange*. As a compound, the word *hupotasso* means *to properly arrange under.*

It is actually a military term depicting *a soldier's obedience and submission to authority.*

In James 4:7, this word *hupotasso* ("submit") signifies one who properly arranges himself under the authority of God and His Word. Most importantly, it pictures the one submitted to authority as being under the covering and protection of a greater authority and who actually *hides behind* the authority of the one to whom he is submitted. This is amazing because this tells us that there is protection in submission.

In a position of submission, you have God's divine protection and the ability to resist the devil. The word "resist" is translated from a form of the Greek word *anthistemi*, which is a compound of the words *anti* and *histemi*. The word *anti* means *against*, and the word *histemi* means *to stand.* When compounded, the word *anthistemi* means *to stand against* or *to stand in opposition.* It demonstrates *the attitude of one who is fiercely opposed* to something or someone and therefore determines to do everything in his power *to resist* it.

Furthermore, the word *anthistemi* means *to defy*, *to stand against*, or *to withstand*, and it depicts a well-thought-out and well-planned resistance. This word was used in ancient Greece to picture the fierce resistance of an enemy, which again signifies that when you're properly aligned under the authority of God and hiding behind Him, He is your fierce Protector that stands against the devil with you.

James 4:7 says when you resist the devil, he will "flee" from you. The word "flee" is the amazing Greek word *pheugo*, which means *to flee*, *to take flight*, *to run away*, *to run as fast as possible*, or *to escape*. It pictures a person's feet running as fast as he can as he *flees* from a situation. This word *pheugo* was used to depict *a lawbreaker who flees in terror* from a city or a nation where he broke the law.

By using this term in this verse, James stated that when you submit to God and align yourself under His authority, you are empowered to successfully resist the devil and anything he brings against you. When you are in that consecrated position of submission, the devil will "flee" from you like a criminal who flees in terror after breaking the law.

When we include the original Greek meaning of all these words, the (*RIV*) *Renner Interpretive Versio*n of James 4:7 reads:

> **It is imperative that you make the decision to properly align yourselves under the authority of God — in a submitted position that actually provides you with protection. Being submitted to His authority gives you the ability to defy, oppose, stand steadfastly against, and withstand the accusing, slanderous, trap-setting behavior of the devil. In fact, he'll be so terrified of you that he'll move his feet as fast as he can to get away from you. Not only will he flee from you, he'll run like a criminal terrified of prosecution — so scared that he'll want to do all he can to put as much space between him and you as possible.**

That is the kind of authority you have against the enemy when you are properly submitted to the authority of God. You are so protected and so empowered, you have the ability to put the devil on the run! So if you are experiencing adverse circumstances in your life and you have eliminated or dealt with the first six possible reasons why sickness has found its way into your life and concluded it must be an attack from the devil — don't give up and throw in the towel. Instead, stay in submission to God, pray, and grab hold of the Holy Spirit's strength to stand tenaciously against the enemy. If you will make the decision not to budge and refuse to faint in the day of adversity, God will cause you to be more than a conqueror!

But the fact remains that numerous Christians fall ill due to unforeseen devilish assaults, and it's crucial to understand how to tackle these occurrences. In the following sections, we'll delve into various instances from Matthew, Mark, and Luke, where illness was sometimes connected with demonic influences, and we'll see how Jesus dealt with it. Before that, however, we'll explore the insights of the Early Church fathers and examine their views on demonic activities, the connection of these nefarious activities and sickness, and the authority we possess to confront demonic powers.

## WHAT EARLY CHURCH FATHERS WROTE ABOUT DEMONS

The origin of demons is a subject of debate, but what is beyond dispute is the historical evidence of demons across all cultures and religions. Every culture has chronicled tales of evil spirits, which demonstrates that the belief in such entities has been present since ancient times.

The Old Testament offers scant insight into the activity of demons, but Jewish literature from the New Testament era paints a more vivid picture. It suggests that once demons possess a person, they unleash chaos within that individual which leads to conditions like unholy physical acts, a devastating loss of self-control, and conditions that seem to mimic dementia and amnesia — all of which wreak havoc on social interactions.[1]

Furthermore, Jewish literature from that period indicates that evil spirits can warp or diminish the senses, affecting hearing, vision, and speech.[2] These types of descriptions are very much in agreement with the accounts of demonic activity found in the gospels.

The subject of demonic activity was so important in the earliest days of the Church that even Early Church fathers commented extensively on this subject. In this section, we will explore their insights and examine specific quotes from their writings and then we will look at various verses from Matthew, Mark, and Luke that chronicle sicknesses that were connected with demonic activity.

As you will see, the Early Church fathers stated clearly that those who walk in God's power possess the strength to crush demons beneath their feet, and at the mere utterance of Jesus' name, these vile entities are compelled to submit and flee away.

## THE NATURE AND ACTIVITY OF DEMONS

We will be specifically looking at the writings of the Early Church fathers Mark Minucius Felix, Lactantius, Origen, and Tertullian — their commentary concerning the activity of demon spirits will be followed by my brief analysis. Christians are empowered to exercise authority over all malevolent spirits, which we will see in the section that follows this one. The quotes below are largely organized by author and the year in which the document was written.

> **"[Demons] cease not, now that they are ruined themselves, to ruin others; and being depraved themselves, to infuse into others the error of their depravity...."[3]**
>
> **— *Mark Minucius Felix* (c. 200)**

This thought-provoking commentary reveals that demons, being inherently corrupt and ruined, find pleasure in spreading corruption and ruin among others. This activity is vividly depicted in the four gospels, and it can still be seen today in those ensnared by the demonic grip of deception and moral ruin.

> **"...Creeping also secretly into human bodies, with subtlety, as being spirits, they feign diseases, alarm the minds, [and] wrench about the limbs...."[4]**
>
> **— *Mark Minucius Felix* (c. 200)**

This insight shows that the presence of demon spirits frequently underlies ailments, phobias, mental disturbances, and physical abnormalities. This idea is echoed in the gospels, where it is noted that spirits of infirmity often lie at the heart of disease and sickness. Those who are noted for healing ministries have observed that, occasionally, both physical and mental health crises vanish following the expulsion of these spirits.

> **"We receive certain initial elements, and, as it were, seeds of sins, from those things which we use agreeably to nature; but when we have indulged them beyond what is proper, and have not resisted the first movements**

**to intemperance, then the hostile power, [demons] seizing the occasion of this first transgression, incites and presses us hard in every way, seeking to extend our sins over a wider field, and furnishing us human beings with occasions and beginnings of sins...."[5]**

**— *Origen* (c. 225)**

The esteemed theologian Origen suggested that every unregenerate individual is innately inclined toward sin. However, through persistent, unreserved submission to this inclination, one can inadvertently open a portal to sinister spiritual activity that allows ordinary human tendencies to be energized by evil spirits, thus transforming a mere inclination into a proclivity or desire and eventually an entrenched addiction and perversion.

An example of a persistent, unreserved yielding to something that can eventually provide an entry point into one's life could be *overeating*. While eating is a normal human function, it can turn into something else if the flesh holds enough sway that it eventually connects a person to a lust for food that is all-consuming. In that way, this habitual persistence in overeating can move the person along an unwelcomed and unintended dark pathway.

Or how about lying? It is *not* a normal human function, yet it may be overlooked when practiced in "smaller quantities" — that is, *until* a lying spirit is entertained and the person becomes "certifiably" demonized in this area of his or her life.

**"...Demons, who are scattered as it were in troops in different parts of the earth, have chosen for themselves a chief under whose command they may plunder and pillage the souls of men."[6]**

**— *Origen* (c. 248)**

Here Origen stated that evil spirits have been unleashed across the expanse of the earth and that they function as troops tasked with the mission of plundering and pillaging humanity. These dark forces inflict harm on multiple fronts — physically, mentally, and spiritually — echoing Paul's vivid depiction in Ephesians 6:12 of demonic forces that are organized and deployed like a formidable army to wage war against mankind.

> **"[Demons] haunt the denser parts of [heavenly] bodies, and frequent unclean places upon earth, and who...because they are without bodies of earthly material...secretly enter the bodies of the more rapacious and savage and wicked of animals, and stir them up to do whatever they choose, and at whatever time they choose: either turning the fancies of these animals to make flights and movements of various kinds, in order that men may be caught by the divining power that is in the irrational animals, and neglect to seek after the God who contains all things...."[7]**
>
> **— *Origen* (c. 248)**

Origen wrote that demons inhabit the lower realms of the atmosphere — essentially sharing the same airspace with humans. This aligns with Paul's words in Ephesians 6:12, where he mentioned that evil spirits dwell in the "air," a word translated from the Greek that indeed depicts the same atmosphere where human beings dwell.

Origen further elaborated on the versatility of these evil entities, asserting that demons have the ability to possess not only humans but also animals. This concept is dramatically depicted in the biblical account of the demoniac of Gadara. In this story, a legion of demons, once they are cast out of the man, find refuge in a nearby herd of swine, as chronicled in the passages of Matthew 8:28-32, Mark 5:1-20, and Luke 8:26-36.

> **"These contaminated and abandoned spirits, as I say, wander over the whole earth, and contrive a solace for their own perdition by the destruction of men.**
>
> **"Therefore they fill every place with snares, deceits, frauds, and errors; for they cling to individuals...[and] since spirits are without [physical] substance and not to be grasped, insinuate themselves into the bodies of men; and secretly working in their inward parts, they corrupt the health,**

**hasten diseases, terrify their souls with dreams, [and] harass their minds with phrenzies....”[8]**

— ***Lactantius*** **(c. 304-313)**

In this passage, we see that malevolent spirits, known as evil spirits or demons, can take residence within humans, and this often leads to ailments, tormented souls, and minds gripped with madness. Such manifestations are evident throughout the four gospels, where Jesus is depicted ministering to individuals afflicted by these sinister forces, as you will discover in the following pages.

**“[Demons] have the power to injure...ofttimes having uttered the greatest howlings, they cry out that they are beaten, and are on fire...they injure... those whom they have in their own power.”[9]**

— ***Lactantius*** **(c. 304-313)**

Here we find that demons inflict suffering and injury on others as they torment those they possess.

## THE AUTHORITY OF BELIEVERS OVER DEMONS

The quotes in the previous section dealt with the activity and operation of demon spirits, but the following compilation of quotes delve into the authority and power bestowed upon true believers by Christ, which grants them mastery over evil spirits. They are arranged according to the authors and the respective years their works were penned.

**“...[Demons] have no power over those who ‘have put on the whole armour of God,’ who have received strength to ‘withstand the wiles of the devil....’”[10]**

— ***Origen*** **(c. 248)**

Obviously reflecting on Ephesians 6:11, Origen stated that every true believer who’s dressed in the armor of God is equipped to withstand the cunning schemes of the devil. The New Testament resounds with the doctrine that Christians are endowed with divine armor that gives them the strength to confront and vanquish the forces of wickedness.

> **"...Demons...and other unseen powers...show that they...fear the name of Jesus as that of a being of superior power...demons...have withdrawn from those whom they had assailed, in obedience to the mere mention of His name."[11]**
>
> — ***Origen* (c. 248)**

Here Origen wrote of the unmatched supremacy of Jesus' name and position. In the words of Acts 4:12, Ephesians 1:21, and Philippians 2:9-10, we discover the unparalleled authority of Jesus and how His name surpasses all other names and powers.

James 2:19 reveals that demons tremble at the mere mention of Jesus' name, and James 4:7 says that evil spirits retreat when they are resisted. Scripture emphatically declares that even the newest believer can use the name of Jesus to unleash a force stronger than any evil and that causes the devil and his minions to flee.

> **"...Under the figure of scorpions and serpents are...evil spirits... [Christ] proclaimed the benefits of His cures, then also did He put the scorpions and the serpents under the feet of His saints — even He who had first received this power from the Father, in order to bestow it upon others and then manifested it forth conformably to the order of prophecy."[12]**
>
> —***Tertullian* (c. 250)**

These quotes echo the promise in Luke 10:19, in which Jesus told His disciples that they — and all believers, including us — are endued with power so mighty that they can trample on serpents and scorpions. Even when evil spirits attempt to strike stealthily like a serpent or create painful predicaments similar to the sting of a scorpion, we as believers have been given the power and authority to keep the devil underfoot and at bay.

## TORMENTING AND SICKNESS-CAUSING EVIL SPIRITS WERE A REALITY IN HISTORY, AND THEY ARE A REALITY TODAY

Throughout this book, we've repeatedly stated that many health challenges Christians face often stem from inadvertently creating opportunities — *entry points* — for the devil to infiltrate their lives. And in a study of the gospels, there's another reason that must be considered, as it is evident that numerous individuals whom Jesus healed were tormented at the core of their illnesses by demonic forces.

The gospels of Matthew, Mark, and Luke share a remarkable similarity in the communicating of events in the ministry of Jesus.

I can't cover them all, but there are more than 25 instances that I plan to cover in-depth in an upcoming book on the healings, miracles, and deliverances that occurred under the ministry of Jesus. The insights are remarkable that each of these gospel writers share on this important subject of physical and mental health challenges linked to demonic forces.

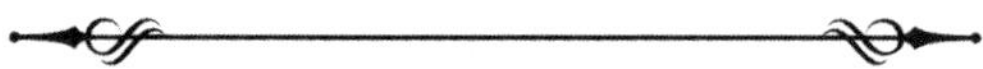

**Even when evil spirits attempt to strike stealthily like a serpent or create painful predicaments similar to the sting of a scorpion, we as believers have been given the power and authority to keep the devil underfoot and at bay.**

In the following sections, I will share an instance of sickness connected to demonic activity — and the deliverance and healing that ensued under Jesus' ministry — from Matthew, Mark, and Luke.

## AN INSTANCE OF SICKNESS CONNECTED TO DEMONIC ACTIVITY IN THE BOOK OF MATTHEW

**And Jesus went about all Galilee, teaching in their synagogues, and preaching the gospel of the kingdom, and healing all manner of sickness and all manner of disease among the people. And his fame went throughout all Syria: and they brought unto him all sick people that were taken with divers diseases and torments, and those which were possessed with devils, and those which were lunatick, and those that had the palsy; and he healed them.**

**— Matthew 4:23-24**

The word "healing" and "healed" in this passage are translated from a form of the Greek word *therapeuo*, which means *to heal*, and it is where we also derive the English word "therapy." When *therapeuo* is used to describe Jesus' healing work — and it is used often — it pictures divine power that takes hold through the cooperative actions of the individual receiving it in much the same way a physical therapist provides guidance and exercises for a patient, but the ultimate progress depends on the patient's participation and adherence to the therapist's instruction.

For instance, when Jesus instructed the sick to "stretch forth a hand" or told the lame to "pick up a bed," He was essentially inviting them to activate this healing power through their cooperation. This word "healed" — again, derived from the Greek word *therapeuo* — reveals that Jesus' approach wasn't simply to touch and move on; rather, He engaged people in the process, encouraging them to take steps of faith, thereby unlocking the power of God to take hold in their bodies.

This teaches us the crucial lesson that if Jesus embraced this interactive approach to healing, we should strive to do the same. Instead of offering a fleeting prayer and moving to the next person, we ought to pause and invite the individual to act in faith — to attempt something he or she previously couldn't do. It is often through such active participation that God's power is activated and healing is actually manifested.

In addition to conveying that Jesus healed "all manner" of sickness and disease, this passage further mentions that many individuals were "possessed with devils." In the original Greek, the word used is *daimonidzomenous*, which has often been inaccurately translated as "possessed with devils." This translation exaggerates the essence of the Greek term, which does not imply complete possession. Instead, it refers to individuals who are experiencing some degree of demonic influence or activity. A more precise translation would be *demonized*, suggesting that these individuals were *demonically affected* either physically or mentally in some manner.

The word "lunatick" (or "lunatic") in Matthew 4:24 traces its roots to the Greek word *seleniadzomai*, derived from the Greek word *selene*, which means *moon*. However, this term is more than a mere reference to the moon; it described an age-old belief tied to the enchanting powers of the moon. The word "lunatic" actually translates to *moonstruck*, and it is a word that was originally associated with occult practices. To understand why this group of infirmed people in Matthew 4:24 are referred to as lunatics, let's delve deeper into how the word "lunatic" was used during the New Testament era.

The Greek word *selene* not only signifies *the moon*, but it also refers to the pagan goddess *Selene*, who was *the goddess of the moon*.[13] She is often depicted in ancient art traversing the sky with the moon in her wake. Worshippers of Selene linked her to romance and childbirth. They believed that sacrifices and prayers to this moon goddess could enhance their romantic affairs and help with an easier childbirth.

Many beseeched Selene's assistance to bring magical love-spells on those they romantically desired or to magically intervene and alienate the pains of childbirth. But the full moon — Selene's high moment of worship — was thought to be a time when her powers were more easily accessed. During one, both men and women would offer Selene sacrifices for outcomes in romance and as a way to seek her help during childbirth.

Furthermore, lunar eclipses were interpreted as the handiwork of witches, whom people believed would call Selene down upon the earth with their spells and incantations to release her wrath. It was also believed if one harbored animosity toward others, he or she could allegedly summon the "bad magic" of Selene to "bring the moon down upon" that person's adversaries. Similarly, breaking an oath to Selene could invite wrath on the one who broke it, which would manifest as bad luck or a curse. Those afflicted by Selene's unfavorable gaze were dubbed *lunatics* — a word that described people with erratic behavior or who were marked with mental illness or a severe state of mental disturbance. This word has carried into modern vernacular as an offensive way of saying someone is crazy, foolish, or silly in the way they act and think.

When a person was deemed a *lunatic*,[14] it meant it was believed that person had either incurred Selene's displeasure or that he had fallen under the influence of evil powers by dabbling in the occult. Signs of such a curse were being demonized or erratic in behavior and having epileptic-type seizures. Again, the sufferers of such a curse were called *lunatic* or *moonstruck*.

Because the word "lunatick" is used in Matthew 4:24, it hints that some individuals had dabbled in prohibited occultic rituals, which resulted in their being demonized. Perhaps they had requested romantic help from the moon goddess, or they had requested the moon goddess's help for a woman in childbirth. But the primary evidence someone had come under the influence of such evil powers was that they became demonized, erratic, or marked with epileptic-type seizures.

While it may be a surprise to you, a significant number of people in Israel meddled with the mystical pagan practices of neighboring nations. Whether it was the cult of the moon goddess Selene or some other cult is not the issue — their flirtation with spiritually forbidden practices inevitably led them on a descent into demonic influence.

This group of "lunatics" referred to in Matthew 4:24 was a group who had become demonized as a result of involving themselves in occult practices, which exposed them to demonic influence. But it's crucial to recognize that individuals who were demonized as a result of their involvement in the occult — even those greatly vexed — were aware that Jesus held the power to bring them freedom. Even today, Jesus continues to deliver people from the lingering effects of participation with occult practices.

This narrative stands as a caution for any Christian who is tempted to meddle in spiritual realms that are forbidden by God. It reminds us that engaging in occult practices can invite malevolent forces into one's life, and for those entangled by such dark influences, true healing may necessitate severing and expelling these sinister powers. As highlighted in Matthew 4:24, many who sought Christ's healing touch needed liberation from the evil forces that they or others had unwittingly summoned through forbidden spiritual pursuits. But importantly, in *each* of these instances, we are told that Jesus "healed" them.

The word "healed" is, again, translated from a form of the Greek word *therapeuo*, typically translated as *healed*, but it embodies healing or deliverance that is activated through the cooperative actions of the recipient. The meaning of this word "healing," as we saw, is so important. Grasping the fullness of this concept is crucial to ministering to the sick and bound if we want to minister as Jesus did two millennia ago.

While multiple Greek words could be used to describe healing, the word *therapeuo* is used over and over again in the gospels to underscore that Jesus' approach wasn't a mere fleeting touch. Instead He remained present with those in need of healing and encouraged them to actively engage with God's power so their healing would manifest. We often lament the scarcity of healing today, but could our hastiness be a hindrance? Are we so eager to move to the next person that we fail to take enough time to encourage each person to cooperate by trying to do what he or she previously struggled to do? Perhaps if we slowed down and fully invested in each encounter, we would witness a greater outpouring of healings.

## JESUS SENT HIS DISCIPLES *AND US* TO EXERCISE THIS 'INFLUENTIAL AUTHORITY' IN HIS NAME — TO HEAL THE SICK AND SET THE CAPTIVES FREE

Mark 3:14-15 says, "And he [Jesus] ordained twelve, that they should be with him, and that he might send them forth to preach, and to have power to heal sicknesses, and to cast out devils." In addition to ordaining them to preach, Jesus also gave His disciples "power to heal sicknesses, and to cast out devils."

The word "power" is a poor translation, for the actual Greek word is *exousia*, which refers to *authority* and *influence* that was effective over both physical illness and the demonic realm. However, it's interesting to note that the *King James Version* includes the phrase "heal sicknesses," which is absent in the original Greek manuscript. There, the emphasis is solely on casting out demons. It's probable that translators added "heal sicknesses" into the text because this phrase is used in Matthew 10:1, even though the original Greek focus here remains solely on casting out demonic forces.

The words "cast out" in Mark 3:15 are interpreted from a form of the Greek word *ekballo*, which is a compound of the word *ek* and *ballo*. The word *ek* means *out*, and the word *ballo* means *to cast, hurl, or throw*. The word *ekballo* conveys the idea of *forcefully expelling or evicting*, which is reminiscent of a landlord who *evicts* an unwelcome tenant from his dwelling. This underscores the fact that Jesus endued the apostles — *and us* — with *authority so influential* that we can remove any malevolent spirits from the afflicted. The plural form of "devils" in this context indicates that we possess such *influential authority* over every form of evil spirit, irrespective of its nature or classification.

## AN INSTANCE OF SICKNESS CONNECTED TO DEMONIC ACTIVITY IN THE BOOK OF MARK

Similar to Matthew, the gospel of Mark offers vibrant narratives showcasing Jesus' healing and deliverance ministry. Within this gospel, a broad array of sicknesses is recorded, and each was miraculously cured by Jesus' touch. However, in this chapter, my focus is to examine illnesses intertwined with demonic influence and explore the profound ways in which Jesus restored health to those who were demonized in some way.

> **But Simon's wife's mother lay sick of a fever, and anon they tell him of her. And he came and took her by the hand, and lifted her up; and immediately the fever left her, and she ministered unto them. And at even, when the sun did set, they brought unto him all that were diseased, and them that were possessed with devils. And all the city was gathered together at the door. And he healed many that were sick of divers diseases, and cast out many devils; and suffered not the devils to speak, because they knew him.**
>
> — **Mark 1:30-34**

Mark 1:30 says, "But Simon's wife's mother lay sick of a fever, and anon they tell him of her."

As we saw in Matthew's account of this event (*see* Matthew 8:14), we find Peter's mother-in-law bedridden and gripped by a severe fever. Mark, in his account, employed the Greek word *katakeimai* to describe her as *lying* in bed. This word, a compound of *kata,* meaning *down*, and *keimai*, meaning *to lay*, pictures her *lying flat*, unable to muster the strength to rise.

Mark further elaborated by saying she lay "sick of a fever." Here Mark used the same identical word used in Matthew's account to depict the severity of her fever. It is the Greek word *puressousan*, derived from *pur*, meaning *fire*. But as *puressousan* it pictures a person *enveloped in an all-consuming blaze*, and it lets us know she had a perilously high temperature. In ancient times, remedies for such severe fevers were scarce, and such conditions could be life-threatening, so her critical state prompted an urgent appeal to Jesus for help.

Mark 1:31 says, "And he came and took her by the hand, and lifted her up; and immediately the fever left her, and she ministered unto them." We often imagine Jesus as gentle and soft-spoken, but the Greek word translated "took" challenges this notion. It is derived from the word *krateo*, which means *to seize* or *to arrest with force* and gives the image of *a firm and commanding grip*. There was nothing delicate about His touch; as He grasped her hand, He simultaneously unleashed divine power to banish the fever. Then He "lifted her up," apparently without granting her the leisure to ponder her healing! The word "lifted" is taken from a form of the Greek word *egeiro*, a word also used for *resurrection* in the New Testament.

Consequently, Jesus didn't merely wish for her recovery, nor did He offer her a moment's hesitation. With decisive action, He seized her hand, releasing God's power with unmatched authority, and then He physically pulled her up and off her sickbed. Instantly, the fever "left" her body. The word "left" is from a form of the Greek word *aphiemi*, which indicates *a complete dismissal* and *an irreversible departure*. So thorough was her freedom from the fever's grip that she rose promptly and attended to those present.

Mark 1:32 tells us, "And at even, when the sun did set, they brought unto him all that were diseased, and them that were possessed with devils." The word "brought" is the Greek word *phero*, which means *to physically bear* or *to physically carry*. Herein we find that there were people so sick they couldn't come to the meeting without physical assistance — in other words, friends and loved ones physically carried them to where Jesus was ministering.

That evening crowds gathered around Jesus as He ministered to people burdened by afflictions described as those who were "diseased" and those "possessed with devils." The word "diseased" stems from the Greek word *kakos*, which conveys a sense of being *grievously, miserably, or wretchedly sick*. On the other hand, the phrase "possessed with devils" comes from the Greek word *daimonidzomenous*, which compellingly suggests not total possession by demons, but rather individuals who were experiencing varying degrees of vexation from evil spirits. Each individual's experience with these different levels of vexation would have varied from case to case. The news of Jesus' healing touch was so great that Mark 1:33 says "all the city was gathered together at the door."

Mark 1:34 says, "And he healed many that were sick of divers diseases, and cast out many devils; and suffered not the devils to speak, because they knew him." We once again find the word "healed," which is derived from a form of the Greek word *therapeuo*.

As we have seen, this word suggests *healing that is accompanied with the recipient's participation*, and it indicates that because of the word "many," this ministry session likely extended over several hours as Jesus worked carefully with each individual. He personally laid His hands upon them to release God's power and then He steadily guided them to cooperate by moving in ways they couldn't before. Patiently, Jesus remained with each person, probably spending substantial time with every individual, assisting each one in experiencing the power of God and achieving the manifestation of healing.

According to Mark 1:34, as dusk descended, Jesus brought healing to those suffering from a multitude of ailments. The original Greek uses the words *poikilais nosois*, which are derived from the word *poikilos*, indicating *a wide array* of conditions, and the word *nosos*, which refers to grave illnesses deemed *incurable* and *hopeless*, often believed to be the result of demonic influence.

But Mark 1:34 also highlights that He "cast out many devils." The words "cast out" once again come from the Greek word *ekballo*. We've encountered this term already and we will see it again when we examine the ministry of Jesus in the gospels to free captive humanity. This word signifies the act of *forcefully ejecting, expelling, or evicting*. Just as a landlord might expel an unwelcome tenant from a residence, Jesus showed no mercy to these malevolent spirits and forcefully compelled them to vacate the lives they tormented.

The text states that there were "many" such instances. This word "many" is from the Greek word *polla*, and denotes *a substantial multitude*. It suggests that Jesus encountered numerous individuals who were afflicted, perhaps knowingly or unknowingly, by illnesses tied to demonic influence.

Due to their ridiculous penchant for theatrics and dramatics, spirits relish the opportunity to put on a grand performance, so in Mark 1:34, it's noted that Jesus "suffered not the devils to speak." A more contemporary interpretation might say that He refused to let them utter a word. The word "speak" is derived from the Greek word *lalein*, which means *to speak*, but it implies engaging in free-flowing conversation.

From my own encounters with demons, it's clear they've got a knack for chattering on endlessly in an attempt to wear you down. It's crucial to silence them, preventing them from unleashing their exhausting tirades and thus preserving the energy of those casting them out. Just as Jesus didn't allow these spirits to voice their theatrics, neither should we let them turn serious moments into their personal stage productions.

## AN INSTANCE OF SICKNESS CONNECTED TO DEMONIC ACTIVITY IN THE BOOK OF LUKE

The gospel of Luke also offers an extensive portrayal of Jesus' healing ministry, with many of the events depicted in the gospels of Matthew and Mark. But given Luke's background as a physician, his narrative often incorporates terminology that is distinctly medical in flavor. There were many instances of Jesus healing those with physical issues; however, my primary aim in this chapter remains to identify those afflictions that are connected to demonic activity.

> **Now when the sun was setting, all they that had any sick with divers diseases brought them unto him; and he laid his hands on every one of them, and healed them. And devils also came out of many, crying out, and saying, Thou art Christ the Son of God. And he rebuking them suffered them not to speak: for they knew that he was Christ.**
>
> **— Luke 4:40-41**

Luke 4:40 says, "Now when the sun was setting, all they that had any sick with divers diseases brought them unto him; and he laid his hands on every one of them, and healed them."

The word "sick" in this verse is translated from a form of the Greek word *astheno*, which serves as an umbrella term for *a wide array of ailments and afflictions*. Intriguingly, Greek literature also employs this word *astheno* to describe individuals plagued by financial woes. This dual meaning offers an insightful connection, illustrating how physical suffering often goes hand in hand with financial strain due to the burden of medical expenses.

The verse continues by mentioning that people with "divers diseases" were also brought to Jesus for a healing touch. Here the word "divers" is derived from the Greek word *poikilos*, which refers to *a multitude* or *a variety*, and it suggests *a broad spectrum of illnesses*. The word "diseases" stems from the Greek word *nosos*, which specifically refers to *incurable, terminal diseases* that, in the context of New Testament times, were believed to be induced by evil spirits.

Luke 4:40 goes on to say, "…He laid his hands on every one of them, and healed them." Throughout the gospel narratives, the image of Jesus laying His hands on individuals occurs frequently. Remarkably, there's not a single account in which Jesus is described as offering prayers for the sick; instead, over and over again, we see Him touch people with His hands.

The word "healed" is once again translated from a form of the Greek word *therapeuo*, which is where we derive the English word *therapy.* This particular Greek word is predominantly used in the Gospels to characterize Jesus' approach to healing. It highlights how, apart from merely laying hands upon individuals, Jesus devoted time to each person, guiding and encouraging them to participate — much like *modern physical therapy* — with the healing power He imparted to them. Acting like a healing therapist, Jesus asked them to attempt feats they previously deemed impossible.

By engaging with Him in this way, divine power would take hold and manifest their healing. I realize that we've touched upon this theme before, yet the gospels of Matthew, Mark, and Luke emphasize it repeatedly. This underlines not only Jesus' method of healing, but also provides a blueprint for us to emulate as we minister to those seeking healing.

Luke 4:41 says, "And devils also came out of many, crying out, and saying, Thou art Christ the Son of God. And he rebuking them suffered them not to speak: for they knew that he was Christ." The word "devils" is the Greek word *daimonoia*, the plural form for *demons*. The words "many" in Greek is *pollon*, and it indicates *a very substantial multitude.*

In modern times, discussions about evil spirits in relation to illnesses are scarce, but Jesus regarded these matters with utmost gravity. Exercising His profound authority, Jesus confronted these vile spirits at the root of some diseases, illnesses, and sicknesses. These spirits were "crying out" — a translation from the continuous form of *kradzo*, which conveys their *relentless wailing, screaming, and shrieking.* However, Jesus did not allow them to persist in their theatrical display. Instead, we find Him "rebuking" them firmly and forbidding them to run at the mouth.

The word "rebuking" is from a continuous form of the Greek word *epitimao*, which is a compound of *epi* and *timao*. As we've seen before, the first part of the word is *epi*, and here it conveys a sense of opposition. The word *timao* refers to someone or something held in high regard or worth. When combined, the word *epitimao* — which is translated as "rebuking" in this passage — conveys *a stern verbal reprimand* or *an assault on one's pride*. In this context, Jesus delivered a powerful verbal assault against the spirits and "suffered them not to speak."

It is important to note that Jesus "suffered them not to speak." Some who engage in casting out demons today believe in allowing demons to voice themselves, but the gospels reveal a different narrative. In the numerous episodes where Jesus expelled demons, we know of just one instance in which He posed a question to a demon and allowed it to speak — as famously recounted in the exceptional case of the madmen of Gadara in Mark 5:9 and Luke 8:30. Jesus understood that demons thrived on attention and melodrama, and to prevent their theatrical antics and to ensure a swift deliverance, He consistently silenced them, cutting short any opportunity for them to seize the spotlight as He cast them out.

## A WORD ABOUT DEMONIC OPPRESSION AND 'GENERATIONAL CURSES'

Before we come to the close of this chapter about how demonic attacks *can be* the source of disease, illness, and sickness, I want to answer questions concerning the following important points:

- *What about demonic oppression, and exactly what is oppression?*
- *What about avoiding places where demonic activity is present?*
- *What about hereditary and generational propensities?*
- *What about 'generational curses'?*

These are very important topics that deserve attention, so let's begin covering them.

There are some people who are "oppressed" mentally and emotionally, but they are *not* demonized, as in the cases we have seen in Matthew, Mark, and Luke. Nevertheless, they wrestle with varying levels of spiritual oppression that cloud their thoughts and emotions and that bind them in an unseen struggle within the confines of their own minds.

But first, what exactly is oppression?

It is crucial to differentiate *oppression* from *depression*. While depression might arise from various factors like setbacks, exhaustion, poor nutritional choices, an unyielding routine, or even an imbalance of chemicals in the brain, oppression is an entirely different beast. Depression often finds its roots within the intricate physiological, or physical workings of our bodies and can sometimes be alleviated by a change of scenery, taking time off, a shift in diet, prescribed medication, or the help of a godly counselor. Typically, the source of depression is physiological and can be alleviated by getting the right kind of help.

But "oppression" is a different matter altogether. The dictionary meaning for the word "oppression" is *the exercise of authority or power in a burdensome, cruel, or unjust manner.* Synonyms for oppression include: *abuse, brutality, coercion, compulsion, conquering, control, cruelty, dictatorship, domination, force, harshness, harassment, hardness, injustice, iron-handedness, maltreatment, overthrowing, repression, suffering, severity, subjugation, torment, and tyranny.*

We find the word "oppressed" used exactly in this way in Acts 10:38 when Peter said, "How God anointed Jesus of Nazareth with the Holy Ghost and with power: who went about doing good, and healing all that were oppressed of the devil; for God was with him."

In this verse, the word "oppressed" is derived from a variant of the Greek word *katadunasteuo*, which is a compound of the words *kata* and *dunamis.* The word *kata* denotes something that is *dominating, manipulating,* or *subjugating.* The word *dunamis* refers to *a power that is explosive.* When compounded, this word means that *oppression is a formidable force that seeks to dominate and manipulate an individual with great intensity.* The word *katadunasteuo* — translated as "oppressed" in Acts 10:38 — was historically used to picture a tyrant, dictator, or a nefarious monarch who forcefully imposed his will upon his subjects. This tyrant controlled every aspect of their lives, from their meals to their abodes and even their earnings, disregarding their desires and subjugating them to his will.

It reveals to us that when an individual is oppressed, their thoughts and emotions come under the sway of *an external spiritual influence* that seeks to distort their self-perception and cast doubt on their present or on what lies ahead of them, dictating the contours of their future. Should these mental strongholds persist unchecked, they grow into deep-seated oppression. Left unopposed, these chains of the mind manifest as despair and produce a sense of hopelessness in a person's mind and emotions. But the good news is that Jesus was, and He still is, anointed to break the bonds of oppression.

In Acts 10:38, we are reminded that Jesus was, and forever remains, anointed with the Holy Spirit and "power." The Greek word for "power" is *dunamis,* which *is explosive, superhuman power that comes with enormous energy and produces phenomenal, extraordinary, and unparalleled results.* This same word is used both in the New Testament and in secular literature to describe *the full might and power of an advancing army.* Such *dunamis* power is explosive and comes with unparalleled results when it is released!

But this verse continues on to say that Jesus went about doing good and healing all who were oppressed of the devil. We have seen the word "oppressed" pictures *the oppressive power of a wicked tyrant who rules over and cruelly tyrannizes his subjects.* In the scriptural context of Acts 10:38, the oppressor is unveiled as the "devil."

The word "devil" is derived from the Greek word *diabolos*, and this Greek word describes one who persistently attacks until he manages to breach a barrier in order to bring destruction, exert influence, and seize control. This name "devil," from the Greek word *diabolos*, also means *to accuse, defame, slander, or penetrate by continuous assault* or *to ensnare with a net* — thus it carries the notion of *entrapment.*

The adversary initiates this oppressive onslaught by bombarding the mind relentlessly, aiming to breach its defenses with unceasing strikes. Once he infiltrates its depths, he seizes control, turning the mind into a prisoner of its own thoughts. As a ruthless dictator, he starts to steer the course of emotions, thoughts, and beliefs, dictating every facet of their existence. He commands his captives, enforcing limits on their actions. He pulls them into a web of inaccurate thinking that entraps them, and, then, like a tyrannical ruler, begins to subdue them mentally and emotionally.

## THE BELIEVER HAS BEEN WEAPONIZED BY CHRIST TO RESIST THIS EVIL AND TO FIGHT BACK!

While this is what the devil attempts to do to people, no believer needs to be a victim. We have been redeemed from Satan's hold on our lives. If he is attempting to exercise control over a Christian, he is violating that believer's Christ-given freedom. But Second Corinthians 10:4 also states that God has equipped us with spiritual weapons that enable us to dismantle any oppressive forces that assail our minds and emotions. That verse says, "For the weapons of our warfare are not carnal, but mighty through God to the pulling down of strong holds."

The words "pulling down" are translated from a form of the Greek word *kathaireo*, which conveys *the notion of meticulously taking something apart, piece by piece, until it's reduced to rubble*. It signifies acts of *dismantling, demolishing, destroying, and disassembling* — much like tearing down a towering structure until no trace of it remains.

The word "stronghold" is derived from a variation of the Greek word *ochuroma*, a word that pictures *an imposing fortress* or *a fortified castle*. This fortress serves as a formidable barrier that is designed to keep *outsiders* on the *outside*, while the same word is also used to describe a dreadful prison constructed deep inside a fortress intended to prevent a hostage or prisoner from escaping. Conceptually, this usage tells us that a mental or emotional stronghold is a place of arrest, captivity, confinement, detention, imprisonment, or incarceration. When you have a mental stronghold, it is like a castle has been built in your brain, and evil spiritual forces attempt to dominate you from that high place like a tyrannical ruler.

Once you believe a lie, it morphs into "your truth," which grants it the power to shape your reality. When you welcome falsehoods that have been seeded into your mind by the adversary, these harmful thoughts solidify into a meticulously defended fiction. Finally, you find yourself captive to it, taken as a hostage to the mental stronghold. It is within the realm of the mind that such strongholds are erected, and it is here that oppression finds its breeding ground.

The adversary is acutely aware that whoever commands your thoughts wields power over you. Should the adversary gain sway over your mind, he knows that he'll be able to dictate what occupies your thoughts and beliefs. This extends to your self-image, which in turn influences your interactions with others and shapes how they perceive you.

From the lofty mental and emotional realm where your thoughts and feelings dwell, those evil forces begin to subdue your thoughts and dictate what you should believe, what you should feel, and what you should or shouldn't expect in your life. Those thoughts entrap you and make you feel as if you are living inside of a prison from which you cannot escape.

Despite the efforts of those on the outside who seek to help, they cannot seem to penetrate it because of the walls that have been formed by the lie. Oftentimes that lie becomes so formidable that when others try to tell them the truth, they are unable to hear it. But the Bible says you have the power to dismantle, disassemble, and, if need be, begin to take apart bit by bit any lie that is working in your mind and emotions.

Second Corinthians 10:5 goes on to say, "Casting down imaginations...." The words "casting down" are a repeat of the Greek word *kathaireo*, which again pictures *taking something apart, piece by piece, until it's reduced to rubble*. It signifies acts of *dismantling, demolishing, destroying, and disassembling.*

The word "imaginations" is interpreted from a form of the Greek word *logismos*, and it is used to denote *the reasonings of the mind*. If a falsehood has taken root in your mind for an extended period of time and now your mind and emotions are being oppressed, it's within your reach to cast down, dismantle, obliterate, shatter, take apart, and topple each of those dominating lies until it is completely gone and your mind and emotions are free.

Second Corinthians 10:5 goes on to say this is why you must be "bringing into captivity every thought to the obedience of Christ." The word "obedience" in this verse comes from a form of the Greek word *hupakoe*, which is a compound of the words *hupo* and *akoe*. The word *hupo* carries the idea of *being in a subservient position*, while the word *akoe* means *I hear*. Together they form an image of someone who not only listens attentively but also follows what is heard with unwavering submission.

To dismantle entrenched mental strongholds requires one to tune his ear to God's Word and then willingly submit to it. By aligning your mind and emotions to God's Word, you start the process that *dismantles* and *shatters* the oppressive lies that have long held dominion over your mind and emotions. If freedom is what you seek, shut your ears to the lies that have been controlling you, and open your ears — your mind and emotions — to what God's Word says about you. This will start the process of liberating you from the oppressive thoughts and emotions that have long attempted to rule your life.

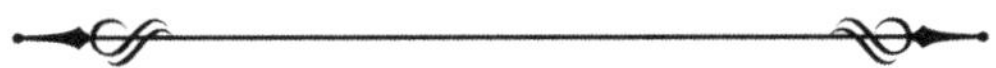

**The adversary is acutely aware that whoever commands your thoughts wields power over you. Should the adversary gain sway over your mind, he knows that he'll be able to dictate what occupies your thoughts and beliefs. This extends to your self-image, which in turn influences your interactions with others and shapes how they perceive you.**

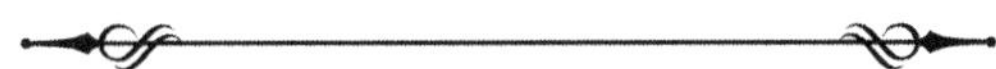

By way of review, if you are depressed, it might naturally be because of life's hurdles, burnout, dietary habits, a monotonous routine, or even a chemical storm brewing in your brain. The roots of depression can be intertwined with both mind and body. A fresh perspective from a change of setting, a well-deserved break, a change in what you eat, or even a counselor or carefully prescribed medication under the guidance of a professional can lighten the load.

Again, depression can affect one physiologically, or physically, but with the right support and intervention, relief is within reach. However, if a person is struggling with "oppression," although relief is also available within reach, it calls for resolution through spiritual means.

## WHAT ABOUT AVOIDING PLACES WHERE DEMONIC ACTIVITY IS PRESENT?

I do not wish to linger excessively on the workings of demon spirits, but I would be remiss not to refer to what the apostle Paul told the Corinthians about steering clear of places where evil spiritual forces are at play and that can result in one becoming spiritually oppressed. As we have seen in the previous section, when a person is spiritually oppressed, or demonized, it produces detrimental results, and for this reason Paul urged believers to stay away from places that reeked of demonic activity.

One such place that early believers were to avoid was pagan temples, where they often went to purchase meat. In First Corinthians 10:14,18-21, Paul wrote, "Wherefore, my dearly beloved, flee from idolatry.... Behold Israel after the flesh: are not they which eat of the sacrifices partakers of the altar? What say I then? that the idol is any thing, or that which is offered in sacrifice to idols is anything? But I say, that the things which the Gentiles sacrifice, they sacrifice to devils, and not to God: and I would not that ye should have fellowship with devils. Ye cannot drink the cup of the Lord, and the cup of devils: ye cannot be partakers of the Lord's table, and of the table of devils."

In this passage, Paul zeroed in on the particular concern of Christians consuming meat bought from temple bazaars, where the remains of sacrificial offerings were being sold for food. Devotees of pagan deities presented prime cuts as offerings to their gods. Following the rituals, a share of this choice meat would be allocated to the temple priests, while the remainder found its way to the public, sold at adjacent temple meat markets. Renowned for its quality, sacrificial meat was deemed the crème de la crème of available meats and caused temple markets to be a favored shopping destination for people.

Paul acknowledged that idols were nothing more than man-made objects completely devoid of power, but he well understood that a demonic presence thrived in these environments of ignorance and idolatry. This is why he admonished believers to "flee" from them. The word "flee" originates from the Greek word *pheugo*, which means *to run as fast as possible*, *to run hastily*, or *to take flight.* Paul instructed his readers *to constantly flee* from such atmospheres with no exception. He was emphatically stating that these places were rife with temptation and potentially spiritually sickening, so going to them should never be tolerated under any circumstances — not then, not now, not ever.

This is why he wrote in First Corinthians 10:19-20, "What say I then? that the idol is any thing, or that which is offered in sacrifice to idols is any thing? But I say that the things which the Gentiles sacrifice, they sacrifice to devils, and not to God: and I would not that ye should have fellowship with devils."

The words "that ye should" originate from the Greek word *ginesthai*, which is a derivative of the Greek word *ginomai* that can at times suggest something that *develops* over time. For example, one may not intend to become an alcoholic, but if his genetic makeup is prone to that disposition, the use of alcohol — over a period of time — may cause him *to become an alcoholic.*

By using alcohol, he has become something that could have been avoided altogether if the use of alcohol had never occurred. But Paul used the word *ginesthai* to sound a cautionary message about the perilous consequences of stepping into spaces that are steeped in evil. He was warning Corinthian believers that merely entering such places put them at risk of entangling themselves with demonic forces — and it could result in temptation, oppression, or numerous other insidious forms of vexation.

Paul additionally wrote in First Corinthians 10:20 that frequenting such places put them in jeopardy of entering into "fellowship with devils." The word "fellowship" is the plural form of the Greek word *koinonia*, from the word *koinos*, which refers to things that are *common* or *mutually shared.* The idea of *commonality* or *connectedness* is intrinsic to the meaning of this word. However, when *koinos* becomes *koinonia*, it more specifically describes *engagement*, *involvement*, *fellowship*, or *participation.*

So when Paul used this word in the context of demons, he was clearly stating that he didn't want his audience to become *engaged* and *involved* or to *partner* with demons as a result of being in evil environments. First Corinthians 10:20 could be interpreted, "...And I would not that ye should have participation with devils [as a result of being in the atmosphere of idolatrous sacrifices and activities]."

Paul perfectly understood there was nothing inherently wrong with the meat itself, but believers venturing into the dark environments to procure it raised the risk of their leaving under the oppressive influence of demonic forces that thrived in those places. Consequently, Paul advised against eating meat sacrificed to idols — not because the meat was somehow demon-affected — but because acquiring it necessitated going into places that were spiritually hazardous.

The apostle John was likewise concerned that his readers stay away from environments where demons operated, and in First John 5:21 he said, "Little children, keep yourselves from idols. Amen."

The word "keep" in this verse finds its roots in the Greek word *phulasso*, a word that basically means *to protect yourself*, *to guard yourself*, or *to shield yourself* from something. It carries the idea to *guard*, *protect*, *secure*, *shield*, or *watch over* in order to protect one from some outside foul force. The tense of the word *phulasso* here doesn't refer to a temporary alertness, but rather to a lifelong determination to remain wide-awake and on course to the very end.

John's use of this word in the context of idolatry and pagan celebrations conveys that we are to guard, protect, preserve, and shield ourselves from places of idolatry where demon activity flourishes. When John charged his readers to "...keep yourself from idols," he was urging them to stay on alert regarding the danger of idolatry. In Greek, the word "from" is the word *apo*, and in this case it implies *intentional distance*. Thus John was saying, "Be very intentional about putting distance between you and idols — or anything that is evil." To this command, he added the word "amen," which means *amen; so let it be*. It is an emphasis marker used to emphasize a statement of great importance.

**The *RIV* (*Renner Interpretive Version*) of First John 5:21 says:**

> **Little children, I immediately order you to withdraw from idols. Those idols — and what they represent — are so evil that you need to seriously guard yourself against them and stay away from them altogether. I'm leaving no wiggle room on this issue. I'm absolutely and emphatically ordering you to immediately put as much space as possible between yourself and idols. They are evil and represent a menace to your life, so you must urgently guard against them. What I'm telling you right now is not open for debate and is not optional. It is an order that I fully expect you to obey. In fact, to underscore the seriousness of what I am telling you, I'm even adding an "amen" to stress the point. I expect you to explicitly obey my instructions on this issue — and do it now!**

The reason I've chosen to highlight all this about evil environments is because many Christians inadvertently give darkness a foothold by being in the wrong environments, mingling with misguided friends, and looking at and listening to things that are spiritually dangerous.

You must always remember that God has positioned you as the sentinel of your own life, and it is crucial for you to be vigilant about where you go, the company you keep, and the images and sounds you allow to saturate your senses. Persistent exposure to evil images and negativity can slowly erode your defenses and potentially lead you into a state of oppression.

## FINALLY...WHAT ABOUT HEREDITARY AND GENERATIONAL PROPENSITIES?

When you step into a doctor's office to see the doctor, one of your first tasks involves diving into a detailed questionnaire that reaches beyond just your personal health. It delves into the history of your parents, grandparents, and other relatives. This investigative journey seeks to unearth any hereditary propensities that might form a pattern of potential health concerns in your life. It is well-known that certain traits and tendencies can be quietly handed down through the generations.

Discovering certain inclinations within your family tree doesn't set in stone that you'll inherit them in your own life. Consider it a cue rather than a command — a gentle reminder to be proactive and vigilant, and do your part to combat any familial tendencies that might try to affect your life. Beyond the good counsel of a doctor, it's vital to engage the transformative truth of your redemption, never forgetting the profound power found in the redemptive work of Christ on the cross.

As we will explore in Chapter Ten, your redemption set you free from the clutches of darkness and the baggage it historically carries. When Jesus' back was ripped to shreds to purchase your deliverance and healing, it encompassed even setting you free from every aspect linked to ancestral traits and inclinations.

When you recognize recurring themes in your life that echo through your family history, it is important to rally every resource at your disposal — whether it be prayer, faith, medication, or any other method you find empowering — to overcome them. Remember, your destiny is not bound by the habits or missteps of those who walked before you.

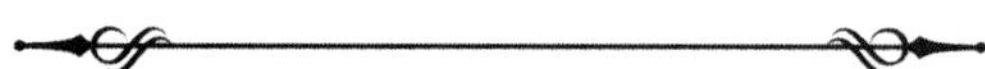

**God has positioned you as the sentinel of your own life, and it is crucial for you to be vigilant about where you go, the company you keep, and the images and sounds you allow to saturate your senses.**

Equally, if someone in your family is displaying an unhealthy pattern in behavior or health that is reminiscent of past generations, refrain from verbally dooming them with your words. Pray for that person and look for open doors of opportunity to speak into his or her life with instruction or encouragement.

Similarly, if any of your predecessors faced heart issues (or other physical maladies), for example, it's not your sealed fate to face the same sufferings. Rather, let it serve as a gentle reminder to eat right, practice good heart health, and take care of your body. Commonsense is not a contradiction to faith.

## WHAT ABOUT 'GENERATIONAL CURSES'?

In contemporary Christian circles, a growing number of believers have come to embrace the idea of generational curses. This concept suggests that the repercussions of ancestral sins ripple through time and affect descendants in ways that manifest as persistent familial struggles. Advocates for this belief often point out patterns such as divorce, adultery, incest, addiction, poverty, or recurring anger as evidence of a curse. Many fear that these patterns will haunt their own lives or even those of their offspring. Some individuals worry that the hidden secrets and past transgressions of their family might cast shadows over their own lives and suggest the eerie persistence of generational curses.

However, while we might inherit certain tendencies from our ancestors — some of which might not be the most uplifting — once the transformative power of Jesus' blood touched our lives, all such unfavorable chains were shattered, as you will see in the next chapter.

I have dear friends in ministry who focus on breaking generational curses. As I speak to them privately, I find that they actually believe the same thing I do, but we simply state it differently. I have appreciation for anyone who helps others walk free of generational propensities of any kind. We must use "every tool in the toolbox" to appropriate what is legally ours in Christ.

Should we find ourselves seemingly replicating our predecessors' behaviors or suffering with their similar health issues, let us not hesitate to act decisively to shatter these chains. When we find ourselves repeating the patterns of those who went before us, it is not enough to attribute our actions solely to a generational curse. We must ask the Holy Spirit to show us if we have learned bad traits from the environment where we grew up, and ask Him to help us change.

If needed, we should get pastoral counseling or professional help to identify areas that need to change, as well as advice about how to change. Instead of simply blaming predecessors for our current predicament, we must courageously accept responsibility for our part, seek forgiveness, and call upon the Holy Spirit to unleash His power to free us of these lingering effects.

We are saved through the precious blood of the Lamb, and our destinies are not shackled by the past. Yet wisdom tells us to use all available means to achieve freedom. Again, if professional guidance is what we need, we ought to earnestly seek it from the most skilled counselors. If medicine is required, then we must faithfully follow the prescriptions of trusted doctors until it is deemed that you no longer need them.

**We are saved through the precious blood of the Lamb, and our destinies are not shackled by the past.**

Every tool at our disposal should be used to secure the freedom that was bought for us on the Cross. Jesus endured immeasurable agony so that we might walk freely in this life, and it is our responsibility to utilize every resource available to claim and experience the freedom that is ours by inheritance.

## IF YOU ARE EXPERIENCING AN ATTACK AGAINST YOUR PHYSICAL OR MENTAL HEALTH...

Throughout this extensive chapter, we've delved into the intricate relationship between demonic influences and illness, and we've explored the impact of oppression and outlined strategies to conquer these challenges. I emphasized the importance of avoiding places where evil forces might thrive and highlighted the necessity of utilizing all available resources to break free from hereditary and generational tendencies.

In the upcoming chapter, we'll uncover the profound cost Jesus paid for your redemption. Then the subsequent chapters will offer invaluable insights and strategies for overcoming challenges that affect both your body and mind. As we navigate this path toward healing and health, you'll find a wealth of actionable advice designed to help you age gracefully, maintain your vitality and mental clarity, and continue thriving in your later years.

Scan the QR code to watch Rick teach more on this subject.

# QUESTIONS TO PONDER AND DISCUSS

1. At times, we open the door to attacks of sickness through the *entry points* discussed in Chapters Two through Eight. Think about one of the ways you've read about so far that has been a breach in your life through which the enemy has assaulted your body or mind. What was that crack, or entry point? Based on what you've read, write down what you can do, or are now doing, to thwart assaults on your life and close those entry points for good.

2. At other times, the attacks we encounter have nothing to do with our mistakes. The devil and his cohorts conspire to throw up roadblocks to hinder God's purposes for our life. But by aligning ourselves with God's authority, we're given all we need to repel every attack and ensure the enemy's retreat. Read James 4:7 in various translations — including the *RIV* as shown on page 253 — and discuss how submitting to God and His Word enables your authority in Christ and assures your victory.

3. Were you surprised to learn of the insight recorded by the Early Church fathers regarding the influence of demon spirits on the physical and mental health of people? Write down one quote that particularly resonated with you, along with a verse of scripture that corroborates or confirms what he wrote.

4. After reading the brief accounts of Jesus bringing deliverance to the suffering by the power, authority, and influence of God, it's clear to see the common thread that *Jesus desires to set the captive free!* In light of the fact that Jesus is the same yesterday, today, and forever (*see* Hebrews 13:8), how does that affect your faith for: 1) *your own total victory, deliverance, and freedom in every area of your life* and 2) *God to work through you in Christ's name to bring His power to others so that they, too, can live free?*

5. How did the sections on *hereditary and generational propensities* and *'generational curses'* also affect your faith and give you hope for your future that in Christ, truly "...old things are passed away; behold, all things are become new" (2 Corinthians 5:17)?

# NINE

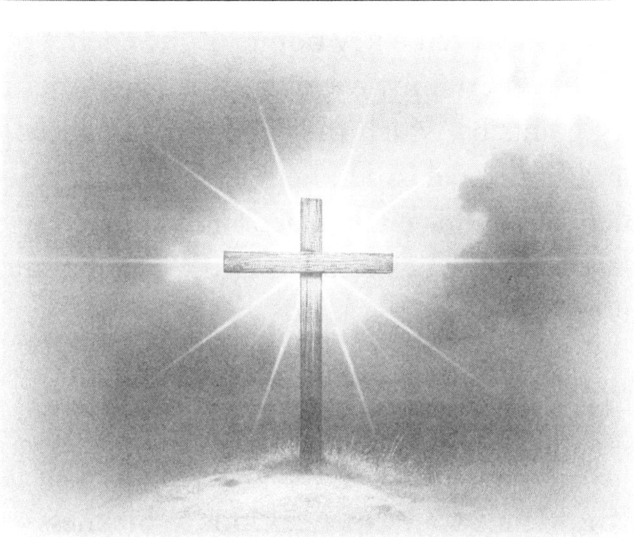

# REDEMPTION AND ITS ROLE IN BOTH YOUR DELIVERANCE AND YOUR HEALING

So far, we have seen seven reasons why Christians get sick. Of course these reasons can apply to those outside the family of God, but my purpose for sharing and expounding on these *entry points* is to reveal why believers often suffer with disease, illness, and sickness that Christ clearly redeemed them from in His death and resurrection.

What exactly happened when Jesus paid the ultimate price to redeem mankind from a life of slavery to sin and suffering? An enormously powerful transaction took place in that divine act, and that is what I'm going to share with you in this chapter. This is not a chapter to miss, for what I share in these few pages is fundamental to your salvation, your deliverance, your healing, and all the blessings that God purchased for you in Christ's redemptive act — blessings that were lost to mankind through Adam's *disobedient* act.

I'm going to review the seven entry points of the enemy that can bring sickness into a believer's life. Certainly, we know there are other reasons, but these are significant entry points by which the devil can access people's lives to cause physical, mental, and emotional issues. Let me encourage you that after reading the previous chapters, if you have taken action to shut every door to the devil, you are already on the path to experiencing the healing and health that was purchased by Jesus on the Cross.

To review, the seven primary *entry points* are as follows:

- The Biggest Culprit Is the Curse
- A Lack of Knowledge Can Open a Door to Sickness
- Disobedience Can Open a Door to Sickness
- Foolishness Can Open a Door to Sickness
- Unresolved, Hidden Issues Can Open a Door to Sickness
- Anxiety, Fret, and Worry Can Open a Door to Sickness
- Devilish Attacks Can Open a Door to Sickness

Over and over again, we have importantly seen that the Garden of Eden was a quintessential paradise that was unmarred by sin, illness, discord, challenges, and death — a place where Adam and Eve enjoyed harmonious communion with God and embraced the fullness of life, precisely as God originally intended for humanity. This blissful existence continued seamlessly until the moment Adam chose the path of disobedience.

Genesis 2:15 tells us that before Adam's transgression opened the door and allowed a deluge of death to come rushing into the earth, God had entrusted him with a crucial duty to "keep" the Garden of Eden. In the original language, the word "keep" encompasses meanings like *to guard, to place a hedge around,* or *to protect,* and it emphasized *a vigilant watchfulness* necessary to fend off any unwelcome intruder.

This specific choice of words underscores that God had already cautioned Adam of possible evil — it was a clear warning about the devil's aspirations to infiltrate that sacred sanctuary. Adam's charge was to stand as a sentinel and ensure that the Garden was impenetrable, and thus forbid any malevolence from crossing its threshold.

According to Genesis 2:17, God told Adam and Eve that they could freely feast from every tree in the Garden of Eden — with one exception: They were not to eat from the tree of the knowledge of good and evil. Yet the serpent lured Eve and seduced her to taste the forbidden fruit. Swayed by the serpent's cunning words, she took the fateful bite. As Adam witnessed his beloved's fall, he apparently chose not to be parted from her, so he, too, reached for the fruit and in doing so sealed their shared destiny. Adam's willful transgression swung the door wide open for death to wash over the world, and it soon shrouded the entire earthly realm in its somber embrace.

In Chapter Two, I gave the example of what happens when a mighty concrete dam is breached. When it surrenders to unrelenting pressure and succumbs to its own fragility, the formidable structure crumbles and unleashes a wild deluge of water, which rushes forth with furious momentum sweeping up everything in its chaotic embrace. The torrent spills over the land, turning serene fields into lakes, swallowing roads, and inundating buildings that stand in its path. Liberated from its concrete prison, the water surges on and leaves behind a wake of devastation — trees are uprooted, edifaces are reduced to rubble, and the once-familiar landscape is reshaped into an unrecognizable form.

This symbolically portrays what occurred in the spirit realm as a consequence of Adam's transgression. When he defied God's command, a spiritual door was flung wide open that unleashed a torrent, as if a barrier had been shattered. A flood of darkness and death surged across the earth and twisted and distorted everything that was originally created to be good. With this gateway for evil unlatched, darkness seeped into every crevice, and its inky tendrils spread across the globe, throbbing with a menacing pulse and radiating an aura of evil as it enveloped the world. Through the breach cracked open by Adam's disobedience, death stormed into the earth realm with ferocity.

Romans 5:12 rehearses the moment of this tragedy: "Wherefore, as by one man sin entered into the world, and death by sin; and so death passed upon all men…." This means that humanity, once vibrant and intimately connected with God in the Garden of Eden, suddenly experienced an irreversible fracture as death not only infiltrated the material world, but also seeped into the essence of the human spirit. Although they were created to be alive to God, Adam and Eve were now filled with spiritual death. Their once vibrant connection to God was tragically severed, and it left them adrift in a state of spiritual disconnection.

In an instant, Adam and Eve found themselves swept away from the embrace of God's Kingdom into a dominion where Satan reigned with an iron grip and where "steal, kill, and destroy" became the dark standard. It wasn't long before this sinister creed took root, and acts of stealing, killing, and destroying began their relentless march across the earth.

Once spiritually alive to God, Adam and Eve were now ensnared by a deluge of death that warped all it touched within the terrestrial sphere and that seeped deeply into their spirits. Through them it spread its insidious influence across the earth as their progeny were born into a world tainted by death and sin. In that egregious moment when Adam transgressed, death enthroned itself within the human spirit and eventually enshrouded the entirety of humankind, unleashing chaos in the world with alarming and relentless tenacity.

Once filled with God's life and covered by His glory, Adam and Eve had originally strolled through the serene paradise of Eden with their steps unburdened by worries or woes. But suddenly they found themselves cast out from this paradise into a world ruled by death that was cold and unforgiving. No longer cradled by Eden's gentle garden, they toiled in the stubborn soil beneath a sky that seemed dark. And where vibrant flowers once flourished, an army of thistles and thorns took their place. Although Adam and Eve were created to live forever in fellowship with God, after death came in they couldn't return to the Garden, and eventually they reverted to the dust of the ground.

In this new kingdom under death's shadow, life's symphony soured into a discordant lament filled with bitterness, chaos, and conflict. It was not long before the darkness took a chilling turn and begin to manifest in actions that were previously unimaginable — like the tragic day Cain, driven by envy and rage, murdered his brother Abel (*see* Genesis 4:8).

That act of violence was but a prelude to a greater decline, for soon death and its twisted nature would manifest as humans not only murdered each other, but became enmeshed in perversions of every kind and enamored with things contrary to the nature of God. When death's rule began, it also brought with it disease, illness, and sickness that never existed until Adam opened the door for evil to rage across the planet.

## SIN BECAME AN INTRINSIC PART OF OUR NATURE

As much as man tried to reform his ways, he could not, for now he was ruled by death at the core of his being. The only way to transform his behavior was to transform his nature at the core — an impossible feat by an act of mere willpower or natural human strength.

Indeed, for such a transaction to occur would require *redemption* — a supernatural act that would retrieve man from the prison of sin he found himself in and set him at liberty to commune with God again as Adam and Eve once did — and that is the subject of this chapter.

But before we get into the subject of redemption, it is imperative to see what Paul wrote about the spiritually dead condition that gripped the entire human race because of Adam's transgression. If you understand every human being's inborn penchant for sinning, you will better see why the human race was in need of *redemption* from the moment of its dreadful fall.

In Ephesians 2:3, Paul wrote before we came to Christ, we "were by nature the children of wrath, even as others." The word "nature" is interpreted from the Greek word *phusis*, which describes *innate qualities* or *inborn instincts*. For example, consider the moment a fish emerges into the world and how it immediately takes to swimming without a lesson or nudge. No one has to teach fish to swim; they instinctively swim because they are fish. It is the *nature* of fish to swim, and that is why they swim.

The apostle Paul used the word *phusis*, translated "nature" to describe the innate inclination in humans from birth to commit sin. *The New Living Translation* of Psalm 51:5 says, "For I was born a sinner — yes, from the moment my mother conceived me." This verse well states that human beings don't require lessons about how to lie, cheat, steal, or engage in wrongdoing. Sinning comes as naturally as breathing because it is woven into the fabric of a lost person's spiritually dead nature.

From the moment we enter the world, we grapple with an inherent propensity for mischief and wrongdoing. This is why even the most adorable infants, whom everyone finds utterly charming, can quickly reveal a penchant for cunning and bouts of tantrums. Picture parents who are captivated by their sweet little one in the high chair and marvel at their child's innocence.

Yet when the meal doesn't meet the child's liking, the same little angel astonishingly flings the food across the room and leaves mom and dad staring in disbelief. They can't help but wonder, *How can our precious baby act out so dramatically?*

How about telling a young child, "Don't touch that," only to observe him waiting for the moment he assumes he's beyond your gaze and can sneak a touch of the "taboo" item? What exactly compels a child to yearn for what is off limits? From the earliest age, humans, like tiny rebels on a quest, have an innate inclination to challenge boundaries and test limits. This innate desire to defy authority is a part of the fabric of human beings that goes all the way back to Adam.

Again, as fish instinctively swim because they're fish, children, starting even in the earliest stages of childhood, instinctively rebel and sin because at the core of their cute little beings, they are *sinners*. They will grow and develop physically, and once they reach a certain age at which they clearly understand their right actions versus their wrong ones — without Christ's intervention as Savior — they will continue to perfect their life of wrongdoing because of their inherently sinful nature.

Due to Adam's transgression, death entered into the spirits of all humans — thus the reason sinning is instinctive to all human beings. It is true that some bad habits can be taught and people can be negatively influenced by a bad environment, but even those raised in the best of circumstances — raised in church, sent to the best school, and given all the right tools for life — sin because humans are born with sin in the core of their nature.

In fact, Paul says that those without Christ are "children of wrath." The word "wrath" in Greek pictures something *contorted* and *distorted* beyond its intended purpose. Such an object is so skewed that it becomes irreparable and deserves only obliteration. This reveals the profound truth that there was nothing in us that could be merely repaired or restored, and that being in the grip of spiritual death, only a complete re-creation would suffice.

For those who claim, "I am not as bad as others," Ephesians 2:3 reminds us that before we were saved, *redeemed*, we were all "even as others." This reveals that, no matter how virtuous one's life may seem in comparison to others, everyone who is without Christ finds himself in the same spiritual predicament. The words "even as others" means that everyone belonged to this collective group of lost humanity before knowing Christ. Some may stumble less than others, but at the heart of every unsaved soul lies an inherited spiritual death — a legacy of Adam's transgression that caused spiritual death to pass into the spirits of all humankind.

## GOD IS RICH IN MERCY AND LOVE

But Ephesians 2:4 tells us, "But God, who is rich in mercy, for his great love wherewith he loved us…."

The word "rich" is translated from the Greek word *plousios*, which depicts *wealth of such magnitude that it defies calculation.* Imagine a treasure beyond vastness, a spectacular display of opulence, and an almost unimaginable profusion of resources — *that* captures the meaning of this word *plousios.* The word *plousios* was employed by Plato in his writings to illustrate the *boundless riches* of the legendary King Midas. Fast forward to the apostle Paul, who used this word in Ephesians 2:4 to declare that God is "rich in mercy." This emphatically means God's mercy is so endless that He possesses a vast fortune of mercy. In fact, in respect to the amount of mercy God possesses, He is absolutely rich with mercy that knows no bounds.

The word "mercy" is translated from the Greek word *eleos*, which can be translated as *compassion* or *pity*. But this is not mere wringing of the hands because of one's pitiful situation. Rather, it depicts *a deeply stirring emotion that drives one to take action*. This means when God saw us in our dire spiritual state, He didn't just wring his hands and say, "Oh, they're such a mess! They are so flawed, so defective, so bent, so twisted, so warped, and so spiritually dead, that there is nothing I can do to help them."

Instead, God was moved with *eleos* — mercy — and He took action to help us. From the wellspring of His boundless mercy, God sent Jesus into the world to accomplish what remained perpetually beyond our reach — it was a demonstration of profound love that brings us to the theme of *redemption*, which we'll explore in the ensuing pages.

In Ephesians 2:10, Paul declared that as a result of God's boundless mercy extended to us in Christ, we are now "his workmanship, created in Christ Jesus…." The word "workmanship" is interpreted from the Greek word *poiema*, and it describes *a poem*, *a product*, or *a thing marvelously made.* It is the very Greek word used to depict a *masterpiece.* This word *poiema* also historically denoted one who had the ability to create *a literary masterpiece.*

Paul used the word *poiema* to illustrate the transformation that occurs upon becoming a child of God. The message is that the moment of salvation marks when God employs His most potent powers and creative efforts to make you so brand new that once He is finished, you become His masterpiece that is skillfully and artfully created in Christ Jesus. This means when you were born again, God put all of His creative, artistic, intelligent genius into your making. And as the greatest writer of all, God wrote a new ending to your story!

**This means when you were born again,
God put all of His creative, artistic, intelligent genius
into your making. And as the greatest writer of all,
God wrote a new ending to your story!**

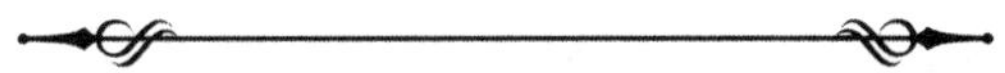

In fact, Paul said you were "created" in Christ Jesus. The word "created" is from a form of the Greek word *ktidzo,* and it describes *bringing forth something entirely from scratch.* This doesn't refer to an object that has been revamped or pieced together from old elements. Instead, it signifies *a pristine new creation* — utterly fresh and unprecedented. It's not about enhancement, improvement, repair, or renovation. It represents the creation of something new, novel, and unique. Those who come to Christ are not a spiritually improved, reformed, or renovated version of who they were meant to be; they are brand-spanking new!

In Ephesians 2:3, Paul described the spiritual dilemma faced by those who have yet to experience the transformative power of Christ, and in the succeeding verses, he painted a picture of God's infinite mercy and the incredible transformation that occurs when one allows Christ to reign supreme in his life. Yet this profound change is only possible through Christ's redemptive work on the Cross. To understand the biblical meaning of the word "redemption," let's proceed to see what it means to be *redeemed.*

## WHAT DOES IT MEAN TO BE REDEEMED?

When I was growing up, we used to sing a song written by Fanny Crosby that was called *Redeemed, How I Love to Proclaim It.* Oh, how I can still picture myself standing in the pew, surrounded by the congregation, as we all exuberantly declared, "Redeemed, how I love to proclaim it! Redeemed by the blood of the Lamb! Redeemed through His infinite mercy — His child, and forever, I am." Then we would jubilantly sing the chorus, "Redeemed, redeemed, redeemed by the blood of the Lamb! Redeemed, redeemed — His child and forever, I am."[1]

I sang that song with every fiber of my being, yet there were many layers to redemption that I had yet to discover. In the New Testament, the concept of "redemption" is expressed through four distinct Greek words: *agoradzo, exagoradzo, lutroo,* and *apolutrosis.* Each of these words offers a unique perspective in that they each share a connection to ancient slave markets. Let's delve into the nuances of these words and keep in mind their shared connection, and then we'll return to each of these four Greek words in a few pages.

## SLAVE MARKETS IN THE ANCIENT WORLD

In antiquity, many large cities had sprawling slave markets — places of unfathomable misery and sorrow. Eager purchasers would meander through the crowded aisles with his eyes scanning for the slave he desired. In these markets, human beings were placed on elevated platforms — auction blocks — where they could be viewed and eventually sold to the highest bidder. Before this buying, selling, and trading commenced, buyers were permitted to "inspect the merchandise."

For example, if a slave was going to be used in menial work that required a great deal of physical exertion, potential buyers might spit on the slaves, strike them, or hurl insults to assess their threshold for endurance. If a slave could suppress his pride, clench his jaw, and maintain composure amidst such demeaning treatment, it was presumed that he could toil in arduous labor without causing issues for his new master. This examination process was similar to taking a vehicle for a ride before committing to buy it. Just as a car buyer wants assurance of the value of what he's acquiring, those in the market for slaves sought to evaluate the "goods" before parting with their money.

Assessing the physical condition of slaves was crucial during auctions, and one important health indicator was the state of their teeth. Shiny, well-kept teeth often implied robust health and could elevate a person's value significantly. Conversely, if the teeth were decayed or rotten, it might lead to fetching a lower price. As a result, potential buyers would tilt back the head of potential candidates, pry open their mouth, and scrutinize the teeth to judge their condition, which influenced the buyer's bidding decisions.

Upon identifying a promising candidate, the buyer would agree to pay the required sum to acquire the individual and thereby transform the purchased slave into the lawful possession of his or her new master. Depending on their physical condition and skills, the price of a slave could range from a mere 500 denarii to an extravagant cost, amounting in the tens of thousands of U.S. dollars — as much as the price of a house![2] Male slaves possessing striking physiques, unique talents, and advanced education, often commanded exorbitant prices. The Romans had a particular preference for male slaves due to their ability to undertake a wider array of physical tasks compared to their female counterparts.

By law, slaves were not permitted to own anything — not even the clothes they wore — and slave owners wielded absolute power over them with the freedom to mistreat, exploit, or even execute them at their discretion. Regarded as mere property, enslaved individuals could be returned to the market when no longer needed to stand again under the auctioneer's gavel to be passed off to a new owner. Furthermore, their owners could choose to lend them to acquaintances or rent them out to others in need of labor.

During the days of the Roman Empire, slavery was prevalent in nearly every aspect of society. Whether enslaved by birth or through a twist of fate, millions of people found themselves bound to slaveowners. In the bustling metropolis of Rome, a staggering one-third of the city's one million inhabitants were slaves. This served as a testament to the relentless conquests of Roman legions, whose victories flooded the slave markets with more and more humans to be bartered and traded as mere goods.

There were primarily two categories of slaves in the Roman world — those that belonged to the government and those that were the private possession of individuals or families. Public slaves, owned by the state, were like the cogs of a mighty machine that powered grand architectural marvels that dotted the empire from horizon to horizon. But private slaves were owned by private individuals or families, and they generally possessed more freedom than public slaves.

Today when most hear the word "slave," an image comes to mind of individuals clad in tattered clothing and assigned to grueling tasks like bricklaying or laboring in fields. This stereotype held true in many cases in the ancient world, yet it doesn't paint the full picture. A significant number of slaves boasted exceptional skills and had high levels of education. Those under the ownership of wealthy masters frequently occupied esteemed roles such as household stewards, financial managers, or secretaries.

There were also slaves who were renowned philosophers, esteemed educators, industrious store managers, and even respected physicians. Thus, slavery transcended the boundaries of low-skilled, uneducated labor and extended to gifted and well-dressed individuals who catered to the upper tiers of society. Some slaves were entrusted with the crucial role of tutoring the offspring of affluent families. Remarkably, some slaves bore such a close resemblance to the general populace that the Roman Senate once pondered the idea of requiring slaves to wear distinctive attire so that it was clear who was a slave and who was not.

## WHAT IS THE SPIRITUAL SIGNIFICANCE OF THESE FACTS?

In Romans 6:17 and 20, Paul vividly reminds us that prior to Christ, we were all bound as "servants" of sin.

The word "servants" is translated from the Greek word *doulos*, which is more accurately rendered as *slave*. This Greek word specifically depicts *the most abject and degrading form of slavery*. It describes an individual who is utterly consigned to a life of bondage and perpetual slavery for the rest of his life. Such slaves existed solely to execute the commands of their owner, and their primary duty was to endlessly satisfy their master's every whim. This pictures one entrenched in the shackles of slavery, their own will entirely eclipsed by that of their master.

By using the Greek word *doulos* to describe who we were before we came to Christ, Paul illustrates the profound truth that prior to finding Christ, each of us was shackled in slavery to sin and the clutches of Satan. We might have fancied ourselves as the masters of our own destinies — believing we held the reins of our lives — but in truth, as we saw in Ephesians 2:2, we were captives that were ensnared in sin's unforgiving grip and our destinies were stealthily manipulated by a sinister, invisible force that controlled and manipulated us, bent on orchestrating our downfall in this life and the one to come.

You can be a Wall Street executive, a renowned architect, a celebrity athlete, or a billionaire businessman, but without the touch of God's grace on your life, your existence remains ensnared in the bonds of spiritual slavery. The truth is that every person, irrespective of prestige, status, or wealth, enters this world shackled by sin and is caught in the snare of spiritual captivity because spiritual death rules him at his core.

Whether people are poorer and less educated or whether they wear sharp suits, boast impressive credentials, drive expensive cars, and live in lavish homes — without yielding their life to Christ, their spirit remains unwashed by His redeeming blood. Until they surrender to the lordship of Jesus and allow His blood to cleanse their spirit, they remain a slave in Satan's slave market.

As we have seen, through Adam's disobedience, spiritual death entered into the spirits of Adam and Eve and all of their descendants. As we have seen, Romans 5:12 says, "...By one man sin entered into the world, and death by sin; and so death passed upon all men, for that all have sinned." With every passing generation following Adam, the chains of spiritual death tightened and led people of all nations, tribes, and ethnicities further into the depths of sin and depravity.

Paul writes about this predicament in Romans 7:14, where he states that we were "sold" to sin. The word "sold" is borrowed from the lexicon of the slave market. It comes from the Greek word *piprasko*, which describes *the complete legal transfer of ownership*. Through this imagery, Paul states that Adam's initial disobedience effectively handed over the entirety of humanity to Satan as a new master and owner. Thus, all of humankind lived under Satan's ironclad authority and were his possessions, all of which occurred as a consequence of Adam's transgression.

Like slaves in a slave market, we stood on the auction block, helpless as Satan slapped our lives around — hitting us, kicking us, spitting in our faces, and abusing us in any way he desired. The master of our chains was relentless and unyielding in his quest to shatter our self-worth and ensnare us with a myriad of issues that would mar us emotionally. When he finished using one kind of bondage and death to torment us, he would put us back on the trading block to be auctioned off again and allow yet another form of bondage to enslave us and begin to leave its destructive marks on our lives.

And so, we found ourselves shuffled from one chain to another in an unending loop of devastation and defeat. Day by day, whether we sensed it or remained oblivious to it, we were auctioned over and over again into the clutches of sin — wholly and completely from the core of our being to every part of our inner being. This is the reason why Paul referred to us as "the servants of sin" in Romans 6:17 and 20.

Our pre-salvation slavery to Satan and his dark kingdom was so entrenched that our nature became filled with rebellion, and the gulf separating us from God widened until Scripture describes us as having become "alienated and enemies" in our minds through wicked works (*see* Colossians 1:21).

Due to all of this, humanity became ridden with guilt, shame, turmoil, disease, illness, and sickness. But Jesus descended into this world where every living person was bound in Satan's grasp, and seeing us as captives that were shackled, guilt-ridden, tormented, and sick, Christ made the decision to pay whatever price was necessary to purchase us from Satan's slave market and reclaim us as His own. With a mercy that knew no bounds and a determination that soared beyond earthly understanding, Christ offered the ultimate price — His own blood — to secure our freedom and to make us His own.

## JESUS CAME TO DELIVER US FROM THE POWER OF DARKNESS

In Colossians 1:13-14, Paul wrote that Jesus' redemptive work delivered us from Satan's slave market. He said, "[God] who hath delivered us from the power of darkness, and hath translated us into the kingdom of his dear Son: in whom we have redemption through his blood, even the forgiveness of sins."

Among a host of important words in this passage, let's focus on the word "delivered." It comes from the Greek word *rhuomai*, which means *to rescue*, *to save*, or *to pluck from peril.* It pictures *someone being whisked away from harm's grasp* and suggests *an urgent deliverance that arrives precisely on time.* This word Paul chose reveals that Jesus embarked on a mission to free humanity from the clutches of the enemy and to rescue them from the devil's iron grip just when all hope seemed lost.

In Colossians 1:13, Paul stated that God delivered us "from" the power of darkness. The word "from" is a translation of the Greek word *ek*, which signifies *a departure or a way out*, and it is where we derive the word "exit." This illustrates that through the sacrifice of Jesus on the Cross, God *plucked us from* and gave us *a way out of* the grip of the "power of darkness."

The word "power" finds its origin in the Greek word *exousia*, which speaks of *authority, dominion, and influence*, and it means that all of humanity was living under the authority, dominion, and influence of Satan and his kingdom. The word "darkness" is translated from the Greek word *skotos*, and it suggests *the pitch-black absence of any glimmer of light*. In this verse, Paul used the word *skotos* to picture the *utter darkness* of Satan's sinister realm.

But then Paul went on to brilliantly declare that the very instant we welcome Christ as the captain of our lives, we are "...translated...into the kingdom of his dear Son." This word "translated" is derived from the Greek word *methistimi*, and it pictures *a transition from one realm to another.* Thus, the moment a person embraces Christ as Lord of his life, he is snatched from the clutches of darkness and transferred into the Kingdom of God. This marks his emancipation from the marketplace of sin and also marks his induction into the family of God.

First John 3:14-15 states that when we were translated from the kingdom of darkness into the Kingdom of God, we "passed from death unto life." The word "passed" is an interpretation of a form of *metabaino*, a compound of *meta* and *baino*. Here, *kata* implies *transformation*, while *baino* signifies *a journey* or *a walk*. When combined, the word *metabaino* pictures *moving from one realm to another* or *a shift in position and environment*.

At the very moment of our salvation, it means we were extricated from death's dominion — rescued from Satan's grasp — and we were transitioned into the Kingdom of God's Son. In the new Kingdom, there is no darkness or death at all, and that means all the toxins of the dark realm were left behind, and we moved into a Kingdom that is to be dominated only by the goodness of God. Thus, when we came to Christ, the power of darkness was broken over our lives!

## YOU WERE *REMARKABLY* SAVED

Hebrews 2:3 (*ESV*) describes this liberation as "such a *great salvation*." The words "such a great" are a translation of the Greek word *telikoutes*, and it denotes that which is *extraordinary*, *grand*, *majestic*, *magnificent*, or *truly remarkable*.

The term "salvation" originates from *soterias*, a variant of *sodzo*, a beloved New Testament term that equates salvation to *rescue from sin and death*, *healing*, *freedom*, *and complete wholeness* in every part of life. In the gospels, it is often translated *heal* or *deliver*. However, it fully encompasses *deliverance, restoration, preservation, and mental soundness*, and without a doubt affirms that deliverance and healing are an intrinsic part of salvation — and that includes complete liberation from the grip of demonic forces.

This is why Hebrews 2:3 calls our salvation "such a great salvation." Through His redemptive work on the Cross, Christ transferred us from the dominion of darkness and legally nullified all claims that the devil once held on us. Thus, our salvation is indeed a "great salvation" or a "grand deliverance"!

## THE FIRST WORD OF REDEMPTION: *PURCHASED* (*AGORADZO*)

But now let's return to the concept of "redemption" as it is expressed through a quartet of Greek terms: *agoradzo*, *exagoradzo*, *lutroo*, and *apolutrosis*. Each of these terms, as previously noted, connects us to the bustling world of ancient slave markets. So let's delve into the *first* of these powerful words, *agoradzo*, and explore its significance for our lives today.

Paul wrote in First Corinthians 6:20, "For ye are *bought* with a price...." This word finds its roots in the Greek word *agora*, which is a word referred to as *the marketplace*. But when transformed into *agoradzo*, it pictures *purchasing something in the marketplace* — and it was the identical word used to specifically describe *buying a slave out of the slave market*.

This word tells us that when Jesus entered the world more than 2,000 years ago, He walked into a vast, grim marketplace of souls where spiritual bondage reigned supreme. Humanity was ensnared, wandering in darkness, held captive under the iron fist of Satan who clutched the hearts of men and women with a fierce chokehold that saturated their very being with chaos and ruin. Entering into this realm that teemed with the pulse of demonic influence and the stench of death, Jesus came to procure our "redemption" for us, and He *bought* us (*see* 1 Corinthians 6:20)!

God sent His own Son right into the very heart of Satan's slave market to pay the price for humanity's freedom. This eternal transaction was sealed with the currency of Jesus' own blood, and it marked the end of our captivity under Satan's dominion. The word *agoradzo* translated as "bought" and "redeemed" in the New Testament illustrates that Jesus offered his own blood to reclaim us from Satan's slave market.

As a result, we who have embraced Christ's sacrifice no longer live under Satan's dominion. We have been legally transferred to the ownership of Jesus. Now as a child of God, we are legally the property of Jesus Christ, and He is our new Master and Owner.

This is why First Corinthians 6:19-20 says, "What? know ye not that your body is the temple of the Holy Ghost which is in you, which ye have of God, and ye are not your own? For ye are bought with a price: therefore glorify God in your body, and in your spirit, which are God's." This means you now legally belong to Jesus — spirit, soul, and body — and your body is the temple of the Holy Spirit. That is why Paul said, "...Glorify God in your body, and in your spirit, *which are God's*" (v. 20).

God's highest plan is for you to glorify God not only in your born-again spirit, but also with your physical body. You have been entirely freed from the grip of darkness and translated into God's Kingdom, and within this new realm, brokenness is healed, fear finds no foothold, anxiety vanishes, poverty transforms into plentiful blessings, and healing and health reign over any form of physical or mental ailment.

When Jesus rescued each of us from the clutches of Satan's grim marketplace, He unshackled us and severed the chains of spiritual bondage once and for all. Unlike the fate of most slaves who were traded repeatedly, Jesus redeemed us once and for all to ensure that we would never face the auction block again.

**Within this new realm, brokenness is healed, fear finds no foothold, anxiety vanishes, poverty transforms into plentiful blessings, and healing and health reign over any form of physical or mental ailment.**

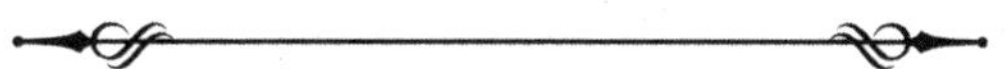

## THE SECOND WORD OF REDEMPTION: *EXTRACTED* (*EXAGORADZO*)

In the New Testament, the *second* word translated "redemption" is the Greek word *exagoradzo.* This word also traces its roots to the word *agora,* the Greek term for a *marketplace.* We find this word in Galatians 3:13, which says, "Christ hath *redeemed* us from the curse of the law, being made a curse for us...."

The word "redeemed" in this verse is a translation of the Greek word *exagoradzo.* It is a compound of the word *ex,* which is a form of *ek,* and the word *agoradzo,* as we saw in the previous section. The word *ex* means *out* and pictures *an extraction* or *an exit*, and the word *agoradzo* again means *to purchase or acquire something in a marketplace setting*. Historically, like the word *agoradzo*, it was also used to describe buying a slave from the market — and thus transferring that slave's ownership to a new master. But when the words *ex* and *agoradzo* are merged to form the word *exagoradzo*, it conveys the liberating of a slave from the market *permanently*, never to return to the old slavery again.

In antiquity, there were benevolent and compassionate slave buyers who acquired slaves for the sole purpose of granting them freedom. Upon being emancipated and attaining the status of freedmen, these former slaves were liberated for life. This word *exagoradzo* conveys the idea of *irrevocable freedom.* It represents *a permanent departure* from the despicable conditions of the slave market and ensures that a former slave would never again face the indignity of being put up for sale. The word *exagoradzo* pictures a permanent *exit* from that stinking, nauseating, disgusting, depraved, and cursed slave market.

Let's look at some instances where Paul employed the word *exagoradzo* to paint a picture of Jesus' redemptive work to permanently remove us from slavery. A perfect example of this word is found in Galatians 3:13, where Paul said, "Christ hath *redeemed* us from the curse of the law…."

In this crucial passage, Paul used the word *exagoradzo* to illustrate that through His sacrificial death, Jesus not only atoned for our transgressions, but He also permanently liberated and extricated us from the shackles of the curse. This means we are no longer bound to live under its oppressive weight because Jesus' sacrifice has severed those chains once and for all.

God's plan of redemption involved sending Jesus, not just to inspect our condition of slavery and to find us in depravity, but His ultimate plan, accomplished in Jesus Christ's death and resurrection, was to pay the price of Christ's blood to purchase us out of that miserable condition and make us His own sons and daughters who are forever extricated — *extracted* or *removed* — far from any curse!

In much the same way slaves in ancient times carried a hefty price tag, this liberation from Satan's grip and our transfer into God's Kingdom came at a significant cost. The price Christ paid for us is described in First Peter 1:19 (*AMPC*), where we read, "But [you were purchased] with the precious blood of Christ (the Messiah), like that of a [sacrificial] lamb without blemish or spot."

## THE THIRD WORD OF REDEMPTION: *RANSOMED* (*LUTROO*)

The *third* word used to describe "redemption" in the New Testament originates from the Greek word *lutroo*. This word illustrates the act of exchanging currency to purchase a slave from the bustling slave market so that a newly acquired slave now belongs exclusively to a new master and owner.

An example of the Greek word *lutroo* is Titus 2:14, which says, "Who gave himself for us, that he might *redeem* us from all iniquity, and purify unto himself a peculiar people, zealous of good works." The word "redeem" in this verse is a translation of this Greek word *lutroo*, which pictures the act of *ransoming* a slave from the chains of a former master and welcoming the former slave into the embrace of a new master and owner.

As we've already seen, if a buyer had his eye fixed on a particular slave, and the auctioneer knew he wished to acquire that exact slave, the cost could soar to exorbitant heights. Aware of a buyer's desire for a specific slave could result in the seller demanding an overwhelmingly steep price. The Greek word *lutroo* that is used in Titus 2:14 pictures the costly price Christ paid to liberate us from the clutches of Satan and bring us under His benevolent ownership and care.

Indeed, to shatter the chains of Satan's dominion — and for us to be legally transferred to the ownership of Jesus Christ — required an immense price to be paid. The price Jesus paid to claim us was unparalleled, surpassing any ransom ever paid for a captive in human history.

It was the price of Jesus' own blood that guaranteed our deliverance and lasting freedom from demonic powers that held us captive and that resulted in our transfer to Christ's ownership. This word *lutroo* — which describes redemption — unmistakably means that Jesus paid the ransom that set us free, and now we are legally the property of Jesus Himself!

## THE FOURTH WORD OF REDEMPTION: *RESTORED* (*APOLUTROSIS*)

In the New Testament, the *fourth* word used to convey the concept of "redemption" is the Greek word *apolutrosis.* This intriguing word is a compound of the Greek word *apo*, which implies *a return* or *a reversal*, and the word *lutroo*, which, as I previously explained, describes *the act of ransoming a slave to grant him lasting liberty and legally transition him to a new master.* But when these two words are compounded to form the word *apolutrosis*, it means *to pay the price required to buy back a slave with the goal of restoring his status.*

God's original plan was never for humanity to be filled with death or shackled by sin, nor to dwell as captives in realms ruled by Satan. This fourth word "redemption" tells us that Jesus offered Himself as the ransom in order to turn back the clock and return us to the former glory God planned for humanity before spiritual death entered the core of human existence. Put simply, Jesus bore the cost to shatter the grip of Satan upon us and ensure our freedom so we would be reinstated as rightful heirs and cherished sons and daughters of God Almighty!

Paul used the word *apolutrosis* in this very way in Ephesians 1:7 when he says, 'In whom [Christ] we have *redemption* through his blood, the forgiveness of sins, according to the riches of his grace.'

By using the word *apolutrosis*, Paul proclaimed that we were rescued from Satan's dark domain and reinstated to a position of rightstanding with the Father that was always meant for us from the beginning. It's no wonder that

Psalm 107:2 resounds with the exhortation, "Let the redeemed of the Lord say so!" Indeed, we have every reason to rejoice and declare that we are redeemed!

**Jesus bore the cost to shatter the grip of Satan upon us and ensure our freedom so we would be reinstated as rightful heirs and cherished sons and daughters of God Almighty!**

Galatians 4:7 says, 'Wherefore thou art no more a servant, but a son; and if a son, then an heir of God through Christ." Romans 8:17 proclaims that we are so entirely restored through the blood of Jesus that we have now become elevated to the status of "joint heirs" with Christ Himself. In addition to Jesus buying us back and setting us free from Satan's dominion, this word for redemption also includes your return to the divine blueprint that God crafted for you from the dawn of creation.

Friend, God designed you to be a free, full-fledged child of God. This intimate relationship with the Father was lost when Adam transgressed, and that is when death entered the world and passed into the spirits of all humanity. As a result, all of humanity from that point on was born into Satan's slave market. But when Jesus paid the price to ransom us, He transferred us from Satan's custody to His own custody, and He lovingly restored us to our intended status as cherished heirs in God's vast family.

There are a number of examples of this word *apolutrosis* that are used in the New Testament, such as Romans 3:24, which says we are "...justified freely by his grace through the *redemption* that is in Christ Jesus." Again, this word indicates we were not just purchased out of slavery, but were completely restored to our pristine state.

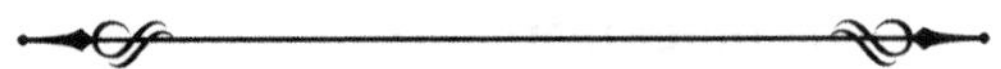

**In addition to Jesus buying us back and setting us free from Satan's dominion, this word for redemption also includes your return to the divine blueprint that God crafted for you from the dawn of creation.**

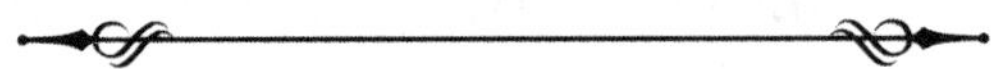

The word *apolutrosis* is also used in First Corinthians 1:30, "But of him are ye in Christ Jesus, who of God is made unto us wisdom, and righteousness, and sanctification, and *redemption*." The word "redemption" here is the Greek word *apolutrosis*, which embodies the idea of being restored to the original status as God's sons and daughters.

The apostle Paul also used the word *apolutrosis* in Colossians 1:14 when he declared, "In whom we have *redemption* through his blood, even the forgiveness of sins." Once more, Paul uses the Greek word *apolutrosis* — here translated as "redemption" — and it signifies our being snatched from the clutches of Satan, transferred to the ownership of Christ, and restored to our original God-given status. *All of this was procured with Jesus' blood!*

## A REVIEW OF THESE FOUR WORDS — *PURCHASED, EXTRACTED, RANSOMED, RESTORED*

When we take into account all these meanings and apply them to our redemption in Christ, we can conclude that the word "redemption" tells us:

- Jesus came into the world, Satan's slave market, because He was looking for us.
- Jesus wanted us and wouldn't be satisfied until the purchase of our freedom and our removal from Satan's clutches were complete.

- Jesus was willing to pay any price demanded to buy, or ransom, us from the slave market.
- Jesus purchased us with His blood, and we were transferred to His ownership and restored to God's original design.

## BREAKING FREE FROM A SLAVE MENTALITY

For believers, the shackles of Satan have been broken, his grip has been shattered, and God's sons and daughters are now living in His Kingdom that is dominated by light and everything good.

Yet many who have been redeemed and are living in God's Kingdom still carry with them the residual of captivity even though Christ has completely liberated them. A new way of thinking that aligns with His Word is required to enjoy the benefits of their liberation and freedom in Christ.

Let's compare this to what happened in antiquity when a slave was suddenly granted freedom. No doubt, when slaves in ancient times were bestowed with freedom, it was a moment of triumph. Yet this newfound freedom came with its own set of daunting obstacles. Although legally freed, many former slaves found themselves still psychologically shackled and living as if they were still in bondage.

For most slaves in antiquity, the very concept of living as a free person was foreign territory, and they were thrust into a world for which they had no "roadmap." While it was exhilarating for them to receive this freedom, it was catastrophic for many who did not know how to live as free men and women. Although legally emancipated, their minds remained ensnared in chains of slavery — a mindset that had been forged through years of oppression that proved difficult to break.

So far in this chapter, we've been talking about slavery in antiquity — but let's fast-forward to consider what happened to newly freed slaves on January 1,

1863, when the *Emancipation Proclamation* was issued in the United States during the time of President Lincoln. This monumental decree came amidst the tumultuous four-year long American Civil War — a fierce battle sparked by the contentious issue of slavery. This war, the most devastating in American history, claimed the lives of more than 600,000 individuals, nearly as many deaths as what occurred in all other American wars combined.[3]

When the bloody conflict of the Civil War concluded, Abraham Lincoln had already signed the *Emancipation Proclamation,* which stated, in part, as follows:

> That on the first day of January, in the year of our Lord, one thousand eight hundred and sixty-three, all persons held as slaves within any State or designated part of a State, the people whereof shall then be in rebellion against the United States, shall be then, thenceforward, and forever free....[4]

In the proclamation, Abraham Lincoln additionally declared:

> ...I do order and declare that all persons held as slaves within said designated States, and parts of States, are, and henceforward, shall be free....[5]

With the stroke of Lincoln's pen, the chains of slavery were officially broken. Every enslaved person in America didn't taste the sweetness of liberty immediately, but the Emancipation Proclamation legally changed the standing of more than 3.5 million of the nearly 4 million enslaved African Americans and marked the beginning of their transition from bondage to freedom. Then the final, formal end to slavery in the United States came with ratification of the Thirteenth Amendment to the U.S. Constitution in December 1865.[6]

As we have seen, slavery dates to ancient times. But the harrowing reality of American slavery was marked by *extreme brutality.* Slaves endured unthinkable abuse and a litany of violent acts that included beatings, whippings, and often mutilations, such as castration, branding, forced piercings, limb amputations — and, all too frequently, death. The torment extended beyond physical anguish, as many enslaved men and women suffered grievously at the hands of their masters, often even atrociously subjected to sexual abuse.

But like the dawn breaking after a seemingly endless dense, dark night, the long-held dreams of slaves to be freed was finally fulfilled as they crossed the threshold into freedom and, in the eyes of the law, became free men and women. For generations, they had dreamed of, prayed for, and awaited this day — and at last, their prayers were answered. Physical shackles fell from them, but the lingering mental and emotional bonds of slavery continued for years as newly freed slaves faced the monumental task of liberating themselves from the continuing effects of enslavement.

In early New Testament times, a slave's emancipation was an uncommon event that occurred sparingly when individual slaves were redeemed by benevolent buyers who set them free. However, a "seismic" shift in history occurred in the United States on January 1, 1863, when, in one bold stroke, a staggering 3.5 million American slaves were granted their freedom *simultaneously*.

Yet making a payment to secure the freedom of a slave, as in the days of antiquity — or signing a legal document to alter one's status and grant him freedom — does not necessarily mean a person will walk free from the mental chains that bind him or obstacles that challenge him. For example, although the chains of slavery were gone in the post-emancipation era in the U.S., life for many who were freed proved to be a formidable challenge.

Those who had been newly freed needed to make their own way instead of working tirelessly to make someone else's way as they had done, profiting their previous owners. For some, that would require additional training if there was a particular trade he or she wanted to practice. It's also likely that a lack of education under slavery now stood as an obstacle that had to be surmounted.

Just because legislation had been passed and signed into law guaranteeing slaves the right to live as free men and women didn't mean opportunities to grow and develop as equal members of society automatically opened to them. Slavery had been evil and oppressive, but a society largely hostile toward those who'd been freed was to be yet another vexing challenge for them to overcome.

But buoyed by an unwavering faith in God, former slaves boldly embraced the promise of freedom, embarking on an extraordinary journey determined to lay down roots — deciding where they would live, work, and raise their families. And with a fierce desire for knowledge, they explored avenues to educate themselves and their children.

Despite beginning with scarce possessions and little financial means after that dark period of history, those who were newly freed seized opportunities to attend school, pursue higher education, and nurture entrepreneurial dreams. They pursued careers in medicine, law, journalism, entertainment, and a myriad of other professions. Many became profoundly successful as educators, pastors, and ministers of enormous churches and ministries. Still others stepped boldly into the political arena to hold public office and help reshape the very society that once enslaved them.

But all of this transformation occurred not just after legally obtaining their freedom, but as a result of their choosing to forge ahead, doing what was necessary to step into their new identity.

## HOW ALL OF THIS RELATES TO YOU AS ONE MADE FREE IN JESUS CHRIST

Jesus came into the world, Satan's slave market, because He wanted us, and wouldn't be satisfied until the purchase was complete and we were made free. He was willing to pay any price demanded to buy us from that cruel marketplace. He gloriously purchased us with His blood, transferred us to His ownership, and legally restored us to God's original design.

Technically, the shackles of Satan have been broken, his grip has been shattered, and we now live in the Kingdom of God that is dominated by light and everything good.

Yet the fact remains that you — like many others whom Christ has thoroughly redeemed — may still be living with the residual effects of captivity that held you physically and mentally before God's grace touched you and liberated you. Like slaves in ancient times and in more recent American history, your salvation was a moment of triumph, but although you have been made free, you may still find yourself psychologically shackled and living in bondage despite your Christ-given freedom. And you will undoubtedly at some point find yourself challenged by the enemy of your soul, from whose kingdom you were liberated.

With the shedding of His Blood, Christ broke the chains of spiritual slavery and all its accompanying effects. The shackles fell from you, but there may be lingering physical and mental effects that try to hang on to your life. For you to step up into the newfound freedom that Christ purchased for you will require you to learn how to "think" as a person whom Christ has freed.

- Just as a set-free slave had to learn all the nuances of what it meant to be free, once you are snatched from the powers of darkness and translated into the Kingdom of God's Son, you must determine to learn what the Bible says about Christ redeeming you and setting you free and what it really means when it says that you are no longer a slave to sin or to its death-dominated consequences.
- Just as a set-free slave had to learn how to think as a free person, once you are snatched from the powers of darkness and translated into the Kingdom of God's Son, you, too, must learn to "think" habitually as one whom Christ has completely liberated from your former shackles. This means you must mentally reject past bondages and spiritually embrace all the benefits of redemption — that is, forgiveness of sin, freedom from guilt and shame, peace of mind, and the healing and health that are yours by virtue of Christ's work of redemption.
- Just as a set-free slave had to overcome a once-entrenched slave mentality, after you are snatched from the powers of darkness and

translated into the Kingdom of God's Son, you must determine to bend your mind to the truths of God's Word, which has the power to wash away any lingering slave mentality from your thinking (*see* Romans 1:16; Ephesians 5:26).

**Once you are snatched from the powers of darkness and translated into the Kingdom of God's Son, you must determine to learn what the Bible says about Christ redeeming you and setting you free and what it really means when it says that you are no longer a slave to sin or to its death-dominated consequences.**

## THE ROLE OF RENEWING YOUR MIND

For you to shed the lingering effects of past bondage, you must embark on what the Bible describes as "renewing the mind," in which old beliefs and wrong ways of thinking are uprooted and replaced with right beliefs and thinking that are aligned with the reality of Christ's work of redemption.

At the moment of salvation, the human spirit instantly undergoes a profound rebirth and becomes entirely new, while the mind and body remain untouched, awaiting the transformative power of God's Word. It's crucial to consciously align your body and mind with your divine birthright as God's child. Every day that you delve deeper into these truths, unraveling the tangled misconceptions handed down by family, teachers and authority figures, religious institutions, tradition, folklore, and society, these erroneous beliefs will dissolve and you will begin to experience the fullness of redemption that Christ secured for you.

This is precisely why God repeatedly urges us to renew our minds. In the following verses we are commanded to submit and subject our minds to truth that has the power to break the lingering effects of slavery that cling to our thinking and negatively affect our ability to walk in healing and health. We are told:

- "...Be ye transformed by the *renewing* of your mind..." (Romans 12:2).
- "...Be *renewed* in the spirit of your mind" (Ephesians 4:23).
- "...Put on the new man, which is *renewed* in knowledge after the image of him that created him" (Colossians 3:10).

In Romans 12:2, the word "renewing" is interpreted from a form of the Greek word *anakainosis,* which is a compound of the words *ana* and *kainos.* The prefix *ana* implies a sense of *renewal* or *repetition* and suggests *a dynamic movement upwards.* The word *kainos* conveys the notion of something *entirely fresh* and *original.* Together, they form a vivid image of *a mind undergoing a transformative renewal — a realigning to its rightful order and put on an upward trajectory* rather than a descent into destruction. It likewise means *to make new* or *to renew* to an original state.

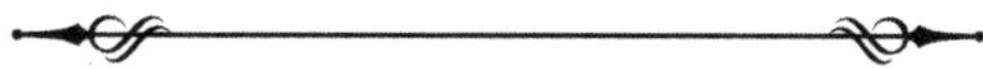

**At the moment of salvation, the human spirit instantly undergoes a profound rebirth and becomes entirely new, while the mind and body remain untouched, awaiting the transformative power of God's Word.**

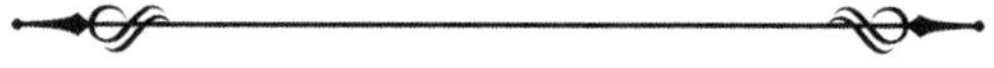

In Ephesians 4:23, the word "renewed" is translated from a form of *ananeoo,* which is another compound word. The first part of the word is the Greek word *ana,* which again implies a sense of *renewal* or *repetition* and suggests *a dynamic*

*movement upward.* The second part of the word is derived from the Greek word *neos*, which is the word for whatever is *fresh*, *young*, or *youthful.* When these two words are compounded, rather than picturing an older mind that is affected by age and life, it instead speaks of a mind that is *regenerated* to be *fresh, young, and youthful* — free from the negative effects of life and thus *renewed* to be as God originally intended it to be.

In Colossians 3:10, the word "renewed" is from a form of *anakainoo*, the same word we just saw that is also found in Romans 12:2, and it pictures *a mind undergoing a transformative renewal — realigning to its rightful order and upward trajectory* rather than a descent into destruction. And it likewise means *to make new* or *to renew* to an original state.

In Colossians 3:10, Paul told us that this mind renewal is connected to "knowledge" — and this is a clear reference to God's Word. In Ephesians 5:26, Paul wrote that the Word of God is like water and that, as we pour the Word of God over every nook and cranny of our minds, like water, it begins to carry away the residual wrong believing and thinking that may have persisted in us from our lives before we came to Christ.

Not only does this "washing of the Word" carry away the remnants of a slave mentality, it miraculously causes the mind to *realign to its rightful order and puts it on an upward trajectory* rather than a descent into destruction. It likewise means *to make new* or *to renew* to an original state. God's Word causes the mind to be *regenerated, fresh, young, youthful*, and free from the negative effects of life — and thus *renewed* to be as God originally intended it to be. When God's Word works in our minds, it *renews the mind* to the original state that God intended for it to be in.

## LIVING IN THE ILLUSION OF BONDAGE — WHY PEOPLE STILL STRUGGLE IN THE STORM

Just as former slaves embarked on an extraordinary journey to embrace their newfound freedom and live transformed lives as citizens, you must determine to understand what Christ did for you at the Cross and then to lay full claim to your new identity in Christ.

There are millions of Christians whom Christ has redeemed, but who are still living and struggling as if they are still held captive. This book especially focuses on disease, illness, and sickness — which Christ absolutely redeemed you from on the Cross, as we will see in detail in the next chapter — but you might find yourself wondering, *If I've truly been liberated from Satan's grip and the evil that accompanies him, including disease, illness, sickness, and all his evil effects, why does it feel as though the storm hasn't yet subsided for me? Why am I dealing with ailments in my life? While I know that forgiveness and peace of mind are promised to me in Christ, I'm puzzled about why physical and mental issues still linger if healing and health are indeed included in redemption.*

I want to respond to these questions by sharing a true story with you. Years ago, in the middle of the night, a friend of mine was jolted awake by the unexpected ring of his phone. The voice on the other end belonged to a police officer, who told him that one of his goats had strayed from his property and had been hit and killed by a car and was lying in a ditch. My friend hastily threw on his jacket and made his way to the site of the alleged accident and braced himself to find his dead goat.

But contrary to what the police had told him, when my friend arrived on the scene, he found that his goat was very much alive. Someone had stolen it, cruelly tied it with ropes, and tossed it into a ditch by the roadside. When my friend saw that the terrified goat simply needed to be freed, he crawled into the ditch and went about freeing the goat, grateful the story had not ended in tragedy.

My friend jubilantly leaned over and loosened the last piece of rope restraining the goat and then gave his freed goat a gentle pat. "Get up!" he said, yet the goat remained sprawled on the ground as if the ropes still held it fast. Undeterred, my friend patted the goat again and said, "Get up!" But the goat lay motionless as though it was still bound. My friend was bewildered by the goat that simply wouldn't get up, so he began to inspect the goat to search for any injury that might be hampering its movement.

That's when he saw that the goat's legs were clenched tightly together, mimicking the posture of being tied up. Suddenly, my friend realized that although the goat was completely free, it still thought it was bound. So my friend pulled the goat's legs apart, gently placed the animal in an upright position, and with another, stronger pat said, "Come on, get moving!" Suddenly the goat seemed to awaken to the exhilarating reality that its legs were free, and it sprang to life and leaped with joy in its liberation. The goat had already been set free, but it was bound by the *illusion* of bondage.

When my friend told me his goat story years ago, I couldn't help but draw a parallel between this goat and many Christians that I knew. There was a time when we were all ensnared by the bondages of Satan, shackled by his destructive grip and living in the domain of darkness. But as the Gospel touched our hearts and we gave our lives to Christ, the Holy Spirit made His home within us and every chain Satan had used to bind us was unfastened and every tether that held us was legally severed.

Yet despite this wondrous liberation, many Christians continue to live as if they are ensnared in captivity, unaware of the freedom that redemption has granted them. They remain in their experience as those who are still captive because the truth hasn't renewed their thinking.

The truth is, in Christ you have been set free! Galatians 4:5 says that Christ came "to redeem them that were under the law, that we might receive the adoption of sons." Galatians 4:7 says, "Wherefore thou art no more a servant, but a son; and if a son, then an heir of God through Christ." In John 8:36, Jesus said, "If the Son therefore shall make you free, ye shall be free indeed." Your freedom is not an illusion; it is a reality.

Now that Christ has set us free, He calls out to us with a clarion voice and tells us, "Get up! Get moving! I have already loosed all the chains that Satan placed upon you. With My blood, I broke every chain that once held you, and I have purchased your freedom in full. Stop living in the illusion of bondage and start rejoicing that you are redeemed!"

If you relate to the story of the goat — and you feel as if you are continuing to live in the illusion of bondages that Christ has already shattered and removed from your life — it's time to align your body and mind with the truth of Christ's redemptive work. It's time for you to get up, get moving, and start enjoying the full benefits of your redemption in Christ, and that includes reclaiming your healing and health!

## A FINAL WORD: YOUR PHYSICAL BODY CAN REFLECT THE MIRACLE OF REDEMPTION

Because you were purchased with the precious blood of Jesus, Paul urged you in First Corinthians 6:20 to "glorify God in your body, and in your spirit, which are God's."

This verse says that you are to glorify God in your "body." Of course we are to glorify God by living a life of holiness, but this indicates that your entire being — body, mind, and spirit — belongs to God and should reflect the miracle of redemption at every level. In respect to healing and health, it means that rather than succumbing to the devil's assaults that affect our bodies and minds, we must employ the power of faith and wisdom to resist physical and mental ailments and attacks, and thereby exalt the profound work of Jesus' sacrifice on the Cross and His intention that you radiate health and wholeness.

Christ has redeemed us from the curse (*see* Galatians 3:13), and a major part of the curse was disease, illness, and sickness. If you are redeemed, it isn't God's intention for any lingering results of the past curse to exericse dominion over your life — and that includes any lingering disease, illness, or sickness. Instead, God desires for you to fully experience and enjoy the healing and health that Christ secured through His redemptive sacrifice on the Cross, along with all the other benefits of redemption!

Now that we have covered what the word "redemption" means, we are ready to delve into the specifics of what Jesus accomplished on the Cross for you and me — for spiritually enslaved humanity. The insights you are about to read in the next chapter are designed to provide you with a solid scriptural base, revealing how Christ secured forgiveness of sins, liberation from guilt and shame, peace of mind, and the promise of healing and health. Get ready to immerse yourself in these powerful truths, which will illuminate the immense price He paid for our sake.

**We must employ the power of faith and wisdom to resist physical and mental ailments and attacks, and thereby exalt the profound work of Jesus' sacrifice on the Cross and His intention that you radiate health and wholeness.**

Scan the QR code to watch Rick teach more on this subject.

## QUESTIONS TO PONDER AND DISCUSS

1. After reviewing the devastation that befell mankind upon Adam's and Eve's disobedience, what does Romans 5:15-19 tell you about the mighty restoration project God planned in order to redeem us back to Himself through the sacrifice of His Son? Use Romans 5:20 to construct your answer. God did a "far-exceeding" work in making a way for us to be *purchased*, *extracted*, *ransomed*, and *restored*. Do you remember the day you embraced Christ's sacrifice for yourself and received the unmerited grace of God that saved you? Would you be willing to write out your testimony or share it with someone else who needs to hear it?

2. Based on what you learned about the four Greek words for redemption — *agoradzo* (*purchased*); *exagoradzo* (*extracted*); *lutroo* (*ransomed*); and *apolutrosis* (*restored*) — what happened to you at the moment you experienced salvation and were delivered from Satan's slave market?

3. To walk out these four redemption words experientially requires that we renew our mind with God's Word and align our thinking with the truth of this "great salvation" acquired for us (*see* Romans 12:2; Hebrews 2:3). Mind renewal doesn't occur if we're only reading the Bible on a "hit-and-miss" basis. Describe your daily time with the Lord in His Word and in prayer — in communion with Him. Does anything need to change concerning the quality time you're spending with your Savior? Remember, this daily routine isn't about rote *works* — it's your *lifeline* to walking in the joy, peace, strength, and victory He provided for you and intends for you to have.

4. Based on your answer to Question 3, what can a believer do to break free from a slave mentality, as illustrated in this chapter regarding slaves in antiquity and, in more recent times in history, in the United States? Give one example of a mental belief or mindset you brought with you into your new life in Christ (*see* 2 Corinthians 5:17). Your spirit was reborn, but your mind and body has yet to be redeemed. What was one wrong belief that you had to

wash away from your thinking with the "water of His Word" (*see* Ephesians 5:26)? (For example, beliefs that God doesn't want to bless people; that He doesn't always keep His promises; that everything that has happened in your life came directly from Him; etc.) What scriptures did you use to perform that mental and emotional "washing"?

5. Consider the true story of the goat that seemed paralyzed because it thought it was still tied up and bound with ropes, although it was completely untied and free. Have you ever behaved similarly in situations where you had perhaps been traumatized — and you still saw yourself as victimized and *bound*? Who gave you that encouraging "pat" to get up and get moving? Was it a pastor, a parent, a spouse, a mentor, or a friend? Write down your own journey of being rescued from a spiritually paralyzing state so you could get up and get moving with your life again.

# TEN

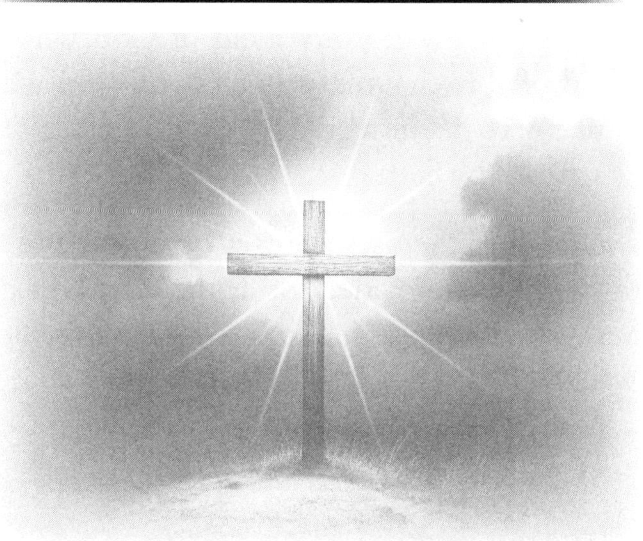

# WHAT EXACTLY DID JESUS' SACRIFICE PURCHASE FOR YOU?

The Bible shows us that healing and health are an inseparable part of what Jesus provided through His redemptive work on the Cross. In fact, healing and health belong to you just as God's forgiveness, freedom from guilt and shame, peace of mind, and everything else belongs to you that was provided in redemption. What Christ endured in His scourging and death on the Cross was literally a deathblow to sin, disease, illness, and sickness — and through faith in His work on the Cross, we can enter into wholeness in every part of our being.

In this chapter, I want to show you that Isaiah, Matthew, and Peter all wrote in agreement that when Jesus died for us, He paid the price to obtain healing and health for us — and healing and health are an inseparable part of what Jesus provided through His atonement.

We can rest in the fact that these gifts are nestled safely in the spiritual bank of Heaven, and they readily await every child of God who will lay claim to them. And at the end of this chapter, we will finally see what Jesus declared about Himself in Luke 4:16-19 in regard to His anointing to deliver and heal anyone who comes to Him by faith.

Yet many Christians find themselves beset by illness and are unaware that healing and health have been provided for at the Cross. Healing is the rightful inheritance of every child of God, and it is God's fervent desire for you to embrace a life of wellness.

**We can rest in the fact that the gifts of healing and health are nestled safely in the spiritual bank of Heaven, and they readily await every child of God who will lay claim to them.**

## A DEEPER LOOK AT ISAIAH 53:3 — 'DESPISED' AND 'REJECTED'

Nearly 700 years before Christ, the prophet Isaiah prophesied about the suffering that Christ would endure and the purpose for it. In Isaiah 53:3-5, the prophet wrote, "He is despised and rejected of men; a man of sorrows, and acquainted with grief: and we hid as it were our faces from him; he was despised, and we esteemed him not.

"Surely he hath borne our griefs, and carried our sorrows: yet we did esteem him stricken, smitten of God, and afflicted. But he was wounded for our transgressions, he was bruised for our iniquities: the chastisement of our peace was upon him; and with his stripes we are healed."

Throughout the Old Testament, no prophecy about Christ's suffering and eventual glorification is as clear as what Isaiah presented. But starting in verse 3, Isaiah said, "He is despised and rejected of men; a man of sorrows, and acquainted with grief: and we hid as it were our faces from him; he was despised, and we esteemed him not."

In the pages of this book, I have repeatedly stated with assurance that Christ paid the price for forgiveness of sin, freedom from guilt and shame, peace of mind, and healing and health. I have also promised that in this chapter, we will delve into passages written by Isaiah, Matthew, and Peter that confirm Christ obtained these for us in His redemptive work on the Cross.

**It is God's fervent desire for you to embrace a life of wellness.**

Because the words of Isaiah are so pivotal in this discussion, we will begin with his prophetic words in Isaiah 53:3. In this verse, Isaiah began by vividly describing that Christ would be "despised" and "rejected" of men. The word "despised" originates from a Hebrew word frequently encountered in the Old Testament that paints a picture of *disdain* and *scorn.*

The gospel accounts of Matthew, Mark, Luke, and John confirm, Jesus was disdained and scorned, vividly illustrating how He was subjected to extreme derision by religious authorities, guards, soldiers, and political figures alike. Various translations of the word "despised" include *despised, disdained, disesteemed, held in contempt*, or *scorned.*

In the span of His three-year public ministry, Jesus was "despised" and treated with contempt nonstop by the religious leaders of His day. Their verbal onslaughts and relentless attempts to undermine Him were unyielding. But their contempt of Him reached its zenith on the night He was betrayed by Judas Iscariot. Upon His arrest in the serene Garden of Gethsemane, Jesus was taken to the residence of Caiaphas, the high priest. It was there that Jesus encountered the brutal hostility of Israel's most revered religious figures. Behind closed doors, these leaders descended upon him like a riled nest of vipers, unleashing their fury with words of venom, spitting on Him in irreverent contempt, and inflicting physical blows upon Him.

Following His interrogation by Pilate and Herod Antipas, Jesus endured unspeakable cruelty at the hands of Roman soldiers. They mocked and cursed Him, striking His face with a reed plucked from Pilate's courtyard. In their brutality, they yanked the beard from Jesus' chin and crafted a painful crown from vines with razor-sharp thorns and forced it onto His head.

As if this torment was not enough, Jesus was led to a whipping post, where two merciless scourgers used their savage instruments to rend His body open with each vicious lash. Of course, ultimately, Christ's hands and feet were pierced with nails that secured Him to the cross they used to crucify Him. These acts of brutality were the bitter fulfillment of Isaiah's prophecy in Isaiah 53:3, which said that He would be "despised" and shunned by the very people He came to save.

But Isaiah 53:3 also prophesied that Christ would be "rejected" of men. The word "rejected" can also mean *abandoned* or *forsaken*. It captures the image of *one isolated, shunned by society, and avoided by those around him.* Despite moments when Jesus drew crowds, His loyal followers were consistently just a "little flock" (*see* Luke 12:32). And of that little flock, we are told in John 6:66 that "many of his disciples went back, and walked no more with him."

There were others who believed in Jesus but would only come to Him by night, as was the case of Nicodemus in John 3:2. We read in John 7:48 that rulers and great men stood aloof from Him, and according to Matthew 26:56, eventually even Jesus' apostles "forsook him, and fled." Thus, we see the complete accuracy of Isaiah's prophecy.

## 'A MAN OF SORROWS' AND 'ACQUAINTED WITH GRIEF'

In Isaiah 53:3, the prophet continued, saying that Christ would be "a man of sorrows, and acquainted with grief." The words "sorrows" and "grief" are also very important for us to understand. For example, "sorrows" is translated from a Hebrew word that is rich with meanings of *physical torment, deep anguish, acute pain, and profound suffering.* It is derived from a root that means *to grieve* or *to be in pain.* It is similar to the Greek word that depicts a scourge that was used by Roman soldiers to torturously rip open the human body and shred it to pieces. Furthermore, the word "sorrows" that Isaiah used in this verse encompasses both emotional and physical torment. Here Isaiah prophesied the violent nature with which Christ would be treated.

Isaiah went on to describe Christ as being intimately "acquainted with grief." The Hebrew word that is translated "acquainted" means *to be acquainted or to know by intimate personal experience and personal knowledge.* The Hebrew word translated "grief" undeniably refers to *physical and mental afflictions of the body and mind — diseases, illnesses, and sicknesses.* While some might attempt to spiritualize this as a metaphorical illness, the Hebrew word clearly points to *tangible physical and mental suffering.* The use of this word "grief" underscores that Christ personally experienced and tasted physical and mental disease, illness, and sickness in His redemptive work on the Cross.

## 'WE HID AS IT WERE OUR FACES FROM HIM'

Then in Isaiah 53:3, Isaiah added that "we hid as it were our faces from him." The word "hid" depicts *an aversion to something so deep that one cannot bear to look upon it.* What Christ endured was so ghastly that when these events occurred, those who were close enough to see it turned their heads to conceal their sight from the horrible rending and tearing of Christ's flesh at His scourging and crucifixion. It was too much for human sight to bear. Isaiah hence prophesied that people would hide their faces from seeing it.

This scenario was cinematized in Mel Gibson's 2004 film called *The Passion of the Christ* — an epic biblical drama that depicts the Passion of Jesus largely according to the gospels of Matthew, Mark, Luke, and John. It is one of the most profound portrayals of Christ's suffering ever produced. As I sat in the movie theater to see it years ago, as the harrowing scenes unfolded before us on the cinema screen, I noticed that I, along with nearly everyone else in the theater, instinctively turned away when the Roman soldiers unleashed their brutal assault upon Jesus. In that moment, I inwardly heard Isaiah's recorded words replay in my mind, "...We hid as it were our faces from him...."

If a cinematic portrayal affected a viewing audience so profoundly, one can scarcely imagine the reality of Christ's suffering witnessed firsthand. In each screening in cinemas worldwide, viewers recoiled from the ghastly spectacle, and every time they "hid their faces," it served as a testament to Isaiah's prophecy that witnesses of Christ's torment would avert their gazes, unwilling or unable to bear the sight of such profound anguish.

For a moment, I must divert us to Isaiah 52:14, where Isaiah prophesied just how torn Christ's body would be in His redemptive work for us. In that verse, Isaiah said, "As many were astonied at thee; his visage was so marred more than any man, and his form more than the sons of men."

The word "visage" in Hebrew describes Christ's visible appearance as a result of the harrowing ordeals He endured. The Hebrew word translated "marred" means that, as a result of His scourging and crucifixion, Christ's human body was in a state of *complete disfigurement.* The words "more than any man" lets us know that His condition was unparalleled, surpassing any suffering endured by another human throughout history.

As you will see in Second Peter 2:24, Peter later wrote that Christ's entire body — from His head to His feet — was covered with a full-body bruise produced by a terrible lashing that not only drew blood but also caused widespread discoloration and swelling of His entire body. Indeed, when we fully grasp the imagery Isaiah and Peter convey, it reveals that Christ's physical form on the Cross was so battered and altered that His human likeness was scarcely recognizable — and this explains why those who witnessed it turned their heads in horror and "hid their faces" from seeing it.

## 'WE ESTEEMED HIM NOT'

But in Isaiah 53:3, the verse continues to say that "he was despised, and we esteemed him not." Here the word "despised" is a repeat of the Hebrew word for "despised" stated at the beginning of the verse, and it emphasizes that despite Christ enduring such profound anguish for our sake, humanity as a collective scorned His sacrifice and looked upon it with *disdain.* It means that in spite of all Jesus endured for each of us, humankind, as a whole, looked upon His sacrifice with contempt and despised it.

In fact, Isaiah said that we "esteemed him not." The word "esteemed" in Hebrew means *to appreciate, consider, esteem,* or *value.* In this case, it conveys a complete lack of recognition. The word "not" in Hebrew is emphatic, which means as a whole this phrase carries the meaning we *emphatically did not esteem* what He was doing on the Cross. This prophecy foresaw that the gravity of Christ's sacrifice would be lost on those who bore witness to it.

In essence, Isaiah's prophecy foretold that at the time of Christ's sacrificial death, those who witnessed it would not appreciate it, consider what it really meant, or esteem what He was doing. This brings to mind the soldiers who callously watched Him die on the Cross while they cast lots for His garments (*see* Matthew 27:35) — or the religious leaders who accused Him of blasphemy, pronounced Him guilty and worthy of death, spit on Him and hit Him, and then mocked and blasphemed Him (*see* Matthew 26:65-68).

Or how about the thief who verbally abused Christ even as He was dying for him and all of mankind so they could be redeemed? Those present during Christ's suffering failed to grasp the monumental act unfolding before them, neither appreciating, considering, nor valuing the priceless gift of salvation they were witnessing as God's plan for man was unfolding before their eyes.

If we stopped here and went no further, the words of Isaiah 53:3 already declare that in His sacrifice for us:

- Christ was despised and treated with contempt.
- Christ was wholesale abandoned and rejected of men.
- Christ endured physical torment, deep anguish, acute pain, and profound suffering.
- Christ personally tasted physical and mental illness, sickness, and disease.
- Christ was shunned by humankind, who turned their faces to avoid looking upon His suffering.
- Christ did it all for each of us, but in the moment He paid that terrible price, humanity as a whole despised Him for it.
- Christ was not appreciated, esteemed, or valued for what He endured for each of us.

## A DEEPER LOOK AT ISAIAH 53:4 — 'SURELY HE HATH BORNE OUR GRIEFS, AND CARRIED OUR SORROWS'

But next Isaiah 53:4 goes on to say, "Surely he hath borne our griefs, and carried our sorrows: yet we did esteem him stricken, smitten of God, and afflicted."

In Hebrew, the word "surely" is imbued with a profound sense of certainty, and it could be rendered *categorically*, *definitely*, *emphatically*, *indeed*, *truly*, or *verily*. This is an emphatic word, which means Isaiah was making an ardent declaration. He was elevating his tone to hammer home an unquestionable truth: "*Categorically, definitely, emphatically, indeed, truly, and verily*, Jesus has borne our griefs." By choosing this potent expression, Isaiah spoke of what is *absolutely certain*, *indisputably and undeniably true*, or *completely unquestionable*.

Then Isaiah added that Christ hath "borne our griefs, and carried our sorrows." In Hebrew, the word "borne" evokes an image of *one who lifts a weight from another's shoulders and chooses to bear it upon himself*. In context, what Jesus lifted from us and took upon Himself is explained by the word "griefs." This word "griefs" in the original Hebrew specifically denotes *physical and mental afflictions of the body and mind* — or physical and mental diseases, illnesses, and sicknesses!

Although some may argue for a metaphorical interpretation and suggest these terms refer to spiritual ailments or weaknesses, the original Hebrew text does not support such a reading. An honest analysis of the text reveals that Christ — in addition to purchasing forgiveness of sin, freedom from guilt and shame, and peace of mind — also lifted physical and mental disease, illness, and sickness from us, and He took it upon Himself on the Cross.

If we stopped here, the original Hebrew text has already gloriously told us, "It is absolutely certain, undeniably true, indisputable, and unquestionable that He [Jesus] has personally lifted all physical and mental diseases, illnesses, and sicknesses from us and has taken them upon Himself..." (*see* Isaiah 53:4).

And then Isaiah eloquently reveals that Jesus "carried" or shouldered the immense load of our "sorrows." The Hebrew word translated "carried" could be rendered as *shouldered*, and it implies an act of *bearing something tremendously heavy* or *lifting a significant burden*. The burden Christ "carried" and "shouldered" for us was our "sorrows." The word "sorrows" is interpreted from a Hebrew word that depicts *physical and mental anguish and pains*.

The precise choice of these words powerfully underscores that through His redemptive act, Christ lifted from us and absorbed into Himself our *physical and mental diseases, illnesses, and sicknesses.* Indeed, it means that He took upon Himself the immense weight of our *physical and mental diseases, illnesses, and sicknesses* — He literally lifted it from us and took it upon Himself at the Cross on our behalf.

## JESUS WAS 'STRICKEN, SMITTEN OF GOD, AND AFFLICTED'

Pausing here to reflect on what all this means, we see that the text could be rendered, "It is absolutely certain, undeniably true, indisputable, and unquestionable that He [Jesus] has personally lifted all physical and mental diseases, illnesses, and sicknesses from us and has taken them upon Himself — absolutely all physical and mental anguish and pain…." But that's not the end of the verse. Isaiah 53:4 continues to say that Christ was "stricken, smitten of God, and afflicted."

In Hebrew, the word "stricken" conveys the notion of having someone or something subjected to *a brutal, harsh, and forceful hand.* In the Old Testament, this word is often used to picture a moment when a person (or people) is visited with severity — and very frequently, the severity manifests as physical disease, illness, or sickness.

Meanwhile, its counterpart, the word "smitten," portrays *someone who physically lays his hands on someone or something else to afflict or severely beat or strike with the intention to destroy.* Notably, this same word is also used militarily to describe a ferocious attack on an adversary during warfare with utter obliteration as the goal. Then on top of all these already intense words, Isaiah added that Christ will additionally be "afflicted," which in Hebrew means *to be utterly crushed.*

Adding all these meanings to this verse, we find that Isaiah 53:4 actually says:

> **It is absolutely certain, undeniably true, indisputable, and unquestionable that He** [Christ] **has personally lifted all physical and mental diseases, illnesses, and sicknesses from us and has taken**

> **upon Himself absolutely all physical and mental anguish and pain as God's forceful hand of judgment came upon Him, and God struck with the intention to completely destroy Him. And God did it with such force that it completely and utterly crushed Him.**

When all of this striking, smiting, and crushing occurred, God was unleashing a mighty blow against the sin and the physical and mental disease, illness, and sickness that Christ had willingly absorbed into His being. God was waging a war against everything Christ took upon Himself on behalf of sinful, fallen mankind — sin, guilt, shame, lack of peace, and every ailment, disease, illness, sickness, and torment — both physical and mental. These were age-old enemies that were unleashed upon the world from the moment of Adam's transgression and that have haunted humanity ever since. Yet at the Cross, God launched an attack that was aimed at eradicating them, and He delivered a decisive and fatal strike against them through Christ's suffering.

## A DEEPER LOOK AT ISAIAH 53:5 — 'BUT HE WAS WOUNDED FOR OUR TRANSGRESSIONS'

Then Isaiah 53:5 summarizes, "But he was wounded for our transgressions, he was bruised for our iniquities: the chastisement of our peace was upon him; and with his stripes we are healed."

In the opening statement of Isaiah 53:5, another part of the prophecy astonishingly unfolds, "But he was *wounded* for our transgressions...." In the original Hebrew, the word "wounded" conveys a sense of *being pierced or deeply wounded*, foreshadowing here with remarkable clarity the future piercing of Jesus' hands, feet, side, and brow. Remarkably, Isaiah captured this vision of Christ's suffering with prophetic precision, seven centuries before the events unfolded.

The Hebrew concept of "transgressions" refers to *violations* of God's commandments and God's nature, and it includes *sin, rebellion, and turning against God* — all of which are a reflection of humanity's flawed nature that was inherited from Adam's initial transgression. Isaiah foretold that Christ would be *physically pierced* and would bear *physical wounds*, shedding His own blood to pay the ultimate price for our sins and acts of rebellion — and that payment of holy, sinless blood was required for Christ to redeem us from Satan's slave market and restore us to God's original intent for our lives.

## HE 'WAS BRUISED FOR OUR INIQUITIES'

Isaiah 53:5 goes on to say, "...[Jesus] was bruised for our iniquities...." The words "was bruised" is a translation of a Hebrew word meaning *to beat to pieces, to crush*, or *to destroy*. Isaiah 53:5 highlights the profound suffering Christ endured on behalf of others and emphasizes themes of substitutionary atonement and redemption. Meanwhile, the word "iniquities" stems from a Hebrew word that encompasses a range of human failings including *guilt, moral lapses, depravity, perversity, and shame.*

This passage reveals that Christ's sacrifice went beyond just *covering* our sins; His sacrifice completely obliterated our iniquities. This includes not just our moral failures, but also the guilt and shame attached to them. Through His redemptive act on the Cross, Christ decimated these burdens entirely, offering freedom from moral failings, all forms of perversity, and the heavy cloak of guilt and shame that once ensnared us.

Thus Christ's redemptive work on the Cross includes the complete removal of all of these things, which means He intends for you to be freed from all associated shame that once hounded you because of past iniquities in your life.

## 'THE CHASTISEMENT OF OUR PEACE WAS UPON HIM'

Isaiah 53:5 further states "the chastisement of our peace was upon him." The word "chastisement" is from a Hebrew word that most often pictures *punishment for past activities.* This illustrates the profound truth that at the Cross, Christ bore the penalty we deserved and paved the way for us to attain "peace." This "peace" is deeply rooted in the Hebrew concept of *shalom*, a word that signifies not just *tranquility*, but an all-encompassing state of *wholeness* and *completeness* in every part of a person's life.

But this word "peace" goes beyond mere tranquility — it also encompasses *happiness, health, prosperity, safety, security, and soundness of mind.* It paints a vivid picture of a life that is abundantly blessed and that is flourishing in every dimension. Thus, when Jesus paid the price for us on the Cross, He was not only bearing our burdens, but also securing our well-being in every way — spirit, soul, and body — and ensuring that we could experience profound *peace of mind* and would *thrive* in every aspect of our lives.

## 'WITH HIS STRIPES WE ARE HEALED'

Next, Isaiah 53:5 adds, "…And with his stripes we are healed." The word "stripes" finds its origins in a Hebrew word that pictures *bruises, welts, and the dark-blue marks left by a severe whipping.* Of course, this is a reference to the scourging that Christ endured to obtain our freedom from all forms of physical and mental disease, illness, and sickness.

The Hebrew word *rapha* is rendered "healed" in this verse, and by understanding it's meaning, it becomes clear that Christ's redemptive act brought about not only the forgiveness of sins, liberation from shame, and mental peace, but also physical and mental healing from all manner of ailments. Christ's work on the Cross provided for the comprehensive restoration of every facet of our existence — spiritual, physical, and mental.

Taking all the Hebrew word meanings in this verse into account, Isaiah 53:5 carries this meaning:

> **But He was pierced and deeply wounded for our transgressions — that is, our violations of God's commandments and God's nature,**

> **including sin, rebellion, and turning against God. He was beaten, crushed, and destroyed for the removal of our iniquities — that is, our guilt, moral lapses, depravity, perversity, and shame. The punishment we deserved for our past activities was laid on Him, and we have been given peace in its place — not just tranquility, but an all-encompassing state of wholeness and completeness in every part of our lives so that we can peacefully thrive in every area. And due to the massive, full-body bruises, welts, and stripes that were laid on Him by a severe lashing of the whip, we are healed from all manner of physical and mental disease, illness, and sickness.**

I encourage you to deeply ponder the various versions of Isaiah 53:3-5 that are listed in Chapter Fifteen. Read them like you've never read them before, and as you do, you will see a chorus of voices — translators and interpreters alike — all converging on the profound truth about the monumental sacrifice Jesus made on the Cross, collectively affirming all that He purchased for you: the forgiveness of sin, freedom from guilt and shame, peace of mind, and healing and health for both body and mind.

## DISPELLING WRONG THINKING ABOUT ISAIAH 53:5

Verse by verse and word by word, we have studied what Isaiah 53:5 means, yet even with the original Hebrew text unveiling its clear intentions a widespread misunderstanding persists, especially surrounding the phrase "with his stripes we are healed." Before we move on to see what Matthew wrote about Jesus taking physical and mental disease, illness, and sickness upon Himself, I would like to biblically dispel this misconception.

Numerous individuals who do not support divine healing in our current era tend to interpret the phrase "by his stripes I am healed" as a so-called "spiritual healing" that takes place at the moment of salvation. However, such interpretation misses the mark for several reasons. First, the notion of "spiritual healing" implies that there was something in us that could be fixed, healed, or mended. But in stark reality, the Bible declares that prior to Christ's work in our lives, we weren't just damaged people who required repair; we were actually "dead" in our trespasses and sins, as stated in Ephesians 2:1.

The word "dead" in Ephesians 2:1 is translated from the Greek word *nekros*, which pictures *a completely dead person* or *a lifeless corpse*. Of course, when a person is dead, there is no heartbeat, no breath in the lungs, and no pulse to feel in the wrists. The clock has quit running and there is no turning it back. Thus, it is impossible to "heal" a dead man. Spiritual death cannot be healed; it requires *resurrection.*

Likewise, when we each came to Christ, we were not spiritually healed; we were *resurrected.* The phrase "with his stripes we are healed" categorically *cannot* refer to spiritual healing that occurs at the time of salvation, because no one who is spiritually dead is simply healed and thereby reconciled to God. No, that person is spiritually dead and his or her nature must become new, or raised to new life (*see* Ephesians 2:1).

For a sinner to awaken to God, a resurrection is required and resurrection is precisely what happens when a person is born again. So the notion that a person is "spiritually healed" when he is saved flies in the face of Scripture. Furthermore, we have already seen that the word "healed" in Isaiah 53:5 is translated from the Hebrew word *rapha*, and this word is only used to describe physical healing.

## ISAIAH'S PROPHECY IS CONFIRMED BY MATTHEW — JESUS 'TOOK OUR INFIRMITIES, AND BARE OUR SICKNESSES'

In this section, we will see that the gospel of Matthew confirms the words of Isaiah 53. In Matthew 8:16, we read, "When the even was come, they brought unto him [Jesus] many that were possessed with devils: and he cast out the spirits with his word, and healed all that were sick." Here Matthew pointed out the fact that Jesus fearlessly dealt with demons, and He physically and mentally healed all who came to Him for deliverance and healing.

But Matthew 8:17 then confirms the words of Isaiah, stating, "That it might be fulfilled which was spoken by Esaias [Isaiah] the prophet, saying, Himself took our infirmities, and bare our sicknesses."

The word "infirmities" in Matthew 8:17 is translated from the Greek word *astheneia*, which is an all-encompassing word for *all types of disease, illness, and sickness.* Mirroring the words of Isaiah, Matthew emphasized that Jesus "...took our infirmities...." We have seen that Isaiah 53:3-5 clearly states that Christ lifted anguish, pain, and every form of physical and mental disease, illness, and sickness from us. Nearly repeating the words of Isaiah, Matthew used the word "bare" which is from a Greek word that likewise illustrates *the act of carrying a heavy load.* By echoing Isaiah's passage, Matthew portrayed Jesus' purpose to shoulder the entire spectrum of anguish, distress, and pain, as well as every conceivable disease, illness, and sickness, with the intention of relieving humankind of these afflictions permanently.

To show how deep Christ intends to free His people from anguish, pain, and every form of physical and mental disease, illness, and sickness, Matthew chose the word *nosos*, which is the Greek word for "sicknesses." This term signifies *a fatal ailment* or one that eludes natural healing methods. It denotes a terminal condition with no conventional remedy. This is significant, for it means Jesus did not only come to relieve minor aches and pains and superficial ailments, but the price He paid when He was scourged and crucified vanquished even the gravest diseases — even those that transcend the boundaries of medical understanding.

**The *RIV* (*Renner Interpretive Version*) of Matthew 8:17 says:**

**All of this was to fulfill what had been spoken by the prophet Isaiah, saying, "He took our physical afflictions, diseases, infirmities,**

**and sicknesses of every kind, and He shouldered our physical conditions for which there was no natural cure."**

## PETER ALSO CONFIRMED ISAIAH'S PROPHECY ABOUT CHRIST'S REDEMPTIVE WORK ON THE CROSS

Reflecting on Christ's sacrifice, Peter personally recalled the unforgettable scene of Christ's suffering. As he penned his letter, he tapped into the well of his own eyewitness account to recall the monumental event when Christ paid the ultimate price to liberate us from the clutches of Satan's bondage. This sacrifice was not just an act of freeing us; it was a glorious transfer into God's Kingdom, a realm dominated by light and overflowing with goodness. As Peter delved deep into his memories to recollect that moment, he wrote, "Who his own self bare our sins in his own body on the tree, that we, being dead to sins, should live unto righteousness: by whose stripes ye were healed" (1 Peter 2:24).

**Matthew portrayed Jesus' purpose to shoulder the entire spectrum of anguish, distress, pain, and every conceivable disease, illness, and sickness, with the intention of relieving humankind of these afflictions permanently.**

In this passage, Peter recounted his firsthand experience of witnessing Jesus dying on the Cross, detailing how in doing so, Christ "bare our sins." The word "bare" is translated from the Greek word *anaphero*, an unusual Greek word that means *to bear up* or *to lift up*. Its usage is deeply significant, as it was often used to evoke the imagery of *a priest whose duty was to present a sacrifice upon an altar.* Peter was well aware of this connotation, and he utilized this word to illustrate that, as Jesus bore the burden of the world's sins on the Cross, He was both the sacrificial Lamb of God and simultaneously assumed the role of the Great High Priest.

In that profound moment, Christ offered His own spotless blood as the ultimate sacrifice for the sin of mankind. This calls to mind Hebrews 9:12, which proclaims, "Neither by the blood of goats and calves, but by his own blood he entered in once into the holy place, having obtained eternal redemption for us." Thus, through His sacrifice, Christ not only atoned for sins, but also became the High Priest who presented His own precious blood for our redemption.

But in First Peter 2:24, Peter additionally wrote that "...[Jesus] bare our sins in his own body on the tree...." The word "in" is a translation of the Greek word *en*, which means *in*, and it is used to emphasize that Jesus bore the weight of our transgressions *in*, or *inside*, His physical form upon the Cross. The word "tree" is derived from the Greek *xulon*, which signifies *anything crafted from wood*. Yet within the Roman context, the *xulon* was used to refer to *altars* fashioned of wood, as well as for *crossbeams* used for crucifixion!

Peter's deliberate choice to include a definite article before the word *xulon* — the Greek word for "tree" — underscores the uniqueness of the Cross. This cross was not just any cross; it was THE Cross, unlike any other. This cross became the sacred altar where Christ's blood was shed to secure everlasting forgiveness for those who seek Him in faith. Indeed, the hideous cross of Christ became a mighty altar upon which our High Priest presented His own spotless blood to obtain redemption for those who embrace Him through faith.

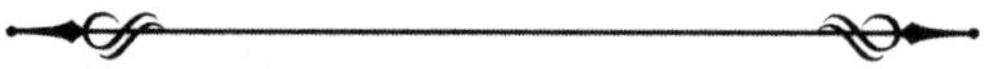

**As Jesus bore the burden of the world's sins on the Cross, He was both the sacrificial Lamb of God and simultaneously assumed the role of the Great High Priest.**

Peter then added in First Peter 2:24 that Christ gave His life on the Cross "that we, being dead to sins, should live unto righteousness." In the original Greek text, the word "dead" is interpreted from a form of the word *apoginomai*, a fascinating compound derived from the words *apo* and *ginomai*. The word *apo* means *away* and signifies *a separation*, whereas *ginomai* in this context means *to emerge*. When compounded to form the word *apoginomai*, it conveys the essence of being *separated from sin* and *emerging* as new and transformed. Before Christ delivered us from the power of darkness, we languished in the grasp of spiritual death, but through faith in Him, Christ's power shattered our chains, we ascended from the clutches of death, and we began a new life filled with righteousness.

First Peter 2:24 goes on to say God's purpose is that we "might live unto righteousness." The word "live" is from a form of the Greek word *zao*, a word that suggests *a sense of vibrancy* as opposed to mere existence. It goes beyond mere aliveness and pictures an energetic life filled with enthusiasm and vivacity.

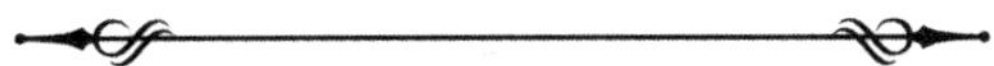

**The hideous cross of Christ became a mighty altar upon which our High Priest presented His own spotless blood to obtain redemption for those who embrace Him through faith.**

Meanwhile, the word "righteousness" finds its roots in the Greek word *dikaiosune*, derived from the word *dike*, which depicts the image of a thorough judicial examination that results in a verdict of *innocence and uprightness*. In the New Testament, the word *dikaiosune* pictures *the approval that God gives* for those who are *right* with Him. Thus, we find in this verse that in Christ, we have been delivered from the power of darkness, and we have emerged as beings that are teeming with spiritual life — and we are to live an energetic life that is filled with enthusiasm and vivacity.

Finally, First Peter 2:24 declares, "…By whose stripes ye were healed." Much like Matthew did in Matthew 8:17, Peter echoed the prophetic words of Isaiah 53:5, which say "with his stripes we are healed." The striking difference lies in their perspectives. Isaiah, writing seven centuries before Christ, foretold of a future where healing is promised through Christ's sacrifice yet to come. In contrast, Peter reflected on this prophecy as a fulfilled reality and affirmed that healing has already been accomplished through Christ's stripes. Isaiah looked ahead to a promise yet to be realized, while Peter invited the faithful to embrace this procured healing as a past-tense event and as a gift already available to every believer.

The word "stripes" is a translation of the Greek word *molops*, which is a word that describes *a full-body bruise* or *a terrible lashing that draws blood and produces discoloration and swelling of the entire body*. This term captures the brutality of a horrific flogging that pierces the skin, draws profuse amounts of blood, and causes the entire body to swell on account of the stripes laid across it.

**Before Christ delivered us from the power of darkness, we languished in the grasp of spiritual death, but through faith in Him, Christ's power shattered our chains, we ascended from the clutches of death, and we began a new life filled with righteousness.**

Peter reached into the recesses of his memory and recalled how Jesus' entire body became completely swollen and discolored from the physical abuse He had endured in His scourging. The vicious and sadistic scourging Jesus experienced literally disfigured His entire body. We have seen that Isaiah 52:14 says His body was marred beyond human recognition. It was discolored, distended, marred, inflamed, and swollen — and all of it paid the price for forgiveness of sin, freedom from guilt and shame, peace of mind, and physical and mental healing and health.

## THE HORROR OF A ROMAN SCOURGING

Because this chapter deals extensively with the stripes that were laid on Jesus' body when He was scourged, I want to tell you exactly what occurred when a person was scourged under Roman rule. In my book *Easter — The Rest of the Story*, I delve deeply into the profound suffering that Jesus endured, but here, I want to touch upon some of that material because it is vital to grasp the immense sacrifice He made to secure healing and well-being for both our bodies and minds.

I really want you to understand what the Bible means when it says "with his stripes we are healed" (*see* Isaiah 53:5). So I ask — do you know:

- What was it like for a person to be scourged at that time in history?
- From what materials were a scourge made?
- How did it impact a victim when the straps of a scourge ripped across his back and body?
- What effects did a scourging have on the human body externally and internally?

When a decision was made by a ruler to scourge an individual, the first step was to strip away every stitch of clothing, leaving the victim's skin fully vulnerable to the lashing to come. This exposure laid bare the entirety of the body to the whims of the torturer and his whip.

Typically, victims were then secured to a stout, stone pillar that stood about two feet high. Their arms were extended overhead, wrists tightly fastened to a metal loop, rendering them immobile and preventing any chance of escape or self-defense. In this confining position, even the most desperate attempts at movement were futile as the iron grip of the clasp securely anchored them to the pillar. Thus the cruelly restrained victims often filled the air with their cries for mercy, pleading for an end to their suffering.

After being bound to the post and splayed across it, the victim was at the mercy of the Roman soldiers, who subjected him to unspeakable torment. One historian from the First Century remarked that the sheer dread of the impending scourging seized the victim in a paralyzing grip, and his body would tense up, muscles coiling in his abdomen like twisted ropes, his face paled as if the very blood had deserted him, and his lips would press into a grim line over clenched teeth, bracing for the initial cruel strike that would begin to rend his body.

The dreaded scourge of the Romans was a fearsome instrument of pain and punishment. The weapon featured a stout, wooden grip, from which dangled an array of leather straps, each stretching between 18 and 24 inches long. At their menacing extremities, these straps boasted tightly bound knots embedded with sharp metal, twisted wire, shards of glass, and jagged bone.

This formidable weapon struck terror into the hearts of many and earned a notorious reputation as one of Rome's most terrifying tools of torment. The mere mention of scourging was often enough to pacify an unruly crowd or break the spirit of even the most defiant insurgent. Hardened criminals, seasoned in their callousness, would shudder at the grisly thought of enduring the merciless lashing from a Roman scourge.

Typically, two Roman soldiers at a time would administer the punishment by scourging, a dreadful duet unfolding as the two tormentors engaged in this brutal ordeal, their whips descending in unison from opposing sides, each tipped with razor-sharp, jagged ornaments. These straps swept across the victim's back, leaving no expanse untouched. Every shard of metal, wire, bone, or glass embedded within the lashes bit hungrily into his skin, burrowing deep to shred the muscle and sinew beneath. Each swing of the scourge rained down upon the victim's battered form in relentless succession.

This brutal punishment began to unpeel the victim's skin entirely until eventually his flesh was flayed off his body. The Early Church historian Eusebius wrote, "They [were] lacerated with scourges even to the innermost veins and arteries, so that the hidden inward parts of the body, both their bowels and their members, were exposed to view...."[1]

With each strike of the whip, grisly straps of leather encircled the victim's body and sank into the tender flesh of his abdomen and upper chest. Every lash left a searing wound and grotesque disfigurement. And although he struggled in vain to wrench himself free, his wrists were shackled unyieldingly to the iron ring fixed into the stone pillar. Trapped in this hellish dance, victims often found themselves crying out in desperation, pleading for compassion to bring an end to their excruciating ordeal.

The trauma inflicted on a person's body in the act of scourging is impossible to overstate. With so many blood vessels sliced open by the whip, torrents of blood and bodily fluids would spill forth from the victim. The heart would thunder with a desperate urgency, as it strived to nourish the ravaged flesh. Yet its efforts were in vain, for this action was comparable to pumping water through an open water hydrant, as there was nothing to stop the blood from pouring through the victim's open wounds.

The significant hemorrhaging led to a steep decline in the victim's blood pressure as well as unquenchable thirst, often causing him to faint from the pain and eventually go into shock. The erratic rhythm of his heart frequently pushed the victim into cardiac arrest.

According to Deuteronomy 25:3, Jewish law allowed for the administering of up to 40 lashes, but it was common practice to stop at 39, as the final stroke often proved fatal. In contrast to the Jews, who were restricted to administering a maximum of 40 lashes, the Romans imposed no such limits.

Thus, when Jesus faced the brutal scourging from Roman soldiers, the count of lashes could have easily exceeded that number. Considering the intense animosity harbored by the Jews toward Jesus and the merciless ridicule He had already endured from Roman hands, it is highly probable that they unleashed a relentless and savage flurry of lashes, surpassing any numerical constraint.

As harrowing as this description is, it serves merely as an introduction to the suffering that was to come, as Matthew 27:26 further narrates, "And when he had scourged Jesus, he delivered him to be crucified."

When we think about the scourging Jesus endured, it is vital that we remember the promise God made in Isaiah 53:5, "But he was wounded for our transgressions, he was bruised for our iniquities: the chastisement of our peace was upon him; and with his stripes we are healed."

In this verse, God declared long ago that the price for our healing would be paid for by the stripes that were savagely laid across Jesus' body.

## YOU ARE HEALED BY JESUS' STRIPES

Peter proclaims that it is through these very "stripes" that we are "healed." The word "healed" is interpreted from the Greek word *iaomai*, a well-known word that means *to cure* or *to be doctored*, and it is often translated as *a treatment* or *a remedy* for a physical or mental sickness.

Peter thusly declares that the stripes borne by Christ serve as *the source* of healing for every believer, and he establishes physical and mental healing as an inherent right for every child of God. The Cross was God's ultimate *cure* and *remedy* for disease, illness, and sickness, and because of the work of Christ, every believer can lay claim to healing and health.

As we have seen, Peter personally witnessed Jesus enduring this vicious torment both in the days leading up to the crucifixion and at the Cross. Peter wrote that it is by His stripes that we *were* healed. This means the price for healing is already paid and has been obtained for every child of God. It is a *past fact* and a *done deal*.

Jesus took that barbaric abuse to provide physical healing for our body and mind. The last part of First Peter 2:24 could be interpreted, "It was by the terrible lashing and stripes laid upon His body that you have been physically healed."

## JESUS CHRIST — THE SAME YESTERDAY, TODAY, AND FOREVER

Hebrews 13:8 is a very foundational verse about the life and present-day ministry of Jesus Christ. It states, "Jesus Christ the same yesterday, and to day, and for ever."

In our fast-paced world, where change is the only constant, we read that Jesus is *"the same."* The Greek word for "same" underscores the *unchanging nature* of Jesus Christ. He is the One we can depend on to be the same, regardless of the times or the spirit of the age. We don't need to refigure who Jesus is, what He thinks, or what His message is, because He is the same — and everything He represents is the same *yesterday*, *today*, and *forever*!

The words "the same" means that if Jesus was the Healer and Miracle-Worker we read about in the gospels, He is still the Healer and Miracle-Worker today, and He will still be the Healer and Miracle-Worker tomorrow. According to Hebrews 13:8, He is the same yesterday, today, and forever. That means whoever He was in the past is exactly who He is in the present, and it's exactly who He will always be to each of us. Therefore, if you discover Jesus of the past, you have also discovered who Jesus is in the present, and you have discovered who Jesus will be in the future, because He is continuously the same.

Before we close this chapter about what Jesus purchased for us on the Cross, we need to go to Luke 4:16-19 to see what Jesus quoted from Isaiah 61 about His own ministry. In that passage, Jesus describes the anointing that was upon Him. Since Hebrews 13:8 declares that He is the same yesterday, today, and forever, it means this very same anointing that was on Jesus in the four gospels is still on Him right now, and it is available to anyone who will come to Him in faith to receive it.

**Whoever Jesus was in the past is exactly who He is in the present, and it's exactly who He will always be to each of us.**

In this book, I am attempting to put weapons into your mental arsenal that will help you combat any doubt that says God is no longer in the healing business. We have already looked deeply at Isaiah 53:3-5, Matthew 8:17, First Peter 2:24, and the subject of redemption, all of which affirm that Christ took our infirmities and sicknesses upon Himself. Yet before we advance to the practical steps of embracing divine healing and health in our lives, Luke 4:16-19 is a crucial piece of Scripture we must explore.

## THE ANOINTING THAT WAS ON JESUS IS STILL ON JESUS, AND IT IS AVAILABLE TO YOU

In the gospel of Luke, chapter 4, a scene full of tension unfolds as Jesus emerged from His time of temptation in the desert. Returning to His hometown of Nazareth, He entered the synagogue on the Sabbath, ready to participate in the sacred readings of Scripture.

When His turn came to read, Jesus unrolled the scroll of the prophet Isaiah, selecting the passage from Isaiah 61:1-2. These verses eloquently speak of the anointing that would rest upon the Messiah. And as Jesus read with authority, He astonished the congregation by proclaiming that these prophetic words are realized in Him.

# CLAIM YOUR FREE RESOURCE!

We would like to send you **free of charge** Rick Renner's message on CD or as an MP3 download, "How To Receive a Miraculous Touch From God."

In His earthly ministry, Jesus commonly healed *all* who were sick and diseased. In this profound message, learn about Christ's love, goodness, and power *today* toward *anyone* who will come to Him in simple faith with his needs.

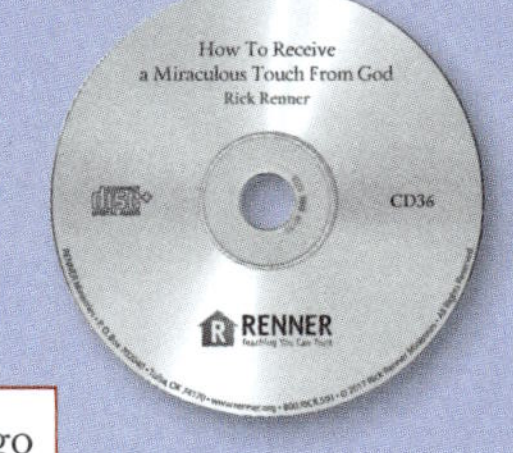

Complete the form below to receive this FREE teaching — or go to **renner.org/claim-your-free-offer** to order. You may mail this postcard postage paid or place it in a stamped envelope and mail your request to the address on the reverse side of this card.

☐ YES, please also send me Rick's FREE monthly Teaching Letter!

Name: ______________________________

Address: ______________________________

City: ____________________ State: ________ Zip: __________

Email: ____________________ Phone: ______________

> **And he came to Nazareth, where he had been brought up: and, as his custom was, he went into the synagogue on the sabbath day, and stood up for to read. And there was delivered unto him the book of the prophet Esaias. And when he had opened the book, he found the place where it was written, The Spirit of the Lord is upon me, because he hath anointed me to preach the gospel to the poor; he hath sent me to heal the broken-hearted, to preach deliverance to the captives, and recovering of sight to the blind, to set at liberty them that are bruised, to preach the acceptable year of the Lord.**
>
> **— Luke 4:16-19**

This bold declaration ignited a fiery anger among the listeners, who, unable to fathom such a claim, were driven into a frenzy. They rose up, intent on silencing Him forever. However, in a miraculous turn of events, Jesus calmly passed through the chaos unscathed, leaving behind the angered throng. Departing from Nazareth, Jesus resettled in Capernaum to begin a new chapter of His ministry.

We read in Luke 4:16-19 of the moment when Jesus took the scroll of Isaiah and began to read: "And he [Jesus] came to Nazareth, where he had been brought up: and, as his custom was, he went into the synagogue on the sabbath day, and stood up for to read. And there was delivered unto him the book of the prophet Esaias. And when he had opened the book, he found the place where it was written, The Spirit of the Lord is upon me, because he hath anointed me to preach the gospel to the poor; he hath sent me to heal the brokenhearted, to preach deliverance to the captives, and recovering of sight to the blind, to set at liberty them that are bruised, to preach the acceptable year of the Lord."

In these verses, Jesus announced He is the Messiah — that is, the Christ, or the Anointed One — and then He vividly described what that anointing upon Him would accomplish in the lives of those who come to Him by faith. Hebrews 13:8 reassures us that Jesus remains unchanging, and His works today are as potent as they were 2,000 years ago. And since He is the same today as He was yesterday, it is vital for us to understand what He was anointed to do in the past in order to fully grasp what He continues to offer to those who seek Him in the present.

Indeed, the words of Hebrews 13:8 irrefutably affirm that the same works Jesus was anointed to perform in the gospels are the same works He is still empowered to accomplish today. In Luke 4:18-19, Jesus spoke of six things He and His anointing came to do, which include five categories of human ailments and frailties that His anointing can change for those who come to Him by faith. As you will see, if this was true of His anointing 2,000 years ago, it is still true of His anointing today, for He and His anointing never change!

### 1. Jesus Is an Economic Game-Changer

*First*, we read in Luke 4:18 that Jesus was anointed "to preach the gospel to the poor." In the Greek language, there are numerous words to picture poverty, but the word "poor" in this verse is drawn from the Greek word *ptochos*. It is a word that transcends the usual depiction of poverty, and it pictures images of *those trapped in the deepest depths of destitution, utterly devoid of resources — a state of despair, indigence, and impoverishment.* But Jesus declared that He was anointed to bring a message that would produce profound economic transformation even for those who languished in the most severe poverty.

Because Jesus is the same yesterday, today, and forever, this tells us that since Jesus was an economic game changer for those devoid of resources 2,000 years ago, He *continues* to be an economic game-changer today for those who suffer in the grip of extreme poverty in our modern world. The anointing to break the stronghold of poverty *was* upon Jesus, and it is *still* on Jesus — and that powerful anointing to this very day unleashes a divine force that shatters the chains of hopelessness for those ensnared in destitution. Because Jesus' nature has never changed, to this day, that anointing provides hope to those who are devoid of resources and lifts them from the depths of scarcity, lack, and impoverishment.

Again, Hebrews 13:8 tells us that Jesus and His anointing have not changed or waned over time. The same divine force that shattered the chains of poverty

2,000 years ago remains just as potent and active today. So if you've been caught in the relentless grip of financial hardship, know that you can turn to prayer with confidence and unwavering faith. Tap into the timeless anointing of Christ, calling upon it to disrupt the cycle of poverty and usher in change in your life, just as it did those many centuries past.

**Since He is the same today as He was yesterday, it is vital for us to understand what He was anointed to do in the past in order to fully grasp what He continues to offer to those who seek Him in the present.**

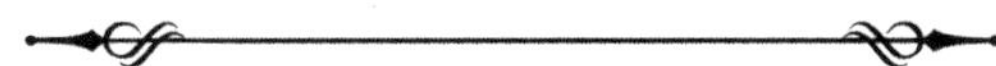

### 2. Jesus Heals the Brokenhearted

*Second*, we read in Luke 4:18 that Jesus was anointed "to heal the brokenhearted." The word "brokenhearted" is translated from a form of the Greek word *suntribo*, which is a word in history that described *the crushing of grapes with the feet* or *the smashing and grinding of bones into dust.*

Taken in context, this word depicts *people who have been walked on by others, those who have been crushed by others*, or *those who feel they have been smashed to pieces by life or relationships.* By using the Greek word *suntribo*, Jesus was declaring, "I am anointed to heal those who have been crushed by others and feel walked on or smashed to pieces by life and relationships."

The word "heal" in this verse is translated from a form of the Greek word *iaomai*, which means *to cure* or *to heal*, and it frequently referred to *a progressive cure*. Unlike instant recuperation, this word depicts *a healing power that progressively reverses a condition over a period of time* or *a sickness that is progressively healed rather than instantaneously healed.*

While the anointing on Christ often yields immediate and miraculous outcomes, this word *iaomai* tells us that 2,000 years ago when Christ's anointing touched people who were deeply crushed by life and were emotionally devastated, the anointing He released moved deeply to start the process of mending shattered emotions and minds. And that invisible anointing worked unabated inside them *until* the person reached full recovery and restoration.

It is fitting that this word "heal" would be used to picture Christ's anointing in a person who bears deep scars and wounds in his emotions and mind. This anointing progressively dissolves layers of pain, one after another, until the individual eventually reaches complete restoration. As a reminder, this is an anointing especially for the "brokenhearted" — for those who have been walked on by others who feel they have been crushed by others; or those who feel they have been smashed to pieces by life or relationships.

Take a moment to reflect on the number of people you know who feel trampled, broken, or overwhelmed by life's challenges and relationships. Our world is filled with individuals carrying emotional wounds and scars in their hearts and minds. Yet Hebrews 13:8 reminds us that Jesus Christ and His healing power remain unaltered. The same anointing that restored the emotionally wounded two millennia ago is just as powerful today, and it is ready to bring complete healing to those struggling with emotional and mental burdens.

Jesus remains constant, and if His power produced emotional and mental healing in people 2,000 years ago, it is equally present today to heal our deepest wounds. So I encourage you to embrace the anointing of Christ and allow it to mend your heart and mind today, just as it healed countless others in times past.

### 3. Jesus Delivers Captives

*Third*, we read in Luke 4:18 that Jesus was anointed "to preach deliverance to the captives." The word "deliverance" finds its roots in the Greek word *aphesis*, which conveys the idea of *complete dismissal*, *unbinding*, *liberation*, or *setting someone free*.

The word "captives" is translated from a form of the Greek word *aichmalotos*, a variant of *aichme*, which is the Greek word for *a spear*. But when the word *aichme* becomes *aichmalotos*, it is not merely a spear, but it pictures *the pointed tip of a spear pressing relentlessly into someone's back.* Consequently, the person who wields the spear holds the power to dictate the captive's path and to steer him or her at his will.

This word "captive" refers to those who are dragged into some kind of bondage by a sinister force that metaphorically holds a spear to their backs. It could be any number of things, including a poor self-image, toxic relationships, stubborn habits, or the overpowering grip of alcohol, drugs, or disease, illness, and sickness. No one wants their lives to be controlled by any of these destructive developments. But this word "captives" includes a wide range of possible meanings, and it unequivocally takes into account anyone who endures the chains of disease, illness, or sickness.

But Luke 4:18 declares that when Jesus came, He came as a herald of emancipation. His anointing unleashed liberation to those ensnared by the devil's grip. The four gospels are testimonials to the power of Christ's anointing, which, 2,000 years ago, brought deliverance to the oppressed, demon-possessed, and all those plagued by various kinds of disease, illness, and sickness. That anointing shattered the spear the devil held against their backs that he intended to use to keep them in bondage. Once touched by the anointing, those individuals experienced an extraordinary and swift liberation, and they stepped into freedom to embrace the life God had designed for them.

Once again, stop and ponder how many people you know who are taken captive by the devil in some area of their lives. Although they long for freedom, the sharpened tip the enemy has pressed into their back drives them with a poor self-image, toxic relationships, destructive habits, or the grip of alcohol, drugs, disease, illness, and sickness, egregiously controlling their lives. As you read this list, you may see yourself in one of these categories and you may be thinking, *The devil has a spear pressed against my back and has been manipulating my life too.*

But once more, let's turn our hearts to the truth found in Hebrews 13:8 — a timeless truth that tells us Jesus Christ and His anointing which liberate those who are bound remains unchanging. The very anointing that broke chains and freed the captive souls two millennia ago continues its transformative work today, completely releasing those ensnared by evil.

As expressed in Acts 10:38, "…God anointed Jesus of Nazareth with the Holy Ghost and with power, who went about doing good, and healing all that were oppressed of the devil…."

**Luke 4:18 declares that when Jesus came, He came as a herald of emancipation.**

The fact that Jesus' anointing shattered shackles and brought freedom to those who were bound 2,000 years ago means that His anointing is still at work to free people today, for Jesus is the same yesterday, today, and forever. Right now His anointing is still available to offer freedom to anyone who is held in any form of physical or mental bondage.

### 4. Jesus Provides Recovering of Sight to the Blind

*Fourth*, we read in Luke 4:18 that Jesus' anointing brought "recovering of sight to the blind." The words "recovering of sight" are translated from a form of the Greek word *anablepsis*, which is a compound of the words *ana* and *blepo*. The word *ana* means *again*, and the word *blepo* means *I see.* As a compound, it means *to see again.* In Luke 4:18, this word depicts *the miraculous restoration of one's sight.* During the New Testament era, the miraculous act of granting sight to the blind was viewed as the utmost miracle, as blindness was believed to be utterly beyond cure.

Yet Jesus returned sight to the blind multiple times, as we read in Matthew 9:27-31; 11:5; 12:22-23; 15:29-31; 20:29-34; 21:14; Mark 8:22-25; 10:46-52; Luke 18:35-43; and John 9:6-7. But because "blindness" was considered to be impossible to remedy, it meant Jesus' anointing was able to heal even the worst of *all* physical maladies. If that anointing could restore sight, people understood that His power could undo *any form* of disease, illness, or sickness that afflicted any human being.

But in addition to miraculously restoring physical sight to the blind, He also gives "sight" to those who have been spiritually blinded by the devil. That word "blind" is derived from the Greek word *tuphlos*, and it doesn't just depict a person who is unable to see; it depicts a person who has been intentionally blinded by someone else. It can picture one whose eyes have been deliberately removed so that he is blinded. The individual hasn't just lost his sight — he has no eyes with which to see.

This reminds us of Second Corinthians 4:3-4, where Paul wrote, "But if our gospel be hid, it is hid to them that are lost: in whom the god of this world hath *blinded* the minds of them which believe not, lest the light of the glorious gospel of Christ, who is the image of God, should shine unto them."

In his writings, Paul used the word *tuphloo* to describe how Satan has "blinded" the unbelievers' minds. This word isn't just about a lack of vision — rather, it depicts one who has had his or her "eyes" removed by another.

This individual hasn't merely lost his ability to see; his eyes have been *removed*. If you have friends or family members who appear unable to see the truth, it isn't that they are naive — they are spiritually *blind*. Satan has "gouged out" their eyes, blocked their view, affected their minds, and they have no spiritual eyes with which to see. But miraculously, when we preach the Gospel to them, the Holy Spirit gives them spiritual eyes to see. Indeed, it's when we shine the light of the Gospel to those whom Satan has blinded that the Holy Spirit miraculously creates eyes for them to see!

Two millennia ago, the anointing on Jesus restored sight to the blind, and since He could do this, it meant there was no known human ailment that could resist the power of His touch. As we reflect on Hebrews 13:8, we are again reassured that Jesus Christ and His healing anointing are unchanged. The same power that gave sight to the blind and that could heal any physical or mental condition continues to heal today. Jesus remains constant, and as He worked wonders then, so, too, does He extend His healing hand to heal all manner of sickness and disease today. He is unchanged, for the same anointing is present right now for all who come to Him by faith.

### 5. Jesus Liberates Those Who Are Bruised

*Fifth*, we read in Luke 4:18 that Jesus' anointing came "to set at liberty them that are bruised." The words "set at liberty" are translated from a form of the Greek word *aphesis,* which is the same word translated as "deliverance" earlier in the verse. It describes *a dismissal, release*, and it can mean *to permanently set someone free.*

The word "bruised" originates from the Greek word *thrauo*, which conveys the idea of *crushing* or *breaking one down*. It pictures *a person whose life has been fractured* or *one whose life has been split up and fragmented.* This word "bruised" also clearly describes those who are oppressed. It can also refer to one who has been shattered by a life experience, by broken relationships, or by the trauma of divorce.

Of course, when we think of oppression, we gravitate to the idea of mental oppression, but oppression can also be felt in the body as one is weighed down by a sinister outside force that tries to crush or dominate it with disease, illness, and sickness.

In the powerful proclamation of Luke 4:18, we see that Jesus was anointed to free those ensnared by life's deepest fractures, both mentally and physically. That anointing which was unleashed over 2,000 years ago shattered the chains of those whose lives had been fractured and shattered, and it permanently freed them from the burdens of past traumas.

Hebrews 13:8 declares Jesus and His anointing are exactly the same today as 2,000 years ago, and that means since He healed this category at that time and His anointing has never changed, then those who are "bruised" in any way, if they will come to Jesus by faith, they can be liberated from their bruised condition today.

## 6. Jesus' Same Anointing Is Available Right Now

*Sixth*, we read in Luke 4:19 that Jesus came "to preach the acceptable year of the Lord." The word "acceptable" is translated from the Greek word *dektos*, and it means *accepted* or *favorable*, and it depicts *a favorable time to receive.*

The use of this phrase means whenever Jesus' anointing shows up, it becomes the most favorable moment in a person's life to receive whatever kind of healing or blessing is needed. And since Hebrews 13:8 says He and His anointing are unchangeable — and because Jesus' power is present through the ministry of the Holy Spirit — it means "right now" is the best moment for you to receive whatever you need His anointing to do in your life!

In Luke 4:19, we see that Jesus' anointing:

- Is an economic game-changer for the poor and will break the relentless grip of financial hardship, disrupt the cycle of poverty, and bring change to their lives.
- Heals the "brokenhearted" or those who feel they have been walked on by others, crushed by others, or smashed to pieces by life or relationships.
- Sets free "captives" who have been dragged into bondage by a sinister force, whether it be a poor self-image, toxic relationships, stubborn habits, alcohol, drugs, disease, illness, or sickness.

- Restores "sight" to the blind, which means Jesus' anointing is so powerful it can restore physical sight (along with spiritual sight) and, since He can heal the blind, there is no sickness known to medical science that He cannot heal.
- Sets at liberty those who are "bruised" — that is, those who have been fractured, fragmented, split up, or are suffering any kind of oppression in their emotions, mind, or body.
- Is available in an "acceptable" time, which means right now, at this very moment, for anyone who comes to Him by faith!

## WHERE DO WE GO FROM HERE?

Having unraveled the profound messages within Isaiah 53:3-5, Matthew 8:17, First Peter 2:24, and now Luke 4:16-19 — where Jesus Himself states that His anointing will accomplish even the "impossible" for anyone who comes to Him by faith — we are now poised to embark on the next part of our journey to discover *How To Appropriate Healing and Health for Your Body and Mind.*

The next chapter is very important, as it gives ways to receive the promised blessings of Scripture. It is my prayer that God will use the principles you are about to read to bring you to a better place physically and mentally. My specific prayer is that the next chapter will assist in helping you walk into the healing and health that the Bible says is God's explicit will for your life!

Scan the QR code to watch Rick teach more on this subject.

## QUESTIONS TO PONDER AND DISCUSS

1. Were you surprised to learn that Jesus not only reconciled you to the Heavenly Father in His act of redemption on the Cross, but He also purchased your peace of mind and your healing and well-being physically, mentally, and emotionally? Using Isaiah 53:3-5, describe in your own words everything redemption encompassed and what it means to you.

2. Regarding the blessing of the redemption purchased by Jesus' crucifixion on the Cross, what steps will you take to honor His death and resurrection by appropriating healing for *spirit, soul, and body*? (Hint: Joshua 1:8 and Proverbs 4:20-22 are keys to receiving from Him what He has freely provided.)

3. From what you now understand about the horrors of a scourging during the time of the Roman Empire, what new meanings do Isaiah 53:3-5, Matthew 8:16-17, and First Peter 2:24 hold for you? If you have traces of emotional trauma from your past, symptoms of sickness in your body, or anxiety that robs you of peace in your mind, in what ways are you now more confident that Jesus desires to remedy those situations in your life and that He has paid the price for you to experience permanent rescue and relief in those areas?

4. From Luke 4:16-19, rehearse the five areas that Jesus' anointing can touch to effect a change? Which one stood out to you as something Jesus wants to change in your life for the better?

5. First Peter 3:15 says, "...Be ready always to give an answer to every man that asketh you a reason of the hope that is in you...." If someone challenged you saying healing, deliverance, miracles, and wholeness and health are not blessings promised to us today, how could you use Hebrews 13:8 to lovingly and effectively counter that challenge? Why not meditate on that verse and write out your own declaration of faith concerning what Jesus and His anointing are doing in your life right now?

# ELEVEN

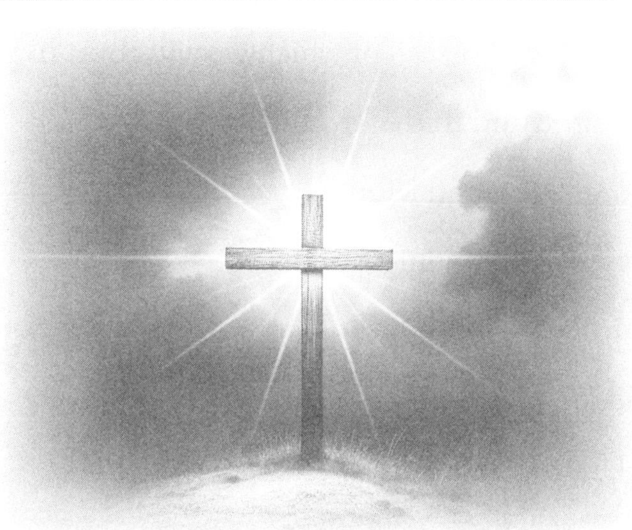

# HOW TO APPROPRIATE HEALING AND HEALTH FOR YOUR BODY AND MIND

Regardless of why a person is struggling with physical or mental disease, illness, or sickness, the fact is that Christ paid the price for him or her to be healed and to live in a state of divine health. Yet despite the fact that healing and health were secured by Christ's sacrifice, numerous people still grapple with physical and mental issues for a multitude of reasons, as we have seen. Although there are many reasons why people get sick, God, in His great mercy, has provided at the Cross everything necessary for them to be healed, healthy, and whole.

If you've taken action to close doors in your life so the devil has no "entry point" to assail your body or mind, it is time for you to take steps to claim what belongs to you as a child of God. In this chapter, we are going to look at how to appropriate healing and health for your body and mind. Because there is a lot of material, I want to provide you in advance with a guide to show you ten points that are important in the process of appropriating the healing and health Jesus purchased for you on the Cross, all of which we will cover in the pages to come.

1. Renewing Your Mind to the Truth
2. Aligning Your Heart and Mouth
3. Holding Fast to Your Confession
4. Letting Patience Do Its Work
5. Asking God for Clarification
6. Staying in Unwavering Faith
7. Laying Hands on the Sick
8. Letting the Gifts of Healing and Working of Miracles Do Their Work
9. Taking Communion
10. Calling for the Elders of the Church To Anoint With Oil and Pray the Prayer of Faith

### 1. Renewing Your Mind to the Truth

We have seen that, unfortunately, countless believers find themselves grappling with illness, despite Christ having already purchased their healing and health at the Cross. It is often the case that seeds of doubt and bad teaching have taken root in their hearts, causing them to doubt and even dismiss that it is God's will for them to be healed and healthy. But most everyone who faces a physical challenge in his body will do all in his power to remedy that situation and be restored to health. This just goes to show that the human condition was not supposed to be one of physical maladies, malignancies, and torments. People instinctively strive to be well for a reason.

Healing is the will of God for you! But you also need to understand that the devil can use others as instruments to sow seeds of doubt regarding the work of Christ on the Cross for your benefit. He knows that if those seeds of doubt and unbelief begin to sprout, he can wreak havoc in your life. He well understands that whoever or whatever controls your mind also controls your life, and that includes your health and well-being.

Consequently, the devil is relentless in his pursuit to infiltrate your mind with skepticism and disbelief. If he succeeds in embedding doubt into your mind, it will open the door for him to wage war on every other facet of your being — and that includes your body and mind.

To protect yourself from wrong thinking and seeds of doubt, it is imperative that you learn everything that belongs to you as a result of Christ's redemptive work on the Cross.

- You need to spend time studying to see what the Bible has to say about healing and health. Read and reread the truths in Scripture that declare it is God's will to heal, and then *keep* reading and meditating on them again and again until these truths are deeply rooted in your mind.
- You also need to study what the Bible — especially the New Testament epistles — has to say about your deliverance from evil powers, and instill in yourself the truth of Hebrews 2:3 that says you have received a "great salvation," or a great deliverance, from those powers of darkness.
- You need to spend time contemplating what "redemption" means and grasp its beneficial consequences in your life. To help you, read and reread what is written about redemption in Chapters Nine and Ten of this book.

You must take an active role to make sure that your comprehension of salvation — and all that it encompasses — is ingrained into your heart and mind. Once the knowledge of salvation and all it entails becomes a part of your thinking, believing, and mindset — to the extent you are convinced beyond a shadow of a doubt what Jesus' death and resurrection purchased for you — it will disarm the enemy from attacking your mind with doubt and unbelief as he has done in the past. If he has no say-so in your mind, it will make it harder for him to have a say-so in your body and mind, or your physical and mental health.

## YOU CAN 'GIRD UP' THE 'LOINS' OF YOUR MIND!

However, if you have any dangling, loose ends of doubt that the devil can latch hold of, he'll use them to entangle and hinder you from appropriating the healing and health that God intends for you to have and enjoy in life.

These dangling and loose ends are referred to in First Peter 1:13 where we are told, "Wherefore gird up the loins of your mind...."

The words "gird up" are a translation of the Greek word *anadzonnumi*, which pictures *runners* who are running in a race. In the ancient world, to run freely and without hindrance, runners would reach down to scoop up the dangling, loose ends of their garments to secure them snugly beneath their belts. If they allowed the dangling ends of their garments to hang loose, they would become tangled in their legs as they ran. Even if they had been maintaining a swift pace and keeping up a good race, these loose ends could at any time thwart their progress. In fact, permitting those loose ends to keep dangling was a sure recipe for defeat, but by tucking them out of the way, it enabled runners to move forward focused, unhampered, and without distraction.

But First Peter 1:13 is not talking about garments fashioned from material. This verse says that we must gird up "the loins of our minds." The use of these words tell us that if we don't remove the loose and dangling ends in our minds — and that includes wrong believing and wrong thinking — those loose and dangling ends will hinder our ability to experience what belongs to us in Christ. If we don't bring correction to those parts of our thinking that have been seeded with doubt and unbelief, we will miss the mark of appropriating by faith what God has provided. That is why we are admonished to grab hold of all those dangling areas in our thinking — to pull them out of the way, remove them, and then replace them with truth that liberates so we can run freely and without distractions.

According to First Peter 1:13, it is crucial to secure the dangling, loose ends of your thinking that the devil might try to use to impede your progress toward healing and health. That means you must intentionally remove wrong believing and wrong thinking and "gird up" the "loins" of your mind.

This removal may include wrong believing and wrong thinking you received from your family, friends, or past church affiliations. If you have repeatedly heard things that are not biblically true and you've therefore mis-learned things concerning divine healing, you must replace those beliefs with the truth.

Just as runners did all they could to eliminate impediments that obstructed or interfered with their race, you must "gird up the loins of your mind" so you can make the progress you need to make in order to cross the finish line of your victory — the manifestation of your healing and restoration to health! You see, if those untethered and unresolved areas of your mind are ignored, the devil will use them to entangle you and send you spiraling far from God's best intention for you.

In His boundless mercy, God transferred you from the dominion of Satan into the realm of His beloved Son. When you embraced Christ's redemptive work on the Cross, it resulted in your liberation from darkness and all its consequences. And when you were moved from the kingdom of darkness into the Kingdom of God, the chains that once bound you *shattered*.

Now if you find yourself not fully embracing healing, health, and numerous other blessings, you need to seek the Holy Spirit's help to renew your thinking to the truth, which is that you've received a salvation *brimming* with deliverance, healing, health, restoration, preservation, and soundness of mind!

Because of what Christ did on the Cross and because of the powerful, indwelling presence of the Holy Spirit in the life of the believer, it means the resurrection power of God is resident in you. Romans 8:11 says that power will "quicken" your body — and that includes quickening it to a state of healing and health when it is violated by disease, illness, or sickness.

**If those untethered and unresolved areas of your mind are ignored, the devil will use them to entangle you and send you spiraling far from God's best intention for you.**

Furthermore, it is vital for you to see and embrace that First Peter 2:24 says you already "were healed" by the stripes of Jesus. When you received Christ as Lord of your life, the healing purchased by those stripes that were laid across Jesus' back activated your physical and mental health. Hence, in God's sight, *you are already the healed of the Lord.* That means if you're experiencing symptoms of a physical or mental malady, either the devil or your self-inflicting actions has robbed you of the healing and health that is yours by virtue of redemption.

This truth of your redemption in Christ and what inherently belongs to you as a result is foundational to everything you will read in this chapter. In other words, if you don't have this fundamental belief straight in your heart and mind, little else will work for you to effect a change in your health or circumstances.

If you are thinking otherwise in any fashion, it's up to you to grab hold of those dangling loose ends of doubt and unbelief and remove them, and then to plant seeds of truth in their place. But I warn you, that if you permit yourself to continue in the vein of wrong thinking and wrong believing, it will affect your ability to possess the fullness of what Christ purchased for you.

## 2. Aligning Your Heart and Mouth

Once those dangling and loose ends are removed and what God's Word says about all that Christ purchased for you has been embedded in your heart, then it's time to take the next important step. That next step is to bring your heart and your mouth into alignment. This is what I call *the heart-mouth connection.*

In Mark 11:23, Jesus said, "For verily I say unto you, That whosoever shall say unto this mountain, Be thou removed, and be thou cast into the sea; and shall not doubt in his heart, but shall believe that those things which he saith shall come to pass; he shall have whatsoever he saith."

In this verse, Jesus taught *the heart-mouth connection* is so formidable that it can bring to pass whatsoever you believe in your heart and declare with your mouth. But notice Jesus said if a person "says" something "and shall not doubt in his heart." In other words, if he really believes what he is saying with his mouth — and doesn't "doubt in his heart" — he will eventually possess exactly what he says.

**In God's sight, *you are already the healed of the Lord.* That means if you're experiencing symptoms of a physical or mental malady, either the devil or your self-inflicting actions have robbed you of the healing and health that is yours by virtue of redemption.**

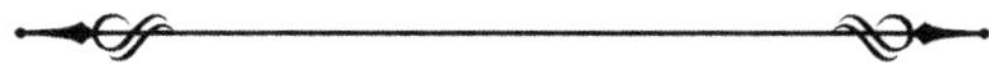

The word "doubt" is translated from a form of the Greek word *diakrinomai*, which means to *differ*, *doubt*, or *waver.* In the context of Mark 11:23, Jesus meant that when an individual's heart harmonizes with his or her own spoken words, it invariably sets things into motion!

The Greek word *diakrinomai,* which is translated "doubt" in Mark 11:23, pictures a person who differs in what he is inwardly believing versus what he is outwardly saying. But according to this verse, when he does *not* doubt (*diakrinomai*) or differ in his heart with what he is saying — his heart and his mouth are beating in syncopation and harmonizing together — that's when results will be forthcoming.

The verse could be rendered, "Whoever shall say…and not *differ* in his heart…." If you say one thing with your mouth, but the reality is that your heart doesn't believe it, or says something else, your heart and mouth are differing from one another, and you are making an empty confession that will not produce what you are saying. Your heart and mouth must be in alignment.

**In the context of Mark 11:23, Jesus meant that when an individual's heart harmonizes with his or her own spoken words, it invariably sets things into motion!**

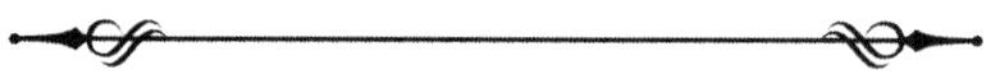

This principle of believing in the heart and confessing with the mouth applies to every sphere of life. But in the context of healing and health for your body and mind, it means if you really believe in your heart that Christ purchased your healing on the Cross — and you put your heartfelt faith together with the confession of your mouth — that combination will detonate divine power that literally brings healing and health into manifestation in your body and mind. *Creative power is released when the heart and mouth get into agreement!*

That is why you must be careful about what you believe in your heart and say with your mouth. When your heart and mouth get "in sync" with each other, it literally makes things come to pass!

In fact, this connection between your heart and speech can produce both constructive and destructive power. For example, the devil is well aware that if he can seed your heart and mind with doubt and unbelief and then coax you into speaking those lies with your mouth, your confession of them will cause those evil things to come to pass in your life. That is why the devil wants to fill your mind with doubt and unbelief. He knows that by enticing you to accept and internalize these doubts and then vocalize them, it's only a matter of time before they manifest into your own lived experience.

***Creative power is released when the heart and mouth get into agreement!*** **That is why you must be careful about what you believe in your heart and say with your mouth. When your heart and mouth get "in sync" with each other, it literally makes things come to pass!**

In Matthew 12:34, Jesus said, "...Out of the abundance of the heart the mouth speaketh." According to Jesus, whatever is in your heart will eventually come out of your mouth. Imagine your heart as a fountain, where whatever it holds will inevitably bubble up through your words. No force, not even gravity, is strong enough to keep what is in your heart from eventually coming out of your mouth. Mark 11:23 says that when beliefs deeply rooted within your heart and mind are transformed into spoken words, they unleash extraordinary power that is capable of shaping reality. Because great power is released when your heart and mouth start working together, it becomes paramount to nurture faith within your heart and to speak words of faith with your mouth, for Mark 11:23 reveals that this heart-mouth combination will ultimately sculpt the world around you.

But as I said before, this principle holds true for anything deeply held in your heart and spoken aloud. When your heart and mouth harmonize with the Word of God, it will produce the blessing of Christ in your life. Conversely, if the adversary persuades you to embrace doubt and unbelief, and you end up intentionally or even unintentionally speaking those words of doubt and unbelief out loud, those corrosive affirmations will bring bad results into your life.

**That is why the devil wants to fill your mind with doubt and unbelief. He knows that by enticing you to accept and internalize these doubts and then vocalize them, it's only a matter of time before they manifest into your own lived experience.**

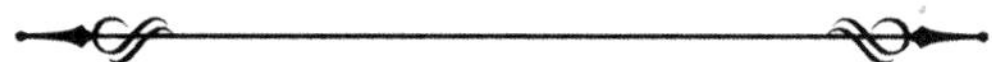

An example of a good heart-mouth combination would be a person who is struggling with some form of sickness. To overcome it, he begins to ingrain in his heart and mind the truth that healing and health belong to Him by virtue of Christ's redemptive work on the Cross. He meditates and meditates on those truths until they come alive inside his heart — and once he is filled with them, as Jesus said in Matthew 12:34, those truths begin to show up in his mouth. And when his heart and mouth get into complete alignment, Mark 11:23 reveals that it will create a conduit through which the healing and health of Christ will flow into his life and become a reality. This means that a person with a heart that is filled with faith in God's Word for healing, and with a mouth that speaks out his faith, will experience an improvement in his health.

On the flipside, let's say another person is also struggling with some form of sickness. However, rather than fill himself with the truth of God's Word about healing and health, he tunes into voices that say it isn't always God's will to heal. This results in him being filled with doubt and unbelief, and he finds himself being inundated with grim forecasts about his condition. According to Matthew 12:34, we know that what fills one's heart is soon reflected in his words. And according to Mark 11:23, when his heart and mouth begin to work "in sync," they manifest as reality. Thus, when a heart and mouth are filled with negativity, it takes root and can summon forth the very health outcomes he fears.

I'm not suggesting you ignore a medical report. Instead, fill yourself so full of God's promises of health and healing that you can face even the toughest medical diagnosis and prognosis with confidence. When you fill your heart with biblical promises about healing and health, and align your words with them, fear loses its grip. Your heart-mouth connection will result in your condition being improved or removed.

**Because great power is released when your heart and mouth start working together, it becomes paramount to nurture faith within your heart and to speak words of faith with your mouth, for Mark 11:23 reveals that this heart-mouth combination will ultimately sculpt the world around you.**

It's perfectly okay to let others know you are seeking healing when faced with illness. Seek the prayers and the faith of others to add to your own — and adhere to your doctor's guidance. However, it's equally important to saturate your heart with God's Word regarding healing and health, and let your faith-filled words echo His promises. As highlighted in Mark 11:23, when your heart and words are in harmony, they have the power to bring forth the healing and health you are seeking.

This is why immersing yourself in biblical promises of healing and health is so crucial. As you attune your mind to God's promises, His Word acts like a purifying stream that gently washes away the doubts and unbelief that the adversary attempts to plant in your thoughts. By making it a priority to saturate your mind with the truth of God's Word, you create a fortress that the enemy cannot breach. And if you're not filled with doubt and unbelief, you won't be speaking and confessing things that are out of sync with God's promises for you.

It is vital for you to choose who or what is going to control your mind. Will it be God and His Word, or will you allow the enemy to seed your heart and mind with doubt and unbelief? You are going to be filled with *something*, so choose the right thing to fill you. Your choice in this matter will determine your success or your failure regarding healing and health, so make sure you choose wisely!

### 3. Holding Fast to Your Confession

Once you have filled your heart and mouth with God's promises about the healing and health that Christ obtained for you in His work of redemption, you must dig your heels into the bedrock of your faith and decide to never budge from your position of faith.

Hebrews 10:23 says, "Let us hold fast the profession of our faith without wavering; (for he is faithful that promised)."

The words "hold fast" are derived from the Greek word *katecho*, which is a compound of the word *kata* and *echo*. The word *kata* carries the force of *something that comes down so hard and so heavily* that it is *overpowering* and *dominating* to the point of being *subjugating*. When this force arrives on the scene, it conquers, subdues, and immediately begins expressing its overwhelming, influencing power.

The second part of the word *katecho* is the word *echo*, which simply means *I have* and carries the notion of *possession*. When *kata* and *echo* are compounded into the word *katecho*, it portrays *seizing something with all one's might and keeping it firmly under one's control* to ensure it never escapes him. Because of the word *kata,* it is the image of someone who finds the object of his dreams and then holds it down — taking control of it, dominating it, even sitting on it — so it doesn't slip away!

The word *katecho* is used in Romans 1:18, where Paul told us about ungodly men "...who hold [or suppress] the truth in unrighteousness." In other words, because these ungodly men didn't like the truth, they "sat on it" or "put a lid on it" in an effort to keep others from hearing the truth and getting set free. But in Hebrews 10:23, this same idea is used positively to describe a believer taking possession of God's promises and refusing to ever let them slip away!

This is the attitude you must have if you want to see God's promises come to pass in your life. Once you've deeply embedded them into your heart and renewed your mind to them, you have to wrap your arms around them and determine to never relinquish them. For example, you must *katecho* God's promises for healing and health so they won't be able to get away from you, and so no one will ever be able to convince you to walk away from them. Hebrews 10:23 could be interpreted, "And let us hold fast to our confession, tightly wrapping our arms around it and embracing it with all our might...."

The words "hold fast" imply there is always a fight to stay on track with God's promises. When it comes to healing, it means you must cling to God's promise with unwavering determination. Without a conscious effort to hold tightly to God's promise of healing and health, either experience or the negative voices of others will try to steal it from you. In times of weariness, it's easier to let God's promises slip away, so Hebrews 10:23 encourages us to grip God's Word tightly and resolutely, refusing to let go of our faith-filled confessions!

The first part of Hebrews 10:23 says, "Let us hold fast the profession of our faith...."

The word "profession" in this verse is derived from the Greek word *homologia*, which is a compound of the words *homo* and *logia.* The Greek word *homo* means *one of the very same kind*, and *logia* is the plural form of *logos*, which means *words.* When these two words are combined, they form the word *homologia*, as used in this verse, and it is translated as the word "profession" in the *King James Version.*

However, the word "profession" inadequately conveys the meaning of the Greek word *homologia.* To capture the meaning of this word, it is essential to consider the meanings of both parts of *homologia.* The first part of the word, *homo*, conveys the idea of *agreement*, and the second part of the word, *logia*, is the plural form of *logos* and means *words*.

Let me give you an illustration of the word *homologia* that will help you understand. I am a writer and have written many books. My words are my thoughts, my convictions, and my beliefs recorded on the printed page. If you read my books and *agree* with what I have written — or you *agree* with my words — in essence, you are in *agreement* and are *harmonizing* with me. Those words are what I think, what I believe, and what I have expressed.

Ultimately, if you *agree* with what I've written, you are *coming into agreement* with *me* as the author. If you take my viewpoint and begin to hold it as your own conviction, it won't be long until you and I are *aligned* in our thinking and believing.

After my words have gotten deeply into your heart and you have fully embraced them, those words will soon become your own convictions. Then when you share that information with others, you will no longer be just repeating — or parroting — what you have read in my book. Instead, you will be speaking from the platform of your own heart about what *you* believe. At this juncture, our ideas are not just parallel — they are united, and we are fluently speaking the same language!

The word "profession" in Hebrews 10:23 is not the picture of a person who simply repeats or parrots what someone else says. Rather, it pictures an individual who has internalized God's Word to such a degree that he aligns himself completely with God's perspective on a matter. This person has immersed himself in the Scriptures so thoroughly that his perceptions mirror God's — he sees, hears, and feels in harmony with what God says about an issue. His heart and God's heart are so unified that they beat in syncopation. Therefore, when this believer "confesses" God's Word, his words are not hollow or superficial; rather, they emerge from a profound well of conviction within his soul.

After a period of meditating and renewing your own mind with the Word of God (*see* Romans 12:2), you will finally begin to see a matter the way that God sees it. You will really believe what God believes. From that place of heartfelt conviction, you then begin to speak and to declare your faith. When a believer internalizes God's Word so profoundly that it harmonizes with his innermost being, his words transcend mere repetition or parroting of familiar phrases. Instead, he boldly articulates his faith from a place of authentic belief!

Many people make the mistake of merely repeating what they've heard someone else say without ever developing any depth of faith or understanding behind their words. They say the right things, but because these words come only out of their mouths — and not from the depths of their hearts — their confession produces no results.

## HOW TO AVOID MAKING MINDLESS, 'MECHANICAL' CONFESSIONS

It's essential that your faith infuses your speech — that your faith and your mouth are connected. A "mechanical" profession doesn't come from the heart and is similar to seedless fruit that is incapable of reproducing. For your confession to be impactful, it must resonate inside the depths of your heart before it comes out of your mouth. So how do you avoid making mechanical, mindless confessions?

- *First*, make certain you have chosen to believe what God says. If it is in regard to healing and health, commit your heart and mind to believing the Word of God, no matter how crazy it may sound to your natural mind.

- *Second*, ask the Holy Spirit to make God's Word real to you — so real, in fact, that should anyone even imply that what God said isn't true, you'd think that person was out of his mind!
- *Third*, pick up your Bible and do some serious study and meditation. Sow that Word into your heart until you and God are aligned on the issue.
- *Fourth*, as that alignment comes into being, it's time for you to open your mouth and start declaring, and continually declare, the Word of God over your body and mind!

We just read the first part of Hebrews 10:23, which says, "Let us hold fast the profession of our faith...." That verse goes on to say, "Let us hold fast the profession of our faith *without wavering*...."

The word "wavering" is rooted in the Greek word *aklines*, which is the Greek word *klino* with an *a* attached to the front of it. The word *klino* means *to bend, bow, or yield*. If you remove the *a* from the word, you are left with the word *klino*, which pictures *a person who is bowed down*. With shoulders stooped and body bent over, this person is so tired he can barely stand. Ultimately, he becomes so exhausted that he throws in the towel and gives up. In fact, the word *klino* comes from the same root word in Greek that describes *a bed* or *a couch*.

But the *a* attached to the front of *klino* as a prefix has a cancelling or negating force. And because the word "wavering" in Hebrews 10:23 has that little *a* attached to it, it reverses the condition and pictures one who does *not* bend, bow, or yield. One expositor says the verse is our instruction to hold fast to our faith-filled confession *without giving in, giving up, bending, breaking, or going to bed on what you have professed*. In other words, this person has too much invested to go to bed on his faith, so he therefore refuses to budge an inch on what he is believing.

Often people let go of their confession of faith for healing and health because the devil or other people tell them, "This thing you're believing for isn't ever going to happen. Surely it would have materialized already if it were ever meant to be. You're squandering your time. Why don't you forget it, let it go, and move on with your life?"

If that describes you and you feel tempted to give up on what you're believing, instead of surrendering, backing down, or giving in and giving up, I encourage you to dig in your heels, drive down your stake, and tell the devil that you are not going to move from your position of faith. It may take awhile for that promise to come into manifestation, but if you will fill your heart and mind with the truth of God's Word about healing and health, renew your mind to it, and hold fast to your confession of faith, God assures that your perseverance will lead to tangible outcomes. With a resolute heart and unyielding will, choose to believe in God's promises despite your feelings, contrary thoughts, dissenting voices, or daunting circumstances. Stand your ground boldly, with conviction, and tell the devil that you are not going to move from your position of faith.

### 4. Letting Patience Do Its Work

We have covered three vital steps to help you start the process of appropriating what Jesus purchased for you at the Cross. In review, they are as follows:

1. Renewing Your Mind to the Truth
2. Aligning Your Heart and Mouth
3. Holding Fast to Your Confession

The next three steps I will give you are filled with a lot of Greek exposition because I want you to really understand what the original text tells us about what we must introspectively do to receive the manifestation of healing and health that belongs to us. Please do not get in a hurry as you read these sections. Read them slowly and deeply take in the words before you.

For these three points, we will go to the book of James to uncover principles that apply to any situation in which you are awaiting an answer to prayer. Every word you are about to read is intended to help you stay on track with your faith until you receive what you are believing to happen in your life. If you are believing for healing and health, or any other blessing that is yours because of Christ's redemptive work on the Cross, the principles you are about to read will be very helpful to you.

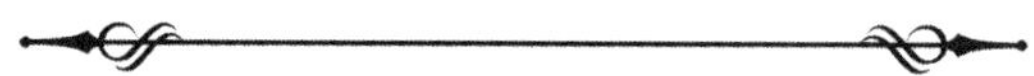

**If you will fill your heart and mind with the truth of God's Word about healing and health, renew your mind to it, and hold fast to your confession of faith, God assures that your perseverance will lead to tangible outcomes. With a resolute heart and unyielding will, choose to believe in God's promises despite your feelings, contrary thoughts, dissenting voices, or daunting circumstances. Stand your ground boldly, with conviction, and tell the devil that you are not going to move from your position of faith.**

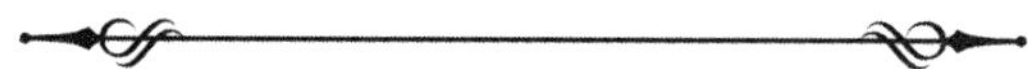

Jesus' brother James wrote this epistle to believers who were experiencing hard times and were tempted to give up. He wrote to encourage them to remain steadfast in their faith, and what he wrote to them also applies in principle to anyone who is believing for something to come to pass in his life. Pay careful attention to what you are about to read, for it holds instructions for you as well.

James 1:3 says, "Knowing this, that the trying of your faith worketh patience."

The word "knowing" is rooted in the Greek word *ginosko*, which means *I know*. But here, it is a participle, which means it would be better translated as *knowing, forever knowing, always keeping in mind.* It depicts continuous and uninterrupted action. Hence, it speaks of what must *always be known and never forgotten.* It means that for anyone who is awaiting an answer to prayer for healing and health, or any other blessing, James is about to tell us something so important that it should *always be remembered and never forgotten.*

Then James 1:3 adds, "Knowing this, *that*...." The word "that" in Greek points the reader to the following important statement, which says "the trying of your faith worketh patience."

The word "trying" is derived from the Greek word *dokimadzo*, which depicts *a test to prove the trustworthiness or claim of a product.* For example, because an advertised product boasts of its merits, someone who sees or hears it takes it upon himself to devise a "test" to see if the product can stand up under pressure and if the claims of the product can be proven true. The use of this word indicates that when you make a declaration of faith — for example, a bold confession that you are going to receive healing and walk in divine health — the devil similarly hears your faith-filled confession, and because you have made such a bold confession of faith, he devises some kind of "test" to see if what you have claimed or confessed by faith can hold up under pressure.

Suddenly, even though you are normally quite physically well, you are hit with sickness, and you may even wonder, *I just made a declaration of faith that I would be healed and healthy. Why am I suddenly hit with sickness?* Such challenges don't come from God's hands but bear the sinister fingerprints of a mischievous adversary who is crafting a "test" designed to sway you from your faith. In respect to healing and health, this principle in James 1:3 lets us know that when we've anchored our faith in God's promises for healing and health — and boldly confessed that healing and health are ours — the devil typically orchestrates an assault in response.

Yet James 1:3 tells us that rather than buckling under this scheme designed to shatter your resolve, it is your opportunity to demonstrate your unwavering commitment to what God promised and to what you have confessed. Rather than crumble, this is your moment to show the devil that you are serious about what you are believing. Embrace this as your opportunity to resist, to stand up, and to never budge from what you believe, claim, or confess. By outlasting the pressure of the test, you will prove that what you claim or confess by faith is indeed authentic, genuine, and true.

## ENDURANCE WILL WORK IN YOUR FAVOR

James 1:3 goes on to say, "Knowing this, that the trying of your faith *worketh patience.*" The word "worketh" is derived from the Greek word *katergadzomai*, which is a compound of the words *kata* and *ergadzomai.* The word *kata* means *down*, and the word *ergadzomai* means *I work*. When these two words are compounded, it means *to work down from the top to the bottom*. It depicts *something that has been thoroughly worked throughout*. Thus, James 1:3 tells us that when a believer decides not to yield under the weight of adversity, but chooses to push back against the enemy's attacks, a heavenly strength is unleashed — a divine empowerment that begins at the top of his head and works its way down to his feet until that believer is filled from top to bottom with it.

The word "patience" in this part of the verse describes the heavenly force that God releases inside you in such a moment. The word "patience" originates from the Greek word *hupomone*, a compound of the words *hupo* and *meno*. The word *hupo* means *under*, and here it depicts *one under a heavy load*. The word *meno* depicts *the resolve to stay put, abide, and not move*. But when these words are compounded to form the word *hupomone,* the word "patience" would be better translated as *endurance*.

This word carries the meaning *to abide, to defiantly stick it out regardless of the pressure mounted against it, to keep a position, to remain in one's spot*, or *to stay put*. It also depicts *staying power, hang-in-there power, the attitude that holds out, holds on, outlasts, perseveres, and hangs in there, never giving up, refusing to surrender to obstacles, and turning down every opportunity to quit*. This word further pictures *one who is under a heavy load but refuses to bend, break, or surrender because he is convinced that the territory, promise, or principle under assault rightfully belongs to him*.

Thus James 1:3 declares that a supernatural power is released in you the moment you choose to push back against the enemy's assault. Rather than face the fight on your own, God joins Himself to the one who chooses to push back against the enemy's attack. He fills that person with the supernatural ability to stay put, to remain in his spot, and to keep his position, and He gives him the ability to maintain the territory he has gained. For those who dig in their heels, stand firm, and refuse to budge despite an onslaught, their decision to stand in faith invites God to provide the fortitude needed to resist the enemy's advances.

This word *hupomone* was also importantly used in a military context to picture soldiers who were ordered to maintain their positions even in the face of opposition. For soliders, the word *hupomone* meant they were to remain at their posts and *to defiantly stick it out regardless of pressures mounted against them.*

This word *hupomone* pictures one who is under a heavy load, but he refuses to bend, break, or surrender, because he is convinced that the territory, promise, or principle under assault rightfully belongs to him. In the context of James 1:3, this word makes the point that when the devil devises a "test" to try to move us away from our confession of faith, *if* we choose to push back against the attack, God joins Himself to us and supernaturally releases *hupomone* into our life — that is, a divine power that gives us the supernatural ability to outlast the assault. The Early Church believed *hupomone* was the "queen of all virtues." They understood that if they had *hupomone*, it was never a question of *if* they would win a fight, but only a question of *when* they would win. Having *hupomone* was the guarantee that they would endure until full victory was achieved.

Let's take this information into your story. If you are believing for healing and health, James 1:3 means when you make a bold proclamation of faith — whether it be for healing and health, or any other blessing — the devil is listening and will likely devise a "test" to see if he can put you under enough pressure to make you back off from what you have confessed. But if you make the choice to push back against the attack, saying, "Devil, if you doubt my resolve, just watch as I cling fiercely to the promises God has made to me," God will step in!

James 1:3 says He will respond by filling you with so much *hupomone* that you will be able to stay put, not budge, hang in there, and never give up, refusing to surrender to every obstacle and turning down every opportunity to quit.

So if an assault comes to challenge your confession of faith, whatever it may be, you must dig in your heels and refuse to budge. If you take this position, God will become your partner in the fight. He will enable you to endure until the fight is finished, and when the pressure lets up, it is entirely possible that you'll find yourself much improved in terms of your healing and health.

Indeed, when the devil sees God has filled you with *hupomone* — that is, *an unshakable resilience that never backs off* — he'll eventually retreat. It's often after such a retreat that the manifestation of one's confession swiftly follows. I cannot tell you how long this process will take, but I can tell you that when God responds to your decision to push back and fills you with *hupomone*, it endows you with all that is needed to stay steadfast until the fight is finished and you are standing healed and healthy or with the answer to whatever it was you were praying about.

## AFTER ENDURANCE DOES ITS WORK...

James 1:4 goes on to say, "But let patience have her perfect work, that ye may be perfect and entire, wanting nothing."

The word "patience" at the beginning of the verse is again *hupomone*, so a better rendering would read, "Let *endurance* have her perfect work...." The rest of the verse says that if you let endurance do its full work, it will make you "perfect and entire, wanting nothing."

The word "perfect" is rooted in the Greek word *teleios*, which describes *maturity* and denotes *one who graduates upward from one level to the next level at school.* Thus, James 1:4 effectively says that when a person chooses to push back against attacks and decides to be unmoving in his stance of faith, this develops him spiritually and puts him on an upward trajectory into higher levels of spiritual maturity.

The word "entire" is interpreted from a form of the Greek word *holokleros*, which is a compound of *holos* and *kleros*. The word *holos* means *complete* or *whole*, and it is where we derive the English word "whole." The word *kleros* refers to *an inheritance received by lot*. When these two words are compounded, it means *to possess everything allotted to one by inheritance.*

James 1:4 thereby states that when a believer allows endurance to work in him, he has found *the key* to receiving the full inheritance that belongs to him through Christ's redemptive work on the Cross. If you have endurance, you have the key to receiving healing, deliverance, prosperity, protection, peace, joy, healthy relationships, and countless other blessings.

The word "wanting" is derived from a form of the Greek word *leipo*, which pictures *a deficiency*, *scarcity*, *shortage*, *shortfall*, or *undersupply*. It describes *one who is in need*, *one who lacks*, or *one who has an insufficiency of some type*. In the context of this verse, it means having *no deficiency* of any type. The word "nothing" is from a Greek word that means *none*, *not even one*, or *not any at all* and, thus, it depicts the image of a believer who has learned the key to having all that one needs, to the point of having *no deficiencies at all, not even one.*

**The *RIV* (*Renner Interpretive Version*) of James 1:3-4 says:**

> **You need to know — really know, and never forget, that difficult situations come to see if you are serious about your stance of faith and if your faith is really all it claims to be or if it will break under pressure. But finally...when those tests let up, and your faith is still standing strong, it will have proven your faith to be real. When you push back to resist the tests that have been sent to break you — that pushback triggers a release of divine endurance that fills you from the top of your head clear to the bottom of your feet! It's a supernatural endurance that will enable you to bear up**

**under any heavy load, and it will give you the ability to stay put, to keep your position, and to never surrender. I'm talking about a power that will enable you to hold on; hold out; never give up; neither bend nor break; outlast; persevere; and stick it out. This power will strengthen you to hold on to whatever promise or territory is under assault.**

**But you're the one who must make the choice to let this God-given endurance do its work. And if you'll let endurance run its full course, it will advance you into higher levels of spiritual maturity. Choosing to let endurance run its full course takes work — but if you'll stick with this process all the way to the end, you'll advance to high spiritual levels in your life. Not only that, but you'll have in your possession the quality necessary to possess your God-given inheritance — ending up with no deficits, shortages, or lack of any kind, and I mean *none whatsoever*.**

## 5. Asking God for Clarification

Anyone who has been waiting a long time for answers to prayer may ask, "I've meticulously followed every suggestion in this book. I've taken a thorough personal inventory to ensure no inadvertent access has been given to negative influences, and I've worked diligently to shut every potential door that was opened. I've rooted my faith firmly in the promises of Isaiah 53:3-5, and I've truly embraced the redemption Christ secured for me on the Cross. My heart and words are in sync as I boldly declare my beliefs. I've resolutely resisted the challenges trying to shake my resolve and have refused to yield to them. I have done all of this to the best of my ability and I've still not received the manifestation of healing and health that I've been believing, confessing, and awaiting. Why?"

For anyone who "feels" that his faith is not working — and does not seem to be able to find anyone who can help him find the answer — James 1:5 gives the best possible advice: "If any of you lack wisdom, let him ask of God, that giveth to all men liberally, and upbraideth not; and it shall be given him."

The word "lack" is rooted in the Greek word *leipo*, and it pictures *a deficiency, scarcity, shortage, shortfall, or undersupply*. It describes *one who is in need, one who lacks*, or *one who has an insufficiency of some type*. My friend, Keith Trump, an American Bible Society scholar, says the word *leipo* was often used by ancient writers to depict a scenario wherein a traveler finds himself on a journey, but he realizes something crucial for his trip was left behind. This missing item is essential to the journey and its absence could make the difference between reaching the destination or not.

Thus, in the context of James 1:5, we can receive this word *leipo* to picture a believer on a faith journey, who discovers that he is in "lack" of the wisdom he needs to complete the trip. Wisdom is not absent because it is out of reach, but because the traveler has unintentionally left it behind at some juncture. But by turning to God, he can easily obtain the wisdom needed — for God is present wherever the person is on the journey to bestow to him the answers needed to advance him confidently on his journey of faith.

In the same way, if your particular journey is to arrive at a place of healing and health, or to receive any blessing obtained for us by Christ at the Cross, you especially need wisdom for why it seems you are not reaching your destination — or for what you need to do, or stop doing, in order to get there. The word "wisdom" is derived from the Greek word *sophia*, and it denotes *insight* or *understanding*. So the first part of James 1:5 essentially means, "If you lack wisdom — answers and insight — about why these principles are not working for you...."

## INSTRUCTION IN RECEIVING WISDOM THAT HAS BEEN LACKING

Furthermore, we are told in James 1:5, "If any of you lack wisdom, let him *ask* of God...." The word "ask" is rooted in the Greek word *aiteo*, which means *to petition* or *to request — always with the expectation of receiving what is being sought.* This means God desires that His children approach Him believing that if they seek His guidance, they'll receive it — He will provide what they need.

It is important to note that this verse says God has one requirement: The person seeking wisdom must ask "of" God. The word "of" is translated from the Greek word *para*, which means *alongside*. It pictures the one *drawing alongside* the heart of God to find the answers he needs. Once in that position alongside God's heart, he is told to make his heartfelt request.

James 1:5 says that God "giveth" to the one who comes alongside His heart to ask for answers. The original text could be rendered, "Let him ask of the 'God that giveth.'" This description of "the giving God" pictures *the benevolent God* or *the God that gives*. In the original Greek text, it is unmistakably presenting God as *the giving God* and that He is pleased to answer any question from those who draw near to His side. However, drawing near is God's requirement for those who seek answers and wisdom. Thus, James 1:5 urges us to come alongside the heart of God, who is generous and who stands ready to liberally supply answers to those who seek His wisdom.

## THE LIBERALITY OF GOD

In fact, God is so generous that James 1:5 goes on to say, "If any of you lack wisdom, let him ask of God, that giveth *to all men*...."

The words "to all men" in the Greek text is *an all-encompassing word* that shows God gives *to all* who meet His conditions of drawing near to Him. Furthermore, James 1:5 says that when God supplies the answers we need, He gives them to us "...*liberally*, and upbraideth not...."

The word "liberally" is derived from the Greek word *haplos*, which denotes something given *abundantly, amply, bountifully, copiously, directly, extravagantly, generously, lavishly, liberally, plentifully, profusely, open-handedly, simply, sincerely, and with no complications.* This means if you are puzzled as to why these faith principles haven't produced fruit in your life so far, if you will come alongside the heart of God and submit your request for answers with expectancy, God will generously give you the answers you need to know.

And James 1:5 says that when God answers you, He "upbraideth not." The word "upbraideth" is rooted in the Greek word *oneididzo.* It means *to berate, to chastise, to criticize harshly,* or *to nitpick.* The word "not" is emphatic. This tells us God is not offended by our honest asking, and He will not be harsh with those who seek Him for answers. God is not a nitpicker who is waiting to scold, rebuke, or point out all one's faults and weaknesses. If you reach out to Him for answers, God will lavishly answer and supply clarity for whatever you need to know. Then James 1:5 concludes with the promise, "If any of you lack wisdom, let him ask of God, that giveth to all men liberally, and upbraideth not; *and it shall be given him.*"

Thus, this passage assures us that God doesn't begrudge those who seek His counsel; instead, He embraces them. For those who come close to His presence to gain the answers they need, God has answers waiting for them.

So if you are among those who ask, "If I have done all these things to the best of my ability, why haven't I received the manifestation of healing and health or other blessings that I've been confessing, believing, and waiting for?" If this question is similar to what you've been thinking and saying to yourself, accept God's invitation to draw near so He can provide the answers you need!

**The *RIV* (*Renner Interpretive Version*) of James 1:5 says:**

**But if — as I'm sure is actually the case — there is anyone among you who lacks insight about why these principles aren't already working, my advice is that you draw near to the side of the giving God to ask your questions with the full expectation of an answer from the One who always generously responds with an open hand to every person who comes to Him. And when you come to Him with your questions, He will not berate, reprimand, or scold you**

**for asking the questions you put before Him — for answers are always generously given to the person who draws near to God to find them.**

## 6. Staying in Unwavering Faith

Regardless of what one is requesting from God, he must ask in faith, and that is why James 1:6 says, "But let him ask in faith, nothing wavering. For he that wavereth is like a wave of the sea driven with the wind and tossed."

The word "ask" is the same Greek word we saw in James 1:5 — the Greek word *aiteo* — which means *to ask, to demand, to petition*, or *to request*, and it pictures one who asks with the full expectation of receiving what was firmly, confidently, and decisively requested. This word *aiteo* does not depict a hope-so attitude that perhaps God will respond, but a firm and full expectation that He *will* answer.

James 1:6 further says, "But let him ask *in faith*...."

The word "in" is a translation of the preposition *en*, which means *in, inside*, or *located inside*, and it gives the impression of a place *in which* this asking is to take place. Here it means *being solidly rooted in* or *from a position of being in faith in* the promises of God's Word. The word "faith" is interpreted from a form of *pistis*, which is translated as *faith* in the New Testament. But the word *pistis* is derived from *peitho*, a word that pictures one who possesses *a rock-solid belief, an absolute confidence, an unmovable conviction*, or *an unwavering confidence.* Thus, real faith is not "back and forth" — up one day and down the next, or indecisive; rather, it is *a rock-solid, unwavering force.*

In light of this, I want to ask, how consistent are you in what you are asking and believing God to do in regard to your healing and health? Are you back and forth — up one day, down the next day, and indecisive — or are you rock solid and unwavering in what you are believing and asking?

James 1:6 continues, "But let him ask in faith, *nothing wavering*...."

The word "wavering" is a translation of *diakrinomenos*, a Greek word that depicts *habitual vacillation*. Since this book is dedicated to the issue of healing and health, I need to again ask, in light of this verse, are you consistent in your asking and believing, or are you vacillating — going back and forth — in your faith in what you're asking and believing?

The word *diakrinomenos*, translated "wavering" in this verse, pictures one who is back and forth, habitually changing his mind about what he believes, what he confesses, and how he prays. And James 1:6 states that any person who is *on again-off again* and who habitually flip-flops in what he asks, believes, or prays is not asking in faith. On the contrary, real faith stands still. It knows what it wants, and it doesn't budge or flinch from its rock-solid position. A person who is asking in real faith doesn't flip-flop back and forth in what he asks or believes.

## WHAT REAL FAITH *DOESN'T* DO

James 1:6 says real faith does not behave "like a wave of the sea driven with the wind and tossed." The words "wave of the sea" are interpreted from the plural form of the Greek word *kludon*, a word that pictures *one wave after another* or *a succession of rising and falling waves.*

My wife and I enjoy watching the waves of the sea. As we watch them, we often comment how the waves swell and grow bigger and bigger until, finally, they peak and then fall, tumbling backward into the sea from which they came. As we continue to watch, we see waves gathering height, volume, momentum, and speed. Then once again, we watch in amazement as they rise and grow bigger and bigger until they finally peak and crash, tumbling right back into the vast sea. Over and over, as the wind maintains its ferocity, this seemingly never-ending process repeats itself.

This is the example James 1:6 gives of a person who is not asking from a position of faith. Rather than being rock-solid and unwavering in what he asks, this person's asking resembles the restless sea, forever in motion, and never steadfast. Although such a person may appear to start in faith, if he habitually changes his mind and rethinks what he's asking or believing, he is, in reality, like a wave of the sea. He is caught in a cycle of doubt and uncertainty. He rises to ask, to believe, and to confess — but then, almost as soon as it seems he's gaining strength, he changes his mind, retracts what he has asked, believed, and confessed, and tumbles back into a state of indecision.

This behavior is completely contrary to real faith, which is not up one day and down the next or continually flipping back and forth in what it asks or believes. In fact, such a continual state of flux starkly contrasts with genuine faith, which remains steadfast, unwavering, and is unswayed by the winds of change or doubt.

James 1:6 adds, "But let him ask in faith, nothing wavering. For he that wavereth is like a wave of the sea *driven with the wind* and *tossed*."

The words "driven with the wind" are derived from a form of *anemos*, a Greek word that depicts *fierce winds* or *turbulence* that has the potential to wreak havoc and destruction. The word "tossed" is translated from a form of the Greek word *rhipidzo*, which pictures *raging currents* of the sea, but it also pictures *a dangerous undercurrent*. Some scholars propose that this word *rhipidzo* is the etymological root for *riptide*, which is a perilous current born from atmospheric turbulence that is capable of pulling anything trapped within its grasp into a relentless pull, potentially causing one to drown as he is forcefully swept far from shore.

By using these words and imagery to caution those whose faith is less than steadfast, James was telling us that those who are easily moved by what they hear and see, and who habitually vacillate in what they believe or say, suffer the threat of being dragged into a state of spiritual bedlam that has the potential to "drown" their faith and make it ineffectual.

Such individuals may not realize the seriousness of such a state of indecision, but this habitual wavering back and forth and vacillating in faith — if it is not halted — can, like a riptide, pull them into an undertow from which it will be difficult for them to break free. Thus, one who falters back and forth in what he asks, believes, and confesses needs to understand that such damaging behavior must be stopped before he or she is sucked into a perpetual sea of indecision.

**The *RIV* (*Renner Interpretive Version*) of James 1:6 says:**

> **But this next point is important, so pay close attention. Whoever is asking must do it with an expectation that God will actually answer him. In other words, he must ask, being rooted in faith (with unwavering confidence). The one who doesn't stick with it, but who habitually changes his mind — who is up one day and down the next, flip-flopping and going back and forth "all over the place" in what he asks or believes — is a lot like the waves of the sea. Just as waves rise, fall, and tumble back into the sea over and over, a doubting person is one who keeps changing his mind again and again. He appears to be making progress, but then, suddenly, he changes his mind again and tumbles back into indecision. He is up and down, back and forth, indecisive, and unstable. And as the waves of the sea are endlessly tossed by ferocious winds, one who doubts is thrown here, there, and all around. A person who can't make up his mind about what he asks and believes doesn't realize the dangerous predicament he's in — for like a dangerous riptide, his doubt and wavering can pull him perpetually into a sea of indecision.**

In fact, James 1:7 goes on to say those who habitually change their minds about what they ask, believe and confess — flipping one way and then another, up and down, and all over the place — are *unable* to receive anything from the Lord. James 1:7 says, "For let not that man think that he shall receive any thing of the Lord."

The words "let not" are a translation of the Greek particle *me*, which here *rules out* the thought that follows. The words "that man" are an interpretation of the Greek word *ekeinos*, which here refers to *the person who vacillates in faith* — going back and forth, up and down, and all around in what he asks or believes — and doesn't know how to "stand still," or stay in the same place in faith without wavering or budging.

James 1:7 continues and says, "For let not that man think...."

The word "think" is from a form of the Greek word *oimai*, which means *to assume, to imagine, to presume*, or *to suppose.* In this case, it means *to wrongly imagine, to wrongly presume*, or *to wrongly suppose* and pictures *fictional thinking.*

Although this person lives in a state of indecision, he has somehow convinced himself that he will receive what he wants from the Lord. But what he wants from the Lord is not clear because this person can't make up his mind about what he is asking. He asks boldly and confidently one moment — but in the next, the "wave" of his faith comes crashing down to riptide level, and he is tossed to and fro in his faith. To believe he will somehow receive an answer when he is indecisive in his faith is *misguided thinking.*

Then James 1:7 says, "For let not that man think that he shall *receive any thing* of the Lord."

The word "receive"' is rooted in the Greek word *lambano,* which simply means *to receive.* Here it depicts *one who graciously receives something that should be freely and easily given.* But James said the person who can't make up his mind about what he asks, believes, or confesses — who is up one day, down the next day, and flipping back and forth in his faith — is unable to receive "anything" from the Lord.

The words "any thing" are translated from the Greek word *ti*, which denotes *the smallest and most minute detail.* It means an indecisive person cannot receive *anything at all* — not because God doesn't want to bless him or her, but because this person doesn't stay in one place long enough to be blessed. *It is hard to hit a moving target!*

**An indecisive person cannot receive *anything at all* — not because God doesn't want to bless him or her, but because this person doesn't stay in one place long enough to be blessed. *It is hard to hit a moving target!***

James 1:6-7 holds important instructions for anyone who needs to receive anything from the Lord — and that includes the healing and health that Jesus obtained in His redemptive work on the Cross. We must simply *ask*, expecting an answer, and refuse to be "tossed about" concerning what we want to receive from the Lord.

## 7. Laying Hands on the Sick

So far in this chapter, we've seen that to appropriate the healing and health that Jesus purchased in His work of redemption on the Cross, you must be dedicated to:

1. Renewing Your Mind to the Truth.
2. Aligning Your Heart and Mouth.
3. Holding Fast to Your Confession.
4. Letting Patience Do Its Work.
5. Asking God for Clarification.
6. Staying in Unwavering Faith.

But now, we will consider the role that laying hands on the sick holds for your own healing and health, and you will also see that God can use you to lay hands on others for their healing and health. But the Bible makes it clear that one way God can deliver healing and health to you is through *the laying on of hands.*

As I was growing up in a denominational environment, throughout my childhood and adolescence, I never once witnessed the laying on of hands. Oh, how I want to make it clear that I am not speaking negatively about my church where I grew up, as they taught me so many wonderful truths from God's Word. As I have repeatedly stated, much of who I am today in God is due to all the wonderful things I received in that church.

However, our church didn't practice this doctrine of laying on of hands or consider it important. We were taught to believe the words of the Bible, but we sincerely didn't understand the importance of the laying on of hands. In fact, I had never even heard about it until years later when I was filled with the Holy Spirit in my mid-teens and introduced to various Charismatic groups. It was in those environments where I first experienced seeing the laying on of hands demonstrated.

But the Bible shows that God has always used hands as conduits for the miraculous exchange of power, blessings, spiritual gifts, and authority. While hands may not possess any supernatural properties on their own, God, in His infinite wisdom, chose them as vessels for spiritual transmission. A divine transaction takes place when a believer lays hands on another person in faith and the Holy Spirit then imparts whatever is needed to the recipient. This includes healing and deliverance to the sick and the oppressed, and so much more.

It is well established in Scripture that God designed human hands to be His instruments through which these blessings would be transferred to another person. But we can also see throughout the Word that this same principle is true concerning God's hands. In the Old Testament, we read often about "the hand of the Lord" coming upon someone. That Old Testament phrase was used to denote a moment when God supernaturally imparted something to a person or a group of people.

I suggest you read my book *Build Your Foundation*, in which I devote an entire chapter to how God used hands to transmit His blessings in the time of the Old Testament. But as you are about to see, this practice of transferring blessing was also very prominent in the ministry of Jesus and throughout the New Testament.

## THE LAYING ON OF HANDS IN JESUS' MINISTRY

Luke 4:40 says, "Now when the sun was setting, all they that had any sick with divers diseases brought them unto him; and he laid his hands on every one of them, and healed them."

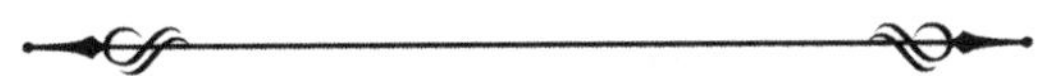

**The Bible shows that God has always used hands as conduits for the miraculous exchange of power, blessings, spiritual gifts, and authority.**

This verse tells us that the entire town left their homes and converged on the place where Jesus was, and they brought to Him all who were sick, diseased, or oppressed. Despite the overwhelming size of the crowd, the Bible says Jesus laid His hands on every single one who needed His healing touch.

At times in Jesus' earthly ministry, Jesus employed a variety of methods to bring healing to those in need. Sometimes He spoke a mere word and healing followed (*see* Matthew 8:5-13 and 15:21-28). However, Jesus recognized the unique significance of physical touch in His ministry. He realized that laying His hands upon the afflicted was a powerful means by which divine power, spiritual gifts, authority, and healing flowed from Him to humanity. His hands, indeed, served as vital instruments through which the miraculous was made manifest.

In Luke 4:40, we see that Jesus wanted to lay His hands on the people who were sick or diseased — because through His hands, a transfer of power would take place that would heal their bodies. Imagine the hours it took as He patiently and willingly moved through the throngs and reached out to lay His hands on each individual in need. But Jesus was willing to do whatever was necessary to be able to lay His hands on the sick and infirm so they could receive the power of God that would make them whole.

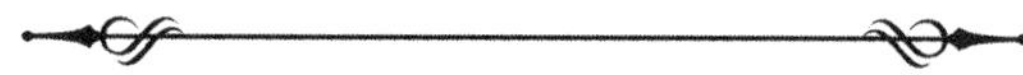

**A divine transaction takes place when a believer lays hands on another person.**

In Mark 6:5, we learn that when Jesus went to His own village, "...He could there do no mighty work, save that he laid his hands upon a few sick folk, and healed them."

Once again, we see Jesus using His hands as conduits of healing and deliverance. When Jesus traveled to His own hometown, He arrived there eager to replicate the miracles He had performed elsewhere — to heal all who came to Him who were sick, oppressed, and diseased.

But the people there were full of doubt and unbelief. They had difficulty receiving His ministry because they had known Jesus all His life, and their familiarity with Him and His family made it difficult for them to see who He really was. They couldn't get past their own familiar view of Jesus to see from a spiritual perspective who He actually was so that they could receive from Him. Yet Mark 6:5 says there was a category of sick people in Nazareth upon whom He laid His hands to impart healing power.

The laying on of hands occurred again and again in Jesus' ministry. He understood the way God had designed the power to flow. He knew it came through His hands. The following are just some examples from the gospels of Matthew and Mark that illustrate how this principle was powerfully demonstrated throughout Jesus' earthly ministry:

- In Matthew 8:3, Jesus *laid His hands* on a man and healed him.
- In Matthew 8:15, Jesus *laid His hands* on Peter's mother-in-law and healed her.
- In Matthew 9:29, Jesus *laid His hands* on blind people and healed them.
- In Matthew 17:7, Jesus *laid His hands* on the apostles and divinely imparted encouragement to them.
- In Matthew 20:34, Jesus *laid His hands* on blind people — and as healing power passed through His hands into them, they were healed.
- In Mark 1:41, as Jesus *laid His hands* on a leper, power passed through His hands, and the leper was cleansed.
- In Mark 8:23, Jesus *laid His hands* on a blind man. Healing power passed through His hands, and the blind man was healed.

As stated in this list, the examples of Jesus placing His hands upon individuals are taken exclusively from the books of Matthew and Mark. We could still go through Luke and John and add many more examples. The gospels are simply *filled* with these accounts.

Moving on to the book of Acts, we find that the laying on of hands continued to be used in the Early Church. Early believers understood that whenever the laying on of hands occurred, some kind of transmission took place. They had grown up learning about this principle from the Old Testament, they saw it in the ministry of Jesus, and they continued this pattern as they walked out those first, early days of the Church. So from the beginning to the end of Scripture, we find the importance of this doctrine of the laying on of hands.

## ALL BELIEVERS ARE TO LAY HANDS ON THE SICK

Before Jesus ascended to Heaven, He told the disciples that particular signs would follow those who believe. Among those signs was the laying on of hands for the healing of the sick. In Mark 16:18, we find Christ commanded all believers when He said, "...They [believers] shall lay hands on the sick, and they [the sick] shall recover." This means that every believer is ordained by God to use his or her hands to deliver His power and blessing to someone else.

The words of Jesus in Mark 16:18 mean that God wants to use your hands. Through your hands, He stands ready to impart His blessing, power, healing, and deliverance to others. You simply must yield by faith and obey His command to lay hands on those who need His touch as His Spirit leads you. In this verse, Jesus Himself tells you, "Your hands are instruments for My power!" If you'll get your hands out of your pockets and start laying them on people, you'll begin to see supernatural activity because God works through the laying on of hands.

When you yield your hands for God to use them as His instruments, you will be amazed at the opportunities that come your way to transfer His blessings to others. Your hands may be used to impart the baptism in the Holy Spirit, healing to the sick, deliverance to the oppressed, an increase of financial blessing, anointings to carry out special tasks, or any of God's many other spiritual blessings that He's so eager to bestow upon those who will receive in faith.

Take a good look at your hands and realize with fresh understanding that they are more than just hands — they are instruments that God wants to use to impart blessings to others. They may look like mere hands to you, but your hands are actually conduits through which all kinds of spiritual goods are meant to be transferred to other people. And as you lay hands on others by the leading of the Holy Spirit, you will begin to regularly see supernatural evidence of God's power and blessing manifested in people's lives because of your obedience.

## YOU CAN LAY HANDS ON OTHERS WHO NEED HEALING, AND OTHERS CAN LAY HANDS ON YOU TO BE HEALED

Not only does God want to use your hands to bring blessings or deliverance and healing to others, but He may use someone else's hands to release the healing and health you are believing to be manifested in your life. If you have done everything else you've read so far in this chapter, but you've never asked anyone to lay hands on you, I encourage you to ask someone who believes to lay hands on you and to pray in faith. It may be that healing and health will be appropriated in your life by the laying on of hands.

But Jesus promised that any believer — including you — can lay hands on the sick and see them get better and better until they are fully restored to health. And God can use any faith-filled believer to lay hands on you for healing and health to be manifested in your life as well. All that is required for a person to be used in this way are three basic criteria:

1. Have a desire for God to heal through you.
2. Lay hands on sick people.
3. Release your faith and believe that God's power will be transmitted through your hands to heal and to impart blessings of all kinds.

Healing the sick is part of your responsibility as a believer (*see* Mark 16:18), and the Holy Spirit is present to impart His power when you lay hands on others in Jesus' name. So rather than look at sick people and only feel pity for them, pull your hands out of your pockets and lay them on sick people by faith in His name — just as Jesus did when He was ministering on the earth!

And if you've already been *renewing your mind to the truth*; *aligning your heart and mouth*; *holding fast to your confession*; *letting patience do its work*; *asking*

*God for clarification*; and *staying in unwavering faith* — maybe now is the time for you to courageously ask a faith-filled believer to lay hands on you to trigger the manifestation of the healing you are waiting for right now.

## NOT ALL HEALING IS INSTANTANEOUS

But it is also important to note that Mark 16:18 says believers will "lay hands on the sick, and *they shall* recover."

The words "they shall" are a futuristic form of the Greek word *echo*, which means *to have*, *to hold*, or *to possess*. The tense used here doesn't picture something that is instantaneous — rather, it refers to something that occurs *progressively* or *over a period of time*. This brings us to the word "recover," which is a translation of the Greek word *kalos*, meaning *to be in good shape*, *to be healthy*, or *to be well*. When we take the meaning of the words "they shall recover" together as one complete phrase, it pictures those who progressively feel themselves getting better and better until, finally, they are well and healthy. This lets us know that all healings do not occur instantly; some of them take place over a period of time.

But Jesus' promise is that if we will lay our hands on the sick, God's power will be released into the bodies of the afflicted. And if we will allow others to lay hands on us, as we engage our faith and believe for His healing power to flow, it can be deposited into our bodies as well. Just as medicine gradually works to reverse a medical condition, the power of God that is deposited with the laying on of our hands on others — or deposited as others lay hands on us — will begin to attack the work of the devil and progressively restore any person to a state of health and well-being again. *This is Jesus' promise!*

### 8. Letting the Gifts of Healing and the Working of Miracles Do Their Work

We've covered many points in this chapter about how to appropriate healing and health for your body and mind. Sometimes healing and health are supernaturally manifested as a result of the working of the gifts of the Holy Spirit, so we must discover what the Bible says to us about the "gifts of healings" and "the working of miracles."

We read about these specific gifts in First Corinthians 12:9-10. These verses say that "to another [is given] the gifts of healing by the same Spirit; to another [is given] the working of miracles."

I want you to notice that the operation of the "gifts of healing" is *plural.* This lets us know that there are different manifestations of this spiritual gift — or various ways that the gifts of healing operate. But the "gifts of healing" and "the working of miracles" are listed separately, highlighting how each one of these operations manifests uniquely, in its own remarkable way.

For example, the word "healing" finds its roots in the Greek word *iaomai*, which means *to cure*, and it can also refer to *treatment* by a physician. This is significant because when a doctor treats a patient, the results are rarely immediate; instead, they may begin a course of medication or a suggested procedure that gradually restores the patient's health. The fact that the Holy Spirit used the word *iaomai* to describe the gifts of healing informs us that, just as medicine works progressively, often a supernatural cure begins with a prayer or with the laying on of hands, but the healing may take full effect progressively or over a period of time. Although the process remains supernatural, the use of "healing" in this context suggests it may occur in stages over time.

An example of a progressive healing is found in Luke 17 when a group of lepers met Jesus as He entered a certain village and sought His healing touch. Luke 17:14 says these lepers were healed and cleansed "as they went." This was a manifestation of a gift of healing — a supernatural touch of the Holy Spirit that generally occurs over a period of time and that ultimately cures a person from his ailment.

Most people would prefer a miracle, which is more often instantaneous, but the fact is that the word *iaomai* is used often to describe many whom Jesus healed, which means there were vast scores of people who were recipients of progressive healing in addition to those whose conditions were instantaneously changed. But whether healing is instantaneous or progressive, the results are nevertheless supernatural.

I tell you this because it is very possible that the touch you receive will be one of a progressive nature. When someone lays hands on you, it is of utmost importance that you inwardly say, *Regardless of how it manifests — instantly or progressively — right now I receive God's healing touch in my life. Just as I believe medicine works to reverse a condition, I release my faith right now to believe that from this moment onward God's power will work in me to reverse this condition until I am made completely whole and free of this disease, illness, or sickness.*

But then after the gifts of healing, Paul went on in First Corinthians 12:10 to list the "working of miracles" as another gift of the Holy Spirit. The fact that he lists it separately from the "gifts of healing" lets us know this gift operates differently from the aforementioned gift. The *King James Version* translates it as "the working of miracles," but the Greek text actually says "the operation of powers."

The word "working" is derived from a form of *energema*, which is related to the Greek word *energeo.* The word *energeo* is the word for *energy*, but when it becomes *energema*, as in First Corinthians 12:10, it depicts *divine activity, divine energy, divine empowerment,* or *divine involvement.* The word "miracles" is from the Greek word *dunameon*, the plural form of *dunamis,* which carries the idea of *explosive, superhuman power that comes with enormous energy and produces phenomenal, extraordinary, and unparalleled results.* It is the very word used throughout the New Testament to depict *mighty deeds* that are *impressive, incomparable, and beyond human ability to perform.* It denotes *miraculous power* or *miraculous manifestations.*

So when Paul wrote about the "working of miracles," he described *a divine operation of supernatural power that comes with enormous energy that produces phenomenal, extraordinary, and unparalleled results.* This divine operation of power overrides natural laws and does quickly, or instantaneously, what would normally take place over a long duration, or perhaps it would never naturally take place otherwise.

When pertaining to the human body, the "working of miracles" usually occurs in a split second — when, for example, a damaged organ or limb is instantly and supernaturally restored. God's power suddenly speeds up a healing process that would normally take place over a long period of time or that would perhaps never naturally occur — but in the blink of an eye, the process is miraculously complete. When the gift of the working of miracles is in operation, the power of God overrides the laws of nature and enables the impossible to miraculously come to pass *quickly*.

As you press forward to appropriate the healing and health that Christ purchased for you in His redemptive work on the Cross, do not dismiss the fact that God may choose to release the healing and health you await through the gifts of healing or the working of miracles. Very often these gifts are manifested in corporate church services, and it is possible that you may be sitting in church when these gifts go to work and you receive either a divine touch that starts the process to progressively heal you, or you may be the recipient of the working of miracles that instantaneously puts your body or mind back in order again. These are manifestations of the Holy Spirit that operate "as the Spirit wills" (*see* 1 Corinthians 12:11).

### 9. Taking Communion

On the eve of His betrayal, Jesus gathered His disciples for a farewell assembly and shared with them what would become known as the Last Supper. With that meal, He served them what we have come to know as Communion. In those sacred moments, Jesus and His disciples entered into covenant with each other. In the same way, when we partake of Communion, we acknowledge our covenant with Christ and, among other important things, we acknowledge what Christ did when He shed His blood and when His body was broken for us.

When Paul wrote of this event in First Corinthians 11, he encouraged us in verse 26 to regularly "take Communion" — that is, partake of the Communion elements — as a way of remembering what Jesus did for us. In Communion, the "cup" represents Jesus' blood that was shed to purchase us from Satan's dominion and to give us forgiveness of sin, freedom from guilt and shame, and peace of mind. The broken "bread" that we share in Communion represents Jesus' body that was broken for our physical and mental healing. As we saw in Chapter Ten, Isaiah 53:5 says, "But he was wounded for our transgressions, he was bruised for our iniquities: the chastisement of our peace was upon him; and with his stripes we are healed."

What Jesus accomplished in His redemptive work on the Cross was so complete and all-inclusive that Second Peter 1:3 says there is not a single part of our beings that remains untouched by this act of redemption. It says, "According as his divine power hath given unto us *all things* that pertain unto life and godliness, through the knowledge of him that hath called us to glory and virtue."

## THE SHED BLOOD AND THE BROKEN BODY OF CHRIST HAS PROVIDED FOR US 'ALL THINGS'

I will briefly divert from the subject of Communion to Second Peter 1:3-4 because I want you to really understand what has been given to you through the shed blood and broken body of Jesus. So let's expositorily explore this passage by looking at the Greek language used in its construction.

When verse 3 says God's divine power "hath given" unto us all things that pertain to life and godliness, these words "hath given" are interpreted from the Greek word *dureomai*, which is past tense in this verse and means He has *amply given*, *bequeathed*, *generously donated*, or *fully supplied*. Then the verse goes on to say that he hath given unto us "all things" that pertain to life and godliness. The word "all things" are from the Greek word *panta,* meaning literally *all things*. It is *all-encompassing* and leaves nothing excluded or untouched.

Peter wrote that God's divine power has given us all things — that is, absolutely everything that touches any part of our beings — that pertain to "life and godliness." The word "life" is derived from the Greek word *zoe*, which indicates *life of all kinds*, but especially *spiritual life.* The word "godliness" is from a form of the Greek word *eusebeia*, which particularly describes what is related to *god-likeness.* This means that Jesus has given us *everything* we need for this present life and our future life, including healing, deliverance, soundness, preservation, wholeness, and eternal salvation. And this also tells us Christ's redemptive work on the Cross has touched every sphere of both temporal and eternal existence.

But then Second Peter 1:4 goes on to say, "Whereby are given unto us exceeding great and precious promises: that by these ye might be partakers of the divine nature, having escaped the corruption that is in the world through lust."

The word "given" here is, again, from a form of the Greek word *dureomai*, which is past tense, and it means God has *amply given, bequeathed, generously donated, and fully supplied us* with "exceeding great and precious promises." The words "exceeding great" in Greek describe something *impressive, magnificent, and stunning.*

The word "precious" is derived from the Greek word *timios*, which means *of great value or worth.* The word "promises" is translated from a form of the Greek word *epangelma*, which describes *pronouncements* or *promises.* As a phrase, it means that God has given and pronounced upon us *impressive, magnificent, and stunning promises* with the covenant He made with us through Jesus.

In fact, Second Peter 1:4 goes on to say that we have become "partakers of the divine nature." The word "partakers" is derived from a form of the Greek word *koinonia*, which is from the word *koinos,* a word that refers to *things that are mutually shared.* This word *koinos* could be used to depict property that *jointly belongs* to two or more people.

The idea of *commonality* or *connectedness* is intrinsic to the meaning of this word. But when *koinos* develops into the word *koinonos* that's used in Second Peter 1:4, it conveys *engagement, fellowship, involvement, participation, or mutual sharing.* So when Peter wrote that we are "partakers of the divine nature," it irrefutably means that through Christ's sacrifice, we have not merely become the sons and daughters of God, but we now are literally partakers of Christ's nature!

But Second Peter 1:4 then adds that as a result of this divine transaction, we have "...escaped the corruption that is in the world...." The word "escaped" is rooted in the Greek word *apopheugo*, which is a compound of *apo* and *pheugo*. The word *apo* means *away* and carries the idea of *separation*, and *pheugo* means *to flee*. But when compounded, this word *apopheugo* means that we have *escaped from* and have been *separated from* the "corruption" that is in the world.

The word "corruption" is translated from the Greek word *phthora*, which describes *corruption*, *decomposition*, *perishableness*, or *anything that is subject to decay.* The use of this word tells us when we were transferred from the power of darkness into God's Kingdom, and we became partakers of Christ's nature, we escaped from and were separated from the corruption that is in the world — all the corruption that is in the world due to Adam's transgression.

At that point in history, the curse stormed into the world, unleashing its destructive force. But Peter stated that when we are born again, we are infused with Christ's nature, and it lifts us beyond the reach of the world's decay and corruption — and that includes being separated from the corrupt effects of disease, illness, and sickness that afflict the body and mind.

God has given us *impressive, magnificent, and stunning promises* through the covenant He made with us through Jesus, and these divine powers touch every realm of our being, physical and spiritual. Those promises include forgiveness of sin, freedom from guilt and shame, peace of mind, and physical and mental healing.

Second Peter 1:4 says that God has given you all these things — things that pertain to life and godliness. This means through Christ's sacrifice, God has provided for your life now and He has provided for eternal life. Life "now" means that if you are facing disease, illness, or sickness in your body or mind, God has given you impressive, magnificent, and stunning promises for your healing.

## THE COMMUNION ELEMENTS OF THE CUP AND THE BREAD REPRESENT CHRIST'S SHED BLOOD AND BROKEN BODY

If you've already been doing what you have read in this chapter so far, and you still haven't seen the results you wish in regard to the healing and health of your body and mind, it might be time for you to obey Paul's admonishment to take the Communion elements as a way to remember that Jesus' blood was spilled for your forgiveness, freedom from guilt and shame, and peace of mind — and that His body was broken for the healing of your body and mind.

Communion — or what many call the Lord's Supper — transcends mere ritual, for as you drink from "the cup," usually, but not always, of some kind of dark-colored juice, you are acknowledging the blood of Jesus that was key to your redemption from the shackles of sin. With each bite of the bread or wafer, you are acknowledging the physical anguish Jesus endured to obtain the healing of your body and mind.

As you drink of the cup and eat of the bread, use it as a moment to release your faith for everything that God has given you through Christ to come flooding into your life. That includes making Communion a moment to open yourself up to receive healing and health into your entire being. Whether you do this privately or in corporate worship with other believers, let the Communion table become a healing table for your life!

## SINCE THE BREAD REPRESENTS CHRIST'S BODY, WE MUST HAVE A RIGHT ATTITUDE TOWARD OTHER MEMBERS OF THE CHURCH — THE BODY OF CHRIST

Alone in the privacy of your own home, with family and friends, or at church, you can partake of Communion. But First Corinthians 11:28-29 tells us that before we partake of it, we should examine our hearts to make sure we are in right relationship with others in the Body of Christ. We saw in Chapter

Six that many are sick and have even died because they have unresolved, hidden issues with others in the Body of Christ. Before you drink the cup and eat the bread, make sure you have laid any issues of this kind at the foot of the Cross and that you have forgiven whomever you need to forgive.

After you have examined yourself and feel you can proceed, reach out to drink of the cup that represents Jesus' shed blood. Stop to thank God for the forgiveness, freedom from guilt and shame, and peace of mind that is yours because of Christ's work on the Cross.

If you've struggled with receiving forgiveness in any area of your life, let this be your moment to open your heart and soul to fully receive the forgiveness that is yours in Christ.

Then reach out to take the bread that represents Jesus' body that was broken for the healing of your body and mind. Stop to thank God for the healing and health that is yours because of Christ's work on the Cross.

Let this be your moment to release your faith and allow God's healing power to invade every part of your being so that you fully receive the healing that is yours in Christ.

You are in covenant with Jesus Christ, and all of these things have been purchased for you at the Cross. Jesus has given you His identity, His authority, His power, His name, His protection, and everything He has is now at your disposal.

As we have seen in Second Peter 1:4, "Whereby are given unto us exceeding great and precious promises: that by these ye might be partakers of the divine nature, having escaped the corruption that is in the world through lust."

The act of receiving or partaking of the Communion elements is powerful, and it is something that we can do every day if needed. Do it now, do it often, and let Communion become a transactional moment when you appropriate the benefits of Christ's redemptive work on the Cross for you.

## 10. Calling for the Elders of the Church To Anoint With Oil and Pray the Prayer of Faith

Before I conclude this chapter about how to appropriate healing for your body and mind, I feel the need to take us to an often-overlooked scripture about yet another important way to obtain healing and health for your body and mind. James 5:14 says, "Is any sick among you? let him call for the elders of the church; and let them pray over him, anointing him with oil in the name of the Lord." In this verse, we find yet another way to receive healing and health for your body and mind.

In this verse, the word "sick" is translated from a form of the Greek word *astheneo*, a word that generally describes *one who is frail in health* or *one so physically weak that he is unable to travel.* It carries the idea of one who is *disabled, faint, feeble, fragile, incapacitated* or *one in such poor health that it would be unthinkable to transport him from one place to another.* In essence, it depicts one who is a *shut-in* or *hospital-bound* or *homebound.* It can also describe people who are strapped in financial need, which is a common predicament when one's body is besieged by illness that necessitates substantial funds for recovery.

It is always best if a sick person can muster the strength to get up and go to a church meeting to receive prayer. In the assembly of the saints, there is a powerful corporate anointing that works wonders. But if a person is so ill that he cannot physically get up and go to the church to receive prayer, James said a person in this predicament should "call for the elders of the church" to come pray for him or her.

I have noted that when illness strikes, people anticipate that the church's spiritual leaders will reach out and offer to visit, pray, and anoint them with oil. Yet James flipped this expectation and suggests that the responsibility falls on the sick individual to initiate this action. Especially as congregations grow larger, it becomes increasingly difficult for spiritual leaders to be aware of every member's health challenges. This is one reason why James advised the sick to proactively request the presence and prayers of church leaders. Instead of waiting for spiritual leaders to assess the severity of every church member's illness, James stated it is up to the sick person to inform the leadership of his condition and to request them to fulfill the conditions of James 5:14.

Again James 5:14 says, "Is any sick among you? let him *call* for the elders of the church...." The word "call" is interpreted from a form of *proskaleo*, a compound of the words *pros* and *kaleo*. The word *pros* suggests a *movement toward*, and the word *kaleo* means *to beckon*, *to call*, or *to invite*. But when compounded, it means *to personally ask, beckon, call, invite, or summon to one's side.* It's important to remember that this doesn't pertain to those with a mere sniffle or some other mild symptom, but to individuals who are so severely unwell that venturing to the church for prayer is not possible. Thus, James 5:14 calls upon them to personally beckon the ordained leaders of the local assembly to come to where they are to deliver passionate, healing prayer.

According to this verse, if one is incapacitated and unable to travel to church to receive prayer, he is to call for the elders of the church to come to him, and the tense used here indicates it's an urgent plea requesting that the elders come and pray. The individual in need of prayer faces the choice of whether to reach out to the leaders or remain silent. If a plea for assistance is extended and met with prayers brimming with faith, James assured us that the outcome will be undeniably positive.

But James 5:14 also specifically says the sick person should call for the "elders" of the church. The word "elders" is interpreted from the plural form of the Greek word *presbuteros*, a word that is traditionally used to refer to the spiritual leaders of Israel, like the influential figures within local synagogues or those who expounded the Law in public gatherings. In the context of the New Testament, it signifies formally designated church authorities. Therefore, it becomes clear that the sick person should reach out to the church's leadership — or to their designated representatives — to come pray and anoint them with oil in the name of the Lord.

**If a plea for assistance is extended and met with prayers brimming with faith, James assured us that the outcome will be undeniably positive.**

When these spiritual leaders arrive at the home of such a person, or at the hospital, James 5:14 says that they are to "pray" over him. The word "pray" is an interpretation of a form of the Greek word *proseuchomai*, which is the most common word for prayer in the New Testament. It is a compound of *pros* and *euchomai*. Here the *pros* depicts a sense of *closeness* or *intimate connection*, while the second part of the word, *euchomai*, means *I beseech* or *I pray* and is derived from the word *euche*, which is a word that originally depicted a person who made some kind of *a vow to God in exchange for a favorable answer to prayer.*

Typically, when such an individual sought a positive answer to prayer, he would set up a commemorative altar to offer a sacrifice called a "votive offering" — a term derived from the word "vow." That altar became a place of *exchange* where the worshipper asked God to do something, but in *exchange* he or she would also offer something to God. Often, the asker made a pledge to live a dedicated life or to give God an offering of praise *in exchange* for a postive answer to prayer.

By using this word "pray," James was stating that when the spiritual leaders come to pray for the sick person, everyone involved is *to draw near to God* as they made their petition, and at the same time, they are *to make a vow* that they will offer God something *in exchange* for a positive answer. In this case, as they ask God to heal, perhaps they "vow" that as a result of the requested healing, they will give God glory and praise Him for what He has done. This word "prayer" — a form of the Greek word *proseuchomai*, again, the most common form of prayer in the New Testament — lets us know that prayer is not just a place of asking. Prayer is *a place of exchange* between God and man.

One of the best examples of this is found in the story of Hannah, the mother of the prophet Samuel. Hannah deeply desired a child but was unable to become pregnant. Consumed by an intense longing for a child, Hannah faced the heartache of barrenness year after year. In a moment of profound desperation and soul-wrenching sorrow, she poured out her heart to God and made a *vow* that she would give back to Him that son in *exchange* for allowing her to become a mother.

On one of her family's annual trips to worship and sacrifice to the Lord in Shiloh, we read in First Samuel 1:10-11 that she prayed, "And she [Hannah] was in bitterness of soul, and prayed unto the Lord, and wept sore. And she vowed a vow, and said, O Lord of hosts, if thou wilt indeed look on the affliction of thine handmaid, and remember me, and not forget thine handmaid, but wilt give unto thine handmaid a man child, then I will give him unto the Lord all the days of his life, and there shall no razor come upon his head."

With earnest sincerity, she vowed, "Should You bless me with a son, I vow to dedicate him to Your service for all his days." God's response to Hannah's vow is seen in First Samuel 1:19-20, "And they [Hannah and her husband, Elkanah] rose up in the morning early, and worshipped before the Lord, and returned, and came to their house to Ramah: and Elkanah knew Hannah his wife; and the Lord remembered her. Wherefore it came to pass, when the time was come about after Hannah had conceived, that she bare a son, and called his name Samuel, saying, Because I have asked him of the Lord."

The reason I share this is, I want you to see that the "prayer" James described depicts a place of *exchange* wherein one gives God his defects, problems, sicknesses, and weaknesses — and *in exchange*, God generously supplies His power, His presence, and His goodness. Thus, James 5:14 means that when we ask God to heal the sick person who has summoned the spiritual leadership of the church to come and pray for him, it is correct for those who pray and for the one who is sick to *vow* to give God glory and praise in exchange for healing the afflicted person.

But James 5:14 goes on to say, "Is any sick among you? let him call for the elders of the church; and let them pray *over* him…." The word "over" is translated from a form of the Greek word *epi*, which means *over* or *upon*, and it depicts the position held by those summoned or hovering over the sick person who is receiving prayer, almost enveloping the person in need with their presence. The use of this word paints a clear picture of individuals gathering closely around, their presence like a gentle canopy of care directly above the sick individual.

James 5:14 furthermore says, "…Let them pray over him, *anointing* him with *oil* in the *name* of the *Lord*." I italicized the words *anointing, oil, name,* and *Lord* for emphasis because each of these four words is important and needs explanation.

- *First*, the word "anointing" is interpreted from a form of the Greek word *aleipho*, a term that refers to *the physical anointing of the body with oil.*

- *Second*, the word "oil" is interpreted from a form of the Greek word *elaio*, which denotes *olive oil.* From the earliest beginnings in the Old Testament to the conclusion of the New Testament and to the present, the substance of *olive oil* has been, and is still, a symbol of the presence and power of *the Holy Spirit.*

  Although the oil itself possesses no inherent healing powers, it has persistently symbolized, in both the Old and New Testaments, the presence of the Holy Spirit and the power of God. The moment the oil is applied in a time of prayer is the moment the sick person is to release his faith for Christ's healing to come into his body.

- *Third*, the word "name" is interpreted from a form of the Greek word *onoma*, which means *a name* or *a reputation.* Not only does Jesus have the *name* that is higher than any other name, and His name is exceptional, good, noble, and superior — but the reputation of His name is above the reputation of all others. Furthermore, Jesus Christ has *a reputation* for healing even the most serious cases of sickness, and when one prays in His name, that person prays in both the *name* and *reputation* of the One who indisputably has the power to heal any sick person.

- *Fourth*, the word "Lord" is an interpretation of the Greek word *Kurios*. Here it denotes the *Master* and *Supreme Lord* or *the One who has ultimate authority in every realm, seen and unseen*, which in this case, includes authority over sickness and disease.

If all the conditions of James 5:14 have been fulfilled, in which the sick person calls for the church elders to pray passionately, James 5:15 says, "And the prayer of faith shall save the sick, and the Lord shall raise him up; and if he have committed sins, they shall be forgiven him."

The word "prayer" is also translated from a form of *proseuchomai*, which we previously encountered in verse 14. At this point, however, the prayer stands retrospectively — a petition already placed before God. But then James added that it is a prayer of "faith." The word "faith" is drawn from a form of the Greek word *pistis*, which is the word for "faith" throughout the New Testament. This isn't a hope-so kind of faith that simply wishes, but it is a *robust, rock-solid, unwavering faith* that believes the One who has been petitioned will positively respond with healing.

The *King James Version* of James 5:15 says the prayer of faith shall "save" the sick. When most people read the word "salvation," they think of eternal salvation and, thus, miss other crucial meanings of this word. The word "save" is interpreted from a form of the Greek word *sodzo*, a word that is most often translated *salvation* in the New Testament. However, this word also importantly depicts *deliverance, healing, liberation, and wholeness* in every part of life. This word *sodzo* also means *to deliver a person or country from enemies* or *to deliver, heal, keep safe, preserve, or keep under protection*. The full meaning of *sodzo* is very broad, and the believers in the Early Church understood this word to contain all these meanings.

By using this word "save" — translated from *sodzo* — James declared that the prayer of faith *will completely deliver, heal, liberate, and return wholeness* to the "sick." But now, the word "sick" is a bit different from the word "sick" previously used in verse 14. This word "sick" is translated from a form of the Greek word *kamno*, and it refers to *a person who has long suffered from an affliction and is extremely weakened from the effects of this disease.*

The use of this word confirms that the person calling for the spiritual leaders of the church to come and pray is one who is so sick he is unable to go to them to receive prayer. While any believer may seek the prayers of church leaders, this passage specifically addresses someone who, because of a long-lasting and debilitating illness, is unable to join a meeting where the collective anointing of God is felt. Hence, he beckons the leaders of the church to come to where he is to anoint him with oil and pray the prayer of faith over him.

In James 5:15 we find that as a result of meeting all these prerequisites, "the Lord shall raise him up." The word "Lord" is again an interpretation of the Greek word *Kurios*, which denotes the *Master and Supreme Lord* or *the One who has ultimate authority in every realm, seen and unseen*, which, of course, includes authority over sickness and disease.

We are promised that after all this has been said and done, the Lord will "raise him up." The words "raise him up" are interpreted from a form of *egeiro*, which not only means *to lift or raise*, but is also the root from which we derive the word "resurrection." Thus, those who have been suffering a long time from the effects of disease will be raised up, out of their debilitating situation. Their condition was so grave that their recovery will seem nothing short of *a resurrection.*

Then James 5:15 adds that "if he have committed sins, they shall be forgiven him." The word "committed" is interpreted from a form of *poieo*, which here carries the notion of *one who has done some kind of sin.* The word "sins" is interpreted from a form of *hamartia*, which is the Greek word primarily translated as *sin* in the New Testament. It pictures *one who misses the mark concerning what is right and wrong*. Because this missing of the mark may at times be unintentional, in ancient Greek texts, it is sometimes translated as the word "mistake," but it primarily carries the idea of one who either *intentionally* or *unintentionally* does what is *wrong* and who is thereby guilty of *sin*.

Because the word "sins" is used in connection with this individual's sickness, it strongly suggests this person may have brought sickness on himself as a result of a repeated failure or fault. We have already seen in Chapters Two through Eight that many diseases, illnesses, and sicknesses are *self-inflicted*, whether through deliberate choices or inadvertent actions that create an "entry point" for the devil to exploit us.

These words in James 5:15 tell us that in addition to healing us, God may speak to us by His Spirit, by His Word, or by the spiritual leaders who have come to pray for us to point out that it may be our own conduct that opened a door to the sickness. Embracing such loving correction can serve as a safeguard and help us break free from a cycle that could invite the return of disease, illness, or sickness.

Then James 5:15 goes on to say that if we acknowledge our conduct is likely the reason why sickness showed up in the first place — and if we seek forgiveness for it — our wrong behaviors that led to that situation will be "forgiven." The word "forgiven" comes from a form of the Greek word *aphiemi*, which means *to discharge, forgive, let go, release, set free, or permanently send away*.

We see the concept of such forgiveness in Psalm 103:12, where it is written, "As far as the east is from the west, so far hath he removed our transgressions from us." This gloriously tells us that God has dismissed our sins from us, and He sent them away, never to be retrieved. Thus, the word *aphiemi*, translated "forgiven" in James 5:15, means *to forgive, to permanently release, and to send away forever.*

**The *RIV* (*Renner Interpretive Version*) of James 5:14-15 says:**

> **Is anyone among you weak, sick, or incapacitated due to illness? Let that person personally call for the ordained leaders of the local assembly to come and passionately petition God on his behalf. Let the leaders hover over him in prayer, anointing the sick person with oil and operating in the stead of Jesus — that is, acting on His behalf and using the authority and reputation of the name of the Lord — the One who has authority in every seen and unseen realm [and that certainly includes authority and mastery over sickness and disease].**
>
> **And the heartfelt prayer of rock-solid, steadfast, unwavering faith will deliver, heal, liberate, and physically save the person weakened from sickness — and as a result, the Lord — the One with supreme authority in every realm, seen and unseen — will raise him up. And if — as the case may be — he has carried out behaviors that have missed the mark of what is right and wrong and are sinful in nature, he will be forgiven and freed from them.**

## 12 EASY STEPS IN 'CALLING FOR THE ELDERS'

Because we have covered a lot of instruction in James 5:14-15 about how to pray for those who are sick at home or in the hospital, and this is a lot of material to grasp, so let me break it down for you into 12 easy steps so you can understand precisely what actions to take in these circumstances.

### Step 1: Define "the Sick"

James 5:15 describes a category of sick people who are so profoundly debilitated that movement from one place to another becomes an insurmountable challenge. Stricken by the severity of their conditions, these individuals find themselves confined to their homes or bedridden, unable to attend church services to ask for healing prayers in person.

### Step 2: The Sick Person Is To Initiate the Invitation

James 5:14 says the responsibility falls squarely on the sick individual to take initiative in informing the spiritual leadership about his condition. Instead of telling the one who is ill to wait for someone else to reach out to him, James emphasized the importance of the sick person making a deliberate effort to summon the spiritual leaders —- or their designated representatives — to come and offer prayers for healing.

### Step 3: Who Are the "Elders" or Spiritual Leaders?

James 5:14 says the sick person is to ask the "elders of the church" to come pray for him. In the Greek, the word "elders" depicts those who are the ordained leaders of the church. This could include the pastor, his team of associates, or appointed individuals who have been entrusted with the responsibility of conducting this ministry under the guidance of the church leadership.

### Step 4: The Spiritual Leaders Are To Come

James 5:14 says that if invited to do so, the church's spiritual leaders, or their designated representatives, are to go to the bedside of the sick, regardless of whether that is at home, a hospital, or in a nursing facility. The Scripture emphasizes that those vested with spiritual authority, or their chosen representatives, are to physically go to the person who has requested them to come and pray.

### Step 5: The Spiritual Leaders Are To Pray

James 5:14 says both the spiritual leaders who come to visit the sick, and the sick person himself, are to pray. The word "pray" implies asking God to move on behalf of the sick and verbally vowing that God will be given all the glory and praise in exchange for a healing touch on the life of the sick individual.

## Step 6: They Are To Pray Over the Sick

James 5:14 says the spiritual leaders, or those whom they have sent as their representatives, are to pray "over" the sick person. This word "over" in Greek pictures them gathering around the sick person, hovering over him, and blanketing him in a chorus of faith-filled prayers.

## Step 7: They Are To Anoint the Sick With Oil

James 5:14 says the spiritual leaders, or those they have sent as their representatives, are called to anoint the sick person with oil. The word "oil" is used symbolically in both the Old and New Testaments to denote the presence of the Holy Spirit. As the anointing oil touches the sick individual, he is to join his faith for healing with the chorus of faith-filled prayers being prayed by those who surround him.

## Step 8: They Are To Pray in the Name of the Lord

James 5:15 says that the spiritual leaders of the church, or those appointed to carry out this ministry, are to offer their prayers in the name of the Lord. The word "name" speaks of *authority* and *reputation*. Consequently, their prayers should be voiced with the authority vested in Jesus' name and with the full knowledge that He has a reputation for healing all manner of sickness and disease. The word "Lord" describes *the One who has power in all realms, seen and unseen*. Therefore, as prayer is offered, those praying are to do so in the authority of Jesus' name, remembering that He has a reputation for healing all manner of disease, illness, and sickness and that His name causes all disease, illness, and sickness to flee.

## Step 9: They Are To Pray in Faith

James 5:15 specifically says that those who gather should pray with a steadfast and unshakable faith — not mere wishful thinking, but resolute confidence. This word "faith" speaks of a deep-seated, immovable trust that God will hear and respond by healing the individual enveloped in their earnest prayers.

### Step 10: The Sick Will Be Saved

James 5:15 says the sick will be "saved." The word "saved" means *to completely deliver, heal, liberate, and to be returned to wholeness.* If all the previously stated conditions have been met, James 5:15 says God's power will be released and the sick person will be delivered, healed, and restored to wholeness.

### Step 11: The Lord Will Raise the Sick Person Up

James 5:15 says that when the prayer concludes, the Lord Himself will raise the sick person from his bed of affliction. The word "raise" in Greek is also the root for the word *resurrection*. This result will be so miraculous that it will appear God has resurrected him from the bed of sickness.

### Step 12: The Sick Person Needs To Take Personal Inventory

James 5:15 says if the sick person has committed any sins that opened the door to this affliction, recognition and repentance are required. This crucial step ensures that past missteps are not repeated. This part of the process is vital, for if past wrong actions are repeated, it could lead to a recurrence of the sickness.

Christ has provided healing and health for your body and mind. As a child of God, it is right for you to lay claim to what Christ did for you on the Cross. But in this chapter, I have provided points that are important in the process of you appropriating the healing and health that rightfully belong to you. For review, they are as follows:

1. Renewing Your Mind to the Truth
2. Aligning Your Heart and Mouth

3. Holding Fast to Your Confession
4. Letting Patience Do Its Work
5. Asking God for Clarification
6. Staying in Unwavering Faith
7. Laying Hands on the Sick
8. Letting the Gifts of Healing and the Working of Miracles Do Their Work
9. Taking Communion
10. Calling for the Elders of the Church To Anoint With Oil and Pray the Prayer of Faith

If you do all these things, it will only be a matter of time until you begin to see a change in your body and mind. Perhaps healing and health will come quickly, or perhaps it will come progressively, but if you do these things — *and stick with them* — it is sure that you will eventually begin to see God's Word take effect inside you as your body and mind begin to get stronger.

But now let's move to the next chapter, where we will see that in addition to taking these ten spiritual steps that we've outlined in this present chapter, there are practical things we can also do to undergird the healing and health that Jesus purchased for us in His redemptive work on the Cross!

Scan the QR code to watch Rick teach more on this subject.

# QUESTIONS TO PONDER AND DISCUSS

1. God has provided so many ways of receiving His gracious provision of healing and health that was made available to us through Christ's death and resurrection. Which of the ten ways discussed in this chapter resonated with you most? Explain which ones have been most successful for you and which require more of your attention and meditation?

2. Did steps one and two — "renewing your mind to the truth" and "aligning your heart and mouth" — reawaken fresh hope in you concerning receiving answers to prayer? These are the basics of faith that we must review and practice over and over again, much like an athlete must stay continually strengthened in the basics of his sport so that he can excel. How did the Greek word for "doubt" (*diakrinomai*) in Mark 11:23 add fresh strength to your faith for receiving from God? Are you *differing* in your heart concerning anything you're confessing and desiring to see come to pass? If so, review the section entitled "Renewing Your Mind to the Truth" and read verses such as Joshua 1:8 to remedy that "heart and mouth" connection. Then put the words of your mouth to work!

3. In the sections "Holding Fast to Your Confession" and "Letting Patience Do Its Work," what did you learn about the Spirit's supernatural support system when you make the decision that you will not turn or budge from God's Word or His promises? According to what you read, why did the Early Church call endurance "the queen of all virtues"? Can you think of an instance in which the force of endurance netted you a spiritual victory? If so, what did you learn from that experience? What could you tell someone else about the benefits of "waiting on the Lord" and increasing your strength, hope, confidence, and expectancy?

4. Before reading this chapter, had you realized the great detail the Bible goes into concerning "the laying on of hands"? Read Mark 16:18 — and especially Jesus' words "they *shall* recover" — and explain in your own words

how a sick person can expect to be well again after a believer lays hands on him or her for healing.

5. Were you surprised to learn from James 5:14 that a believer who is so sick that he's homebound must initiate the call for the church elders to come and pray for him? Read the *RIV* of James 5:14-15 on page 419 and ponder the richness of God's goodness and grace in not only raising back up to health the person who was sick, but also forgiving him completely of sin and wrongdoing. What are your biggest takeaways from the 12 steps contained in this small passage in James 5?

# TWELVE

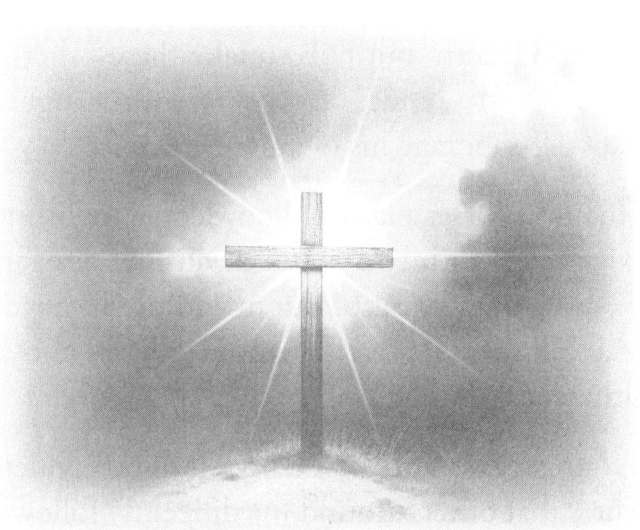

# THE ROLES OF DIET, EXERCISE, SUPPLEMENTS, DOCTORS, MEDICINE, AND A BALANCED LIFE

This book has highlighted the importance of understanding what Christ secured for us through His sacrificial act on the Cross. Indeed, He paid the ultimate price for our sins, liberating us from guilt and shame, granting us peace of mind, and offering us healing and health. Embracing these profound truths and allowing them to renew our minds is essential in knowing how to fend off threats to our well-being and live vibrant lives. Psalm 119:89 says, "For ever, O Lord, thy word is settled in heaven." This means that what Christ has done for us is forever settled!

Yet alongside these spiritual insights that profoundly influence our existence, there are tangible and practical steps we can take to enhance our healing and health. Some mistakenly assert that by merely claiming promises from the Bible, they can achieve flawless health and an enduring life. If one lays claim to God's promises of healing and health, but fails to take these other practical steps, he can foolishly create an "entry point," as we've seen, through which the enemy will enter and thusly self-sabotage his own well-being.

We have seen that the curse; a lack of knowledge; foolishness, unresolved or hidden issues; anxiety, fret, and worry; and devilish attacks are all contributors to assaults on one's healing and health. But in addition, I have learned firsthand that not taking practical steps to care for one's health is also a contributor to a wide array of health issues.

When I was a younger man, I believed myself to be invincible and neglected the practical measures that others around me diligently followed. But over time, I came to realize — often through tough experiences — that attending to one's physical needs is as crucial as nurturing one's spiritual self. In this chapter, we will specifically look at the role of diet, physical exercise, supplements, doctors, medicine, and a balanced life as practical measures to take against disease, illness, and sickness.

Let's begin by delving into the pivotal role that diet plays in maintaining, nurturing, and restoring healing and health to the body.

## THE ROLE OF DIET

A friend of mine recently had to remove all the pipes in his mother's house because they were thoroughly clogged from years of her pouring leftover cooking grease down the kitchen drain. The pipes were completely clogged and impenetrable. Faced with this monumental plumbing disaster, my friend found that the only solution was to dismantle and replace the entire network of pipes. But as he recounted the saga of dripping, greasy woes and the effort required to remove them, I privately thought, *If her pipes are so thoroughly choked with grease, what must her arteries look like?*

That experience got me pondering the age-old saying, "We are what we eat." If that is true, and I think that it largely *is* true, it's hardly surprising that a multitude of people are grappling with difficulties these days because their plates are piled high with foods that are mere shadows of nutrition, void of real sustenance.

I recently stumbled across an astonishing fact that despite America's distinction as the most overweight and obese industrialized nation globally, many Americans are paradoxically undernourished. Despite their high caloric intake, many are deficient in essential nutrients. In effect, they are "starving" on a diet rich in empty calories, nearly barren of nourishment. Alarmingly, more than half of individuals with obesity suffer from nutritional shortfalls — micronutrient deficiencies. The seriousness of this situation has intensified to such a degree that some authorities see it as a looming national-security threat.

I hold no judgment against anyone with less-than-stellar eating habits, for as I was growing up, my precious mother, who led me to Jesus, influenced my life, and worked with me in the ministry for decades until she went to Heaven, had no idea what a healthy diet was or anything about nutrition in the earlier years of her life. For that reason, we Renner kids grew up knowing little to nothing about eating good, nutritional food. While my parents always ensured our plates were full, what we ate wasn't exactly the epitome of healthy and nourishing.

In our household, our culinary experience revolved around canned and frozen vegetables, a parade of starchy delights like chips in every conceivable flavor, and an overflowing supply of cookies, pastries, cakes, and syrup-doused pancakes. Margarine was a staple, and nearly every kind of meat we ate emerged sizzling from a sea of delectable, golden grease. Our meals also featured TV dinners and canned tamales, with fried hamburgers, french fries, and fried SPAM®, as well as crispy bacon which made regular appearances on our dining-room table — not to mention the twice-weekly ritual of really greasy goulash. The "crown jewels" of our dining table were my mother's lavishly breaded and fried pork chops, accompanied by her legendary fried potatoes. She'd round off our meals with slices of pineapple upside-down cake and expansive trays of fudge. Even as I reminisce about it, I can still nearly taste all of it right now!

And I must add that a journey to my mother's mother's house — my Grandma Ettie — was exciting as well because she would always make me one of her legendary peanut butter and jelly sandwiches. Oh, I remember how those sandwiches were covered with such a generous spread of peanut butter and luscious grape jelly that the sandwich actually bulged out the sides of the slices of white Rainbow bread. Each bite was delightfully messy and utterly irresistible.

My father's upbringing was very similar to my mother's when it came to food and "nutrition." For example, visiting Grandma Renner's house in the mornings was like stepping into a breakfast wonderland. Her unrivaled knack for crafting the heartiest, most indulgently flour- and grease-rich gravy was nothing short of amazing. We would lavishly drench her colossal biscuits with this creamy concoction to create a symphony of salty flavor with each bite. Then as noon rolled around, Grandma treated us to delectable sandwiches loaded with mayonnaise, followed by heavenly slices of cantaloupe crowned with mountains of white sugar that sent us into a spiral of high-energy followed by a mid-afternoon crash.

What I'm getting at is that throughout my childhood, we were ignorant about what was a nutritious diet. Our palates were tantalized by foods bathed in grease or loaded with sugar. Concerns about excessive carbohydrates or sugar or consuming foods damaging to our organs or bereft of nutrients never crossed our minds. We generously heaped onto our plates almost everything that, by today's standards, would be considered harmful to our health. And as mentioned earlier, nearly every dish prepared on our kitchen stove dripped with grease.

Denise's family, on the other hand, ate only nutritious food that was mostly grown in their own large garden in the backyard of their house on a small farm, where they lived in the countryside. Their garden overflowed with crisp green beans, plump tomatoes, vibrant-colored carrots, succulent cucumbers, sweet corn, peppers of all kinds, colorful squash, luscious cantaloupe, and juicy watermelon — and they even grew sunflowers so they could eat nutritious sunflower seeds. Oh, and I must not forget to mention the fresh milk that was delivered every morning to their home — or the fresh eggs they retrieved from their own chickens every morning from the small chicken coop in the backyard. They almost never drank soft drinks or had very much of anything that contained white sugar.

I'll never forget the first time I went to meet Denise's family before we got married. When we sat at the table in their kitchen to eat lunch, I was shocked to see so many fresh vegetables on the table. I'm talking about fresh green beans, fresh okra, and fresh corn on the cob right from the garden — all in one meal. Very often they didn't even add any meat to the table because it was already full of so many wonderful treasures they grew in their own garden — along with healthy milk, butter, and homemade cornbread. This was the world Denise's family thrived in — a stark contrast to my own weekday servings of bologna sandwiches slathered in generous dollops of Miracle Whip® that were accompanied by a crunchy chorus of multiple bags of Fritos®.

The reason I am telling you this is, when Denise and I first married, it was a difficult merger of two totally different dietary styles. To be honest, it was a shock to my system when I came to realize that I actually married a rabbit! I vividly recall the day I casually mentioned my craving for a snack, and Denise, with a sparkle in her eye, handed me a lone stalk of celery. Suffice it to say, it didn't quite match my vision of snack-time indulgence. I couldn't believe all the green things Denise ate and wanted me to eat. As a newly married man, I wondered, *Does Denise think I am going to eat like a rabbit for the rest of my life?*

When I looked at what she prepared for our evening meals, I shuddered inside to eat it. It was all unfried, nearly free of the carbohydrates that I had grown up loving, and instead of giving me soft drinks that I usually drank, she gave me a glass of bland and tasteless water. Day after day, I looked at the plates she set before me that were full of garden goods, but I longed for fried foods and carbohydrates. Nevertheless, Denise was determined she was going to reset my dietary course and make me eat lettuce, radishes, and other endless greens for the rest of my life.

## *'WE ARE WHAT WE EAT'*

Since it's largely true that we are what we eat, it is important to really think about what we are pouring into our bodies. We must make it our mission to fuel our bodies with lively, nutrient-rich foods that elevate our well-being and bolster our long-term health. But if navigating the world of proper nutrition feels like setting sail into unknown waters, why not seek the expertise of a healthcare provider to help steer your course? If you don't know how to eat right, you can find a nutritionist or medical professional to help you. Today there are many resources at your fingertips, many of which are online and free. These tools can help chart your path to a nutritious dietary lifestyle and help you transform your eating habits for the better.

Pouring leaded fuel into a car designed for unleaded gasoline is like tossing a wrench into a finely-tuned machine — it's a recipe for disaster. Not only will it wreak havoc on your engine, but it will also have your wallet crying out for mercy as repair bills skyrocket. To ensure your car operates smoothly down the highway for miles to come, it's crucial to feed it with the right fuel. You might have all the optimism in the world and believe your vehicle that takes unleaded gasoline can sip leaded fuel without a hitch, but your thinking will be proved wrong as you face untold automotive woes.

Similarly, if you choose to fuel your body with the wrong kinds of foods, it's not just your arteries that might suffer the consequences; your entire system will eventually bear the brunt of your choices. You might chuckle at the thought of consuming unhealthy foods and playfully declare your intentions to stay strong and healthy as you continue to indulge in toxin-laden meals. However, laugh as you may, if you persist in this dietary rebellion, sooner or later your body will send you a stark wake-up call — a costly struggle with health issues that will demand attention. You might find yourself urgently seeking prayers for healing or lying beneath the glaring lights of an operating room while a surgeon works diligently to unclog your arterial plumbing.

You need to understand that when you eat wrong foods, it is like inviting a silent architect into your life to craft a foundation for a myriad of chronic ailments, such as heart disease, diabetes, and various obesity-related conditions. Regularly eating unhealthy foods even increases the risk of certain cancers. A poor diet impacts one's mental health, saps energy reserves, and compromises overall wellness. And those who feast on junk food — laden with excessive fats, inflammatory oils, and sugars — often find themselves facing not only immediate discomforts but also enduring persistent challenges, including weight gain, diabetes, and a host of other health predicaments.

**You might chuckle at the thought of consuming unhealthy foods and playfully declare your intentions to stay strong and healthy as you continue to indulge in toxin-laden meals. However, laugh as you may, if you persist in this dietary rebellion, sooner or later your body will send you a stark wake-up call — a costly struggle with health issues that will demand attention. You might find yourself urgently seeking prayers for healing or lying beneath the glaring lights of an operating room while a surgeon works diligently to unclog your arterial plumbing.**

With the growing concerns of excess weight and obesity, the digital world is now filled with guidance for crafting a healthful eating regimen. Today a plethora of specialists stand ready to assist in tailoring a personalized dietary blueprint that best suits your needs. As research continues, it emphasizes the benefits of prioritizing specific nutrients, welcoming particular food categories, and nurturing holistic eating practices to boost well-being and to help prevent common diseases. I advise that when charting the course for your nutritional journey, seek out a vibrant mixture of food choices that embraces all the essential food groups.

In my youngest years, the idea of healthy eating wasn't exactly my cup of tea. As I told you earlier, when Denise and I got married and she tried to force me to eat nothing but garden vegetables, it was a miserable experience for me.

Denise flourished with this type of diet, but I found it completely uninspiring, bland, and monotonous. Personally, I loved Mexican dishes, Chinese cuisine, and everything fried. So when I eventually realized the importance of eating healthy and set my will in the direction of eating for health, I began to crave food that was delicious and enjoyable to me as well as nutritious.

Remember, there are all kinds of eating plans available today to choose from, but the most beneficial ones will emphasize whole, minimally processed foods. But I discovered that it's crucial to carve out a dietary journey that helps you balance portions from each food group, to opt for ingredients that are effortlessly accessible at your local grocery store, and to indulge in a variety of foods that bring you joy. Above all, you must seek a dietary rhythm that speaks to your taste buds, aligns with your lifestyle, and respects your wallet.

A nutritious and well-rounded diet — as well as proper sleep, movement, and hydration — fuels your body, ensures that you have the energy to stay active from morning to night, delivers essential nutrients for growth and repair, and empowers you to remain strong and healthy.

The following is not meant to be comprehensive, but many experts suggest the following for a well-rounded diet that fuels every system and organ in your body, including your skin.

- A heart-friendly diet brims with colorful fruits, vibrant vegetables, wholesome grains, and low-fat dairy. This type of palette is said to keep your blood pressure and cholesterol in check, thus lowering the odds of heart disease. Additionally, indulging in a twice-weekly serving of oily fish like salmon or trout might just be your heart's best friend.
- A calcium-rich diet helps fortify your bones and teeth against the ravages of time and slows the creeping effects of osteoporosis. While dairy is a well-known source for calcium intake, there are also plenty of other sources to consider.
- Remember also that your body needs vitamin D, which is important in guiding calcium's journey into your system, and it also provides amazing immune defense. Let the light of the sun bathe your skin whenever you can and then fill your kitchen with vitamin D-rich delights like oily fish, eggs, and dairy. The intake of calcium and vitamin D supports bone strength and overall health.

Fuel your body with the right nutrients, and it will thank you with vitality and longevity. Just like a finely tuned engine, your body will hum along smoothly and efficiently. However, if you continually fill your "tank" with the wrong foods, you're essentially sabotaging your own machinery. Over time, this misguided fueling practice will inevitably lead to unwelcome repercussions, undermining even the divine healing and health won for you through Jesus' sacrifice on the Cross.

## AN EVENT I'LL NEVER FORGET

Many years ago I attended a large healing service that deeply impacted me. Allow me to paint a picture of this memory that is forever carved into my mind and one that illustrates how, at times, we unwittingly pave the path for our own health challenges. My memory stems from a sizable healing meeting I attended that was filled with individuals who were invited to step forward for healing prayer.

From my vantage point in my seat located on the side of the auditorium, I gazed down at the scene unfolding below. A line had begun to snake across the floor near the platform that was comprised of people waiting patiently for their moment of prayer. That day I was in shock when I saw the physical sizes of the people who were coming forward for prayer. Having grappled with my own weight issues, I have nothing but empathy for those on similar journeys.

Yet as I watched that day, the sheer magnitude of their frames was shocking to me. Many among them were so large that independent movement was a challenge, so they required the aid of motorized scooters, wheelchairs, walkers, and crutches to carry them to the front to receive prayer. These individuals were not just overweight; they faced the challenges of morbid obesity. As I stood watching, I kept thinking, *If these are people of faith, this is a disheartening reflection of a faith that overcomes the world.*

Once more, I offer no criticism for those grappling with the challenges of weight, as I, too, have battled with this in my past. Journeying through my own experience, I've come to realize that God's grace is ever-present and is waiting to heal those who seek Him with unwavering belief. At the Cross, Jesus bore our diseases, illnesses, and sicknesses, yet as I observed many seeking prayer in that meeting that day, it became evident to me that much of their suffering stemmed from dietary choices.

While some face conditions that contribute to weight gain, I realized that a lack of discipline or a lack of knowledge of proper nutrition was at the root for many who were in line for prayer. If they had simply eaten correctly, most of them would have been well. An adjustment in dietary choices would have proven miraculous for them. Jesus always stands ready to heal, but for one to "keep" healing sometimes requires a transformative change in diet, exercise, and other habits. Jesus is the Great Shepherd; He died for His flock to be well, and He stands ready at all times to heal — even if a health issue is self-inflicted.

But I must importantly mention that many people also suffer from various types of eating disorders that include anorexia nervosa, bulimia nervosa, binge-eating disorder, avoidant or restrictive food-intake disorder, pica, rumination disorders, and other specified feeding and eating disorders.[1] At any given moment, countless individuals grapple with eating disorders. While disorders such as anorexia nervosa and bulimia nervosa predominantly affect women, they are not confined by age or gender and spare no demographic.

These disorders often manifest as an intense obsession with food, weight, or body shape, along with a deep-seated anxiety regarding eating and its perceived repercussions. The behaviors typical of eating disorders include strict food restrictions, avoidance of specific foods, episodes of binge-eating, self-induced purging through vomiting or misuse of laxatives, and compulsive exercising. These actions can dominate one's life with an intensity that mirrors an addiction and can consume one's thoughts and dictate behavior.[2]

Such eating disorders frequently coexist with various psychiatric conditions, such as mood and anxiety disorders, obsessive-compulsive tendencies, and challenges related to alcohol and substance use. An effective treatment plan should encompass psychological counseling, behavior modification, nutritional guidance, and attention to any other medical issues. Some must also consider that evil spirits may have found an "entry point" into their soul and their situation therefore necessitates deliverance. But often, those who grapple with these disorders will resist treatment, deny their condition, or feel anxious about altering their eating habits. With medical and spiritual support, they can be healed, they can learn to eat correctly, and they can achieve renewed emotional, mental, and physical well-being, but it is up to them to decide they are ready for it.

Regardless of one's reason for struggling with excess weight, obesity, or eating disorders, it's vital to enlist the guidance of a nutritional expert or a medical professional to help map out your journey to wellness. But that's not all you'll need. Surround yourself with a supportive community — ideally a faith-based group — that will offer encouragement, resilience, and unwavering support as you strive toward wholeness.

On my path to overcoming weight-related hurdles, I was fortunate to be enveloped by a circle of family and close friends who acted as my personal cheerleaders and celebrated each milestone of my progress. While it's certainly possible to navigate this path alone, it is significantly more challenging, so if you are in a situation where you recognize your diet needs to be corrected or adjusted, I urge you to find and embrace a network of individuals who will keep you accountable and uplift you as you embark on this transformative journey.

My prayer is that as you journey toward a life filled with healing and health, you will recognize the importance of feeding your body a wholesome diet that allows you to fully enjoy what Jesus secured for you on the Cross. Embracing healthy eating habits helps close the door to any "entry points" the adversary might use to sow chaos into your health. But if you are struggling in this area and resist addressing the root causes of your issues and refuse to cooperate with the Holy Spirit to bring correction, you will keep that "entry point" open and find yourself caught in a relentless cycle of illness.

If you know you need to make changes in the area of your diet, take heart, for God's plan for your healing and health goes beyond a temporary fix. Christ's sacrifice on the Cross purchased your complete restoration and healing — and He desires to help you through that restoration process so you can live free of past struggles and embrace a future filled with vibrancy, strength, and wholeness.

## THE ROLE OF PHYSICAL EXERCISE

This area of physical exercise is another one I can speak to personally because of what I have overcome to embrace exercise — as well as a healthy diet — as a part of my lifestyle. During my youth, our family was part of a church that embraced the joy of sports with enthusiasm. We gathered for softball tournaments, competitive football games, energetic basketball showdowns, and even participated in a church bowling league. My father, an athlete through and through, was passionate about any sport that involved a ball, his enthusiasm bounding from one game to the next.

However, I never liked sports, and I detested being dragged into any game that required my participation to throw, catch, hit, kick, carry, or bowl a ball. From my earliest days and well into adulthood, I avoided sports *and* any form of physical exercise. I'm sharing this with you because I want you to understand that much like my ignorance of healthy eating, before I finally decided to start exercising, I was completely ignorant about this subject as well. For years, I conveniently leaned on the verse First Timothy 4:8 as my trusty shield against exerting myself to exercise: "For bodily exercise profiteth little...." Although I twisted its intent to suit my sedentary lifestyle, it was more about creative justification for my actions, or lack of actions, than any sincere scriptural interpretation.

But after my family had a heart-to-heart talk with me about my expanding physical size and declining health, I realized shedding the nearly 100 pounds that I needed to lose wasn't just about changing my diet — it was going to come about by my embarking also on the journey of exercise.

Having avoided gyms my whole life, I had no idea what steps to take to fundamentally change this aspect of my life and catapult me into a life of increased physical health and strength. Thankfully, God led me to a trainer who would guide my trembling steps. The very thought of exercising filled me with dread, partly because of my large size and lack of fitness that seemed to be insurmountable obstacles. But more so, I also struggled with back pain, probably due to my overweight condition, and I feared injury while I was exercising. Anyone who has stood on the precipice of such a daunting lifestyle overhaul will understand the apprehension that accompanies the first steps on this path.

But the trainer God gave me in the beginning was compassionate and understood my struggle. Rather than pushing me too fast, he gently guided me with small, manageable steps — encouraging a tiny triumph each day. Over time, he meticulously nurtured my confidence and showed me that I was capable of achieving far greater feats. But fast-forward many years to the present, and I can tell you that today physical exercise has become a cornerstone of my life. Three times a week, I eagerly visit the gym, where I continue to engage in sessions with a trainer. Not only has my apprehension vanished, but I have wholeheartedly embraced this as a benefit in my life, and I have discovered that physical exercise not only positively affects my body, but it enriches my spirit, my mind, and overall well-being.

Today I relish my time at the gym where three times a week, I dive into high-octane intensity workouts, with my trainer leading the charge. I have embraced the HIIT routine: a protocol of explosive, anaerobic movements interspersed with brief intermissions — all the way to delightful exhaustion. In this balance of vigorous bursts and restful pauses, my trainer hovers nearby to help motivate me with compassionate encouragement that helps fuel my resolve to push my limits and embrace an exhilarating workout.

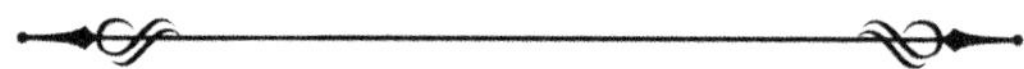

**Anyone who has stood on the precipice of such a daunting lifestyle overhaul will understand the apprehension that accompanies the first steps on this path.**

In First Timothy 4:8, Paul said, "For bodily exercise profiteth little...." In the First Century when Paul wrote this verse, the word "exercise" was translated from the Greek word *gumnadzo*, a word that portrayed *naked athletes who exercised, trained, and prepared for competition* in the athletic games of the ancient world. Stripping down to bare skin was considered essential for shedding any barriers that might otherwise disrupt an athlete's fluidity of motion.

This act of disrobing signified a commitment to casting off every obstacle and dedicating oneself wholeheartedly to the discipline of athletic rigor. The term "exercise" here extends far beyond a casual round of sit-ups; it evokes an image of someone fully immersing themselves into the strenuous, all-consuming pursuit of physical mastery.

In the First Century when Paul was writing this verse, such physical exercise was deemed *honorable*. Yet Paul wrote that it "profiteth little." The word "little" is derived from the Greek word *oligos*, which here means *small in number*. However, in this context, it more accurately conveys the idea of something that is *short-lived*. Paul employed this term to emphasize the transient nature of physical fitness — it benefits us only during our earthly existence. But Paul acknowledged its value when he said that exercise "profiteth." This word, from the Greek *ophelimos*, signifies what is *advantageous*, *beneficial*, or *profitable*. Thus, Paul underscored that physical activity offers real benefits, even if they are temporary.

Interestingly, in the First Century, when Paul penned these words, exercise was seen not just as a path to *physical improvement*, but it was deemed necessary for *mental clarity* and as an aid for *spiritual advancement*. I find this interesting because, through physical exercise, I have discovered that my mind becomes sharper, my spirit more attuned to hearing the voice of God, and I experience significant spiritual growth. But when we travel to do ministry and our intense travel schedule does not provide time to exercise, I find myself to be sluggish physically, mentally, and spiritually. In addition to making the body feel better, exercise really does contribute to mental and spiritual clarity.

When Paul extolled the virtues of exercise, describing it as *ophelimos* — *advantageous, beneficial, and profitable* — he knew exactly what he was talking about. His insight was not merely theoretical; it was a practical truth integral to his life and mission. If Paul had not possessed exceptional physical fitness, his extraordinary mission would have been unattainable. His ministry demanded a level of physical vitality and activity that only a fit individual could muster. For example:

- Paul *walked* from Antioch Pisidia to Iconium (Acts 13:51).
- He *walked* from Iconium to Lystra (Acts 14:6).
- He *walked* from Lystra to Derbe (Acts 14:20).

- From Derbe, he *walked* back to Lystra (Acts 14:21).
- From Lystra he *walked* back to Iconium (Acts 14:21).
- From Iconium, he *walked* back to Antioch Pisidia (Acts 14:21).
- From Antioch Pisidia, he *walked* throughout the whole region of Pamphylia (Acts 14:24).
- Then he *walked* all the way to Perga (Acts 14:25).

For a brief period, Paul and his team traveled by ship to Antioch (Paul's home base). But then:

- They *walked* to Phenice and Samaria (Acts 15:3).
- From there, they *walked* to Jerusalem (Acts 15:4).
- From Jerusalem, they *walked* back to Antioch (Acts 15:22).
- From Antioch, Paul *walked* throughout the regions of Syria and Cilicia (Acts 15:41).
- He *walked* back through the cities of Derbe (Acts 16:1) and Lystra (Acts 16:1).
- Then he *walked* to Phrygia (Acts 16:6) and *walked* throughout the region of Galatia (Acts 16:6).
- After that, he *walked* to Mysia (Acts 16:7) and then *walked* all the way down to Troas (Acts 16:8).

After Paul saw a vision of a man in Macedonia calling to him for help (Acts 16:9), he took a ship from Troas (Acts 16:11). His ship ported in the city of Samothracia (Acts 16:11) but departed the next day to Neapolis (Acts 16:11). From there, Paul and his associates sailed to Philippi (Acts 16:12), a chief city in that part of Macedonia. After that:

- From Philippi, Paul *walked* through Amphipolis and Apollonia (Acts 17:1).
- Then he *walked* to the city of Thessalonica (Acts 17:1).
- From Thessalonica, Paul *walked* to Berea (Acts 17:10).

*Paul then took a ship from Berea to Athens (Acts 17:14).*

- But from Athens, he *walked* to Corinth (Acts 18:1).

*Then Paul sailed from Corinth to Syria (Acts 18:18).*

- And from Syria, he *walked* to Ephesus (Acts 18:19).

*From Ephesus, he sailed to Caesarea (Acts 18:22).*

- From there, he *walked* to Antioch (Acts 18:22).
- From Antioch, he *walked* all over the regions of Galatia and Phrygia (Acts 18:23).
- Then he *walked* along the upper coastlines to Ephesus (Acts 19:1).

Considering the vast distances Paul covered during his ministry — trudging the eastern and northeastern Mediterranean lands — it is evident that he spent significant amounts of time walking in addition to starting churches and preaching. The Gospel's path was paved with his footsteps, and his journeys not only demanded spiritual zeal but also the robust stamina of an athlete. This was a man familiar with physical exercise, so when he said that exercise *profiteth*, his words carried the weight of experience and credibility.

I've had the privilege of visiting numerous locations where Paul carried out his ministry and have witnessed firsthand the extensive network of uneven roads and paths that he traversed on his journeys. The landscapes are not just rugged; they are blisteringly hot, making long-distance travel incredibly challenging in these regions. Some skeptics argue that Paul was frail and frequently unwell, but I find this notion utterly absurd. Anyone familiar with these terrains would understand that such a feat would be beyond the capabilities of someone who lived that much of his life in poor health.

To embark on journeys as Paul did — trekking thousands of miles over hills and valleys, fording powerful rivers, and navigating desolate territories — demands a person be in peak physical condition — in other words, someone who was accustomed to vigorous exercise.

I encourage you to explore Paul's own words in Second Corinthians 11:23-28, where he detailed the arduous landscapes he braved to complete his mission. Additionally, my book *Apostles and Prophets,* specifically pages 278-302, delves into the physical demands on Paul as he fulfilled his ministry.

If Paul hadn't taken the time to care for his body — his God-given fleshly instrument with which he served the Lord — and maintained it in peak condition, performing what he was destined to do might have remained unfulfilled. We have seen that any tool left untouched will corrode and become useless over time. Similarly, while Christ has achieved healing and health through His sacrifice, letting your physical being languish in idleness leads to decline.

On the other hand, the benefits of regular exercise are so remarkably appealing that they're nearly impossible to overlook. It's easy to misunderstand First Timothy 4:8 and use it as a reason to skip physical activity, but in truth, this passage underscores that even though physical exercise is temporary, it is fruitful, advantageous, and crucial — not only for bodily health, but also for sharpening the mind, advancing spiritually, and serving the Kingdom of God.

I urge you to ponder that if you maintain your current level of physical activity, where will you be in five or ten years? Will you remain agile and ready to serve a higher purpose, or will you find yourself slowing down or even stopping due to lack of mobility? Your answers to these questions are important, as they will determine how long and how well you will run your race.

The Mayo Clinic website cites the following seven benefits of physical exercise,[3] which I expounded on to demonstrate the importance of physical activity as a lifestyle.

**1. Exercise helps control weight.**

Engaging in exercise is a powerful ally in the battle against unwanted extra weight and can also be your steadfast partner in maintaining weight loss. Each time you move, calories are set ablaze, with more vigorous activities fanning the flames brighter and stronger.

While making regular pilgrimages to the gym is wonderful, there's no need to fret if your schedule doesn't allow for extended exercise sessions daily. Instead, embrace the philosophy that every bit of movement counts. Integrate bursts of activity into your routine — opt for the stairs over the elevator, turbo-charge your cleaning tasks, and, if safe to do, park farther from the entrance to a place of business than you would normally park.

Remember, the secret ingredient to reaping the rewards of an active lifestyle is movement and consistency. So I encourage you to look for ways to add physical movement to your everyday routine.

**2. Exercise combats health conditions and diseases.**

In addition to standing on the promises of God's Word for healing and health, think of exercise as your earthly ally in the quest to fend off heart disease and high blood pressure.

Regardless of where you find yourself on the scales, engaging in physical activity acts as a catalyst to enhance your levels of high-density lipoprotein (HDL) cholesterol, affectionately known as the "good" cholesterol, while reducing harmful triglycerides. This dynamic duo keeps your blood coursing seamlessly through your veins, effectively reducing the risk of heart and cardiovascular ailments.

In addition to helping improve cognitive function and being associated with a lower risk of an early death, engaging in consistent physical activity and exercise can thwart or keep in check a multitude of health issues, such as:

- Stroke
- Metabolic syndrome
- High blood pressure
- Type 2 diabetes
- Depression
- Anxiety
- Many types of cancer
- Falls

It's also important to note that, although exercise does not prevent arthritis, it can reduce the symptoms, improve mobility, and help manage pain in those with this condition.

**3. Exercise improves mood.**

When the weight of the world feels too heavy on your shoulders or the stress of the day clings like a stubborn shadow, consider the liberating power of movement. Dive into physical activity of some sort, whether it's a jog, a walk, a rejuvenating gym session, exercising to a video online, or doing some form of physical activity around the house. Physical exercise, although it can be a challenge to get started, can be so empowering once you determine to do it.

Science reveals that physical activity releases brain chemicals (neurotransmitters) designed to regulate mood, reduce stress and symptoms of anxiety, and promote relaxation. Moreover, as you embrace regular exercise, you might find a renewed admiration for yourself, a spark of confidence lighting up what might have been a dim self-image.

**4. Exercise boosts energy.**

If you notice yourself gasping for breath after a brief stroll, a trip to the grocery store, or even while doing chores around the house, it's time to embrace the power of regular exercise! Engaging in physical activity can enhance your muscle strength and elevate your stamina. When you exercise, you're gifting your tissues with essential oxygen and nutrients and it helps your cardiovascular system to operate with greater efficiency. As your heart and lung health flourish, you'll find yourself brimming with energy and ready to take on the hustle and bustle of daily life with newfound strength.

**5. Exercise promotes better sleep.**

If you find yourself tossing and turning at night, incorporating regular physical activity into your routine might just be the "lullaby" you need. Exercise not only ushers in sleep more swiftly, but it also enhances its quality and depth.

Personally, after going to the gym three times a week, after each session, I find myself drifting more quickly to sleep, and my sleep is more restful. However, a word of caution: Avoid exercising too near your bedtime, as the energy surge you often get from exercising might keep you awake longer than you'd like.

**6. Exercise puts a spark back into your romantic life.**

If you're finding that exhaustion due to a lack of fitness is dampening your enthusiasm for physical closeness, engaging in regular physical exercise can be a game-changer, as it boosts your energy reserves and can enhance your confidence in both your body image and your love life. The advantages of exercise are abundant, and one of the most rewarding gains could be the rejuvenation of intimacy with your spouse.

**7. Exercise can be a fun social event.**

Engaging in physical activity offers a wonderful opportunity to relax, soak in the outdoors, or participate in activities that bring you joy. It's also a fantastic way to bond with family or friends in a social atmosphere. Exercising is much more enjoyable when shared with someone else. For instance, when I head to the gym, I go with a friend, whose companionship not only keeps me accountable, but it motivates me and makes the whole experience more enjoyable.

It's amusing to me that I'm speaking to you from personal experience about the wonders of physical exercise, considering I was an adamant opponent of it for more than half a century!

Yet now, breaking a sweat has become a cherished part of my regular routine — a testament to the delightful transformation that can occur if we choose to align ourselves with God's plan to run our race and finish our course in life strong. My transformation has reinforced in my heart and mind the crucial truth that to experience health and longevity, we must get our bodies in motion.

While God's promises offer us healing and health — promises that were purchased by Jesus on the Cross — it is incumbent on us to make the most of them. Do we want to live 40 quality years of life — or do we want to live 80 or more years of meaningful life that is replete with purpose and the strength to fulfill it? Embracing physical activity is our tangible contribution to nurturing the life that God has given us.

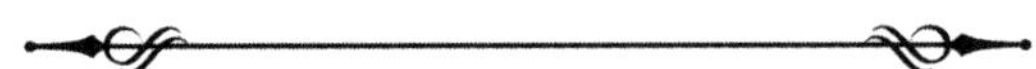

**Embracing physical activity is our tangible contribution to nurturing the life that God has given us.**

Without our active participation, we might miss out on the full measure of healing and health that God intended for us to have. So let's lift our hearts and our feet, and let's commit to moving our bodies in a way that leads to prolonged health and longevity.

## THE ROLE OF SUPPLEMENTS

It's truly astonishing that a person who once cringed at the idea of exercise is now singing the praises of physical fitness and an active lifestyle. Equally amusing is the fact that I am now about to speak to you about the inclusion of vitamins and other supplements in your daily routine. Allow me to share why I find this so amusing by telling you a bit about my childhood and its surprising *lack* of vitamins and other supplementation to our not-so-nutritious diet.

During my childhood, our family medicine cabinet was a treasure trove of home remedies, stocked with concoctions for every conceivable ailment, whether it was the sniffles, the flu, or a pesky headache. We were always prepared for whatever health hiccups might come our way. However, one thing you wouldn't find amidst that sea of medicine was vitamins. My mother, who worked alongside a doctor, was influenced by his firm belief that vitamins were nothing but an expensive waste of money. Consequently, our household was so skeptical about vitamins that we basically deemed them a frivolous expense.

The only vitamins I ever remember taking as a child were Flintstone® vitamins. When they first came on the market in 1968, we Renner kids thought they were really neat because each "vitamin" was molded to look like characters from the Flintstones cartoon and they tasted just like candy. Right there in the bottle were *Fred Flintstone, Wilma Flintstone, Pebbles Flintstone, Barney Rubble, Betty Rubble, Bamm-Bamm Rubble*, and *Dino.* It was the whole cartoon family in a bottle, and the multi-colored Flintstone vitamins went along really well with our sweetened cereal in the mornings that we redundantly covered with *heaps* of grainy white sugar!

Conversely, while Denise grew up nestled in a household where fresh vegetables graced every meal, hers was also a home where fistfuls of vitamins were religiously consumed every dawn and dusk. Shortly after Denise and I were wed, I visited her parents' home and embarked on a quest for a water glass. I accidentally opened the wrong cabinet door and was greeted not by glasses, but by an army of vitamin bottles, standing in endless rows. My eyes widened in disbelief at the sheer volume of vitamins in front of me. The thought flashed through my mind, *Who would squander so much money on such inconsequential tablets and capsules?* This was years before the vitamin craze really caught on, which means Denise's family were pioneers in the realm of vitamin enthusiasm, and they embraced a passion for supplements long before it became a trend.

As the years rolled by, Denise and I found ourselves blessed with the friendship of those whom many revere as "giants of faith" and leaders of influential healing ministries. During countless lunches and dinners we shared with them, I often marveled to see these titans of faith and healing reach into their bags, purses, or pockets to extract fists full of vitamins. And when I say "fists full," I am not exaggerating. Over many years, I have witnessed these champions of faith and leaders of healing and health using vitamins and mineral supplements to strengthen and undergird their physical health. They knew something I didn't about stewarding the physical life bestowed on us by God to care for and nurture!

Since I was never vitamin friendly and Denise really wanted me to be, very often when this happened, I could see her casting a playful near-wink my way, a silent testament of her steadfast belief in the power of vitamins — a belief she had persistently tried (and spectacularly failed) to instill in me.

I will not give you the names of these titans of faith who are avid consumers of vitamins and mineral supplements, but I will tell you that not only do they use vitamins and supplements as preachers and teachers, they often seize the moment at meals to teach those around the table about how important it is to replenish the body with nutrients that are depleted due to age and other factors.

And I now see their point. If your car's oil level runs dangerously low, do you blindly continue to drive and ignore inevitable damage that will result from your negligence? Or do you replenish that vital fluid to ensure a smooth journey and the longevity of your vehicle? Similarly, when your air conditioner falls short on antifreeze, do you simply pray and believe for a miracle to maintain a cool breeze in your home, or do you summon an expert to restore its efficiency? It's all about providing what's needed to keep everything running optimally — be it your car, your cooling system, or even *your body.*

The truth is that if our diets were abundant in nutrient-rich foods and untouched by the loss of essential nourishment, the need for quality vitamins and mineral supplements would diminish. But in our modern age, much of our food has been stripped of its natural bounty. By choosing foods that are grown naturally and that retain their God-given nutrients, we could naturally satisfy our dietary needs. And if we eat a well-balanced diet that is filled with lean proteins, whole grains, fruits, and vegetables, it would lessen our need for vitamins and supplements, as our nutritional requirements would be beautifully met by what we consumed.

However, in today's atmosphere where food is grown commercially, it often falls short of the natural richness that it once held. And as time progresses, our bodies gradually lose critical nutrients vital for maintaining health and extending our lifespan. Consequently, incorporating vitamins and supplements into our daily routine grows increasingly crucial. Yet despite their potential advantages, it's important and wise to seek advice from a healthcare expert to help us tailor the types and amounts of vitamins and mineral supplements to our individual needs.

While I'm far from being a vitamin connoisseur (and could use a nudge to make a habit of taking them regularly), it's undeniable that our bodies crave the replenishment of depleted essential nutrients. Again, ideally, a diet replete with nutrient-rich foods would naturally supply us with these vital vitamins and minerals, nourishing us from the inside out. But because most of our food supply is lacking these nutrients, quality vitamins and minerals and other supplementation act as the unsung heroes in various metabolic processes and ensure our health and bodily functions remain in top form.

When your body runs low on certain vitamins, it falls into a state of deficiency, which can lead to a myriad of health issues. Each vitamin plays a crucial role in maintaining our bodily harmony. But as you delve into the world of vitamins and mineral supplements, it's essential to remember that more isn't always better — and overconsumption can even lead to toxicity, which is why it is important to consult with a professional as you begin the process of incorporating vitamins and supplements into your lifestyle.

The following is a guide to the essential vitamins that our bodies require to thrive and operate at their best. In this list, you will discover the benefits each one brings to our system and what can happen when our bodies are deficient in them.

As I write the following information with the insight I have received from respected members in the medical community, I am awestruck by God's brilliance in designing nature to provide all of these needs so perfectly.

- **Vitamin A** plays a crucial role in shaping and preserving resilient soft tissue, protective mucous membranes, and vibrant skin. A deficiency of vitamin A can dim your vision, sometimes even leading to blindness, and may spell trouble for your skin, heart, lungs, tissues, and immune system.

- **Vitamin B6** (also called *pyridoxine*) is an essential nutrient that assists in the production of red blood cells and supports the brain in performing its functions efficiently. This vitamin is also a key player in the myriad of chemical reactions occurring within our body, particularly those involving proteins. Consequently, as your protein intake increases, so does your body's demand for pyridoxine.

  When your body has a deficiency of this particular vitamin, it can lead to anemia, a condition where your supply of red blood cells drops too low. This deficiency can leave you feeling as if you've run a marathon with no finish line in sight, and thus leave you in a state of exhaustion and weakness. Senior adults might find themselves running low on this vitamin, which happens when their diets fall short or when their bodies no longer absorb nutrients as efficiently as earlier in life.

- **Vitamin B12** plays a significant role similar to its fellow B vitamins and acts as a key player in metabolism. Beyond its metabolic duties, it serves as an essential architect in the construction of red blood cells and as a steadfast guardian of both the central and peripheral nervous systems, affecting neurological function, as well as being necessary for DNA synthesis. When your body has a deficiency of red blood cells, your tissues and organs miss out on vital oxygen, and this oxygen deficit means your body operates less efficiently. Signs of a B12 deficiency can manifest as muscle weakness, neuropathy (numbness, walking difficulties), glossitis (affecting the tongue), nausea and other gastrointestinal symptoms, unintended weight loss, irritability, fatigue, and a racing heart.

- **Vitamin C** serves as a powerful antioxidant and plays a vital role in maintaining the health of teeth and gums. Its properties enhance the body's ability to absorb iron and sustain robust tissues. Moreover, it is a crucial component in the body's arsenal for healing wounds efficiently. A deficiency of vitamin C can show up as bruising or bleeding easily, tender or bleeding gums, loose teeth, sluggish wound healing, fatigue, anemia, weakened immunity, and tiny red spots on the skin. When vitamin C deficiency becomes extreme, it can lead to a condition known as scurvy.

- **Vitamin D** is a remarkable nutrient that can be produced by some people simply by soaking up some rays of the sun! Just 10 to 15 minutes of basking in sunlight three times per week is often sufficient to fulfill the vitamin D quota for some people. However, those residing in less sun-drenched regions might struggle to produce adequate levels of this vital vitamin — and age and other factors can affect the production of this vitamin as well. Relying solely on dietary sources to obtain sufficient vitamin D can be a challenging endeavor. That is why it's best to be routinely tested on the levels of this vitamin in the body. This dazzling vitamin plays a pivotal role in helping your body absorb calcium, which is an essential mineral for building and maintaining sturdy teeth and bones.

Additionally, vitamin D is crucial in keeping blood levels of calcium and phosphorus in harmonious balance — as well as *supporting the immune system*, *helping blood-sugar management*, *promoting heart health*, *assisting in the regulation of hormones*, and *positively affecting cognitive function* — underscoring this "super-vitamin's" importance in your overall health. A deficiency of vitamin D may lead to fatigue, susceptibility to infectious diseases, and bones that are fragile, frail, and prone to bending or bowing during development.

- **Vitamin E** serves as a powerful antioxidant and plays a pivotal role in the creation of red blood cells, as well as aiding in the effective use of vitamin K by the body. A deficiency of vitamin E can dim one's ability to see in the dark or to feel subtle vibrations. As the deficiency progresses more significantly, it may manifest as an unsteady gait, pronounced muscle enfeeblement, and a restricted ability to gaze upward.

- **Vitamin K** plays a crucial role in ensuring that our blood clots as it should, and thus it can prevent uncontrolled bleeding. Emerging research additionally indicates that this vital nutrient may also contribute significantly to maintaining strong and healthy bones. A deficiency of vitamin K hampers the body's ability to produce essential clotting factors, which can lead to a heightened chance of bleeding and bruising.

  The gravest concern stemming from vitamin K deficiency is hemorrhaging, a complication that can affect individuals of all ages. In newborns, this condition can be especially dire, sometimes proving to be fatal.

- **Biotin** plays a vital role in the intricate dance of our body's inner workings and orchestrates the metabolism of proteins and carbohydrates while also being a key player in the creation of hormones and cholesterol. A deficiency of biotin is uncommon, yet when it strikes, it can manifest as a skin rash, thinning hair, elevated cholesterol levels, and potential heart issues.

- **Niacin (Vitamin B3)** is a member of the B vitamin family and plays an important role in nurturing radiant skin and supporting resilient nerve function. When taken in higher doses, it also serves as a helpful ally in reducing triglyceride levels, promoting overall cardiovascular wellness. A deficiency of niacin can gradually lead to a troubling trio of symptoms: skin inflammation, cognitive decline, and digestive disturbances. If left unchecked, these issues can become life-threatening. Additionally, individuals suffering from niacin deficiency often find themselves lacking in essential nutrients such as protein, riboflavin (another B vitamin), and vitamin B6.

- **Folate** teams up with vitamin B12 in a dynamic duo to craft red blood cells. This vital nutrient is essential for spinning the intricate web of DNA, the master architect behind tissue growth and cellular operations. Pregnant women in particular should ensure they have an ample supply of folate. Thankfully, an array of foods now come enriched with a version of folate — folic acid — to help bridge any nutritional gaps. A deficiency of folate can lead to feelings of tiredness, a lack of strength, troublesome mouth ulcers, and issues affecting the nervous system.

- **Pantothenic Acid (Vitamin B5)** is essential for food metabolism and helps transform what we eat into usable energy. Additionally, it acts as an architect in the body's production of hormones and cholesterol and ensures our internal systems run smoothly. A deficiency of this vitamin is rare, but it often appears in those suffering from malnutrition. A person with this deficiency is likely missing several other essential nutrients. Research shows that those afflicted with this deficiency may experience persistent fatigue, headaches, a general sense of unease, shifts in personality, numbness, muscle cramps, prickling sensations, abdominal discomfort, nausea, and difficulties with muscle coordination.

- **Riboflavin (Vitamin B2)** teams up harmoniously with its B vitamin companions. It plays a crucial role in fueling body growth and orchestrating the creation of vibrant red blood cells. A deficiency of riboflavin often accompanies a lack of other B vitamins and can manifest as a sore throat, mouth lesions, lip inflammation, a swollen tongue, eye irritation, skin issues, and anemia.
- **Thiamine (Vitamin B1)** plays a crucial role in transforming carbohydrates into the fuel your body craves. Ensuring an ample intake of carbohydrates becomes especially vital for expectant and nursing mothers. Thiamine is also a key player in maintaining a healthy heart and supporting vibrant nerve cells. A deficiency of thiamine can lead to a spectrum of unwanted symptoms, stretching from mere weariness to complete paralysis.
- **Choline** plays an important role in the harmonious operation of the brain and nervous system. Without adequate levels of this vital nutrient, one might experience liver inflammation, a foggy mind, and a diminished attention span.
- **Carnitine** transforms fatty acids into energy and fuels the body's inner powerhouse. A deficiency of carnitine may reveal itself through a variety of concerning indicators. Infants and young children might experience profound challenges such as serious brain malfunctions (*encephalopathy*). People of all ages can be critically deficient and experience an enlarged or feeble heart (*cardiomyopathy*), episodes of

vomiting, diminished muscle strength, and dangerously low levels of blood sugar (*hypoglycemia*).

Even if we stand on the promises of God's Word for healing and health, lifestyle stressors and other factors, including the passage of time and aging, inevitably leave us with dwindling reserves of crucial nutrients. We must see to it that our faith in God's promises goes hand in hand with practical steps to ensure we're not lacking in these vital nutrients. While I'm no specialist in the world of vitamins and supplements, I can tell you that under the careful guidance of a healthcare professional, incorporating these into our lives can help restore what our bodies may be lacking.

## OTHER NEEDED ELEMENTS TO REPLENISH YOUR BODY

In addition to vitamins, it's crucial to ensure that you're receiving enough **magnesium** — an essential mineral that plays a significant role in our well-being. Astonishingly, studies reveal that 30 to 50 percent of individuals over the age of 70 consume inadequate amounts of this mineral. This deficiency is associated with a myriad of health issues, ranging from sleep disturbances to cardiovascular complications, strokes, Type 2 diabetes, and depression. Magnesium works its magic by relaxing the smooth muscle of the vascular wall, keeping muscles flexible, and, for those who tend to live anxiously "on edge," even helping to lower blood pressure.

Additionally, your body also needs a healthy dose of **omega-3 fatty acids**, which are essential nutrients discovered in the depths of the ocean and in fields of flax. These underwater and terrestrial treasures are contributors to cognitive vitality. Studies focusing on the elderly and the middle-aged hint at the potential heart-health benefits these fatty acids offer. This includes supporting healthy lipid levels, and it's even linked with reduced cardiovascular risk, especially through lowering triglycerides. Since we lack the innate ability to produce omega-3s ourselves, we must intentionally seek them out — whether through a serving of fatty fish or a flax-enhanced food or as a supplement brimming with concentrated goodness.

Don't forget the important role of **fiber**. As you age, your digestive system may change (slower digestive function and changes in gut bacteria), which can lead to constipation and bloating. But when taken regularly, fiber offers a bounty of health perks that can ease digestion and potentially promote weight loss by helping balance blood sugar and also providing the sensation of satiety when consumed. Not only can it reduce the risk of diabetes and certain cancers, especially colorectal cancer, but research shows that those who consume plenty of fiber are also less prone to heart disease. Embracing fiber is like giving your digestive system a tune-up that ensures everything runs smoothly while also protecting your overall health.

Your body also needs an adequate intake of **calcium**, which plays a crucial role in supporting bone strength, aiding nerve function, and facilitating muscle movement. It is vital in helping to reduce bone loss with age, supporting the prevention and management of *osteopenia* and *osteoporosis.*

You also need to ensure that you're getting sufficient **protein**, as it plays a key role in muscle development and helps counteract the gradual decline in muscle mass. As people age, their protein requirements are higher relative to those for younger adults because older people become less efficient at using protein to build and maintain muscle. Protein also aids in recovery from illness and upholding a good quality of life. Moreover, protein supplies the essential amino acids that our body requires for cell growth and repair. It also helps stabilize blood sugar levels and is vital for both building and retaining muscle.

And don't forget the importance of **hydration** — of keeping your body well-hydrated. As we journey through life, the inclination to drink water dwindles, and it often results in dehydration. This lack of adequate fluid intake is especially risky as we age, for it can lead to lightheadedness and dizziness and increase the likelihood of falls.

Next, it's noteworthy to consider hormonal balance in the body. In men, testosterone levels tend to surge during the teenage years and early adulthood. As time marches on, however, these levels gradually wane, usually by about one percent each year after the age of 30 or 40. In the golden years, it's common for testosterone to dwindle due to the natural progression of aging, and it can result in potential shifts in sexual health, increased weight, and even emotional fluctuations. Some research suggests that **testosterone-replacement therapy** might offer a helping hand in managing these changes.

As women gracefully journey beyond the threshold of 50, they may encounter a myriad of health challenges that are influenced by low estrogen, progesterone, and testosterone and there may be the need for **balancing hormones**. This delicate dance of hormones within the body is influenced by a mélange of health conditions, medications, and lifestyle and environmental factors and, if out of balance, can lead to uncomfortable symptoms and heightened health risks.

The waning of estrogen, progesterone, and testosterone in women is commonly an issue as they age, yet the disruption does not stop there. Imbalances in cortisol, insulin, and thyroid hormones can also add symptoms of fatigue, weight changes, and cognitive difficulty while a decline in estrogen and progesterone often beckon the arrival of hot flashes, fatigue, and the silent thief of decreased bone density. Consulting a medical professional for potential **hormone-replacement therapy** may help women and men maintain their health and greatly improve their quality of life.

Again, I wish to remind you that when the oil in your vehicle dips into the danger zone, a simple refill of oil ensures you're cruising the roads without a hitch. Similarly, when your air conditioner starts gasping for antifreeze, you don't hesitate to call in an expert to bring it back to its breezy best. These actions are vital for keeping both your car and air conditioning system running like a dream. It's much the same way with your physical body. Your body is a magnificent creation, a gift from God, and maintaining its harmony requires more than just faith. It's about embracing the wisdom of how to care for it. Looking after yourself isn't a sign of unbelief; it's an acknowledgment of the body's needs. So be vigilant and proactive in supplying your body with the essential nutrients it craves, ensuring it operates smoothly and efficiently throughout your life.

## THE ROLE OF DOCTORS AND MEDICINE

For some, the idea of stepping into a doctor's office stirs up apprehension. This unease can escalate into a pronounced psychological condition known as *iatrophobia*.[4] This term is rooted in the Greek words *iatros*, which means *doctor* or *healer*, and the Greek word *phobos*, which means *fear*. As the word *iatrophobia*, it pictures *those who harbor an intense dread of doctors or medical procedures*. It paints a picture of individuals for whom the very thought of a medical setting invokes significant anxiety.

When someone suffers even slightly from *iatrophobia*, they might shun medical care despite being severely ill or exhibiting symptoms of a serious condition. This dread can stem from previous medical experiences, past traumas, or even just an aversion to doctors' offices, needles, or medical procedures in general. It's astonishing how many individuals grapple with anxiety about visiting healthcare professionals, medical settings, and injections to the extent that they forgo treatment that could easily alleviate their troubling symptoms.

For many, the mere thought of entering a doctor's office can ignite a wave of anxiety so intense that it compels them to delay essential annual checkups, medical screenings, and vital diagnostic exams. This fear prevents them from receiving timely care, and their failure to address minor health issues, which could have been easily treated, can potentially evolve into more formidable challenges. Some dread the prospect of painful procedures, others fear an unwelcome diagnosis, and then there are individuals who view the medical field suspiciously and are influenced by unsettling stories from others who have had a bad experience.

Growing up, my family's close ties with the medical world were thanks to my mother's longstanding role as an assistant in a doctor's office. This connection made doctor visits feel as routine to us as a trip to the grocery store. We saw doctors as more than just practitioners; they were heroic figures who were esteemed in our home. Our faith in medicine was visible by a well-stocked medicine cabinet at home that brimmed with remedies for every conceivable ailment — be it a pounding headache, a stubborn cold, or the creeping aches of the flu.

In contrast, Denise's home was a world apart. Her family had deep convictions about the healing powers of vitamins and natural remedies and rarely found the need to darken the door of a doctor's office. Her father, a pioneering spirit in his own right, embraced alternative medicine and naturopathy long before these practices became mainstream. I remember him lounging comfortably in his recliner, surrounded by a fortress of journals dedicated to natural healing. Having grown up in a household that held traditional medicine in high esteem, I often found his ideas and suggestions rather unconventional and occasionally baffling.

While some of these remedies indeed proved effective, they were a far cry from the straightforward medical treatments I was accustomed to as I grew up. Raised under her father's skeptical gaze, Denise developed a cautious disposition toward conventional medicine, viewing it through a lens of doubt. This deep-seated skepticism meant that for Denise, mustering the courage to see a doctor required a determination similar to bracing oneself for battle — starkly different from the ease with which I could seek out medical counsel.

I also know people who have a similar aversion to medication and who avoid it completely. They fight sickness for long bouts when a simple medication could help them get well much quicker. Some Christians feel that using medication is a signal that they are not standing firm in faith, but it is possible to use medication and to simultaneously release one's faith for it to do its job effectively and quickly — in addition to receiving God's blessing of healing and restored health.

Romans 14:23 reveals the principle that "whatsoever is not of faith is sin." In this verse, Paul emphasized the importance of acting according to one's convictions. If a person cannot pursue a particular course of action with a clear conscience, it is better to hold back or wait until he can act with confidence and faith.

When applied to decisions about doctors and medication, this principle suggests that if you are unsure about a treatment and cannot proceed with conviction, it might be wise to wait prayerfully or to seek alternatives.

Conversely, if ignoring a specific medical path "violates" your conscience, or you know inside you're simply avoiding a situation that needs to be confronted, following that path may be necessary. It is important to act in a manner that aligns with your inner moral compass, and it's okay to seek counsel from others who are spiritually seasoned and sensitive — or even to get a second opinion medically.

Based on Scripture, I believe that Jesus stands firmly opposed to disease, illness, and infirmity, and we have seen that a significant part of Christ's work of redemption was dedicated to eradicating these afflictions from our lives. And we certainly see His opposition to such afflictions in His earthly ministry as recorded in the gospels.

However, if someone finds himself grappling with physical or mental challenges, and a medication prescribed with expertise can swiftly usher in a positive change — and if his conscience is at peace with this path — there is no harm in embracing medical aid. In fact, God's aversion to sickness is so profound that we should use every available resource in our battle against it.

I am reminded of when Timothy had some kind of physical issue with his stomach, and Paul told him, "Drink no longer water, but use a little wine for thy stomach's sake and thine often infirmities" (1 Timothy 5:23).

Let's explore this verse in the light of Timothy's circumstances. In the city of Ephesus, Timothy was the most prominent leader of the church, and he was steering it through a tempest of trials. Faith was under siege, and unrelenting persecution coerced many believers to forsake their convictions for the sake of survival. As the senior leader of the church of Ephesus, Timothy's charge was to stand resolute and unwavering. Yet Second Timothy 1:7 reveals that he wrestled with a spirit of fear that could have been the fountainhead for anxiety, unease, and apprehension.

But if we go back to First Timothy, which was composed in the days before the fierce persecution began, we discover earlier hints that Timothy was already grappling with anxiety and that it was taking a toll on his health. At that juncture, the church was growing and Timothy found himself caught in a whirlwind, and the strain of challenges seemed to weigh upon him. Amidst the stress and strain, Paul advised him, "Drink no longer water, but use a little wine for thy stomach's sake and thine often infirmities" (1 Timothy 5:23).

Remember that Paul was a preacher of the Cross and all its benefits, which included forgiveness of sin, freedom from guilt and shame, peace of mind, and healing and health for the body. Nevertheless, Paul acknowledged with this statement the significance of using other means available when tackling issues of the body or mind. Perceiving that Timothy was laden with emotional struggles that were producing digestive issues, Paul gave him the counsel, "Drink no longer water, but use a little wine for thy stomach's sake and thine often infirmities."

The words "drink no longer water" originate from the unique Greek word *hudropoteo*, which appears only here in the New Testament, and it is rarely found in other ancient texts. This rarely used word depicts *a committed teetotaler* — someone resolutely abstaining from all forms of alcohol. Timothy's aversion to any form of alcohol appeared so profound that he shunned it altogether, even when, according to the medical beliefs of that time, just a modest sip might have calmed his stomach and aided his digestion. It's conceivable that Timothy witnessed firsthand the negative effects of alcohol, leading him to take to heart the warning that a leader should be "not given to wine" (*see* 1 Timothy 3:3), thereby choosing complete abstinence. Additionally, Timothy may have been believing for a miraculous healing of his stomach woes and shunned any medical assistance because he placed his faith wholly in divine intervention.

Paul's words to Timothy, telling him to "use a little wine for thy stomach's sake," were not an open invitation to indulge in alcohol. Paul wasn't promoting casual drinking; rather, he was advising Timothy to utilize an available remedy to help with his ailment. Although Christ's work of redemption at the Cross secured the promise of healing and health, sometimes the realization of that promise unfolds more slowly than we hope. Timothy seemed to be in one of those waiting periods, and as he awaited a miraculous intervention, Paul's counsel was to "use" other available means to soothe his stomach and to bring relief to his digestive woes.

The term "use" means *to engage* or *to make use* of something. Again, Paul was not advocating casual or social drinking. Instead, he advised the modest use of wine purely for its health benefits regarding digestion. In fact, the words "a little wine," are rooted in the Greek word *oino oligo.* The Greek word *oinos* means *wine* and the word *oligos* means *a very small amount.* As the phrase "a little wine," it pictures *a very minor quantity of wine.* Timothy was known for his strong opposition to alcohol consumption, which prompted Paul's recommendation to employ merely a dash of it for its therapeutic effects, specifically to aid his digestive health.

Historically, it was believed that a mild mixture of wine blended with water could serve medicinal purposes and alleviate stomach and digestive complaints. Thus, Paul was acting in accordance with the medical beliefs of his day when he suggested Timothy incorporate a slight measure of wine mixed with water, as a type of medication, to ease his stomach and digestive discomforts.

Denise and I don't personally drink any alcohol, and to affirm that Paul wasn't promoting casual or social drinking, we see in First Timothy 5:23 that he advised Timothy to partake for the sake of his stomach. In the original Greek, the word used is *dia*, which more accurately means *on account of* your stomach. This subtle distinction highlights that Timothy's health issue was tied to his stomach or digestive system. The phrase "thy stomach" comes from the Greek words *ton stomachon*, referring explicitly to the stomach and, by extension, the whole digestive process. Furthermore, Paul observed that Timothy frequently faced other health challenges, described as "often infirmities."

The word "often" is translated from the Greek word *puknos*, which suggests *frequent recurrence*. Meanwhile, the word "infirmities" is derived from the Greek plural form of *astheneia*, which denotes *physical ailments* and *general physical weaknesses*. Together, the words "often infirmities" sketches an image of *recurring physical challenges*. The coupling of these words suggests that Timothy's health troubles were predominantly rooted in his stomach and digestive tract — ailments potentially exacerbated by the elevated anxiety, ceaseless worry, and stress that hounded him during this phase of his life for a variety of reasons.

As noted earlier, it is possible that Timothy was holding out for a miraculous healing without the aid of medications. But until divine healing showed up, Paul recommended using a natural remedy to help as he awaited healing to manifest.

In addition to Paul's advice to Timothy about using medical assistance for his stomach's sake, let's consider the relationship between Paul and Luke, whom Paul affectionately refers to as "the beloved physician" in Colossians 4:14.

The term "physician" is derived from the Greek word *iatros*, which unquestionably denotes *a medical doctor*. This reveals that before embarking on his spiritual mission, Luke was a cherished figure in the medical field. Beyond this, we learn that Luke was a constant companion on Paul's journeys, which enabled him to chronicle the book of Acts with remarkable precision — he had a firsthand account of Paul's every move due to their shared travels. But what I wish to highlight is that Luke, the beloved and cherished doctor, walked alongside Paul through many phases of his life and remained a faithful companion across numerous seasons.

What motivated Luke to remain so faithful by Paul's side?

The reasons are manifold, yet chief among them was likely Paul's history of enduring severe beatings and torture for the sake of the Gospel. Luke's presence served not just as companionship but also as a means to provide medical aid, ready to offer care until the manifestation of healing was realized. I affirm again that we hold a firm belief that Christ's sacrifice purchased both healing and health.

However, what action would you personally take if you suffered a significant injury, like colliding with barbed wire or inflicting a deep wound on your arm? At first, you would fervently pray for healing, but if immediate healing and relief for a bleeding wound did not materialize, wouldn't you instinctively take steps to ease the pain and stop the blood flow?

Paul endured countless beatings and torturous moments, yet each time he rose more resilient than before, as he drew upon an extraordinary supernatural strength to heal and mend whatever was broken. The power of the Holy Spirit enabled him to keep moving forward against all odds, and with each ordeal, Paul unleashed his faith and believed for complete restoration so that he could continue onward with his mission.

By reading Paul's personal narratives in Second Corinthians 11, we find a story of relentless trials and persecutions. Take, for instance, Second Corinthians 11:24, where Paul recounted "of the Jews five times received I forty stripes save one." This wasn't just a punishment; it was a brutal testament that he endured, not once, but five times. Yet remarkably, after each severe thrashing, Paul would rise again, undeterred and steadfast, continuing his God-given mission with unwavering resolve.

Paul's commitment to his God-given assignment was so profound that no adversity could veer him off course. His determination was buoyed by a seemingly supernatural resilience that prevented these harrowing episodes from becoming insurmountable obstacles. Instead, each challenge became a mere hurdle he pushed aside as he forged ahead, ever committed to completing the work he felt called to accomplish.

In Second Corinthians 11:25, Paul added, "Thrice was I beaten with rods...." This brutal punishment was one of the cruelest forms of torment in ancient times. Curiously, the book of Acts does not provide a detailed account of such a beating endured by Paul, but this experience was obviously etched in his memory. Yet despite such a harrowing ordeal, Paul refused to surrender, and instead seized the power that was afforded by his faith and forged onward with his mission.

In Second Corinthians 11:25, Paul additionally wrote that "once was I stoned." This significant episode from Paul's life is recorded in Acts 14:19. After a fruitful mission among the Gentiles in Lystra, Jewish agitators journeyed from Iconium who were determined to disrupt Paul's work. Their efforts were so persuasive that they turned the entire city against him. In a fit of rage, the people of Lystra stoned him and "...drew him out of the city, supposing he had been dead" (Acts 14:19).

In the grim ritual of stoning, those who carried out the sentence would hurl jagged stones with precision toward the victim's head, seeking to inflict a lethal impact. The assault would relentlessly continue until the victim's skull succumbed to the barrage, ensuring certain death. Once life had unequivocally departed, the remaining stones would be discarded, and the lifeless body would be unceremoniously dragged beyond the city's bounds, left as food for scavenging dogs and wild creatures. Therefore, when Acts 14:19 recounts that the inhabitants of Lystra "supposed" Paul was dead, there is no reason to think he was not dead at that moment.

According to Acts 14:20, after Paul was left for dead, the disciples came and stood near his corpse, and "he rose up." Is it possible that these disciples joined hands and prayed for Paul's resurrection? In Second Corinthians 12:1-4, Paul shared an extraordinary experience of entering into Heaven, where he encountered indescribable wonders that he was not granted permission to disclose. Could this heavenly experience have occurred during that deadly moment in Lystra when stones rained down upon him?

As stones were being hurled on Paul, he could have surmised, "Well, I guess this is the end of the road for me." If he had chosen that thinking, the stones would have possibly claimed his life. But I am convinced that amid the onslaught, a defiant spark ignited within him, as if he were declaring to himself, *I'm not done with my ministry yet, so if they kill me, I'll just have to be resurrected!* Paul encountered numerous such divine interventions that defied the odds.

Yet among these remarkable experiences, certainly there were occasions when having Dr. Luke by his side was a cherished comfort. As Paul awaited healing and recovery from the beatings he endured, the presence of a kind-hearted physician friend was likely a source of strength. Can you see that it is likely Dr. Luke's gentle medical hands provided relief until full healing unfolded?

If Dr. Luke assisted Paul, it wouldn't have been a sign that Paul's faith in the miraculous nature of God's touch was shaken. In fact, as Luke lent his medical expertise, it's easy to envision both men praying for healing in tandem with every applied remedy.

Picture the absurdity, however, if Paul had turned to Dr. Luke with stoic resolve and said, "Although pain rages in me and you could immediately help me, I refuse your help because I will only receive divine intervention. Despite the fact that you could ease my pain and stop my bleeding, I reject your assistance."

Pain can be taxing on the mind, clouding one's focus and making it difficult to concentrate. Luke's medical help could provide relief that would enable Paul to focus more strongly on God's promises. Thus, Luke's medical interventions could help to move Paul into an even more profound state of faith. As he awaited the full manifestation of healing, I'm sure he was grateful for the presence of a dearly beloved doctor friend who was ready to assist him in any possible way.

Reflecting on Paul's advice to Timothy about using a little wine for his stomach's sake and also Paul's interactions with Dr. Luke, we see that Paul witnessed miraculous healings and also embraced the support of medical professionals and natural remedies when necessary. He believed in miracles and simultaneously embraced the need for a doctor's care and for medicine as aids on the journey to health. I invite you to consider these perspectives when contemplating the role of doctors and medicine in your own life.

## THE ROLE OF A BALANCED LIFE

As we draw to the close of this chapter, we will now see how living a balanced life is also a cornerstone for healing and health. Time and time again in this book, we've acknowledged that Christ's redemptive work on the Cross purchased the forgiveness of sins, liberation from guilt and shame, peace of mind, and healing and health. However, by straying from a commonsense approach to life, one can sabotage the blessings of healing and health that God intends for him to experience.

I'll once again share insights I've learned in my own life to underscore the importance of embracing a balanced lifestyle. Then I'll give you a New Testament example of one whose health was possibly jeopardized because of an imbalanced lifestyle and an overly busy schedule.

It was, and is, ingrained into our particular group of Renners that we do not just "surrender" to sickness. A steadfast refusal to succumb to illness and a fierce commitment to "simply power through" any trace of physical frailty was forged in the spirit of my grandfather, a German immigrant who toiled relentlessly to carve out an education and meaningful existence in the New World. He passed this mindset to my father, who then infused it within my sisters and me.

Thus, from a young age, my siblings and I were taught to dismiss any notion of frailty and to stride forward, irrespective of fatigue or discomfort. As a result, my sisters and I are tireless workers, and over the years, this mentality has resulted in my having short patience with people who go "too easy" on themselves when they could be accomplishing more with their lives.

I'm deeply grateful for the work ethic my father imparted to me — a guiding principle that merges with the teachings of Jesus, particularly in John 15:16, where He told His disciples to "go and bring forth fruit." This verse deeply impacted my life so much that one of my foremost prayers every day is that I will be fruitful and productive and yield lasting results. And as I lay in bed each evening when the day draws to a close, I reflect on my day to assess whether or not I've been fruitful and productive. The industrious spirit my father instilled, intertwined with my conviction drawn from Jesus' words in John 15:16, has created in me a commitment to a life brimming with purpose and that leaves no room for idleness.

All of this is good in a measure, but as the years passed from my childhood and young adulthood, I failed for many years to see the need to take a pause or rest along the way. I likened myself to a perpetual engine, tirelessly whirring without the need for downtime. Even the mightiest of industrial machines demand maintenance and periodic rest, yet I stubbornly denied such needs until middle age. Alas, in my late 50s, I faced a physical collapse so profound that rest was no longer a choice, but a necessity. That jarring wake-up proved to be a vital course correction that ultimately prolonged my life and invigorated my productivity. Yet as time marches on, I must honestly admit that the temptation to fill my days to the brim and to push past sensible boundaries is still one I have to overcome.

In all sincerity, I confess that I still grapple with an insatiable desire to test the limits of human potential. The call I have from God is very serious to me. It deeply affects my desire to be fruitful and productive, and it significantly influences the way I navigate life. The fleeting nature of time is very real to me, and this awareness urges me to use every moment to its fullest. And in my desire for peak productivity, I sometimes find myself ensnared by the trap of overextending myself — trying to squeeze an endless array of tasks into an unrealistic time frame.

Although I can maintain a "relentless" pace temporarily, the inevitable consequence is the toll of exhaustion and illness. I must honestly admit that these moments of exhaustion and illness are not a matter of a lack of faith but, rather, of a lapse in practicing balance and common sense.

Since I'm being transparent, let me give you a recent example from a trip to the United States, during which I was slated to speak at a staggering 56 events in 32 days. First of all, the journey from Moscow to our initial stopping point in the U.S. was a marathon in itself, taking us a grueling 56 hours door to door, due to travel restrictions during that period. Rather than taking a day to catch my breath upon arrival, I dove headfirst into the first of my commitments without a pause — a relentless tempo that persisted throughout the entire trip.

It was a Herculean task to fulfill every engagement on the itinerary, and as the days wore on, the strain became more intense and the task more difficult. Nevertheless, each morning I summoned every ounce of my resolve, pulling myself up by my bootstraps, determined that I would joyfully fulfill every obligation. Despite exhaustion that was mounting day by day, I powered through it all until I completed every single commitment I had set out to achieve.

As I embarked on the grueling 56-hour journey back to Moscow, I noticed an all-too-familiar sore feeling in my throat — a familiar sign that I had pushed myself beyond my limits. The reason I saw it as a "familiar" sign is, I have frequently experienced a bout of sickness after a long and unrealistic schedule. Such a bout of sickness had absolutely nothing to do with a failure of God's promises for healing and health but was a sign that I had once again pushed my physical body beyond its limitations.

You see, in my relentless pursuit of productivity and my eagerness to assist as many people as possible in the shortest span of time possible, I still struggle with pushing myself beyond my limits. Time and again, it has left me besieged with a sore throat and a stubborn cold. Again, this is not an issue of a lack of faith; it is an issue of failing to use commonsense.

I still grapple with committing to an overly ambitious schedule, but, thankfully, I'm surrounded with a loving family and caring ministry team who loves me enough to remind me, "You're taking on too much in too short a time. It's time to reel it in and focus on what's feasible." I usually resent it when they tell me this, but later I'm thankful that they stepped in to help me. Now I am finally moving at a pace that is more realistic. But to show you what a realistic pace is to me, let's move on to the next paragraphs where I'll share a little insight from my life.

Every year I aim to write four substantial books, typically ranging from 350 to 850 pages each and some of which are accompanied by companion workbooks, and each year it is my goal to reach this four-book target. Alongside these extensive projects, I churn out a steady stream of content weekly, contributing to various ministry publications. I sit in front of a TV camera and film about 700 different television and media programs annually, and each new TV series we launch is accompanied by many documents that I prepare. From the programs, we also produce comprehensive study guides that follow along with each program.

Monthly, I appear as a guest for numerous online interviews, some sporadically, others regularly, while also participating in key meetings with our top ministry leaders scattered across the globe. I speak at about 50 percent of the church services at our physical Moscow Good News Church, and I play a leading role in our online Moscow Good News Church, a vibrant online community with more than 250,000 regular participants.

Beyond these commitments, my ministry takes me across the world to minister and speak at churches, conferences, and gatherings throughout Russia, Europe, America, and beyond. Between these engagements, I meet with key government and religious figures in Moscow and make it a priority to hit the gym three times a week for exercise. In addition to these responsibilities, I treasure my roles as husband to Denise, father to Paul, Philip, and Joel and their wonderful spouses, and I am a proud grandfather to our eight precious grandchildren.

In the last week of December every year, I sit down to review what I accomplished that year. I encourage you to do this as well. When you write down what you did, or didn't do, it helps you to be honest about your level of productivity. As a part of my review, I list all my accomplishments to gauge whether I've been genuinely effective and fruitful. Simply being busy isn't my aim. It is to produce fruit that remains — to produce teaching people can trust that strengthens the Church and gives glory to God. But as the year draws to a close and I write out my annual assessment, no matter how much I have achieved, I usually find myself lamenting that I hadn't been able to do more, and I try to figure out a way to use my time to be more productive in the upcoming year.

I don't know what you accomplish in a single year, but what you just read above is much more balanced and realistic than what I tried to do in my earlier years. Please do not compare your annual output to mine, as we are all at different stages and different levels of fruitfulness. Second Corinthians 10:12 says it is not wise to measure ourselves by others or to compare ourselves to others.

But it is important that every person finds his own balance — his own pace, including periods of rest — so that he can be fruitful and productive in a way that does not throw off his physical, mental, and spiritual equilibrium. As I said earlier, my temptation is to try to accomplish more in a time frame than is realistic, and when I have failed to resist that temptation, it has repeatedly thrown off my physical, mental, and spiritual equilibrium.

A life lived out of balance not only affects our productivity and our everyday schedules, it also strains our relationships and can take a toll on our physical, mental, and spiritual health. This is why, since the dawn of creation, God emphasized and also modeled the importance of rest. Genesis 2:2-3 says, "And on the seventh day God ended his work which he had made; and he rested on the seventh day from all his work which he had made. And God blessed the seventh day, and sanctified it: because that in it he had rested from all his work which God created and made."

To reaffirm the need for God's people to devote a day to Him in which they can rest, God gave the principle of the Sabbath in the Ten Commandments. In Exodus 20:8-11, God said, "Remember the sabbath day, to keep it holy. Six days shalt thou labour, and do all thy work: but the seventh day is the sabbath of the Lord thy God: in it thou shalt not do any work, thou, nor thy son, nor thy daughter, thy manservant, nor thy maidservant, nor thy cattle, nor thy stranger that is within thy gates: for in six days the Lord made heaven and earth, the sea, and all that in them is, and rested the seventh day: wherefore the Lord blessed the sabbath day, and hallowed it."

Many debate the role of the Sabbath for a New Testament believer, and we will not delve into that discourse in the pages of this book. But what is abundantly clear is that God has ordained a day of rest — a sacred interlude for halting one's routine in order to especially worship the Lord and to rejuvenate one's body, mind, and spirit.

The notion of "rest" is a deeply personal affair, varying from one person to another in the way it is carried out. Recognizing what defines rest for you is essential, and it is just as imperative to refrain from projecting your interpretation onto others. Take, for example, the idea of lounging on a sun-drenched beach, an idyllic retreat for some. But for me, that would be a torturous, misery-making ordeal. For Denise, a visit to the mall is restful, but for me, a venture to the shopping mall is similarly torturous and leaves me exhausted rather than refreshed.

Conversely, immersing myself in the quiet halls of a museum, surrounded by ancient artifacts, breathes life back into me — while Denise might find it an exhausting effort despite her best intentions to accompany me there. Denise and I have divergent definitions of "rest," and we have had to learn how to negotiate our various styles of rest into our combined schedules.

Balance and rest are inherently personal pursuits, so it is vital that you discover what restores equilibrium for you. To perpetually work without some kind of reprieve is self-abuse. To neglect rest is treating yourself like a mechanical machine that neither demands rest nor requires care, but this lifestyle ultimately leads to an inevitable breakdown. I know this all too well, having pushed myself beyond my limits repeatedly over the years.

Today, I have a far more balanced existence, where my life remains both productive and rewarding. If you glanced at my daily and weekly schedule, you might wonder where "rest" fits into the picture. Yet I have discovered a rhythm of work and rest that works for me, and Denise has identified her own rhythm of work and rest, and together, we've crafted a harmonious blend that supports each other. This decision has resulted in the sustenance of our vitality and strength, and it enables us to fulfill the endeavors to which we feel called versus being "diluted" in both our efforts and our fruit because we're spreading ourselves too thin.

**What is abundantly clear is that God has ordained a day of rest — a sacred interlude for halting one's routine in order to especially worship the Lord and to rejuvenate one's body, mind, and spirit.**

Allow me to share a story from the New Testament that highlights the possible perils of an unbalanced lifestyle. This narrative features Epaphroditus, one of the Paul's dearest friends — a faithful minister with steadfast dedication to his calling. But despite Christ's redemptive work on the Cross that provided healing and health, Epaphroditus found himself in the throes of a serious illness. The account in the book of Philippians suggests that his ceaseless and relentless work in the ministry led him to overextend himself, and it ultimately compromised his well-being. Could it be that his tireless devotion and desire to do too much too fast inadvertently opened an "entry point" for the enemy to try to bring him down and take him out?

In Philippians 2:25, Paul wrote about Epaphroditus, saying, "Yet I supposed it necessary to send to you Epaphroditus, my brother, and companion in labour, and fellowsoldier, but your messenger, and he that ministered to my wants." I emphasize this verse, as it unveils the profound importance of this person in Paul's journey — a genuine brother, cherished colleague, steadfast comrade, and devoted minister who commanded Paul's deep respect.

In Philippians 2:26, Paul continued, "For he longed after you all, and was full of heaviness, because that ye had heard that he had been sick."

When Paul discovered that the news of Epaphroditus' illness had reached the ears of the Philippians, he understood that it would pierce their hearts and weigh heavily upon their spirits. The seriousness of Epaphroditus's condition evoked a fear that they might never again witness the warmth of his smile or be graced by the melody of his laughter. Again, the term "sick" finds its roots in the Greek word *astheneia*, which encompasses a broad spectrum of *physical frailties* and *weaknesses*. But as we delve into the following verse, it becomes clear that this malady afflicted him so severely that it had brought him to the very brink of death.

Philippians 2:27 adds, "For indeed he was sick nigh unto death: but God had mercy on him; and not on him only, but on me also, lest I should have sorrow upon sorrow."

In Greek, the word "indeed" serves as an emphatic exclamation to highlight the profound gravity of the situation. Again, the term "sick" is from the Greek word *astheneia*, which embraces a spectrum of *physical frailties* and *weaknesses*. The word "nigh unto" is an interpretation of the Greek term *paraplesion*, which is a compound of the words *para*, meaning *beside*, and *plesion*, which is the Greek equivalent of a *neighbor*. But when compounded, the word *paraplesion* pictures someone who resides in close proximity to a neighbor.

In this case, Epaphroditus was living close to "death." The word "death" is derived from a form of the Greek word *thanatos*, which signifies either *death* or *a death sentence*. As a complete phrase, it means that Epaphroditus "was so sick that he was living right alongside death." He was so sick that he was living as a neighbor to death, and it seems that a death sentence was hanging over his life. Epaphroditus was so perilously close to death that he was practically its next-door neighbor.

But Paul then wrote that "…God had mercy on him…." The word "mercy" is from the Greek word *eleeo*, which depicts *a heart-wrenching emotion that compels one to action.* This tells us that driven by deep compassion, God intervened to bring about Epaphroditus' recovery from a perilous situation. The specifics of his healing — whether through miraculous means, faith and prayer, or a combination of spiritual and medical efforts — is not disclosed in the text. But what is certain is that Epaphroditus lingered under the grim shadow of death for quite some time before finally regaining his health.

The narrative refrains from revealing the precise reason for Epaphroditus' illness, yet Philippians 2:25 paints a picture of him as a steadfast laborer, passionately committed to his ministerial duties. Experts tend to interpret the scriptures where he's mentioned as suggesting that his unwavering dedication, potentially compounded by stress and insufficient rest, might have ushered in the illness that threatened his life. This was not a trivial ailment, but a severe condition that brought him to the brink of death. However, through divine intervention, he was granted recovery and was able to return to resume his essential ministry work.

In this story, we see the example of a devoted servant of God who grappled with physical ailments, even though Christ secured his healing and health on the Cross. It appears that Epaphroditus was stricken with illness brought on by the relentless pressures and stress of his work. By doing too much of a good thing with no pause, it appears that he opened the door to an attack. But he found the path back to health through a mixture of faith, fervent prayer, likely medical aid, and much needed rest.

If you have overdone it for too long and now your health is jeopardized in some way, God's mercy is also present to restore you. If God will do it for me, and if God will do it for Epaphroditus, God will also do it for you. But once you are restored, it is vital that you learn — as hard as it may be to learn it — to find a rhythm of work and rest that is balanced for your life. It is vital that you discover what lifestyle works best to bring equilibrium to your life.

If you ignore this word of caution, sooner or later the devil will discover a way to slip into your life, targeting your body, emotions, or mind with the aim of dragging you down and snuffing you out. Instead, why not adopt a proactive and preventative approach? Cultivate a lifestyle of balance, where you're empowered to achieve much while also ensuring you get the necessary rest along the way. Your body will express its gratitude, your spouse will be appreciative, your friends and other relationships will cherish you more, and you'll enjoy happiness and health throughout your life.

## IN CONCLUSION

In this chapter, we've looked at the roles of diet, exercise, supplements, doctors, medicine, and a balanced life. Each of these subjects is so expansive that they could each command an entire book. My aim here has been to guide you gently through these topics and to encourage you to not only lean on the cornerstone of faith in Christ's redemptive work on the Cross, but also to remember the crucial roles these practical elements play in our lives.

In the next chapter, we will see how to stay strong and healthy as you age, and we'll look at making the choice to consistently live in divine health. While we believe in God's promise of healing and health and to live long and strong, the fact is, aging is a reality that everyone eventually faces. But in the following pages, we'll discover what God says about our golden years, and we'll see examples of biblical characters who lived long and strong to the very end. You will see that this testimony can be yours too!

(Please note there is no QR code for this chapter.)

# QUESTIONS TO PONDER AND DISCUSS

1. Of the main areas covered in this chapter, which one interested you the most — the role of *diet, exercise, supplements, doctors and medicine*, or *a balanced life* — and why? Also, which of these areas resonated with you the most as something you need to change?

2. What short-term steps will you take in the days ahead to begin shoring up any weak areas of your life (e.g., making a new grocery list consisting of healthier food items; scheduling medical checkups you need to make appointments for; considering supplements you need to add to your daily routine; and/or making a new *work, rest, and sleep* schedule)? What are your long-terms goals (e.g., weight-loss if you need to lose weight; fitness goals if you need to tone muscle, increase stamina, or just get back in shape)? What steps can you begin taking now to reach those goals?

3. Do you know someone who is on an unhealthy trajectory because of a poor diet, lack of exercise, etc. and needs a wake-up call in this area to recover himself or herself from future consequences of an unhealthy lifestyle? Would you be willing to pray for this person to have an open mind and heart to receive revelation concerning the potential dangers of his or her present course, as well as what to do about it? If so, what verses of Scripture will you use as you present this person's needs before the Lord?

4. Name two practical things you learned in this chapter — takeaways that you will act on to improve your health and well-being — such as the need for B12 and magnesium in your diet or the need to find your own rhythm of work and rest?

5. Were you surprised to learn that the apostle Paul traveled with Luke the physician? Paul had perhaps more revelation of Christ's redemption of His Church than anyone, including the revelation that Christ secured our healing from every disease, illness, and sickness. Yet a medical doctor, also a

believer, was Paul's near-constant companion. Do you imagine that in all Paul's physical sufferings and perils due to persecution and the hardships of ministry that Dr. Luke never bandaged a wound or practiced his trade in any way to bring relief to the apostle? What does this tell you about utilizing the assistance available to you when you have physical symptoms of sickness or injury *while* you believe for supernatural healing and recovery at the same time?

## THIRTEEN

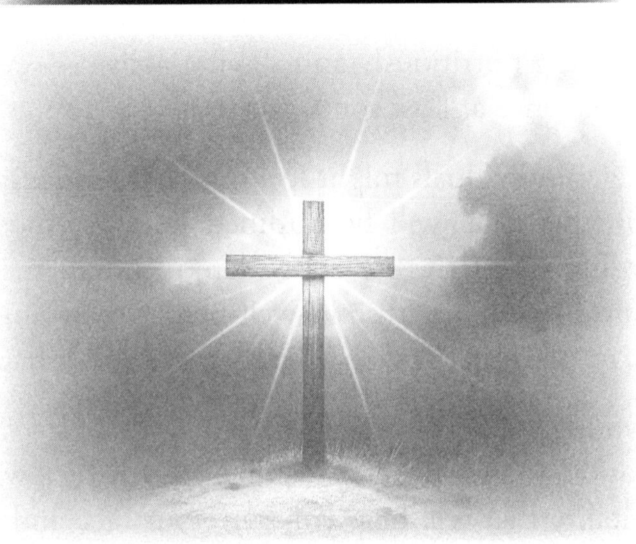

# STAYING STRONG AND HEALTHY AS YOU AGE (MAKING THE CHOICE TO LIVE IN DIVINE HEALTH)

In this chapter, we will focus on staying strong and healthy as we age. Since we're all aging day by day, this chapter is important whether you're in young adulthood, middle age, or of a more mature age. No matter where you are in life, you can glean something concerning God's will for your health and vitality as you grow older.

We have seen over and again that Jesus paid the price for our forgiveness, freedom from guilt and shame, peace of mind, and for the healing and health of our body and mind. However, as we age, it is normal for the human body to begin to show signs of wear, tear, and age. Even if we embrace God's promise of healing and health and His blessing to live long and strong, it doesn't change the fact that aging is a reality everyone faces. No matter how diligently one tends to his well-being — eating nutritiously and staying active — even those that are robust in health experience at least some age-related factors as they get older.

As I said, younger individuals might feel this chapter doesn't apply to them. However, the principles that will be outlined here are most effective when adopted earlier in life. While it's never too late in life to make some positive changes in the care of your health and well-being, there might come a time when a complete, revolutionary overhaul in life is more difficult.

And if you're young when you adopt the principles of stewarding your spiritual, mental, emotional, and physical well-being, you're sowing into a future of strength and vitality that will help you run your race and fulfill your God-appointed course.

So no matter your age or station in life, please take the time to read every word and let this chapter guide you toward making wise choices. These decisions will help you maintain a fit and healthy body as you grow older — but if one does not lay hold of the promises and power of God, a time will come when gravity begins to take its toll as things that once stood firm and sturdy begin to drop, muscle tone begins to relax, and momentum seems to slow a bit. These things eventually come to us all, but they don't have to come prematurely or with full force if we're sowing in the direction of maintaining our strength and vigor for the future.

Some individuals reach their senior years showing few obvious signs of aging, and often it is due to the fact that they have released their faith believing they would not experience the typical effects of wear and tear associated with aging. Others are simply blessed hereditarily with exceptional health. But even if you are in good health and firmly grip the benefits of redemption that include healing and health, the aging process frequently requires a little help along the way.

James said we show our faith by our works (*see* James 2:18), and that principle certainly applies here.

When I say "help along the way," I am referring to many of the things I've already covered in this book — commonsense measures that keep your mind and body, *and your life*, running smoothly as you age with grace. I'm talking about such things as:

- Having regular medical checkups to determine what kind of maintenance is essential for your aging body.
- Taking supplements to rejuvenate or enhance energy levels, in addition to maintaining a lifestyle of a healthy diet, exercise, and adequate rest.
- Making sure you're not neglecting eyecare, dental care, etc., including obtaining any necessary corrective eyewear and hearing assistance — or even undergoing cataract surgery or other procedures to ward off diminished capacity in some area.

None of these things detract from the profound influence of Christ's redemptive work. On the contrary, accepting Christ's redemption can actually enable us to handle the challenges of growing older with elegance and grace. Nevertheless, it's an unmistakable reality that as the years roll on, our bodies might start to display the inevitable traces of time.

Isn't it true that most things that age require attention? For example, consider a brand-new car that operates smoothly at first, but as the miles tick by, it needs care and maintenance to stay in pristine condition. Oil must be changed regularly. If you drive on tires for too long, they become bald and lose their tread, and brakes also need periodic replacement.

Even if your brand-new car came with a manual outlining its operation, and it was purchased with a warranty that guarantees its operation, it doesn't negate the fact that wear, tear, and aging impact its performance.

To keep a car in good shape, routine maintenance is essential. Is it a lack of faith to provide maintenance for your car? You can continue driving without ever changing the oil, brakes, or tires — essentially neglecting all care and maintenance. However, this approach will inevitably result in breakdowns, significant issues, and costly repairs that could have been avoided with proper upkeep. Routine maintenance is not only essential — it is economically a good decision.

Similarly, when you build a new house, it shines brightly when you first settle in, and you delight in the experience of living in your dream home. However, as time passes, even the most magnificent home begins to reveal signs of aging. Keeping a home in excellent condition requires a steady financial investment to ensure everything functions well. This includes replacing carpets, refinishing wood floors, repairing or upgrading furniture, giving the kitchen a fresh update, and enhancing the garden or landscape — the list goes on.

Just as a neglected car will eventually break down if it is not maintained, a house will suffer if one does not give it attention and care. Over time, the air conditioner or heating system may fail, carpets will become worn, and plumbing issues might arise — all due to a prolonged lack of essential maintenance. Avoiding the care required for a home, much like neglecting a car, can lead to serious problems and expensive repairs that could have been prevented with regular upkeep along the way.

But in regard to the aging process, as one grows older, he may notice changes in his hair color, wrinkles forming on his face, and blood vessels bulging more noticeably on his hands. To help the body look and feel its best, it's crucial to take care of it, address any concerns, and occasionally adjust what isn't functioning or appearing as you desire. For those who can afford it, cosmetic surgery can tighten the skin and reduce visible wrinkles. Hair coloring is an option to temporarily cover grey or white hair, and regular exercise or walking can help to maintain mobility and counteract the stiffness that often comes with aging.

Or, on the other hand, you could just nestle into your favorite armchair with a remote control in hand, sitting motionlessly for hours watching TV except to get up and walk to the kitchen or to the bathroom. You could dismiss any desire to move physically because you don't want to put out any exertion. However, just as a car left unattended falls into disrepair and as a house not taken care of falls into decline, the choice to sit and do nothing will eventually lead to a serious deterioration in your health. Neglecting your body's needs results in stiffness, a lack of mobility, elevated blood pressure, persistent aches in your legs and back, and other issues that could have been avoided or remedied by taking an alternative route.

The truth is that just as any physical house demands care and upkeep, so does the body that you inhabit. Let me give you an example. Years ago when we built a fabulous church building in Moscow, those who came to the dedication were speechless at how beautiful and glimmering it was when the doors first opened. But it didn't take too long for wear and tear to begin to show up. To keep that spectacular look, a meticulous maintenance plan was essential. Simply reminiscing about its former glory or wishing for its perpetual splendor would have been a mere fantasy. To keep anything nice and updated requires money and repair.

Today that church building is several decades old, and tens of thousands of people have come through its doors over the years, which brings a lot of wear and tear — but this building nevertheless remains spectacular. Ensuring its upkeep doesn't come cheap, but it remains nice because of a plan devised to keep it in shape. At times this careful plan does require us to spend money on the building that we'd rather not spend. Someone might even argue that to maintain and update this building is too expensive. But it's always expensive to keep good things in good working order.

Neglecting maintenance and watching a building fall into disrepair will lead to even higher repair costs that dwarf any early maintenance or updating expenses. It's far wiser to fix it along the way than to let it fall to pieces and then shell out a fortune for restoration. Any building owner must come to grips with the reality that caring for property is a fundamental aspect of ownership.

## YOUR BODY IS A 'HOUSE' — YOUR PROPERTY AND GOD'S

Your body is a dwelling place or a "house" not only for you, but also for the Holy Spirit (*see* 1 Corinthians 6:19). Just as it takes attention, care, intention, and finances to keep a physical building in good shape, effort is required to keep your body in good condition.

Just as you would devise a meticulous maintenance plan for a car or a physical home or building, you must cultivate a plan for your physical well-being that will account for the normal wear and tear of time and aging. A part of that plan should include good dietary choices, exercise routines, and other essential factors that we will see in the pages ahead.

While aging often brings its own set of health challenges, embracing both practical wisdom and faith can help you overcome many of these hurdles. As you delve into the following pages, you'll discover stories of biblical figures who defied the typical effects of aging, maintaining sharp minds and robust bodies well into their twilight years.

Nevertheless, we must acknowledge that many age-related health concerns can be traced back to earlier lifestyle choices. As I said previously, it's crucial to adopt healthier habits sooner rather than later to avoid unnecessary struggles. And as I've emphasized throughout this book, I harbor no judgment for those who've stumbled along the way, for I've faced my own share of past missteps and have learned to rise above them. I've personally discovered that by embracing the grace of God and allowing the power of the Holy Spirit to help us, we can conquer even the challenges that we inadvertently brought upon ourselves.

I want you to know that your body can be in top-notch condition for years to come, but you must embrace the fact that God has made you the steward of your body, and it is your responsibility to take care of it. If you do, you'll be blessed, but if you fail to do this, you will not experience the healing and health that God wants to be yours even into your senior years.

## CARING FOR YOUR BODY IS A COMMAND OF SCRIPTURE

We saw on pages 145-146 that in First Thessalonians 4:4 Paul wrote, "That every one of you should know how to possess his vessel in sanctification and honour."

This verse is so pivotal to our well-being that I feel compelled to visit it once again. In this verse, the word "vessel" is a metaphor for the *human body*. The Greek word uses the word "vessel" to picture our body as *a finely crafted tool.* Imagine for a moment an assortment of instruments and tools that are stored in your garage — in a space where climate remains more constant and consistent than outside.

But despite this climate-controlled environment, if those instruments and tools lay dormant and are not used, they will nevertheless begin to rust and lose their functionality. Due to a lack of use, an instrument or tool can be rendered unusable — therefore, the secret to keeping an instrument or tool in good working order is to regularly use it.

Paul likened your body to a finely tuned instrument, one that demands both your care and constant use to maintain its symphonic potential. Here's another way to think about it. Instead of imagining your body as a tool in the garage, picture it as a grand piano in a silent, climate-controlled room. Despite the perfect conditions, neglect would lead it to gather dust and lose its resonance.

**I've personally discovered that by embracing the grace of God and allowing the power of the Holy Spirit to help us, we can conquer even the challenges that we inadvertently brought upon ourselves.**

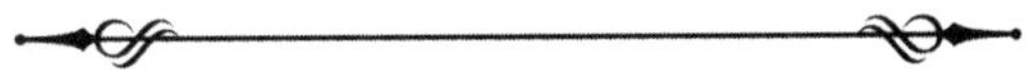

Similarly, while the body doesn't necessarily need climate control, it vitally needs other elements in order to function properly. For example, without movement or nourishment, the body, like this piano, risks falling into disrepair — its once harmonious functions would become discordant and frail. In all of God's creation, the human body stands unrivaled in its brilliance, yet its splendor requires diligent and devout care to remain vibrant. To disregard this necessity is to invite a slow, inevitable descent into deterioration.

You might find yourself less than thrilled by the idea of savoring balanced meals, cutting down on portion sizes, or breaking a sweat with exercise. Yet skipping these habits is like ignoring the mounting interest on a debt that becomes overwhelming in the future. If you don't do it, later you'll be sorry because the price tag of negligence will far outweigh the effort you should have made earlier. When you prioritize your body's care, you are giving yourself a gift for your future. And as the pages of time turn, it becomes increasingly important to nurture and maintain your body's engine to ensure it runs smoothly for years to come.

Let's return again to First Thessalonians 4:4, where Paul said, "That every one of you should know how to possess his vessel in sanctification and honour." The words "every one" are translated from the Greek word *heskatos*, which means *every one of you without exception*. This highlights the universal relevance of Paul's instruction — it is meant for everyone and that means *you* are included.

The word "know" is interpreted from a form of the word *eido*, which means *to be aware* or *to perceive*, and in this verse it conveys the essence of having *a personal awareness*. The word "possess" in this verse is translated from a form of the Greek word *ktaomai*, which suggests *control* or *management*. Hence, the verse means that *every one of you without exception should become aware of how to control and manage his body*.

Thus, the verse conveys that every single person should gain awareness of how to govern and manage his or her own body. With this statement, Paul called each believer to cultivate a personal understanding and mastery over the body entrusted to him or her by God, and this underscores the fact that we have divine stewardship and a responsibility to care for and maintain our mental and physical self.

Paul continued and said we must learn to manage our bodies with "sanctification and honor." In Greek, the word "sanctification" refers to *something set apart by God for sacred purposes*, implying that it is *holy* and *special*. This tells us that in God's view, the body of a believer is holy and special. The Greek word for "honor" conveys the idea of something of *immense worth*. Therefore, Paul was encouraging everyone to develop a personal consciousness in governing and tending to his own body and to recognize that it is holy and special, that God has set it aside for His purposes, and that it is *valuable*.

So I ask you, *are you treating your body as holy, special, and valuable, or are you neglecting it through inadequate care?*

If you're already in your senior years and you acknowledge that you've made mistakes in caring for your body, it's not too late to make a recovery. Christ's redemptive work on the Cross includes your healing and health, even today — and if you will apply from your heart what you read in Chapter Eleven about how to appropriate healing and health, it is entirely possible for you to experience a turnaround in your body.

It's important to never forget that your body is the only one you have in this life, so it's crucial to treat it with respect and as the precious dwelling place of the Holy Spirit. Don't let your body become stiff like a rusty and unusable tool in the garage — or discordant like a piano that has been ignored for too long. If you've made past mistakes, consider this moment a fresh start.

So purpose yourself to utilize what God has given you and maintain it well so your body can serve you for a lifetime. If you do not self-correct, when the enemy exploits these weaknesses in your body, it will be up to you to acknowledge that neglecting your health provided an "entry point" for attacks against your health. *You have a key role to play in staying in shape!*

If you've made mistakes, be honest about it and ask for cleansing and forgiveness. First John 1:9 says, "If we confess our sins, he is faithful and just to forgive us our sins, and to cleanse us from all unrighteousness." According to First John 1:9, if you align yourself with God regarding your past actions or inactions and confess them as sin, you will receive cleansing and forgiveness. From that point on, refrain from looking back and let the Holy Spirit lead you in cultivating a new self-awareness about how to control, manage, and steward your body for God's glory.

## PRAYING EMERGENCY PRAYERS

When we get into trouble or have some kind of emergency — be it turmoil in the family, financial upheavals, health crises, relationship challenges, or any other predicament — when calamity seems to enfold us and emergencies tower like giants, we discover the profound truth that reaching out to God in faith summons His presence and help. And very often when people get into trouble with their health, they turn to God for help. Thankfully, emergency help is promised in Hebrews 4:16, where the Bible says, "Let us therefore come boldly unto the throne of grace, that we may obtain mercy, and find grace to help in time of need."

The words "help in time of need" are a translation of the Greek word *boetheia*, an old word with a military connotation. In the time of the New Testament, this word specifically depicted the urgent cry from a soldier who had fallen, who was besieged, ensnared, or wounded in conflict. When he cried out in a time of need, a fellow soldier who heard his cry for help would swiftly mobilize and move to liberate his fellow warrior. When that nearby soldier heard that cry for "help in time of need," he spared no effort to do whatever was necessary to deliver his fellow soldier and to rescue and bring him back into a place of safety, security, and protection.

In Hebrews 4:16, the word *boetheia* paints a vivid picture of *divine intervention*. It describes how, when we find ourselves in distress and call upon God with unwavering faith for assistance, Jesus — like a Mighty Warrior — swiftly springs into action. With determination, Jesus charges forth to protect and liberate us from our troubles. For those who lift their voices in faith and seek help in time of need, they can rest assured that Christ will spring into action and provide the urgent assistance they require.

God's faithfulness knows no bounds and extends even to those entangled in self-wrought troubles. Consider individuals ensnared by family strife, financial instability, health emergencies, relationship woes, and countless other challenges — predicaments often created by their own actions or inactions.

Yet in His boundless mercy, God responds and moves to liberate them when they call out in faith during their time of need. I have personally experienced such grace, and I am sure you have too. No matter the origins of one's difficulty, Jesus remains the steadfast Shepherd who answers cries for "help in time of need."

I include this in a book about healing and health because Christ also intervenes to mend your mind and body when they are in jeopardy. But stop and think how glorious it will be when God's people experience such robust mental and physical health that they never have a need to pray emergency medical prayers again.

Imagine the glory of God's people thriving so abundantly in mind and body that the need for urgent healing prayers is a rare occasion. Or imagine a Christian leading a life rich in longevity and perpetually sustained by the health and healing that Christ achieved through His sacrifice on the Cross. While it is undoubtedly awe-inspiring when healing comes to those who have faced health challenges, imagine the splendor of a believer who dwells in constant divine wellness and whose life is untouched by any mental or physical ailment.

What holds more wonder? A prayer answered in the face of urgent medical need, or a life so fortified by healing and health that medical emergencies become a foreign concept? Both hold profound power, yet a life flourishing in the healing and health that Christ has secured uniquely magnifies His name!

## THE STRESS OF LIVING IN NONSTOP EMERGENCY SITUATIONS

When life morphs into a relentless cycle of medical turmoil, where each day demands the intervention of a mental or physical miracle just to survive, the result is an existence steeped in despair. Enduring crisis after crisis is an arduous burden. But to illustrate my point, imagine facing turbulent financial waters, where every morning your fervent hope rises, desiring a miraculous reprieve, only to be crushed by the incessant tide of bills at the end of the day. Have you ever found yourself in that position?

If you have, you surely understand how such relentless pressure can turn life into a grim endurance test. Occasionally, these periods are the result of our own choices, but there are also moments when they seem like direct attacks from forces determined to derail you. When divine intervention finally arrives, and an unexpected windfall materializes to temporarily lift you over the looming obstacle you're facing, your heart overflows with gratitude. However, this momentary relief often acts like a "band-aid" — a short-term solution that covers the immediate need but fails to secure your future stability. Once more, you're swept into a vortex of anxiety, pleading for another miraculous intervention to carry you through.

Living amidst the relentless turmoil of perpetual crises is a formidable challenge. Over the years of our ministry, we've navigated the shifting terrains of financial plenty and scarcity. In times of abundance, it's been easier to stay focused on our God-given mission. In darker hours when we've experienced scarcity, we've raised our voices in faith and sought divine intervention. Time after time, we've witnessed the steadfast mercy of God to meet our needs, and it allowed us at last to exhale a sigh of relief.

But the roller coaster of financial stress — marked by relentless ups and downs — is notoriously hard to endure. Often such dilemmas in one's personal life (or, likewise, in an organization) spring from his or her own missteps, be it ill-considered choices or inadequate planning. Yet in moments of divine intervention, when unexpected financial support arrives, hearts swell with gratitude to God and to those He used to help.

In contrast, when individuals, businesses, churches, or ministries live in financial stability — which renders urgent and emergency monetary prayers a rarity rather than a routine — they are able to shift their focus from survival to *growth*. Dwelling in the realm of God's abundant and unfaltering provision brings extraordinary honor to His name and showcases His steadfast faithfulness. *What a testimony!*

Undoubtedly, the stories of God's intervention are wondrous and deserve to be shared, yet the most profound testimony is when one can give witness to God's unwavering faithfulness and constant provision, which transforms life's tumultuous roller coaster of ups and downs into a journey free of stress.

While miracles are awe-inspiring and necessary at times, they are not meant to be a constant lifeline. It is not God's intention for anyone to remain in a perpetual state of tension and emergency. Eventually a time comes when you must move from living in emergency to emergency into a higher state. God does not wish for you to live in this nonstop pressure cooker for the rest of your life.

**When individuals, businesses, churches, or ministries live in financial stability — which renders urgent and emergency monetary prayers a rarity rather than a routine — they are able to shift their focus from survival to *growth*.**

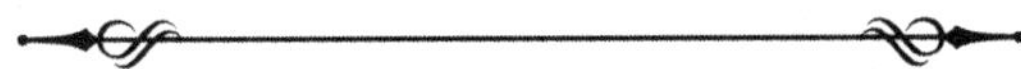

In Psalm 37:25, we read, "I have been young, and now am old; yet have I not seen the righteous forsaken, nor his seed begging bread."

What a powerful testimony! Yet it seems few people today lay claim to it. Such a statement demonstrates God's absolute faithfulness, and it brings honor and glory to His name.

## MANNA IN THE WILDERNESS

During Israel's journey through the barren wilderness, miraculous provision appeared in the form of "manna" — a mysterious gift from the heavens. When the Israelites were in need of God providing emergency food, manna settled like dew upon the earth, and neither its origins nor its supernatural delivery were understood by anyone. Every time the Israelites gathered this sustenance and tasted its mysterious texture, they were indulging in a divine wonder beyond earthly reasoning.

Indeed, in a spectacular display of mercy, God bestowed this otherworldly nourishment upon them as a testament to His care in their dire moments of need. Although other foods existed at their disposal, none could compare to the manna's miraculous essence that fulfilled needs beyond the capabilities of mere earthly fare. This extraordinary sustenance was a marvel that met every requirement, as if it was tailored to their souls.

God lavished manna upon His people, as is recounted in Psalm 78:23-25, where it's written that God "opened the doors of heaven, and had rained down manna upon them to eat."

Determining the exact quantity of manna that cascaded from the heavens during those 40 years is beyond our grasp. But with the consensus among biblical scholars suggesting the Israelites numbered around 3,000,000, it is estimated that they required approximately 4,500 tons of manna daily to be sustained. Imagine a daily harvest of 4,500 tons for every day spanning those 40 years.

This would mean an astounding total of around 65,700,000 tons of manna supernaturally appeared over the course of that epic journey!

Imagine waking up every day to a city blanketed in 4,500 tons of fragrant manna, a miraculous feast gifted freely to anyone willing to step outside and gather it. The alluring scent would drift through the streets and draw people from their homes like moths to a flame. Such an astonishing event would spark an international frenzy — scientists would descend from every corner of the globe to analyze its wonders, while journalists would scramble to capture the essence of this edible enigma. Major news outlets would buzz with excitement, chronicling every detail of this extraordinary phenomenon.

Yet for the children of Israel, this daily spectacle became as routine as the sunrise, a testament to the everyday supernatural miracles they experienced in their exodus journey, with God at the helm. A whole generation of young ones came into the world and grew up with the belief that it was perfectly normal for 4,500 tons of manna to materialize out of thin air each morning (*see* Exodus 16:35).

The manna descended with such clockwork precision and unwavering consistency that eventually, the Israelites scarcely marveled at its arrival. In a gradual fade from wonder to familiarity, the miraculous became mundane, its divine splendor blending seamlessly into their everyday existence. The extraordinary nature of this heavenly sustenance slipped into obscurity, and it began to be seen as a normal, regular occurrence.

And when the next generation entered the Promised Land, the daily manifestation of manna ended. For 40 years, God had intervened and met their emergency need, but a time came when the provision stopped. Joshua 5:12 tells us, "And the manna ceased…neither had the children of Israel manna any more; but they did eat of the fruit of the land of Canaan that year."

In time, the wondrous supply of manna ceased, and God beckoned His children to embrace a more elevated way of life. God stopped feeding them hand-to-mouth and required them to use their faith to conquer the Promised Land and take the fruit for themselves. I've shared this to remind you that while God stands ready to greet you repeatedly with miracles of healing and health,

His ultimate desire is for you to step into a realm of divine wellness — where you enjoy a vigorous and enduring life brimming with vitality. Overcoming physical and mental challenges, and fully living in a state of incessant divine health, is a magnificent testament to God's glory!

Indeed, instead of navigating from one health crisis to another and crying emergency prayers for God to intervene time and again, God desires for you to conquer illness and embrace a state of divine wellness, where vitality and healing predominently prevail over sickness. However, much like the Israelites, this transition will demand a shift in your mindset. Beyond resting on the bedrock of God's promises, you must take concrete steps and adhere to them with dedication so you can enter a sustained realm of divine health in your life.

## PREVENTION AND MAINTENANCE ARE TWO KEYS TO ENSURING GOOD HEALTH FOR THE LONG HAUL

As of the time of this writing, the latest statistics reveal that the United States alone currently spends over $4.9 trillion each year on health care.[1] A significant portion of this comes from the federal government, which invests more than $1.9 trillion annually in various health programs.[2] In fact, *for every four dollars the federal government spends, more than one is dedicated to health-related expenses.*

During a conversation about these statistics with a prominent physician in the U.S., I was stunned when he said, "It's astonishing when you realize how many of our health problems can be traced back to poor diet, obesity, lack of exercise, chronic stress, and unresolved emotional struggles. While medicine is vital and often lifesaving, much of what it does is manage the complications of conditions that could have been prevented."

He went on to say, "If people embraced a healthier way of living — consuming nourishing food, engaging in regular physical activity, getting good rest, managing stress effectively, and even letting go of grudges and practicing forgiveness — many illnesses would be reduced dramatically. We could not only ease the suffering of individuals, but also relieve much of the financial strain that burdens families and the nation alike."

This is why in addition to renewing your mind to the biblical truth that Christ purchased healing and health for you in His redemptive work, if you wish to move into a lifestyle of consistent divine health, you will also need to do some natural things that contribute to a state of prolonged health and longevity. Trust me, it's almost never too late to begin this journey — I've embarked on much of it myself in my later 50s and 60s. Starting later is far better than never beginning, and I chose to embrace tangible steps to honor and care for the "temple" the Lord has given me.

As I have mentioned throughout this book, in my late 50s, my family, driven by love and concern, staged a heartfelt confrontation with me regarding my escalating weight and declining health. Over time, I had gradually ballooned to 320 pounds, and my mobility was slipping away. The signs were all too visible, yet accepting this reality was a bitter pill to swallow. Nevertheless, my loved ones made it abundantly clear that failing to shed the excess pounds and alter my lifestyle would undoubtedly hasten my journey to an early grave. With their invaluable support, along with that of a dedicated doctor, a compassionate counselor, and a relentless physical trainer, I embarked on a transformative journey to reclaim my life.

Facing the challenge of my limited mobility due to excess weight, I decided it was time to embark on a journey of change. Slowly but surely, I began shedding pounds, which gradually opened the door to engaging in light physical activities. As the scale tipped downward, it empowered me to integrate more exercise into my daily routine, driving me toward the goal of revitalizing my mobility. Acknowledging my fear of injury, my physical trainer approached our sessions with remarkable patience and kindness. Step by cautious step and over time, I found myself embracing an increasingly active lifestyle.

Forgive me for being redundant, but I find myself compelled to share this once again to emphasize the crucial truth that it's almost never too late for transformation. In my own case, doctrinally I was aware that healing and health was mine, thanks to Jesus' sacrifice on the Cross. However, I sabotaged my own well-being by neglecting self-care. Despite my understanding that Jesus died for my forgiveness, freedom from guilt and shame, peace of mind, and healing and health, I had unwittingly compromised my health.

So in my late 50s, I embarked on a journey of change that has since become a continuous quest for improvement. I've dedicated myself to doing everything possible to nurture my mental and physical well-being so that I may enjoy a long and strong life and fulfill all of the will of God for my life. Now as I age, if I am at home and not traveling, I go to the gym three times a week and work with a physical trainer to continually work on my mobility.

Through my journey, I've also discovered that even those in peak mental and physical condition often find their stores of essential vitamins and nutrients dwindling with age. Thankfully, these vital elements can be easily replenished through the use of supplements with a professional's oversight.

Moreover, I've learned that maintaining a balanced diet, staying active, and addressing underlying stressors and worries can significantly reduce or even mend the damage done to our bodies. Previous chapters in this book highlighted how poor dietary choices can wreak havoc on your health. However, many issues could be rectified with a thoughtful approach to eating. And regular physical activity not only alleviates stiffness, but also keeps our bodies flexible and agile.

Each year, besides committing to a balanced lifestyle of exercise and healthy eating, I also dedicate time to a comprehensive health evaluation, ensuring that my body — this instrument that God gave me — stays in prime condition. Opting for a doctor's visit doesn't signify a deficiency in faith — *quite the opposite*. I approach these annual physicals brimming with confidence and trusting in a favorable outcome. After my latest examination, the doctor couldn't help but chuckle in astonishment. "I wish my medical report looked like yours!" he exclaimed. Intrigued, he asked, "How are you maintaining such health at your age?" My response was straightforward, "I follow promises of healing and health found in God's Word, and I'm committed to nourishing my body with wholesome food and with regular exercise."

Beyond our annual visits for thorough health assessments, my wife and I ensure we're regulars in the dentist's chair to keep our smiles vibrant and robust. We believe that a smile is a cherished gift we bestow upon the world, so we're committed to maintaining our oral health — like polishing a precious gem. If a tooth needs attention, we don't procrastinate, swiftly handling repairs, as our whole body is part of our sacred duty to maintain and cherish. We also seek out chiropractic adjustments when necessary, ensuring everything stays aligned and harmonious.

Not long ago, I went for my annual eye checkup, and when my eye doctor pointed out the unwelcome arrival of cataracts, I didn't hesitate to book the surgery needed to clear my vision — taking action like a meticulous homeowner addressing wear and tear. Again, just as you would tend to your car or house, you need to intentionally care for and nurture your body. If a window is dirty, you clean it, so when the doctor told me I had cataracts, I knew it was time to take action to have them removed. Just as I would use my faith for healing, I used my faith to believe the surgeon would perfectly remove the cataract and my vision would be improved.

Whether *inside* the doctor's office or *outside* the doctor's office, we need to be spiritually engaging our faith. While I hold a steadfast belief in divine healing and health, I also understand the importance of proactive attention, ensuring that my body receives the necessary care and fine-tuning it deserves throughout life's journey.

Many people feel a pang of apprehension when it comes to visiting the doctor, even for routine checkups. Yet consider how diligently a responsible car owner visits the mechanic for a tune-up, an oil change, or a tire replacement. Ignoring these services is a sure-fire way to meet with costly and avoidable car troubles. Regular maintenance checks not only preserves the car's health, but also delivers peace of mind and ensures everything runs smoothly.

Similarly, making time for a yearly medical checkup or consultation can offer valuable insights into one's health, allowing adjustments and interventions where necessary. This proactive approach replaces anxiety with assurance. Unfortunately, some people's lives have been cut short — not from a lack of opportunity to enhance well-being, but from neglecting that opportunity.

But beyond merely fine-tuning your physical self, it's also essential to harness the power of your mind to maintain sharpness. As you'll discover in the following pages, the latest research defies common assumptions and reveals that the golden years of mental productivity are, in fact, between the ages of 60 and 80. I urge you to avoid jesting about growing older — about forgetfulness, Alzheimer's, dementia, aches and pains, poor movement or mobility, and low motivation, etc. These topics aren't humorous and can be detrimental to your mental and physical health. Keep in mind that your words hold power — use them wisely to affirm that your mind and body are vibrant, sharp, and agile as ever.

As the years have passed, I've noticed a remarkable blossoming of my mental prowess, aligning perfectly with the latest findings on aging. My cognitive foundation has expanded so vastly that I now reach conclusions with unprecedented speed and confident certainty. In fact, my mind has become so finely honed that my productivity has reached unparalleled heights. I write more books in a year than most people could dream of reading in the same time frame.

Just as a vintage wine deepens in flavor as it ages, my intellect has ripened and flourished with the passage of time. This isn't boasting — it's a celebration of God's work in my life. I believe it reflects God's ultimate desire for us to flourish both mentally and physically throughout our lives. After all, how does it glorify God if we fade into cognitive decline? Instead, by maintaining our mental acuity until the very end, we inspire others to hope for a life of continued purpose and productivity.

Psalm 92:13-14 says, "Those that be planted in the house of the Lord shall flourish in the courts of our God. They shall still bring forth fruit in old age;

they shall be fat [healthy; vital] and flourishing." This is God's will for our lives *till the very end* of our lives!

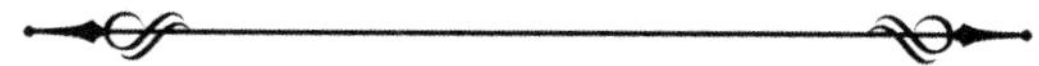

**Some people's lives have been cut short — not from a lack of opportunity to enhance well-being, but from neglecting that opportunity.**

## HOW'S YOUR SOCIAL LIFE?

A remarkable discovery has emerged in recent years that has shed light on one of the key catalysts for living a prolonged life and maintaining robust mental well-being. Amidst a plethora of factors — such as diet, exercise, climate, sleep, and stress reduction — social interaction shines as a cornerstone in the pursuit of longevity and health.[3] Essentially, human beings crave companionship, and those who regularly nurture social ties are statistically inclined to enjoy longer and healthier lives.

Among decades of study, evidence consistently points to social connectedness as essential for enhanced physiological function and diminished risks of physical ailments. This need for social engagement is so intrinsic that since the early 1900s, research has indicated a deficit in social bonds can amplify the likelihood of mortality by more than 50 percent.[4] Moreover, more recent studies have indicated that isolation is a significant risk factor to a myriad of health challenges, including depression and the deterioration of mental acuity.[5]

This underscores the vital importance of nurturing connections with others, especially as we journey through the later stages of life. Isolation is a silent thief, often robbing individuals of their mental and physical well-being. It presents an invaluable opportunity for families and faith communities to embrace and support the elderly, fostering an environment where they can thrive in meaningful relationships. I witnessed this firsthand with my own mother, who passed away during the COVID-19 pandemic after enduring prolonged isolation. She was in a rehabilitation facility that did not allow any visitors for a prolonged period of time, and she experienced a loneliness that I believe hastened her passing.

Understand that especially for those in their golden years, it is crucial to take an active role in maintaining social ties. Whether it's reaching out with a phone call, stopping by for a visit, or simply staying in touch, these interactions not only provide you a chance to share your lifetime of wisdom and care for others, but they also fortify your own well-being and longevity. This is another reason why involvement in a church or small group is so vital as one ages. The assembly of the saints is as important for the older saints as it is for younger saints. Science shows that, regardless of age, social interaction strengthens one's health and prolongs life.

So I pose this question: How deeply are you woven into the fabric of others' lives? Are you engaging with your church community? Are you actively participating in fellowship, or are you at risk of drifting into solitude, a state that might pave the way to an untimely end? To enjoy a vibrant and long life, nurturing strong social bonds is essential.

As time marches on, no matter how diligently you adhere to the rules of healthy living, you may one day find yourself gazing into the mirror, observing the inevitable arrival of wrinkles or the shifting hues and thinning of your hair. But rather than resign yourself to dwelling on the passage of time and its physical manifestations, why not embrace a daring leap of faith to strive for greater deeds as the years advance?

Take Caleb as your example. As you will see in the pages before you, at the venerable age of 85, Caleb was imbued with such vigor in both mind and body that he sought one of the most formidable endeavors of his life. Instead of succumbing to thoughts of weariness and age with a resigned, "I'm too old for this," he chose to shine brightly until the very end. If Caleb, a figure from the Old Testament era, could do this without the indwelling presence of the Holy Spirit, then surely, as a New Testament believer blessed with the Holy Spirit residing within, you possess the power to do at least the same.

So when fatigue begins to creep in and whispers to you about your age or your deficits, don't succumb to the murmurings of time. Instead, embrace the powerful message found in Romans 8:11 that says, "But if the Spirit of him that raised up Jesus from the dead dwell in you, he that raised up Christ from the dead shall also quicken your mortal bodies by his Spirit that dwelleth in you." Since the power of the resurrection resides inside you, why not ask the Holy Spirit to infuse your being with supernatural energy and empower you to transcend the limitations of wear, tear, and age. He will quicken your mortal body and you'll be able to outdo and outwork even those who are younger than you.

It's worth highlighting that as we grow older, ensuring a good night's sleep becomes increasingly crucial as well. Those who burn the midnight oil often face physical setbacks. This is because during the stages of deep sleep, several key processes are hard at work —- our brains are flushing out toxins, muscles and tissues are being repaired, and our immune system is recharging and powering up.[6]

Although the liver is constantly working as a detoxifier, it works most efficiently during sleep, so consistently staying up late or cutting sleep time disrupts the body's circadian rhythm, metabolism, and hormone regulation, notably insulin.[7] Thus, sinking into sufficient and consistent slumber is essential as time passes. Many find that the days of surviving on merely 4-6 hours of sleep per night are long gone, realizing that to preserve their health, they need the restorative benefits of 7-8 hours instead.

And besides these concrete, natural steps you must take to ensure the maintenance and upkeep of your mind, body, and health, remember to keep your mouth filled with God's Word and to let your tongue be the rudder that guides your life all the way to a gloriously victorious conclusion.

## MENTAL DECLINE AND ALZHEIMER'S

If you are younger, please pay heed to what you are about to read and respond wisely by taking precautionary measures after reading this material. Although many cases of Alzheimer's disease have traditionally been linked to genetic or hereditary factors, there is growing evidence linking insulin resistance and poor metabolic health with Alzheimer's, leading some researchers to call it Type 3 diabetes.[8]

This suggests that lifestyle choices made earlier in life could have potentially diverted or altered for some the course of this cognitive affliction. (Of course, while it's clear that lifestyle factors strongly influence risk, we know that Alzheimer's is multifactorial in its cause, and not all cases are naturally preventable.)

For years, countless individuals consume nutrient-poor diets without any immediate indication of their detrimental impact on brain health. Much like an assassin lurking in the shadows, poor eating habits stealthily compromise the brain's ability to metabolize insulin. Over time, this insidious process erodes neuronal function, impairing vital cognitive abilities, such as learning and memory. Thus, it is possible that one key to altering the trajectory of Alzheimer's may lie in reshaping our nutritional choices before the silent damage takes hold.

Growing evidence suggests that the brain's insulin imbalance also plays a role in various types of dementia,[9] which manifests as memory lapses and a deterioration in cognitive function among the elderly. When someone experiences insulin resistance, it impairs how the brain cells utilize glucose, leading to alterations in amyloid-beta and tau proteins linked to dementia's onset.[10]

Although Alzheimer's and dementia are influenced by a multitude of factors beyond our control, naturally speaking, there are certain elements within our grasp that we can modify. These include our diet, blood pressure, body weight, and stress levels.[11] Scientific evidence highlights the benefits of consuming nutritious foods, engaging in regular physical activity, keeping blood pressure in check, and stimulating the mind to help prevent Alzheimer's and various types of dementia.

While a definitive cure for Alzheimer's remains elusive, these strategies can influence the advancement of the disease and also mitigate insulin resistance. Proper insulin levels crucially regulate blood sugar by facilitating glucose entry into cells, influencing metabolism, nerve cell health, neuronal communication, and other cognitive functions. Fundamentally, it suggests that in many instances, Alzheimer's and dementia are conditions we sometimes bring upon ourselves, and it raises the possibility that this grave issue might be averted through good lifestyle habits earlier in life.

It is interesting that in Russia (where my family has lived for decades), people have an innate culture of walking everywhere. For example, it's not uncommon for apartment buildings to lack elevators, compelling people to take the stairs. And because the older population does not drive, they walk long distances nearly everywhere they go. This lifestyle naturally encourages the use of one's legs as a primary mode of transportation, keeping the population physically engaged.

Our Moscow-based ministry has one of the largest ministries to senior adults in the world — a ministry that has impacted hundreds of thousands of elderly individuals. In our work with senior adults over many decades, we've never encountered a diagnosed instance of Alzheimer's among them. When I shared this with a renowned doctor from the United States, it left him astonished, but he said, "It stands to reason given their nutritious diets and active lifestyles."

I am not insinuating that all dementia or Alzheimer's cases are dietary related, but it is astonishing how deeply foundational habits like mindful eating and consistent exercise can transform our well-being. It's equally astonishing the grace of God and our ability to change the course of our future no matter where we are on the path of life. And if you have eaten poorly or are concerned that you've been a contributor to someone else eating poorly — and now he or she is facing mental issues that may be related to past dietary and other lifestyle habits — remember that God's power is more than enough to undo whatever has been done.

God's power is more than capable of undoing the consequences of our past mistakes! The redemptive work of Jesus on the Cross offers redemption not just for sins, but also for the mistakes we've previously made. Instead of shouldering the blame for the physical or mental challenges that arise, it's time to unleash your faith in Christ's healing power to work miracles for anyone who is ill-affected. Jesus is Lord over every condition, and that includes dementia and Alzheimer's.

But all this highlights the importance of nourishing your body with wholesome foods, staying active, keeping your blood pressure in check, committing to a healthy body weight, and staying socially connected to others as you age. By embracing a practical and mindful approach to your well-being, evidence strongly shows that many health problems can be prevented, delayed or better managed.

## FAITH OVERCOMES THE WORLD

We've discovered that by leading a life of balance, embracing common sense, and nurturing our faith, we can defy many of the burdens imposed by life's inevitable challenges, such as aging and gravity's pull.

As stated earlier, the path to longevity is paved with good habits, such as nourishing our bodies with healthy foods, engaging in regular exercise, staying active, keeping our minds vigilant, building strong connections with others, and embracing faith as a catalyst for personal growth.

When we feel our body speaking limitations to us, instead of resigning ourselves to the idea that "I'm too old to embark on new ventures," we should fill our heart and mind with the promises of God's Word concerning health and longevity. We must keep our mouths filled with God's Word and let our tongue be the rudder that guides our lives all the way to a glorious and victorious conclusion.

Remember that First John 5:4 says, "For whatsoever is born of God overcometh the world: and this is the victory that overcometh the world, even our faith."

Notice that the word "overcometh" appears *twice* in this verse, but actually it's reapeated *three* times because the word "victory" is the same word in Greek. In each instance, the word is from a form of the Greek word *nikao*, which means *to conquer*, *overcome*, or *prevail*, and it also denotes *victory*.

The word "world" is translated from the Greek word *kosmos*, and it denotes *the world and everything in it*. This verse speaks the profound truth that those who are born of God possess an intrinsic power to triumph over the world. Deep within each believer lies an unstoppable, victorious spirit that empowers them to rise above challenges and claim victory — and this mighty force is none other than our faith!

So instead of giving up and retreating to the background when the burdens of time weigh heavily upon us, we must unleash the strength of our faith to triumph and persevere until our life's final moments. In the upcoming pages of this chapter, I will share inspiring biblical stories of individuals who defied the boundaries of age, refused to yield to their advancing years, and lived lives of victory and resilience to the very end.

But this also reminds me of a more contemporary, personal story of a very dear friend in her senior years who injured her back and consequently found herself immobile for many months. Her back was so injured that the doctor forbade her to move without assistance, and when she did attempt to walk, it was with the help of a walker. But the doctor had no idea how ferocious and tenacious her faith was. One day when a therapist came to her home to help her get up, the therapist told her, "Now we don't want you to actually try to walk... just take it easy...realize that this slower pace is what you're probably going to live with for the rest of your life."

But my remarkable friend, with her unwavering conviction, replied, "I refuse to accept a future where my days are spent on my back in a recliner or shuffling with a walker. I'm going to be up and moving freely and normally because God has a plan for me that is not finished. His plan does not include me living the rest of my life lying in a chair and walking with a walker."

It wasn't long until my friend was out of that chair, the walker was gone, and she was driving her car as if she never had an injury to her back. While medical care and therapy were instrumental for a short season, had she succumbed to her condition and prognosis, she might have found herself permanently relegated to that chair.

However, fueled by a fierce determination to be active and mobile, she chose a different path. Refusing to let that injury define her life or to heed the discouraging words of her therapist, she resolved to rise above it. She is an example to me personally of the commitment we must each make as we get older not to just give in to the aches and pains of life.

We must choose to use our faith to get up, get moving, and live overcoming and productive lives to the very conclusion of our lives — *long and strong*!

## PROMISES OF STRONG HEALTH AND LONGEVITY IN OLDER AGE

Typically, middle age is seen as the period stretching from the early 40s to the mid-60s. In many nations, reaching 64 years old has traditionally marked one's entry into senior citizenship. In the United States, the government has designated age 65 as the official threshold for senior status. According to the 2020 census, more than 55 million Americans, accounting for almost 17 percent of the population, have crossed this milestone and are now considered elders in the eyes of the nation.[12]

Surprisingly, those between the years of 65 to 69 are more frequently employed than the teenage crowd. An impressive 32 percent of individuals beyond the traditional retirement threshold maintain jobs and reap various benefits in the process. Often in retirement, people begin to sit around not knowing how to fill the hours and face a diminished sense of purpose. Many times, their health deteriorates and declines so quickly that they pass from this life soon after retirement. Thus, having a job provides people a purpose for living.

- The average life expectancy in the United States for women is 80.2 years.
- The average life expectancy in the United States for men is 74.8 years.
- An unexpected twist in the American narrative is the remarkable surge in centenarians. Over the past 30 years, the count of citizens aged 100 or more has almost tripled.
- It is projected that by 2050, no fewer than 400,000 Americans will be celebrating their century-old status.
- Presently, the world is home to an estimated 722,000 centenarians (people 100 years or older).
- By 2054, the worldwide centenarian population will reach nearly 4 million.
- If Jesus doesn't return before 2100, this number is predicted to increase to more than 25 million.[13]

All this underscores the undeniable truth that our lifespans are stretching further than ever. Yet this shouldn't catch us off guard, for the Bible eloquently speaks of extended years for those who fulfill certain conditions.

Unfortunately, some nurtured in conventional churches were mistakenly taught that God's promise of life was capped at merely 70 or 80 years of age, and they base that thinking on Psalm 90:10, which says, "The days of our years are threescore years and ten; and if by reason of strength they be fourscore years, yet is their strength labour and sorrow; for it is soon cut off, and we fly away."

At face value, this verse does appear to say that a person's lifespan is between 70 (threescore and ten years) and 80 (fourscore years). However, we must consider the audience for whom this passage was originally intended. Psalm 90:10 was written to the children of Israel, who rebelled and lost their privilege to enter the Promised Land, and who were thereby destined to wander the rest of their lives in the wilderness.

Rather than let this disgruntled generation wander in misery for decades on end, God placed a limit on their years, declaring essentially, "This particular rebellious generation will live no more than 70 to 80 years because I do not want them to wander in misery for years on end."

Thus, the lifespan of 70 to 80 years mentioned in this verse was a boundary set by God's compassion for one specific generation, and it was not a universal decree that applies to all His people for all time. In fact, when the next generation of Israelites, who honored and adhered to God's laws, finally made their home in the Promised Land, many of them lived well beyond the 70- to 80-year lifespan referenced in Psalm 90:10. This scenario emphasizes the importance of knowing who God is speaking to in Scripture and why He is saying what He is saying.

## LONG LIFE FOR THOSE WHO LOVE AND OBEY THE LORD

The fact is, the Bible is filled with promises of a long, vibrant life for those who walk with the Lord. Longevity is His blessing to the obedient and faithful. Consider this promise in Psalm 91:16: "With long life will I satisfy him, and shew him my salvation."

The word "long" in this verse is translated from a Hebrew word that speaks of length, and it implies *longevity* or *a life that stretches generously over time*. The word "life" denotes *days*, and as a phrase, the words "long life" depict *long days* or *a very long life*.

In Hebrew, the word "satisfy" means *to have enough, to have plenty of,* or *to be fully satisfied.* If you want a verse to claim longevity, Psalm 91:16 is your verse because it guarantees long life to those who abide in the shadow of the Almighty (*see* Psalm 91:1), and it is God's promise that you can live until you reach *the point of satisfaction.* This Hebrew word could describe how a person feels after eating a big meal and is "full" and "satisfied" as a result. This tells us that God wants us to live a life that is *full* and that leaves us *satisfied.*

Although some may think this is a fairytale, it is not. This is God's own Word and what He promises in Psalm 91:16. If you're struggling to believe it, you are thinking wrongly, and you need to renew your mind to the truth. It's time you raise your level of faith to align with God's Word and His will, and begin to declare that you will aim for the maximum number of years and live until you are fully satisfied. God desires for you to bask in every drop of His goodness throughout your life's journey, and His wish is to showcase you as a testament to His boundless power and grace.

In fact, Psalm 91:16 goes further to tell us what God wishes for our lives. He wants us to know and to experience the fullness of His salvation. The verse says, "With long life will I satisfy him, and shew him my salvation." The word "salvation" is translated from a Hebrew word that means *deliverance, healing, prosperity, wholeness, and everything else that is packed into salvation.*

And notice that God wants to "show" us His salvation. The word "show" means more than to see from a distance. It means *to see and to personally experience.* It means that in context of longevity, God wants to us to live until we are satisfied to move on, and He wants us to see and personally experience *deliverance, healing, prosperity, wholeness, and everything that is packed into salvation* all the way to the end of our life!

The use of the word "show" in this verse is the equivalent of God saying, "I wish to display the wonders of My salvation to you as you grow older." Here the word "salvation" refers to the entirety of God's blessings — an outpouring of health, clarity of mind, prosperity, and success. God intends for you to savor every facet of His goodness throughout your lifetime — His desire is to make you a trophy of His grace and His power!

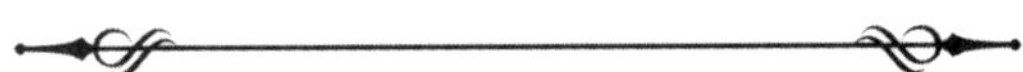

**God desires for you to bask in every drop of His goodness throughout your life's journey, and His wish is to showcase you as a testament to His boundless power and grace.**

God does not wish for His children to exit this world in a state of brokenness or illness. He promises that (if we fulfill His instructions) our days can be marked by resilience and vitality. Can you think of a more profound way to glorify God than to walk to the end of your life with strength and wellness and to bring honor to God until your very last breath?

## A LIST OF GOD'S PROMISES GUARANTEEING LONGEVITY

The blessing of longevity is promised throughout the Scriptures. Countless verses celebrate God's gift of longevity — far more than we could possibly delve into within the confines of this chapter. However, to truly embrace this truth, I invite you to immerse yourself in the following 20 biblical promises.

As you reflect upon these passages, allow the Holy Spirit to transform your understanding and reveal God's yearning to bestow upon the obedient a life that is rich, fulfilling, and long.

In **Exodus 20:12**, we find a powerful promise connected to the fifth of the Ten Commandments. That verse says, "Honour thy father and thy mother: that *thy days may be long* upon the land which the Lord thy God giveth thee."

It may sound simple, but this verse means honoring our parents comes with a reward. God promises those who honor their father and mother will enjoy a longer life.

**Deuteronomy 4:40** says, "Thou shalt keep therefore his statutes, and his commandments, which I command thee this day, that it may go well with thee, and with thy children after thee, *and that thou mayest prolong thy days upon the earth*, which the Lord thy God giveth thee, for ever."

This verse categorically means if we obey God's Word, our lives are going to go well — things will go well with us — and our obedience will benefit our children and grandchildren. Living a life of obedience will "prolong your days upon the earth"!

**Deuteronomy 5:16** says, "Honour thy father and thy mother, as the Lord thy God hath commanded thee; *that thy days may be prolonged*, and that it may go well with thee, in the land which the Lord thy God giveth thee."

In this verse, we discover once more that bestowing honor and respect upon our parents not only brings harmony and prosperity into our lives but also sows the seeds for longevity.

**Deuteronomy 5:33** also says, "Ye shall walk in all the ways which the Lord your God hath commanded you, that ye may live, and that it may be well with you, and that *ye may prolong your days* in the land which ye shall possess."

This passage underscores that by following God's ways and adhering to His commandments, including the New Testament commandment of walking in love, we unlock the promise of a life richly blessed and extended with longevity.

**Deuteronomy 6:1-2** then adds, "Now these are the commandments, the statutes, and the judgments, which the Lord your God commanded to teach you, that ye might do them in the land whither ye go to possess it: that thou mightest fear the Lord thy God, to keep all his statutes and his commandments, which I command thee, thou, and thy son, and thy son's son, all the days of thy life; and that *thy days may be prolonged*."

This verse promises that if we walk in the ways of the Lord, our lives will flourish, and our days will be lengthened. This is a promise for anyone who lives with a reverential fear of God and who lives in obedience to His commands.

In **Deuteronomy 30:19-20** we read that Moses called upon the people to make a choice between life and death. If they chose to live in obedience to God's Word, He promised that they would experience blessings in life, including longevity. Moses wrote, "I call heaven and earth to record this day against you, that I have set before you life and death, blessing and cursing: therefore choose life, that both thou and thy seed may live: That thou mayest love the Lord thy God, and that thou mayest obey his voice, and that thou mayest cleave unto him: for he is thy life, *and the length of thy days....*"

Here we find that God prolongs life for those who choose to walk in His ways and keep His commandments.

**Deuteronomy 4:40** says, "Thou shalt keep therefore his statutes, and his commandments, which I command thee this day, that it may go well with thee, and with thy children after thee, *and that thou mayest prolong thy days upon the earth,* which the Lord thy God giveth thee, for ever."

By embracing and adhering to the statutes and commandments of God, prosperity is promised to us and to our descendants. By following God's statutes and commandments, not only do we set the stage for a flourishing life, but we also extend our days upon the earth with God's gift of longevity.

**First Kings 3:14** says, "And if thou wilt walk in my ways, to keep my statutes and my commandments, as thy father David did walk, *then I will lengthen thy days.*"

This passage beautifully reminds us that a life devoted to following God's way is rewarded with the blessing of longevity.

**First Kings 3:24** says, again, that God promises peaceful and long life to those who hear, receive, and obey His commands. It says, "And if thou wilt walk in my ways, to keep my statutes and my commandments, as thy father David did walk, *then I will lengthen thy days*."

This scripture also echoes God's assurance of peace and extended years for those who embrace, heed, and follow His decrees. This passage serves as a reminder that a life dedicated to walking in alignment with God's guidance is graced with the gift of a fulfilled and prolonged life.

**Job 5:26** says a long life is promised to the obedient. It says, "Thou shalt come to thy grave in a *full age*, like as a shock of corn cometh in his season."

This verse means you will die mature and old and that you will live fully and vibrantly until your final days. Here we find it is God's blessing to the obedient when they live to a full, mature age and reach their greatest fruitfulness at the end of their lives. God's intention is for us to arrive at the twilight of our lives, not broken and sick, but at the pinnacle of productivity.

**Psalm 92:13-14** says, "Those that be planted in the house of the Lord shall flourish in the courts of our God. They shall still bring forth fruit in *old age*; they shall be fat and flourishing."

In other words, if you live in the house of God, even as you age, your life will continue to bear abundant fruit and remain vibrant and vigorous. God promises you a long life that is fruit-producing to the very end.

**Psalm 103:2-5** says, "Bless the Lord, O my soul, and forget not all his benefits: who forgiveth all thine iniquities; who healeth all thy diseases; who redeemeth thy life from destruction; who crowneth thee with lovingkindness and tender mercies; who satisfieth thy mouth with good things; *so that thy youth is renewed like the eagle's*."

The words "youth is renewed like the eagles" alludes to the majestic renewal of an eagle's vigor as it ages. This imagery beautifully illustrates one of God's blessings bestowed upon the faithful — a rejuvenated spirit and enduring vitality that persists even into one's twilight years.

The book of Proverbs has many verses with a promise of longevity for those who walk in obedience to God's commands.

**Proverbs 3:1-2:** "My son, forget not my law; but let thine heart keep my commandments: *for length of days, and long life*, and peace, shall they add to thee."

This is another promise of longevity. But this verse says length of days, long life, and peace are added to life if one keeps God's commandments.

**Proverbs 3:13:** "My son, forget not my law; but let thine heart keep my commandments: *for length of days*, and *long life*, and *peace,* shall they add to thee."

This verse also promises length of days, long life, and peace to those who remember God's commandments and keep them.

**Proverbs 3:16:** "*Length of days* is in her [wisdom's] right hand; and in her left hand riches and honour."

Thus, we find that aligning one's life with divine wisdom bestows the dual gifts of longevity and prosperity. Those who choose to walk the path of obedience to God's commandments are promised a scepter of enduring life in one hand, while the other carries the treasures of wealth and respect. These are blessings that are promised to the obedient.

**Proverbs 4:10:** "Hear, O my son, and receive my sayings; *and the years of thy life shall be many.*"

Here, again, we are reminded that by heeding God's instructions and living in alignment with them, our lives will not only be extended with longevity, but will also be blessed abundantly.

**Proverbs 9:11:** "For by me *thy days shall be multiplied*, and *the years of thy life shall be increased.*"

The words "thy days shall be multiplied" don't merely speak of more days, but of days that are multiplied with productivity, while "the years of thy life shall be increased" promises a gratifying, long existence.

**Proverbs 10:27:** "The fear of the Lord *prolongeth days:* but the years of the wicked shall be shortened."

Those who do not live with the fear of the Lord and who therefore do not live in obedience to His commands will live a shorter life. Conversely, those who embrace the fear of the Lord and walk in His ways are blessed with longevity.

We are also told in the New Testament that living in obedience to God's commands results in blessing and longevity.

**Ephesians 6:1-3** reminds us of God's promise in the fifth of the Ten Commandments that says, "Children, obey your parents in the Lord: for this is right. Honour thy father and mother; which is the first commandment with promise; that it may be well with thee, and thou mayest live long on the earth."

Here God emphasizes His desire for us to enjoy a life filled with ample good days and extended years, yet this divine blessing is intricately connected to the respect and honor we bestow upon our parents.

**First Peter 3:10-11** says, "For he that will love life, and see *good days*, let him refrain his tongue from evil, and his lips that they speak no guile: Let him eschew evil, and do good; let him seek peace, and ensue it."

The words "good days" refers not only to the quality of days, but also to the longevity of one's life. Peter herein stated if a person fully intends to have a life that is full of gusto and zest, a life really worth living, and wishes to experience really good days, times, and seasons, he must make sure his tongue refrains from speaking evil.

I want you to understand that the Bible is rich with verses extolling the virtues of a life blessed with longevity and productivity, more than we could possibly include here. These scriptures vividly illustrate God's unwavering promise of a long life — and also one that is deeply satisfying and fruitful — to those who fear Him and faithfully follow His commandments.

## HOW YOU THINK AND BELIEVE ABOUT AGING WILL AFFECT HOW WELL AND HOW LONG YOU LIVE

When I was a boy, I remember looking at people who were about 60 years old and remember thinking that they looked really old. Often, I'd find myself seated beside one of my six living grandmothers during a Sunday service. There, I'd gently cup her hands in mine, tracing the raised veins in her hands with my finger, amazed at how I could push the vessels one way or the other and how easily her wrinkly skin moved when I pressed against it. I was particularly fascinated by the liver spots that covered ever-increasing sections of the skin on her upper hand.

I remember thinking that she was so old, but actually, as I look back on it now, I realize she was probably only in her late 60s. But back in those days, we were incorrectly taught that Psalm 90:10 only promised 70 years of life — maybe 80, if we were lucky — so around the time people began to reach 60 years of age, they began to act and think as if they were coming to the end of their lives.

We can see from the scriptures I just listed that God repeatedly promises longevity to all those who fear and love Him and who obey His commands. The fact is that you can live much longer than 70 or 80 years if you walk with Him, keep His commandments, and do what is necessary to take care of your body. Medical science now remarkably states that if certain conditions could be met to drastically slow down the aging of cells, it could be entirely possible for the human body to live up to 1,000 years,[14] which is interestingly just about how long people lived before the Flood.

What this tells us is that the way most people have been thinking about "aging" and "old age" needs to change. Proverbs 23:7 says that as a person thinks in his heart, "so is he." If you believe you're old and past your prime, you'll likely start behaving that way sooner than you should. However, if you see yourself as having more miles left on your journey, you'll likely experience more energy and enjoy a longer and more vibrant life. How we think about ourselves determines what we become, so you need to know that the way you think really is going to affect what you experience in life.

I'm not dismissing the inevitability of aging; it's a truth everyone faces. In our time, many strive to defy it, and there's certainly no harm in utilizing every available means to preserve one's youthful glow. But despite the arsenal of creams, potions, and surgeries at our disposal to ward off time's advances, the march of age brings physical changes. It's no wonder the cosmetic surgery industry is booming, as people eagerly open their wallets to not only reverse the passages of time but also to "remodel" what they perceive as imperfections in their appearance.

As noted earlier, if you can afford it and you wish to do it, do what you can to give yourself a fresher and more youthful look. But no matter what precautions one takes with his or her eating habits or exercise routines, eventually gravity does its work, and things that once stood sturdily in place begin to sag.

Although we may employ various strategies to sidestep the ticking clock, the march of time is unrelenting, and sooner or later, everyone faces the undeniable trademarks of aging. However, our mindset toward aging plays a crucial role; thinking young can infuse our actions and spirit with youthful vitality. So I encourage you to make the decision to see yourself as vibrant. What you think will really affect how you believe and behave.

Thankfully, thinking about "aging" and "old age" is beginning to change in our times. As we saw in the statistics earlier in this chapter, people are living longer, more productive lives. But we need to renew our minds to what the Bible promises in regard to longevity — and the truth is that God promises a long and satisfying life to the faithful and obedient. He does not limit His blessings to 70 or 80 years. Instead, Psalm 91:16 declares that God's perfect will is for you to fully experience *salvation* — that is, *deliverance, healing, prosperity, wholeness,* and everything else that is packed into salvation — and to live until you are completely full, satisfied, and ready to move on to Heaven.

I want to remind you of Moses' words to the children of Israel, "I call heaven and earth to record this day against you, that I have set before you life and death, blessing and cursing: therefore choose life, that both thou and thy seed may live: That thou mayest love the Lord thy God, and that thou mayest obey his voice, and that thou mayest cleave unto him: for he is thy life, and the length of thy days..." (Deuteronomy 30:19-20).

Just as Moses urged the people to heed God's instructions so they could live a full life marked with blessings and longevity, I implore you to cast aside the mindset of "old" thinking and choose life and longevity as God promises. If you do, you and your offspring will experience length of days, and the end of your life will become some of the most productive years of your life!

Proverbs 23:7 says our thoughts shape who we are. So let me ask you: How do you perceive yourself? Are you viewing yourself as antiquated, past your prime, and out of touch, or do you see yourself as seasoned, well-prepared, and on the cusp of your most fruitful years?

*How do you see yourself?*

## SUPERNATURAL AGE-RENEWAL IS ALSO A PROMISE FROM GOD

For those who choose to walk with God and obediently follow His commandments, you have an additional promise of renewal in your life, even while you are aging. Psalm 103:5 says, "[God] satisfieth thy mouth with good things; so that thy youth is renewed like the eagle's."

There is no medical procedure, no series of treatments, no healing cream or supplement that can compare with the divine regenerative power of the Spirit of God. His strength is unmatched, and He gives it to those who are His own. Isaiah 40:29-31 declares, "He giveth power to the faint; and to them that have no might he increaseth strength. Even the youths shall faint and be weary, and the young men shall utterly fall: but they that wait upon the Lord shall renew their strength; they shall mount up with wings as eagles; they shall run, and not be weary; and they shall walk, and not faint."

In today's shifting landscape, the way we perceive "aging" and the concept of "age" is evolving for the better. We're fortunate to witness countless modern-day examples of individuals who are reshaping their perspectives and who are embracing the reality that life's later chapters can be jubilantly long and exceptionally productive.

These individuals are proving that one's golden years can indeed shine the brightest!

A significant factor in this transformation is the burgeoning "Baby Boomer" generation, born between the close of World War II and the mid-1960s. As they advance in years, this significant category finds itself faced with the necessity to continue working, often due to financial reasons.

Yet in doing so, they have shattered preconceptions and demonstrated that age is no barrier to excellence. In fact, their extensive experience often surpasses that of younger people and reaffirms that seniority can be a profound asset.

In today's world, longevity is more than just living — it's about thriving. People are not only celebrating more birthdays, but also extending their careers in ways previously unimaginable. The entertainment industry sees seasoned veterans gracing the stage and screen far beyond conventional retirement.

Meanwhile, professionals in various fields are extending their duty, serving at restaurants, retail stores, and checkout counters with their experience and wisdom. Corporate leaders are steering their companies with time-tested expertise, and pastors and ministry leaders are shepherding their communities with enduring passion and vigor well into their later years.

## AGE IS A PLUS, NOT A MINUS

As Denise and I fly around the world to do our ministry, we frequently comment to each other about how the age of flight attendants is older and how they continue to deliver impeccable service with grace and professionalism. This trend of vibrant longevity crosses many spheres, and it is being carried out by those who are doing their jobs in a first-class and top-notch manner. In years gone by, reaching a particular age would have signaled a retreat, a transition into retirement, and a handing over the reins of work to younger generations. But thanks to groundbreaking studies on aging, we now understand:

- A person's most productive age is from 60 to 70 years of age.
- A person's second most productive stage is from 70 to 80 years of age.
- A person's third most productive stage is from 50 to 60 years of age.

As individuals navigate through their 50s and 60s, they often find thoughts of retirement creeping into their minds. However, recent studies suggest that if you fall into this age range, pushing retirement to the back-burner might be wise. You see, your peak years are just around the corner, nestled between your 60s and 70s.

In fact, when you're between 60 and 70, it means you're in the best mental stage of your life. Even more amazing is that the second-best mental stage is between 70 and 80. So perhaps it's time to shift your focus from *winding down* to *revving up,* for your best days are ahead of you!

You are never too old to begin something new, and there are many stories of people who achieved great things later in life. For example, Yuichiro Miura was the oldest person to climb Mount Everest at the age of 80. At 72 years old, Edwina Brocklesby became the oldest British woman to complete an Ironman triathlon, and she stated that she didn't even start exercising until her 50s. Even the oldest person to begin elementary school, Kimani Maruge, enrolled at 84 years old. He wanted to learn how to count money and how to read so he could read the Bible.[15]

Retired Lt. Col. James C. Warren, at the age of 87, became the oldest person in the world to receive his pilot's license. He is a former navigator of the Tuskegee Airmen, the first African American military aviators in the United States Armed Forces.[16] And Leila Denmark was an American pediatrician in Atlanta, Georgia. She was a co-developer of the whooping cough vaccine and the world's oldest practicing pediatrician until her retirement after 73 years, at age 103. Interestingly enough, she also volunteered her time at a local church.[17]

Imagine if these stalwart visionaries had thrown in the towel earlier; their crowning achievements might never have been realized. Had they chosen early retirement, they might have missed the most illustrious phase of their career. And if any of them decided to go with the status-quo mindset of inevitable decline at their age, they never would have achieved the amazing feats — as well as the physical and mental benefits — merited unless they pushed past the prevalent expectation that old age must certainly mean the onset of deterioration. The truth is, many miss their most fruitful and productive phases because they choose to step back too soon.

Trust me when I say that I'm not implying there's anything wrong with deciding to retire a bit earlier in life. For some, retirement is exactly what they need. Yet evidence suggests that if you choose this path, you might bypass the most fruitful phase of your life. Believe it or not, the golden years between 60 and 80 could be your most impactful. At 60, you start to tap into your true potential, and this journey can stretch well into your 80s.

So if you're 60 or beyond, you're about to enter your prime years. My hope is that you ponder these insights, seek guidance, and ask the Holy Spirit whether your path is truly complete or if more awaits you. Should you feel you're stepping away too soon, embrace the divine strength within you and affirm that your brightest days are still ahead!

Many individuals who opt for early retirement do so with excitement, envisioning a life of leisure and opportunities to explore new interests. However, they often find themselves unexpectedly ensnared in monotony and dissatisfaction.

The absence of a clear purpose can lead to feelings of depression and frustration, with physical health following a downward spiral. The human body and mind resemble a finely tuned instrument; when used regularly, it flourishes, but left idle, it gathers "rust" and loses its vigor. When someone is overwhelmed with unstructured time, lacking meaningful activity, it can take a toll on both mental and physical wellness and actually hasten the aging process.

In search of relief from the monotony, some retirees take up part-time work to occupy their hours. Yet these positions are often below their skill level and abilities, and although they are grateful for the distraction from inactivity, there remains a yearning for something more fulfilling. When people still possess untapped reservoirs of talent and energy, such jobs can feel diminishing, as they are acutely aware of their potential to contribute far beyond mundane tasks.

I am thinking of a ministry friend, who once confided in me his plan to retire and pass his leadership torch to a younger successor. At the time, he was in his early sixties — radiating with vitality and brimming with intellectual fervor with many productive years still ahead of him. I challenged him, "What's next on your horizon? How much golf can you play to fill your hours? How do you plan to spend the next quarter-century of life in front of you?" I am grateful that he embraced my advice wholeheartedly. He remained in his calling, and the next season of his ministry became the most bountiful chapter of his ministry, bursting with unmatched spiritual harvest.

## THE BEST IS YET TO COME!

It is a grave mistake for those who are a little older to conclude that they're irrelevant due to age. If you haven't used your mind to its fullest capacity, and your body is in trouble due to ill health, perhaps taking a slower approach is needed to get back in shape. However, the evidence clearly celebrates age as an asset, not a minus. Having age means you've had time to grow and gain priceless experience.

If whispers in your mind suggest you're too old, out of date, or irrelevant because of your age, pray and see if there are things you need to do to grow and to remain relevant. However, if you recognize these thoughts as the devil's whispers aiming to undermine your confidence, you need to dismiss them outright. Nothing would delight the devil more than convincing you to leave the playing field and sit on the sidelines just as you're coming into your most productive years. The adversary knows well that in the years ahead lie your most profound potential, blessings and achievements yet to unfold.

Psalm 84:7 tells us that God's plan is for us to go from strength to strength and not to dwindle into weakness or frailty. Again, thankfully in our day, many are beginning to change the way they think about age. Today we are surrounded by an older category of leaders who are living testaments to vitality and who are courageously redefining what it means to grow older and to stay relevant.

These trailblazers are not simply defying expectations; they are setting a new standard for the rest of us. They are demonstrating that through God's grace, it is possible to live a long life, run a strong race, and become more valuable all the way to the end of their lives. Their examples encourage us that we can shine ever brighter as we age.

So don't buy the lie that you are capped at 70 or 80 or that age should push you to the sidelines. If you believe that you'll live and serve for 70 or 80 years, that's probably what you will get. But if you aim at a longer productive life — for example, living into your 90s — you'll come a lot closer to it. Jesus said, "...All things are possible to him that believeth" (Mark 9:23).

Your beliefs shape much of what lies ahead. Set your expectations low, and "low" will likely be your result. But set your sights for greater things, and you'll come closer to reaching them. What you believe will determine so much for you, so make sure you're believing for the right things.

I encourage you as you age to stay spiritually vibrant, stay on track with God's Word, stay filled with the Holy Spirit, and stay engaged in God-given relationships that enrich you along the way. And by all means, take care of yourself and stay physically fit. Remember that in Mark 12:30 Jesus said, "Thou shalt love the Lord thy God with all thy heart, and with all thy soul, and with all thy mind, and with all thy strength...." This verse calls you to honor God with every facet of your being — spirit, soul, and body.

**Nothing would delight the devil more than convincing you to leave the playing field and sit on the sidelines just as you're coming into your most productive years. The adversary knows well that in the years ahead lie your most profound potential, blessings and achievements yet to unfold.**

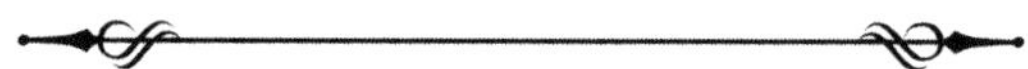

To lead a long and fruitful life, you need to ask God to help you remain spiritually vibrant, nourish your body with wholesome food, stay active, exercise regularly, and make sure your body and mind don't become like a rusty tool that is no longer usable. All these elements contribute to your longevity. Your most productive years will probably be your latter years. You need to get your mind renewed and in line with God's promise of longevity for those who love and obey Him.

Consider some dear friends of ours, who in their early 60s, faced the pivotal decision of whether to retire or embark on their inaugural business venture. They chose the latter, creating a venture that ultimately blossomed into one of the nation's foremost developers and purveyors of innovative ice-cream flavors.

By opting to dive into the arena rather than watch from the sidelines, they transformed their decades of experience in the dairy industry into an era of remarkable productivity. This bold move at a time when many step back led them to establish one of the most significant dairy enterprises in the United

States. Their success not only marked their personal triumph, but also enabled them to support Gospel missions across the globe.

Whenever I reflect on my own age, my thoughts invariably drift to these two friends. As I write these words, I find myself standing on the cusp of nearly the same age at which they bravely embarked on their entrepreneurial adventure. It often crosses my mind, "Their most productive years began precisely at the age I'm reaching now."

Witnessing how their lives have flourished, fueled by age and experience, it fills me with expectation that my most bountiful chapters lie in the years ahead. We have years behind us of walking with God and learning what to do and what not to do, and as a result, we're on the brink of our most fruitful era yet. Our age is not a minus — it's a remarkable asset and plus that propels us forward!

So instead of thinking your best season is behind you, renew your thinking to believe that your golden era of productivity and creativity is before you. For those of you who've been blessed with age, it's not the moment to bow out and yield to the stereotypes of growing old.

Rather, it's an opportunity to redefine what it means to be aging and to step into a season rich with potential and success. With the accumulated wisdom and experiences of a lifetime behind you, you are more ready for triumph than ever before.

Contrary to what most people believe, our latter years are meant to surpass even the brilliance of our younger years. Referring to God's people, the psalmist said, "[Growing in grace] they shall still bring forth fruit in old age; they shall be full of sap [of spiritual vitality] and [rich in the] verdure [of trust, love, and contentment]. [They are living memorials] to show that the Lord is upright and faithful to His promises…" (Psalm 92:14-15 *AMPC*).

*The best is yet to come!*

## PATRIARCHS IN THE BIBLE WHO LIVED LONG AND STRONG

If you look through the pages of the Old and New Testaments, you'll discover an inspiring number of figures who lived and served productively into their twilight years. Some walked with God from childhood, others found Him along the winding paths of adulthood, yet all of them remained fruitful well into the later years of their lives.

The pages of Scripture overflow with stories of those who dedicated their latter years to service, and their lives serve as witnesses that it is possible to live long and strong and productively until later in life.

It would be impossible to recount every story, but in the pages that follow, we'll focus on the examples of Enoch, Noah, Abraham, Moses, Caleb, Daniel, and the apostle John to see how they continued to serve God with devotion and passion into their senior years.

### Enoch: A Promise Coming to Pass at Age 365

The first example is Enoch, a remarkable man of unwavering faith. As a young man, Enoch received a promise that he would be spared from the sting of death. Clinging to this promise, Enoch remained steadfast through the passage of years, his trust unfaltering even as age crept upon him.

True to the promise He received, Enoch was eventually whisked away from the earthly realm without ever facing death. This extraordinary story serves as a powerful reminder that the fulfillment of divine promises knows no age limit.

There were many things that could have been recorded about Enoch's life, yet the Bible highlights the profound truth that Enoch *walked with God*. Genesis 5:22-24 says, "And Enoch walked with God after he begat Methuselah three hundred years, and begat sons and daughters: and all the days of Enoch were three hundred sixty and five years...."

By steadfastly holding fast to God's promise, Enoch witnessed an extraordinary extension of his years, and he became the first to experience what no one else had ever experienced. Genesis 5:24 says, "And Enoch walked with God: and he *was not*; for God took him."

There may have been times when Enoch might have pondered whether God's promise would ever see the light of fulfillment. But unwavering in his faith, Enoch clung tightly to this sacred promise, and he was miraculously snatched from the world, bypassing the grasp of death entirely.

This remarkable death-escaping story of Enoch is also mentioned in the New Testament. Hebrews 11:5 says, "By faith Enoch was translated that he should not see death; and was not found, because God had translated him: for before his translation he had this testimony, that he pleased God." Notice that the words "translated" or "translation" appear three times in this verse. In each instance, it is the Greek word *metatithimi*, which signifies the act of *relocating something from one spot to another*. The repeated use of this word tells us that Enoch was lifted from the earthly realm and *relocated* to Heaven.

In Hebrews 11:5, it intriguingly says that Enoch "was not found." The Greek word used here is a form of the word *heurisko*, which means *to find* or *to discover by diligent search or investigation*. Thus, when the text states Enoch "was not found," it tells us that despite the fact that people made diligent searches and carried out intense investigations to find him, Enoch could simply not be located. He vanished, taken by God Himself, and there was not a single trace of him left on the earth.

But Hebrews 11:15 also says, "...For before his translation he had this testimony, that he pleased God." The word "before" is the Greek word *pro*, which means *earlier* and implies that Enoch had been given a "word" from God earlier in his life that he would defy mortality. Clinging to that promise, Enoch lived his life in anticipation and trust until the extraordinary day when God fulfilled it and spared him from death. We do not know how much earlier God made

His promise to Enoch, but Enoch waited and waited. And so it was, after 365 years, God's promise finally became a reality in his life.

In the end, God's promise to Enoch came to pass and he never died. To this day, Enoch remains very much alive in Heaven, a testament to his faith and God's promise. Remarkably, even though his son Methuselah boasted an earthly life spanning 969 years before passing away, Enoch's life surpasses his by millennia. He has been living in God's glorious presence for an incredible 5,000 years, and that means Enoch holds the extraordinary title of the longest-living man in existence!

So how long have you been waiting for your promise from God to come to pass? While you might feel like an eternity has passed, I assure you, you haven't quite crossed the 365-year mark just yet! So take courage from Enoch's example, and hold tightly to God's promise and trust that it can still happen in your life, even if you're well into your senior years.

**Noah: A Mission Starting at 500**

Noah is an example of a man who only received his assignment when he reached the ripe age of 500. Born into a lineage of devout believers, it wasn't until his half-millennium birthday that he grasped the monumental task given to him by God — the construction of the Ark. At 600 years old, Noah led his family of eight into the Ark, where they survived the deluge that engulfed the world, they emerged after the waters subsided, and finally they embarked on the formidable task of replenishing life on the earth. Noah's story is one of a man who lived a life full of fruitful purpose, even into the very last of his senior years.

When Noah reached the age of 500, he not only embraced fatherhood (*see* Genesis 5:32), but also experienced a profound spiritual awakening that opened his spiritual ears to hear the voice of God. Similarly, you might view your latter years as a time of winding down, but this could very well be the chapter where your soul ignites with its most vivid spiritual awakening. For Noah, his monumental task arrived when he reached 500 years old, reminding us all that our latter years are not for retreat. Instead, embrace them, for like Noah, this might be your moment to truly tune into God's plan and embark on the most significant phase of your life.

As years add wisdom to your life, the perfect moment can arise to embark on a project inspired by God's instructions to your heart. With a life full of experiences, you've honed your skills and deepened your understanding, and you are ready to savor the precious time that remains.

With all that you've learned in life, the truth is that this last stage holds the potential for unparalleled growth and impact. Yet it's essential to cast aside the doubts of older age and irrelevance and step forward with faith to embrace the calling God has placed before you. Boldly proclaim, "This chapter of my life will be the most fruitful yet. My journey isn't over until I've fulfilled everything God has asked me to do and I've achieved every victory awaiting me!"

**You might view your latter years as a time of winding down, but this could very well be the chapter where your soul ignites with its most vivid spiritual awakening.**

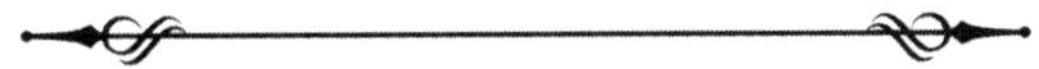

Noah likely had this mindset, for Genesis 6:13-22 tells us that when God commanded him to construct the Ark, he obeyed without hesitation in spite of his maturity in years. The colossal endeavor spanned nearly a century and demanded the dedication of Noah and his family. According to Genesis 7:6, Noah was 600 years old when the Flood engulfed the earth. Genesis 8:1-3 says after judgment was complete, God caused wind to pass over the entire planet, which seems to have set certain weather conditions into motion, initiating the evaporation phase of the water cycle. That Heaven-sent breeze pushed the water in specific directions as God set in motion restoring the earth and "starting over" with a mere eight undefiled souls — led by the direction of Noah who was, again, a mere 600 years old!

We read in Genesis 9:1 that "God blessed Noah and his sons, and said unto them, Be fruitful, and multiply, and replenish the earth." Emboldened by God's directive, Noah and his family started the monumental task of repopulating the world. They descended into the valley that stretched below the resting place of the Ark. Genesis 9:20 tells us Noah took on the role of a farmer, and the family established their roots in a new world. Genesis 9:28 recounts that Noah's life after the Flood spanned an additional 350 years! The sum total of Noah's earthly life was an astounding 950 years, and at the end of it, he peacefully took leave of this world.

Although the Bible does not explicitly mention it, one can easily imagine that when Noah was assigned the task of building the Ark at the ripe age of 500, he might have questioned whether he was too advanced in years for such an undertaking. Having already traversed half a millennium of life, it's conceivable that the effects of age were making themselves known, as they eventually do to all of us.

Yet regardless of any doubts or concerns he may have harbored, Noah decided to set aside the constraints of his age and faithfully heed God's command. Because of Noah's determination at 500 to embrace the challenge ahead, humanity is still here today. Noah's story stands as a witness to the potential of living purposefully, no matter how "senior" one may be in life.

### Abraham: A Promise Fulfilled at Age 100

Abraham serves as a striking illustration of a former pagan, an unbeliever, who astonishingly found God at 75 years old. Despite discovering his calling late in life, he embraced his heavenly mission with unwavering resolve. Even though his spiritual path was strewn with errors and missteps, his dedication remained unshaken, and he steadfastly pursued the fulfillment of God's promises. His faith-driven odyssey was fraught with challenges, and it took a quarter of a century before God's promise became reality — just as he approached his *one hundredth* year!

At the senior age of 75, Abraham had a life-altering encounter with God, proving that the discovery of a higher calling isn't exclusive to the young. Hailing from Ur of the Chaldees, a region of opulence and grandeur, Abraham and his wife flourished amid riches and prestige. Securely ensconced in his golden years, Abraham might have seemed an unlikely candidate for such a task. Yet it was at this seasoned stage that he crossed paths with God and embarked on an extraordinary journey of faith. Despite being senior in years, he embraced a new destiny that not only reshaped his own life but left an indelible mark on history.

Acts 7:2-3 tells us of the moment when Abraham had an unexpected celestial encounter with God that altered the entire trajectory of his existence. Those verses describe how the glory of God manifested to Abraham, and enveloped him in God's presence. At that time, Abraham was living in the land of Ur of the Chaldeans, and he was engaged in the worship of many gods as was customary among his people. Yet *suddenly*, God's glory enveloped him, and it marked the significant turning point of his life. In this divine moment, God called upon Abraham to start a journey of faith and promised that he would become "a great nation" (*see* Genesis 12:2).

This promise from God seemed utterly impossible. Abraham was 75 years old, and his wife Sarah, herself advanced in years, faced an unfathomable challenge, because she was barren (*see* Romans 4:19; Hebrews 11:11). Yet amidst the doubt, God's voice rang clear to Abraham, and as recounted in Genesis 15:6, Abraham placed his faith in God's Word.

For those who find themselves in the twilight of their years, let this true story be an inspiration to you. Should God give you a task that appears beyond reach because you are in your in latter years of life, remember you are never beyond the age of realizing God's plan. Instead of relegating yourself to a spectator's seat and dismissing yourself due to age, seize God's promise with conviction. Believe fervently and with expectancy and watch as the seemingly impossible becomes reality.

For Enoch, Noah, and Abraham, the answer did not come quickly to them for a variety of reasons. Abraham and Sarah waited a quarter of a century before witnessing the fulfillment of God's promise. They might have easily muttered, "This is dragging on too long. We're past our prime. It's never going to happen. We're just too old and time is running out."

Yet they opted to anchor themselves in faith and to continue believing steadfastly. In a similar vein, if you find yourself in the twilight of life, like Abraham, hold firmly to God's promise for you. Stay rooted in the place where God has called you, engage in the tasks He has entrusted to you, embrace the promise He has instilled in you, and remain unwavering. Even though you may feel you are in the sunset years of your life, God is not out of pay days, and He has not forgotten you or your faith in Him!

The Bible bestows upon Abraham the illustrious title of "father of faith" and marks him as the progenitor of the Hebrew nation. His life's journey is so pivotal to our spiritual heritage that the Old Testament devotes a substantial 14 chapters solely to narrate his story (*see* Genesis 12-25).

When Abraham reached the age of 75, he was enveloped by the presence of God, who revealed Himself in a blaze of glory. With unwavering trust, Abraham embraced God's call, yielded to His authority, and followed His commands, even though he didn't understand how any of it would come to pass. Despite not grasping how the promises would unfold, he emerged as the "father of many nations."

Genesis 25:7-8 says, "And these are the days of the years of Abraham's life which he lived, an hundred threescore and fifteen years. Then Abraham gave up the ghost, and died in a good old age, an old man, and full of years; and was gathered to his people." The word "score" pictures a span of 20 years, so when the Bible states that Abraham's life spanned 100 plus 3 score and 15 years, it is indicating that he lived to the ripe old age of 175.

One can't help but imagine the quiet moments Abraham and Sarah shared as they aged, pondering the deepening lines of their own faces and the persistent creaks in their bones, all while the promise of God seemingly lingered in the air. With Abraham nearing the century mark and Sarah not far behind, it would have been unsurprising for them to exchange a resigned glance and whisper, "Even if a miracle graces us with a child, aren't we too old to become parents? How will we chase after an active child with bodies our age?" Yet their spirits remained unyielding, and they allowed God to write through them a new chapter of human history.

So if you find yourself navigating senior years and the thought of surrender flits through your mind, remember the ripple effects of perseverance and that the destiny of others hinges on your steadfast action in the face of doubt. *Too much is at stake for you to give up!*

Through their unwavering faith and steadfast obedience, Abraham and Sarah found themselves blessed with a miraculous gift from God — a child that seemed impossible by earthly standards. Genesis 25:8 recounts that Abraham thrived until his last breath, living to the venerable age of 175, imbued with vigor and strength. His life reminds us that no matter how advanced in years we may feel, the potential for extraordinary accomplishments remains boundless. Abraham's story illustrates that with faith, you can always be a supernatural fruit-producer, regardless of how "senior" you may feel you are at this stage in your life.

### Moses: Ministry Beginning at Age 80

Moses is yet another story of someone whose encounter with God occurred in the senior years of his life. Although he appeared to drift aimlessly — lost in deserts both literal and metaphorical — it was in his advanced age that he was called to greatness. At 80, he heard God beckoning to him, and he was entrusted with the extraordinary mission of freeing the Israelites from the oppressive grip of Egyptian captivity.

Upon Moses' birth, his parents sensed the extraordinary nature of their son. In defiance of Pharaoh's command to cast newborn Hebrew boys into the Nile River's murderous embrace, they sought refuge for him in secrecy (*see* Exodus 2). Crafting a tiny ark from bulrushes, his mother placed him gently into the river waters, trusting that God would direct the currents of the Nile to carry him to safety. The river guided that little ark to a fateful encounter with Pharaoh's own daughter. Drawn to the infant nestled among the Nile's reeds, she claimed him as her own, adopted him, and raised him as her royal son.

From the tender age of three months until he turned 40, Moses grew up within the opulent walls of Pharaoh's palace, surrounded by his identity as an Egyptian prince under the guardianship of Pharaoh's daughter. Acts 7:22 says, "And Moses was learned in all the wisdom of the Egyptians, and was mighty in words and in deeds." Although he was steeped in the vast knowledge and rich traditions of Egypt, seeds of truth sown by his mother during his early, impressionable years lay dormant inside him until they blossomed unexpectedly when Moses, at the cusp of 40, became attuned to his true identity.

By the age of 40, Moses had ascended to legendary status within Egypt, a figure of renown and reverence. The historian Josephus recounts that Moses had attained the pinnacle of Egyptian education, distinguished himself as a formidable warrior, and amassed a litany of remarkable accomplishments long before he identified himself with the people of God.

But rather than revel in the lofty position of being called the son of Pharaoh's daughter or enjoy the temporary pleasures of sin or bask in the wealth and treasures of Egypt, "By faith he [Moses] forsook Egypt, not fearing the wrath of the king: for he endured, as seeing him who is invisible" (Hebrews 11:27).

Driven by unforeseen events, Moses found himself fleeing from Egypt and venturing into the untamed wilderness. It seemed as though destiny had led him into oblivion. It seemed that he didn't just lose his way, but everything he once held dear had also been taken from him. For the next four decades, Moses roamed the desolate wilderness, living a humble life as a shepherd — but God had not finished writing his story.

When he reached the venerable age of 80, standing on the precipice of what many might call his senior years, Moses stumbled upon an extraordinary encounter with God in the form of a burning bush (*see* Exodus 3). Although he was 80 years old, and it seemed his greatest achievements thus far had passed forever into the forgotten annals of history, he discovered that God had a magnificent plan set to unfold at the senior age of 80 years, and he obediently launched into the most formidable period of his life.

Moses was such a mighty prophet that Deuteronomy 34:10-12 says, "And there arose not a prophet since in Israel like unto Moses, whom the Lord knew face to face, in all the signs and the wonders, which the Lord sent him to do in the land of Egypt to Pharaoh, and to all his servants, and to all his land, and in all that mighty hand, and in all the great terror which Moses shewed in the sight of all Israel." But to think, this great phase of Moses' life started at the age of 80 years!

We read in Deuteronomy 34:7 that "Moses was an hundred and twenty years old when he died: his eye was not dim, nor his natural force abated." According to this verse, Moses' eyesight was clear, he possessed mental acuity, and he was physically strong all the way to the end of his 120-year life. Rather than being old, sick, weak, and decrepit, he lived long and strong to the very end.

God is not a respector of persons (*see* Romans 2:11; Acts 10:34), and if Moses experienced his most remarkable achievements in his latter years, it's entirely possible for your latter years to be just as fulfilling. Remember, at the age of 80 Moses embarked on his most extraordinary journey. So if you are in your senior years, instead of lamenting, "My best years are behind me and I'm too old to start a new project," start declaring, "God has a plan for me and my best days are in front of me. My senior years are going to be my most productive years."

God's promise and power will quicken your body and mind and set you on a new trajectory so the years that remain can be the most fruit-producing years of your life. God wants you to press forward into your senior years with hope and faith to accomplish His plan for your life. If Moses could finish his race with unabated strength and health, so can you!

## Caleb: A New Challenge at Age 85

Now we come to the story of Caleb. Throughout his journey, his dedication never wavered, but instead, his story is one that shone brighter with age. It was in his later years that he achieved remarkable strength and productivity that outshined the outstanding feats of his younger days. *This can be your story too!*

According to Numbers 13:6, Caleb traced his roots back to the tribe of Judah and was recognized as a devout follower of God from his youth. In Numbers 14:24, God spoke to Moses about Caleb and said, "But my servant Caleb, because he had another spirit with him, and hath followed me fully, him will I bring into the land whereinto he went; and his seed shall possess it."

Caleb was different from the others in Israel in that he served God wholeheartedly and passionately. Caleb had "a different spirit" from the other ten spies that Moses had sent to evaluate the Promised Land. Numbers 13:28 tells us all twelve of the spies who explored the new territory came back and said, "... The people be strong that dwell in the land, and the cities are walled, and very great: and moreover we saw the children of Anak there."

The children of Anak were enormous giants. In fact, they were so massive that Numbers 13:33 says that ten of the twelve spies went on to say: "And there we saw the giants, the sons of Anak, which come of the giants: and we were in our own sight as grasshoppers, and so we were in their sight." Although the ten spies with a fearful report acknowledged the land was beautiful and filled with amazing fruit and fertile pastures, they were paralyzed by the looming figures of the Anakim. Their hearts consumed by fear, these ten spies brought back what was regarded as a daunting and "evil report" and didn't believe the people of Israel were sufficient to overcome the giants they saw there.

Because those particular ten spies were fearful, faithless, and saw themselves as grasshoppers compared to the size of the giants, God did not allow them to enter the Promised Land. But the remaining two spies, Caleb and Joshua, were of a different spirit. They didn't deny that there were giants in the land, but they fixed their eyes on the magnificent fruit and the amazing God they served, and they said, "We are well able to overcome it" (*see* Numbers 13:30).

Caleb was 40 years old when he was sent as a spy into the land of promise. He and Joshua were the only two spies who returned with a faith-filled report. For the next 45 years of his life, Caleb remained courageous, faith-filled, and stayed on track, and this lifestyle of unwavering faith was used to shape the next 45 years of his life. At the age of 85, the time came for the Promised Land to be parceled out to the various tribes of Israel. Unbowed by the weight of his years, Caleb boldly advanced to claim his inheritance. While many might have dismissed someone of 85 as too advanced in age for such a new and huge assignment, Caleb reminded Joshua of his unwavering loyalty since the age of 40 (*see* Joshua 14:7).

Although he was 85 years old, Caleb wanted in on the action that was about to happen. The daunting senior age of 80 had no affect on him, as he was as bold and confident as he had been at the age of 40. As he retold the account of the spies who went in to survey the land, he reminded Joshua, "Nevertheless my brethren that went up with me made the heart of the people melt: but I wholly followed the Lord my God. And Moses sware on that day, saying, Surely the land whereon thy feet have trodden shall be thine inheritance, and thy children's forever, because thou hast wholly followed the Lord my God" (Joshua 14:8-9).

Caleb continued rehearsing to Joshua what happened more than 45 years earlier when he said, "And now, behold, the Lord hath kept me alive, as he said, these forty and five years, even since the Lord spake this word unto Moses, while the children of Israel wandered in the wilderness: and now, lo, I am this day fourscore and five years old"(Joshua 14:10).

Despite being in his later years, Caleb remained sharp and vigorous, showing no intention of slowing down or stepping away from his pursuits. God had given him the strength to continue through all of Israel's wanderings in the wilderness — and for 45 years, he maintained a consistent walk of faith and stayed on track with God. In Joshua 14:11, Caleb declared, "As yet I am as strong this day as I was in the day that Moses sent me: as my strength was then, even so is my strength now, for war, both to go out, and to come in."

In essence, Caleb proclaimed that, at the age of 85, his vigor was undiminished from when he first ventured forth at 40 years old when Moses sent him out to survey the land with the other spies. Rather than just relaxing and riding out the remainder of his years, Numbers 14:12 tells us that he said, "Now therefore give me this mountain, whereof the Lord spake in that day; for thou heardest in that day how the Anakims were there, and that the cities were great and fenced: if so be the Lord will be with me, then I shall be able to drive them out, as the Lord said."

Remember that the Anakims were fearsome giants, the titans among titans, and they lived in the towering mountain that lay in Joshua's sights. While the mere thought of these imposing figures sent shivers down the spines of other men and caused their hearts to quake with terror, Caleb stepped forward with a fiery resolve. With the wisdom of 85 years etched into his spirit, he boldly declared, "I might be 85 years old, but I want a new assignment. Give me that mountain — the big one filled with the biggest, most ferocious giants of all, where the cities are fenced up to the heavens. That's the one I want. The Lord will be with me, and we will drive them out!"

Remarkably, Caleb had reached the age of 85 and was more than twice the age since his adventurous days as a young spy four decades prior. Can you imagine his body not feeling the weight of those additional 40-plus years? Inevitably, he might have faced the common aches and pains that accompany such advanced age. While the Scriptures offer no insight into any physical discomforts he may have experienced, it's reasonable to assume that an 85-year-old would encounter some age-related issues. However, Caleb's fervent spirit and unyielding determination transcended these limitations, and he refused to let time's passage impede the triumph he so fervently pursued.

If you are in your senior years, I advise you to take Caleb as a prime example of making the choice to do the impossible all the way to the end of your life. There are still mountains God wants you to claim. So if you are in your senior years, know that you can flourish like Caleb flourished in his senior years. Rather than sit on the sidelines, it's time to boldly declare, "God give me that mountain! I'm ready for a big assignment!"

## Daniel: He Held a Job Until His Mid 90s

Daniel defied every conceivable challenge and flourished until he was nearly a 100 years old. Seventy years of his life took place in the grip of Babylonian captivity, but in the midst of those seven decades, he served as a royal advisor and high-ranking official to nine different royal administrations!

Daniel and three of his friends were taken captive from Jerusalem to Babylon and found themselves in that challenging new world somewhere in their mid-teens. Although Daniel had many opportunities to compromise in the new pagan environment, he refused to bend in his convictions.

Here we find that when you purpose in your heart to do right and to do what is honorable to God, He will cause His blessings and favor to come upon you. Indeed, God's favor enveloped Daniel and his companions, gifting them with unparalleled knowledge and wisdom across a spectrum of disciplines, and it gave them distinction in a land far from home.

Over the course of 70 remarkable years, Daniel rose to become the trusted advisor to nine distinct royal regimes. As recorded in Daniel 1:21, his influential counsel extended into his old age, enduring "even unto the first year of King Cyrus." What makes his journey extraordinary is that it all began 70 years earlier under the reign of King Nebuchadnezzar. From that initial appointment, Daniel's wisdom and insight made him indispensable, and he helped guide a course of rulers until the era of King Cyrus arrived seven decades later.

Daniel faithfully dedicated his service to King Nebuchadnezzar for the entirety of the king's formidable 43-year rule. However, even the mightiest kings meet their end, and Nebuchadnezzar eventually passed from the world into legend. The Scriptures remain silent on the details of the rulers who ascended the throne between Nebuchadnezzar and Belshazzar. Yet the ancient historian Berosus recorded the stories of each Babylonian sovereign. In each reign, Daniel's wisdom and counsel were revered, and he remained a steadfast pillar at the heart of the royal court, his role as an advisor undiminished through the changing tides of leadership.

According to historical records, Daniel served the following rulers:

- *First*, he served in the administration of King Nebuchadnezzar.
- *Second*, after Nebuchadnezzar died, his son Evil-Merodach took the throne, and he was the third king of the Neo-Babylonian empire, mentioned in Second Kings 25:27-30 and Jeremiah 52:31-34. Daniel served as his royal adviser and high official.
- *Third*, Daniel served as a royal adviser and high official to Neriglissar, who ruled for three to four years. He is briefly mentioned in Jeremiah 39:3,13.
- *Fourth*, after Neriglissar, Daniel served as a royal adviser and high official to Laborosoarchod, Neriglissar's son, who ruled for only a few months and seems to have been assassinated by a gang of conspirators.
- *Fifth*, Daniel served as a royal adviser and high official to Labashi-Marduk, who was relatively young when he became king and only ruled a short time.

- *Sixth*, Nabonidus was next to rule as king of Babylon, and like those before him, Daniel served as his royal adviser and high official, but for less than a year.
- *Seventh*, the last of the Babylonian kings Daniel served as a royal adviser and high official was Belshazzar, the eldest son of Nabonidus and grandson of King Nebuchadnezzar II. At that time, Daniel was in his 60s.
- *Eighth*, when he was in his 60s, Daniel served in Belshazzar's administration and interpreted the handwriting on the wall, but King Darius the Mede took over the kingdom. Daniel served as a royal advisor to Darius all the way into his 80s — another proof that our senior years are meant to be our best years. Daniel 6:28 says, "So this Daniel prospered in the reign of Darius, and in the reign of Cyrus the Persian."
- *Ninth*, Daniel went on to serve King Cyrus the Great.

Numerous scholars believe that Daniel lived well into his centennial years, defying the usual norms of frailty and mental decline. Rather than succumbing to the ravages of age, he exhibited an unwavering vivacity of mind, and he continued to serve a series of rulers with distinction well past his 90s.

Daniel's steadfast commitment to righteousness and honoring his faith endowed him with divine favor and allowed him to remain remarkably fruitful and industrious even throughout his advanced years. In his exceptional story, he held prestigious roles and provided counsel and wisdom as a royal advisor and acted as a high-ranking official across nine different royal regimes over the course of seven decades.

As Daniel aged over a period of 70 years, it was inevitable that fresh-faced challengers would emerge, eager to tarnish his reputation in hopes of sliding into his influential seat beside mighty kings. Observing the silver threads of his hair or the deepening lines etched upon his face, they might have pondered, "What keeps him going so long and so strong?" Daniel himself might have mused, "Am I too old to keep contributing or should I back out and give this position to someone younger?" Yet his story reveals that Daniel not only maintained his relevance until the very end, but also outlived nine rulers as he etched a legacy of godly productivity into Babylonian history.

Instead of telling yourself, "I'm too old to make a difference," choose to look to Daniel as your inspiration. Grab hold of God's power that can sustain your body and mind, and make the decision to impart what you know to be a benefit to others. Your potential to be impactful and productive remains boundless, even as time progresses. Consider how your accumulated wisdom and experience equip you like never before — and treat this phase of your life as a precious chance to flourish until the very end.

### John: A Ministry Until His 100s

The story of the apostle John began in the days of his youth when he walked alongside Jesus as one of the 12 disciples. His unwavering service continued through the years and endured until the 90s or early 100s of his extraordinary life. According to the annals of church history, John was considered the youngest among the disciples, and he started his walk with Jesus at a tender age. The apostle John is a prime example of someone who lived long enough to receive insights and knowledge from the Lord much later in life.

Historical records reveal that the apostle John enjoyed a remarkably long life, and that he is distinguished as the longest-lived of the apostles. At about the age of 92, his journey took a dramatic turn when he was apprehended and exiled to the rugged island of Patmos by order of Emperor Domitian. This remote and inhospitable island became John's new home, where the venerable leader endured a solitary existence within the confines of a cave.

One day in the isolation of that cave, John was unexpectedly caught up into the realm of the Spirit, and he beheld Christ in all His splendor. On this remarkable day, Jesus — rightly declaring Himself the "King of kings and Lord of lords (*see* Revelation 19:16) — entered that desolate cave, unveiling a vision of Himself to John more profound than he had ever experienced.

As previously mentioned, John was about 92 years old when he experienced this divine encounter that transcended anything he had known before. This revelation surpassed all previous insights and experiences he had accumulated in all the previous years of his life. In the solitude of that cave, John beheld Jesus in a manner that was unparalleled, and it altered his understanding entirely. Although he recalled Jesus' face and voice from earlier years and remembered resting against Him during the Last Supper, the revelation of Christ now before him was magnificent beyond any previous memory.

John was so empowered by the Spirit that he outlived Emperor Domitian, and he was released from Patmos. John traveled back to Ephesus, where, despite being in the senior years of his life — well into his mid-90s — he resumed his role as a spiritual leader for the burgeoning churches of Asia.

It was during his most senior years, after his amnesty from Patmos, that he took up his quill to compose the gospel of John, as well as the epistles of First, Second, and Third John and the book of Revelation. Defying the expectations of age and refusing to move into obscurity, John poured his Spirit-inspired words onto parchment. Some scholars believe he continued to be a vibrant force in his ministry until he reached the age of 105 or 106.

## THERE'S AN ANOINTING FOR YOUR DECADES

John serves as a remarkable illustration of how certain anointings, insights, and revelations are reserved for the more seasoned chapters of our lives. Each decade ushers in new experiences, revelations, and spiritual empowerments. It's crucial that we embrace longevity with determination, eager to uncover those truths and the wisdom earmarked for our more senior years. As we journey through our 60s, 70s, 80s, and beyond, each year and decade unveils distinct new insights and revelations. Personally, I've witnessed with each passing year as

I get older that I am able to see with clarity and perspective what was elusive in my younger years. I look forward to what additional years of walking with God will enable me to better see in the time to come.

Had John's life ended sooner, he would have missed the revelation he encountered in that cave on Patmos. And his post-Patmos years blossomed with such abundance that had his life come to a close there, the most fruitful chapter of his ministry might have remained unwritten. But John lived long and strong all the way to the end of his life. In his most senior years, he gained revelation and entered an unparalleled season of productivity. He flourished in ministry until, possibly at 106, he finally passed from this life and went to Heaven.

Let's face it, as an elderly gentleman residing on Patmos, nestled in a less-than-cozy cave amidst rather harsh climatic conditions, there must have been moments when John felt the twinges and pangs of his advancing years and challenging environment. It would have been easy for him to cry out, "Lord, I am old and weary, ready to depart this earthly life and to look upon Your face. Please, free me from these bleak surroundings and let me come home to Heaven."

Yet John adopted the steadfast resolve of a true warrior, he firmly resisted the burdens he felt, and he outlasted his adversaries and returned to the fullness of his ministry once he was granted amnesty at the time of Domitian's death. And when he returned to Ephesus, he returned as a man filled with new revelation that he set himself to impart to others.

I want you to understand that as we age, we may feel aches and pains related to age, but we are more prepared to receive greater insight and revelation. The fact is, God has great things waiting for you in the days and years ahead — but you must reach those days and years before you'll be ready to receive them. So don't grow weary, give up, and die prematurely. Let John be your example to stay physically fit, spiritually vibrant, and on track with God's Word and His Spirit.

*Again, the best is yet to come!*

## MAKE IT YOUR GOAL TO LIVE AND DIE IN GOOD HEALTH

After reading the stories of biblical characters who lived long and strong and were productive in their senior years, you might find yourself thinking, *Sure, those were legendary figures from the Bible, and here I am just an ordinary person wrestling with the physical and mental challenges that accompany aging.*

I'm not ignoring the reality of aging, nor the challenging transitions it often entails. However, instead of conceding defeat, choose to harness your faith to defy the odds, committing to be as vibrant and industrious as possible while you have breath in your body. Remember, the biblical figures we've learned about each had to decide between yielding to death and to circumstances and pressing toward fruitful productivity in their later years. Every Bible character we studied in this chapter faced choices to surrender to death and to circumstances or to keep pressing on toward longevity and late-life productivity.

I encourage you to strive to live in such a way that when it's time for your final farewell, those who've journeyed with you will exclaim, "Their life was a testament to the truth of God's Word! They were active, vibrant, and productive to the very end. Much like Moses, they were strong and sharp to the very end."

*That kind of testimony gives glory to God!*

Scan the QR code to watch Rick teach more on this subject.

## QUESTIONS TO PONDER AND DISCUSS

1. Have you ever viewed the upkeep and care of your body in the same light as maintaining your house or apartment or your automobile? There's a principle of stewardship at work here — what you expend time, money, effort, and energy on to nurture and maintain will generally last longer and bring you joy and reward. Explain why the care of your spiritual, physical, mental, and emotional health and well-being honors God — and why it *dis*honors Him to neglect this responsibility. First Corinthians 6:19-20 says, "...Know ye not that your body is the temple of the Holy Ghost which is in you, which ye have of God, and ye are not your own? For ye are bought with a price: therefore glorify God in your body, and in your spirit, which are God's." Can you recall another Bible verse that deals with this subject?

2. Have you ever lived from "miracle-to-miracle," constantly praying for God to intervene in your circumstances because of instability in some area of your life? Perhaps your situation was caused by someone else, or maybe it was your own indiscretion that brought on your troubles. Rehearse one incident of God's faithfulness to rescue you and the ways you transformed to bring more stability and peace to your life afterward. If you're in that situation right now, be assured God will be merciful again — but as you envision yourself on the other side of your trouble, write down things you can change to avoid revisiting that situation, or a similar situation, in the future.

3. Are you at a place in life where you're simply looking for things to do to avoid monotony — or do you burn with vision from God for this season of your life? What vision or passion from your earlier years lies dormant that you might need to stir up? If you can't think of anything, be assured that as long as you're alive, God isn't finished with you yet. Ask Him to show you the next steps in His plan for your life and write down your impressions to share with a loved one — a family member, a close friend, or a seasoned believer you trust.

4. Of all the Bible patriarchs in this chapter who lived "long and strong" — Enoch, Noah, Abraham, Moses, Caleb, Daniel, and John — which one were you most intrigued by and why? Which one resonated most with you — what things do you have in common with that Bible figure? Think about it: God has written a book about *your* life (*see* Psalm 139:16). Just as these men in Bible history were real people who faced real struggles and trials of their faith, yet they overcame — God is expecting you to "make history" and bring change to your life, family, *and generations* through your own journey of faith.

5. Do you have any goals for how you'll age and what you'll accomplish in God's plan for your life over the next decade? What are they? Write them down, as well as any ideas or thoughts that come to mind as steps you'll take and how you'll get them done. (For example: "I'll work out 3-4 days a week for 30-40 minutes"; "I'll walk 3-5 miles per week"; "I'll schedule checkups with my primary-care provider and a nutritionist, naturopathic provider, or integrative-medicine specialist"; "I'll attend certain social activities at my church"; "I'll visit nursing-home residents or the homebound"; "I'll contact family and friends I've lost touch with"; "I'll start that project that has been on my heart, and I'll spend 3-5 hours per week on it until it's done." Write it all out prayerfully, big things and small things — the possibilities are endless!)

# FOURTEEN

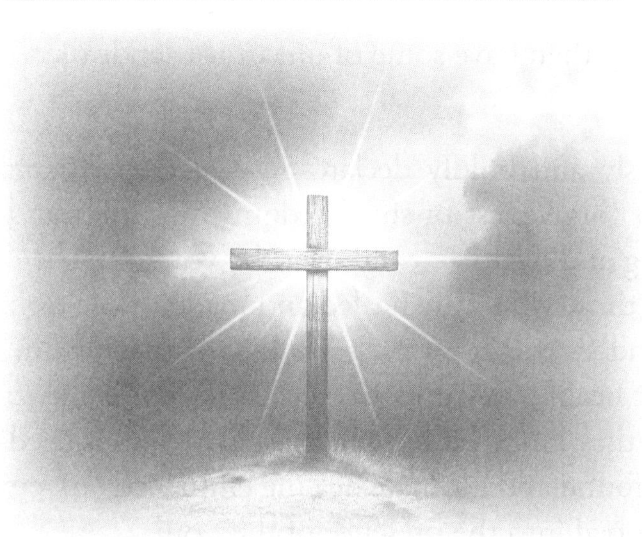

# HEALING IN HEAVEN — UNLESS JESUS COMES FIRST, EVERYONE WILL DIE

In the Introduction to this book, I shared how our ministry is blessed with the opportunity to receive countless prayer requests, many of which come from individuals seeking healing for themselves or for loved ones or friends. In response to our faith-filled prayers of agreement with them, we regularly hear from people who reach out again to let us know they (or those they know and love) received healing or grew progressively better after we prayed with them. Oh, how we love to hear those praise reports!

But there are others with whom we agreed in prayer for healing who are still waiting for the answer to come, and in some cases those individuals have waited so long that it seems to them as if the answer is endlessly delayed. As I also explained in the Introduction, in recent years, some of the most faithful church members in our congregation in Moscow fell ill and then passed away as a result. This loss led some to ask the question: "If Jesus has paid the price for our well-being, why then have some of our dear friends died because of disease and sickness?"

Let me joyously and boldly declare once again that Christ has paid the ultimate price for forgiveness of sin, freedom from guilt and shame, peace of mind, and healing and health — and over the years, we have received *reams* of testimonies from those who were healed and made whole from various kinds of disease, illness, and sickness. Yet there have been those who, despite believing in the promise of healing, left this world before their time. In such moments, while the healing they longed for might not have been realized as they no doubt envisioned, a profound and ultimate healing embraced and enveloped them the moment they stepped into the presence of the Lord.

Such was the story of a cherished member of our congregation, a devoted wife, mother, and a faithful assistant to Denise in her expansive outreach to Russian-speaking women. This precious woman was like a daughter to Denise, so when she was diagnosed with an aggressive form of cancer, Denise stood firmly in faith with her for healing. However, it wasn't long before the cancer spread to various parts of her body. Astonishingly, against all odds, the tide turned, the doctor declared her free of cancer, and we watched her regain strength, weight, and carry on joyfully and victoriously.

However, the cancer later resurfaced, and after a prolonged battle against it, a day came when she closed her eyes and was ushered into the presence of the Lord. When she died, there was a sense of loss, but it was also a victory to know that her battle with cancer was finished, and at long last, she was healed and made whole in Heaven.

Naturally, people asked, "She fought so bravely — why, then, did she not see her healing fully realized?" I cannot answer why she didn't receive the manifestation of healing on Earth, but now that she is in Heaven, I am certain she knows the answer to that question. But what is glorious is that the instant her spirit departed from her physical body, she was transported into the Lord's presence where she now has a wholeness far greater than we can even begin to imagine. She can now fully comprehend Paul's words in Philippians 1:21 that "to die is gain" and in Philippians 1:24 that to "depart, and to be with Christ, is far better."

The instant this woman transitioned from this world into the radiant presence of the Lord, every trace of cancer vanished as if it had never existed. In Heaven, ailments, calamity, disabilities, handicaps, heartbreak, and sickness of any sort is nonexistent. In Heaven, even before our spirits are reunited with our bodies in the resurrection, we are immediately made whole — thus, the reason this chapter is titled "Healing in Heaven." I want you to know the Bible teaches that even when it may seem that a battle is lost in this realm, it transforms into triumph the very moment one enters Heaven.

For this reason, believers can look into the face of death with a bold expectancy for what awaits beyond the veil. Death, far from being an end, acts as the gateway into a magnificent future. With this understanding, we can approach our departure from this earthly life with unwavering confidence, courage, profound peace, and triumphant victory. In the pages in this chapter, you will discover that for a Christian, death is a "portal" into the presence of the Lord. While no one wants to pass that threshold prematurely, upon crossing it, we are liberated from the effects of corruption and are instantly brought into a glorious state of complete wholeness.

But the truth is that death is a reality people try to avoid — to the point that the words "died" and "death" have almost disappeared from many people's vernacular. Terms like "died" and "dead" have become replaced by more gentle expressions like "passed" or "passed away."

The stark finality of the word "death" prompts many to sidestep it, finding comfort in the more palatable phrasing "passed away." But despite our linguistic gymnastics, the reality remains unchanged that each person eventually transitions from this earthly stage (dies) into some future eternal home.

If Jesus doesn't comes in our respective lifetimes for the rapture of His Church, we will all physically die. We long for the rapture of the Church, and it is possible that we may be the generation who escapes death as we are caught up to meet the Lord in the air. However, if this event does not happen in our lifetime, it means a funeral lies in our future.

A day will come when each of us, if typically buried, will be laid to rest in a coffin. Family and friends will come to our funeral service, the casket lid will be closed for the last time, we will be lowered into a grave that will be covered with dirt, and grass will eventually grow on top of it. This is the universal fate we all shall share, unless we are blessed to experience Christ's glorious return for the Church within our lifetime.

## THE FLEETING NATURE OF LIFE

Coming to grips with mortality is something that Christians should be able to do better than anyone else. But what is so glorious that I want you to see is that the moment we pass into Heaven, we arrive there completely whole.

James, who was the senior leader of the Church in Jerusalem, pondered life's transient quality in his writings. In James 4:14, he asked, "...For what is your life? It is even a vapour, that appeareth for a little time, and then vanisheth away."

James likened our physical existence to a "vapor." The word "vapor" is translated from the Greek word *atmis*, which was employed by thinkers like Aristotle, Herodotus, and Plato to convey *the ephemeral nature of a breath, a fleeting mist, a wisp of steam*, or *a transient vapor.* By invoking this imagery, James aimed to remind his audience, ourselves included, that our lives are merely a fleeting moment, a short-lived blink in the vastness of time.

James added that our earthly existence "appeareth" for a brief moment before fading into history. The term "appeareth" is derived from the Greek word *phaino*, which means *to emerge*, *to radiate*, or *to become seen*. On one hand, this choice of word serves as a reminder that our lives are meant *to shine brightly*, *radiate*, and to leave an impression on the world around us. But it conversely reminds us that even the most luminous life will eventually cease. No lighted candle burns forever. In fact, James noted that each person's time eventually evaporates "like a vapor" or mist. No matter how lengthy or impactful one's life may be, it is a short glimmer in the context of time immemorial.

That's why James elaborated with the phrase "for a little time" that our existence is as fleeting as a moment. In Greek, the word *oligos* is used to capture this essence of anything that is *few in number*. Here it signifies a scant span of time — a handful of years, at most — emphasizing the brevity of our days. Essentially, it paints a picture of a brief chapter in a book or a swiftly closing window in the grand narrative of time. As Psalm 103:15-16 says, "As for man, his days are as grass: as a flower of the field, so he flourisheth. For the wind passeth over it, and it is gone; and the place thereof shall know it no more."

When we are younger, in some ways we live in an optical illusion. Because time passes slowly and a year feels like an eternity, those who are younger feel as if they will live forever. But as the years slip by, the mirage fades and reality reveals itself, showing life as a fleeting passage. In fact, James 4:14 observes that life's fleeting essence eventually leads to a moment when our existence simply "vanishes." James wrote, "…It is even a vapour, that appeareth for a little time, and then vanisheth away." The words "vanisheth away" are derived from the Greek word *aphanidzo*, which paints a picture of *something that was once visible but suddenly disappears from sight*.

James 4:14 in the *RIV* (*Renner Interpretive Version*) says:

> **…Let me ask you…this life of yours…what is it, really? Isn't it in reality a mere breath, mist, or passing vapor that becomes visible**

**only for a relatively brief time? And then —*poof*— it evaporates, passes from the scene, and is gone?**

In today's world, there's an endless fight against the march of time. People try to avoid aging, often seeking eternal youth through elixirs and the artful work of a surgeon's hands. While there is no fault in aspiring to preserve the visage of youth, the reality is that Father Time is a persistent artist. Eventually, silver strands weave their way into our hair, wrinkles etch stories on our faces, and once-thick hair may thin and disappear altogether.

To lead robust and extended lives, we must pay special heed to our skeletal and muscular systems, as they can lose their vigor without devoted care and targeted exercise. Keeping these crucial structures in top form allows us to preserve their vitality and ensure our enduring strength.

There are many age-related realities that eventually show up with age. But when it comes to growing older, despite one's best efforts to use cosmetic procedures, consume a nutritious diet, and engage in vigorous exercise, gravity inevitably has its way, and what once stood firm inevitably begins to droop. No matter how one attempts to dodge the passage of time, the reality is that everyone must eventually face the undeniable effects of aging.

James 1:11 likened every person's life to a blossoming flower that eventually wilts. He wrote, "For the sun is no sooner risen with a burning heat, but it withereth the grass, and the flower thereof falleth, and the grace of the fashion of it perisheth…" (James 1:11).

The words "burning heat" are derived from the Greek word *kauson*, which gives the imagery of *an intense, searing heat* that ultimately wilts plants. Meanwhile, the word "sun" comes from the Greek word *helios*, which pictures *the sun, its light, its warmth*, or metaphorically, *the zenith of the day's brilliance and heat*. As for "withereth," it traces back to a form of the Greek word *xeraino*, which signifies the process of *drying, parching, shriveling*, or *gradually fading away*.

The phrase "grass of the field" springs from the Greek word *chortos*, which encompasses the notions of *grass*, *hay*, *vegetation*, or *any kind of flower*, including one that flourishes in a meadow. Meanwhile, the word "flower" finds its roots in the Greek word *anthos*, vividly depicting *a radiant and blooming blossom*.

These words serve as a reminder that, similar to a magnificent flower in full bloom, human life on this side of the veil is intended to fully blossom and bloom; however, it is transient and "falleth" — it cannot last. The expression "falleth" is derived from the Greek word *ekpipto*, which means *to fall away* or *to fall off*, and it captures the moment when a flower's petals gently fall, one by one, to the ground, as its life draws to a close with the changing season.

The word "grace" is translated from the Greek word *euprepeia*, which captures the imagery of *a flower's exquisite form*. Meanwhile, the word "fashion" is derived from the Greek word *prosopon*, which is actually the word for *the face*. Although this verse speaks of the appearance of a flower, it metaphorically mirrors the transformation human aging brings, which is first subtly seen in one's face as he or she approaches the latter years of life. As time marches on, one's facial appearance begins to change, serving as a reminder that his or her earthly journey is drawing to a close, much like a blossom in the meadow gently yielding its fullness to the final passage of time, thus ending its last season.

The *RIV* (*Renner Interpretive Version*) of James 1:11 reads:

> **For just as the scorching heat of the sun eventually shrivels and wastes away the grass of the field, a time eventually comes when every blossoming flower wilts, and its lovely appearance comes to an end....**

As Christians, we should be able to gracefully face the truth that eventually every person takes a final bow and the curtain call of his life takes place for the last time. Even the most famous and notable people from the annals of history — Alexander the Great, Julius Caesar, Cleopatra, Herod the Great, and the succession of leaders across all the ages — ultimately bade this life farewell. No one is so great that he has escaped death, except for Jesus, who alone triumphed over death, never to die again.

## TO BE ABSENT FROM THE BODY IS TO BE PRESENT WITH THE LORD

But while we might attempt to dodge the truth of life's finality, escaping it is impossible unless you are alive and among those who will be raptured when Jesus comes back for the Church. Your inability to sidestep physical death as a believer will eventually transition you to your heavenly home with the Lord. However, for those who depart this life without Christ, there will come an eternal prospect in hell that is unimaginable.

When it comes to the passing of believers, Paul provided a comforting word in Second Corinthians 5:8, saying, "We are confident, I say, and willing rather to be absent from the body, and to be present with the Lord." In this passage, Paul employed the words "absent" and "present" to illustrate a Christian's experience following physical death. The word "absent" is derived from the Greek word *ekdemeo*, which is a compound of the words *ek* and *demos*. The word *ek* denotes *out*, and it is where we drive the word "exit." The word *demos* signifies *a comforting or familiar place*, like a physical home where one feels a sense of belonging. Thus, the word *ekdemeo*, translated here as "absent," conjures the image of *someone departing from their familiar home where they have always felt a sense of belonging.*

Through this choice of words, Paul conveyed that when a true believer passes away, he departs from his body, which was his temporary earthly dwelling. But Paul further explained that at the precise moment of death, an authentic Christian is instantaneously "present" with the Lord. The word "present" is a translation of the Greek word *endemeo*, a compound of the words *en* and *demos.* The word *en* means *in*, as in being "in" a specific location, while the word *demos*, once again, refers to *a dwelling place.* By selecting this specific word at this juncture, Paul expressed that upon dying in faith, a person's spirit leaves its earthly body — its former home — and immediately finds itself *in a new home* in the presence of the Lord.

Thus, Scripture unequivocally teaches that when a true Christian passes away, his spirit promptly leaves the physical form that housed it and is whisked away into the presence of the Lord. Although his mortal, corruptible body lies as an empty shell, his spirit finds its new home beside the Lord. In this sacred place, surrounded by a community of those faithful who have preceded him in death, he patiently awaits the glorious return of Jesus, when the Savior will resurrect his mortal body from the earth as a then glorious, immortal vessel — a wondrous event that will happen just prior to the Church's rapture.

At that time, there will be a miraculous reunion as the spirits of the faithful are joyously rejoined with their renewed, resurrected bodies. (I write about this in-depth in my book *The Rapture, the Antichrist, and the Tribulation — An End-Times Countdown and What Happens Next.*)

But regardless of the physical issues believers face on the earth, no affliction of any kind accompanies those who go to Heaven. These earth-bound physical and mental issues remain with the dead body when it is buried in the earth, and they disintegrate with the body as it perishes over time. Then one day in the future when Christ returns for the rapture of the Church and the resurrection of the righteous whose bodies lay buried, those bodies will be raised, miraculously changed, and reconnected with the spirits of the righteous. All these miraculous events will transpire at the moment of the resurrection of the bodies of the righteous dead and the glorious catching away of the Church (*see* 1 Thessalonians 4:15-17). But the instant the body dies, the human spirit is immediately in the presence of the Lord, and that is the moment he is instantly made complete and whole.

How could it be possible for anything that reeks of death or physical or mental defect to exist in the presence of the powerful, radiant, healing presence of God Almighty? Remember that when Jesus walked the earth, disease, illness, and sickness fled at His touch. Additionally, God is Light, and in Him is no darkness at all, so in Heaven — which is permeated with His all-consuming Light — it simply isn't possible for any hint of anything imperfect, dark, diseased, or misaligned to exist.

## EVENTUALLY THE TIME COMES TO SET SAIL AND BREAK CAMP

In his letter to the Philippians, Paul eloquently shared his perspective about death. In Philippians 1:23, he wrote, "For I am in a strait betwixt two, having a desire to depart, and to be with Christ; which is far better."

Notice that Paul described himself as caught in a "strait betwixt two." Here Paul used the Greek word *sunecho* to convey the sensation of being *pressed from opposing sides*. This term paints a picture of *a person being tugged back and forth*, much like a competitor in an intense game of tug-of-war, with arms stretched by the relentless pull of opponents.

Yet intriguingly, the Greek word implies that the person subjected to this tugging is the one who holds the power to decide the victor in this contest of forces. Paul grappled with two compelling desires vying for his heart. On one side, the allure of departing to be with Christ tugs at him earnestly, while on the other, he feels the tug to remain in his earthly life to complete the unfinished tasks of his ministry.

This compelling tug of Heaven is seen through Paul's words in verse 23 where he expressed a "desire to depart." The word "desire" originates from the Greek word *epithumia*, a compound the words *epi* and *thumos*. Here, the prefix *epi* is an intensifer, and the Greek word *thumos* speaks of an *intense passion*, often suggesting *a surging or burgeoning emotion*. But when these words are combined to form *epithumia*, the new word pictures *someone who is fervently passionate and utterly consumed* by a desire. Through his choice of words, Paul vividly conveyed the exhilarating notion of departing from this earthly realm to unite with the Lord. For Paul, the concept of death transcended the usual perception of life's conclusion; it was instead the expectation of a joyful departure, marking the beginning of the next chapter in his endless voyage.

The word "depart" is translated from the Greek word *analuo*, which pictures *the image of a ship gracefully unfurling from its dock, finally unshackled, and setting sail to journey to its final destination.* Thus, Paul imagined that when he shed the chains of earthly existence, he would finally set sail on a spiritual journey destined to carry him home to Heaven.

In his eyes, death wasn't an end, but a vibrant beginning — a new and thrilling chapter that lay before him. Eager and filled with excitement, he eagerly awaited for the moment that this departure would take place.

But hold on a moment — there's a deeper layer to the word *analuo* ("to depart") that's key to grasping this passage in Philippians 1:23, "For I am in a strait betwixt two, having a desire to depart, and to be with Christ; which is far better."

Historically, the word *analuo* wasn't just about leaving; it was a strategic term used by the military to describe the pivotal moment when troops broke down their camps, packed up their tents, gathered their gear, and set their sights on advancing to conquer new territory. This vivid metaphor sheds new light on how Paul envisioned the concept of death, turning it into a decision to leave past victories behind and to boldly march toward new horizons.

Having weathered countless earthly conflicts, Paul found himself eager to dismantle his earthly encampment and move onward and upward to Heaven. His heart, mind, and imagination were thoroughly enraptured by the promise of Heaven, and he felt an intense yearning to take leave of this world to join Christ — a longing so profound that he found himself caught in a "strait betwixt two." On one side, he felt a magnetic pull to set sail, break camp, and move onward and upward to be with Christ — but on the other side, he felt a tug with almost equal force to remain a little longer in life to fulfill tasks still unfinished.

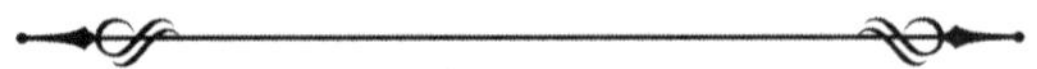

**For Paul, the concept of death transcended the usual perception of life's conclusion; it was instead the expectation of a joyful departure, marking the beginning of the next chapter in his endless voyage.**

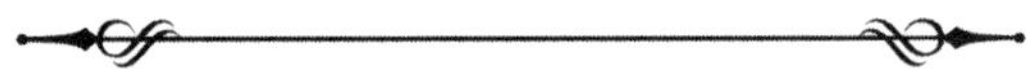

Even though Paul eagerly yearned to leave this earthly life and be united with Christ, he was conscious that his journey was not finished, and leaving at that juncture would mean abandoning his ministry while it was yet unfulfilled.

Despite his intense longing to fold up his earthly dwelling and set sail into the eternal embrace of the Lord, he realized in his heart that vital tasks still awaited him on the earth for the sake of the Kingdom. This conviction is why he expressed in verse 24, "Nevertheless to abide in the flesh is more needful for you."

## DEATH IS A DEPARTURE

Several years passed, and eventually Paul understood the moment had come to bid farewell to his earthly life. He had preached, taught, and eagerly anticipated the rapture of the Church, yet as he sat in prison and awaited his own execution, it seemed clear that he would lay down his life as a martyr for his faith before the rapture occurred.

With the day of his execution coming closer, he wrote these poignant words: "For I am now ready to be offered, and the time of my departure is at hand" (2 Timothy 4:6).

Let's be clear about what Paul meant when he spoke of being "offered" and about his "departure."

The word "offered" finds its roots in the Greek word *spendo*, which gives the imagery of a ritual of pouring out wine upon an altar during times of celebration. For Paul, who had devoted every breath to serving Christ since his conversion, his entire existence had symbolically flowed like a drink offering as he had lived his life dedicated wholly to his Lord.

But now, with his blood literally on the brink of being spilled out, Paul embraced this as a jubilant and festive occasion. He saw it as a an opportunity to present Christ with the ultimate and most profound sacrifice he could ever bestow. Rather than dwelling on the notion of loss, Paul turned his gaze to the joyous moment ahead — a final, supreme act of devotion to celebrate the depth of his offering.

The word "departure" is translated from the Greek word *analuo*, which is a form of the same word that we saw earlier in Philippians 1:23. This word pictures a ship that is poised to harness the wind for its journey toward a final harbor. Alternatively, it evokes an army's readiness to dismantle their camp, bundle up their gear, and advance toward unexplored horizons. Rather than viewing his death as the end, Paul embraced the notion of a "departure." For him, it wasn't an end, but an elevation, a moment to catch the winds of the Spirit and ascend. He was poised to take down the tents of his earthly life and move upward in the Lord's embrace.

Rather than being consumed by the dread of death, Paul embraced the prospect of leaving this world, eager for his encounter with the Lord. In Second Timothy 4:8, he expressed his anticipation, proclaiming, "Henceforth there is laid up for me a crown of righteousness, which the Lord, the righteous judge, shall give me at that day: and not to me only, but unto all them also that love his appearing."

Paul was acutely aware that his final moments were approaching rapidly, knowing that his beheading was close at hand. Yet instead of dwelling on how his life would end or fearing the sharp bite of the blade upon his neck, his spirit took flight toward the notion of "departure" — a *transition*, not an end.

Paul's death transpired following the calamitous Great Fire of Rome in July of 64 AD, yet before the curtain fell on Nero's reign in 68 AD. Clement I wrote that Paul "had borne his testimony before the rulers," and he "departed from the world and went unto the holy place, having been found a notable pattern of patient endurance."[1]

Meanwhile, Ignatius of Antioch chronicled that Paul met a martyr's fate. Tertullian noted that Paul was "crowned" as he made his departure from his earthly confines. Eusebius chronicled that Paul's death occurred during the Neronian persecutions. Sulpicius Severus stated that Paul was beheaded, and Lactantius testified that it was Nero's orders that ended Paul's life.

According to the writings of Jerome, Paul was martyred for his faith and was eventually laid to rest along the Ostian Way.[2] The site of his execution is believed to be at the *Abbey*, where, intriguingly, the very column upon which he was executed is safeguarded within the church there. After his execution, his devoted friends transported his remains to the Ostian Way. There, they buried Paul in a tomb belonging to a Roman woman by the name of Matrona Lucilla, and they erected a marker near the roadway in his memory. In the Fourth Century, the Emperor Constantine honored this site by constructing a church dedicated to Paul's sacrifice. Early in the Nineteenth Century, the magnificent Basilica of Saint Paul Outside the Walls was built on this site as a testament to Paul's legacy.[3]

An ancient Christian tradition recorded that the moment Paul faced his beheading, as he approached the site of his execution, he gazed upon the half column where his head would soon rest and where the soldier stood poised with the sword destined to sever his head from his body. Instead of retreating in dread, Paul, with a heart brimming with joy, rushed eagerly to the column, where he voluntarily placed his head upon it. He welcomed the blade as the final moment when he would be joined to Christ.

While others might have feared death, he embraced it with open arms. Remember, it was Paul who wrote in First Corinthians 15:54-55, "Death is swallowed up in victory. O death, where is thy sting? O grave, where is thy victory?"

## A STORY FROM MY YOUNGER YEARS

Let me tell you a story about an event in my young life that impacted me at an early age and helped me to form a serious approach to life. When it was time for me to get my first job as a junior high-schooler, I heard about a job opportunity at the nearby cemetery, a place not far from my family's home. The elderly caretaker was seeking a young hand to keep the cemetery grounds neatly mowed.

I ambled over to the cemetery and knocked on his door. When the door opened, I mustered my courage and said, "Good day, sir. I've heard there's a position available here, and I'd like to be considered." The caretaker gave me a thoughtful once-over and posed a few probing questions. Satisfied with my responses, he nodded and instructed me to commence work the following Monday. Thus began a chapter that would influence the story of my life.

The following Monday afternoon marked the beginning of my brief stint at the local graveyard — a milestone, as it was my first real job. Each day, as soon as the final school bell rang, I'd sprint down the hallway, tuck my textbooks into my locker, and make a beeline across town to the cemetery. Once there, I'd grab hold of the lawnmower and set off on my daily quest to maneuver it across the seemingly endless green expanses of the cemetery that awaited grooming. Five days a week, I found myself living and working among the dead!

Every day, I guided my mower and trimmer around both fresh and older tombstones, tending to the weeds that grew perpetually around the gravestones and mausoleums. I particularly liked the oldest part of the cemetery where the limestone markers stood as silent, indecipherable witnesses to forgotten lives. When it was time to welcome another body to a final resting place in that cemetery, I was there, and played my part in setting up a tent that loved ones stood under during gravesite rites, and then later I helped take it down. I was on-site to help dig the grave, and I helped gently lower the casket into the earth before it was covered with layers of dirt.

When the flowers wilted that loved ones had placed on the graves, I was the one who gathered up the dead flowers and threw them away. My job was to keep up the neat appearance of that cemetery, working among the dead day after day. Yet those days spent amidst tombstones had a profound impact on my youthful years. It was as if God used that time to prompt deep reflections within me about the gravity and fleetingness of life itself and to question what legacy my own life might bequeath once I "set sail" and "broke camp" in my own journey.

During my tenure at the cemetery as a teenager, I encountered countless graveside ceremonies, each marked by a unique demonstration of human emotion in the face of death. For those without the comfort of salvation or the assurance of a secure eternity, these moments overflowed with raw, unrestrained sorrow.

In stark contrast, I noticed a prevailing sense of peace among those who knew Christ and were convinced of the eternity in Heaven for the deceased. Believe me when I tell you that there is a vast emotional difference in response to death for the saved and unsaved. Those who know Christ have hope, but those without Christ are plunged into a chasm of despair when a loved one or friend dies.

As I'm sure is true with you, Denise and I have found ourselves bidding farewell to cherished grandparents, parents, close friends, and beloved ones. As we've gazed upon their faces one last time as they lay in their caskets, we have found comfort in the promise of James 2:26 that says "the body without the spirit is dead" and in Second Corinthians 5:8 that reassures us that when an authentic believer is "absent from the body," he is "present with the Lord." Thus, the body that lies in the casket is but an empty shell, a former home, for the deceased, who now basks in the presence of the Lord in Heaven.

Regardless of what contributed to their deaths, whether it was the slow wane of age or the swift touch of illness, we hold fast to the faith that at the moment of passing, their physical issues were exchanged for wholeness. We know that the moment they pass into the presence of the Lord, they are healed and made whole beyond what this world can offer.

We may wonder why some were not healed here on earth, but we are assured that in the presence of the Lord, they now hold the answer. And we are assured that if we need to know the answer, one day the Lord will see to it that we know it too. But rather than give up the fight because healing comes to us immediately in Heaven, our task is to fight the good fight of faith to the end.

Our faith remains unshaken in the full redemptive work of Christ that includes forgiveness of sin, freedom from guilt and shame, peace of mind, and healing and health. Each premature or even timely death only fans the flames of our dedication to spread these truths and help others to renew their minds to the blessings Christ has bestowed upon us.

Rather than throw in the towel and surrender, we are even more determined to do our best to help others to deal with every issue — visible or hidden — to make sure they are not hindered from receiving what Christ died for them to receive.

## EVERYONE'S EARTHLY JOURNEY COMES TO A FINAL CONCLUSION

No matter how diligently someone tends to his well-being, there comes a time when he gracefully reaches a ripe old age that signals his journey's conclusion. It's often amusing to me how surprised we are when an elderly person departs this world. I find myself pondering, *Did we believe they would outlast time itself?* They journeyed through the seasons of life with strength and grace, and left behind an example of a life well-lived for us to celebrate. The truth, however, remains unchanged that regardless of our efforts to nurture our health and extend our days, unless the Lord comes in our lifetime, each of us will inevitably leave this realm to the enter the next.

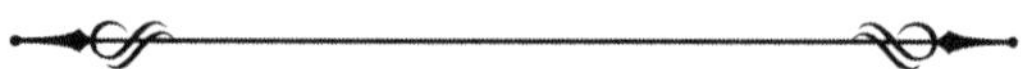

**Regardless of what contributed to their deaths, whether it was the slow wane of age or the swift touch of illness, we hold fast to the faith that at the moment of passing, their physical issues were exchanged for wholeness.**

That even includes extraordinary individuals who had great healing and miracle ministries, like Kathryn Kuhlman, Kenneth E. Hagin, and Oral Roberts, whom I mentioned in the first chapter of this book as having a profound influence on my life. These spiritual giants, as transformative as their earthly ministries were, are now in Heaven, eagerly anticipating the glorious return of Jesus when they will accompany Him for the resurrection of the saints and the rapture of the Church. At that moment, their earthly bodies that lay in their graves — along with those of all the righteous dead — will be miraculously raised, transformed, and reunited with their spirits. *But right now...*

- The body of Kathryn Kuhlman, a vessel that God mightily used to bring divine healing to countless lives, is buried at Forest Lawn Memorial Park Cemetery in Glendale, California.
- The body of Oral Roberts, a man of faith and power that God used to bring healing to an entire generation, who founded the university that bears his name, and whose life and ministry dramatically influenced the modern Church, is buried in Tulsa's Memorial Park Cemetery.
- The body of Kenneth E. Hagin, a man that God healed and raised up to teach faith to an entire generation and whose ministry bears

his name, is buried at Floral Haven Cemetery in Broken Arrow, Oklahoma.

I emphasize their names alone because each of them imprinted an unforgettable legacy on my life. They each were mighty instruments through which God's healing power touched countless lives. These remarkable individuals, who were used by God in immense spiritual power, have since stepped into Heaven.

But a time is swiftly approaching when both the righteous dead and the living will be roused by a mighty shout and the triumphant sound of a trumpet, and the dead will be raised, the living will be caught up, and all of them will be miraculously transformed — a miracle surpassing even the greatest miracles achieved through their extraordinary ministries!

If you are among those who know someone who lost a battle to disease, illness, sickness, and you've asked, "If Jesus has paid the price for our well-being, why then have some of our dear friends died because of disease and sickness?" I want to again joyously and boldly declare once again that Christ has paid the ultimate price for forgiveness of sin, freedom from guilt and shame, peace of mind, and healing and health.

If you know someone who was believing for a healing but left this world before his or her time, the healing that person longed for was manifested the moment he or she stepped into the presence of the Lord.

**Rather than throw in the towel and surrender, we are even more determined to do our best to help others to deal with every issue — visible or hidden — to make sure they are not hindered from receiving what Christ died for them to receive.**

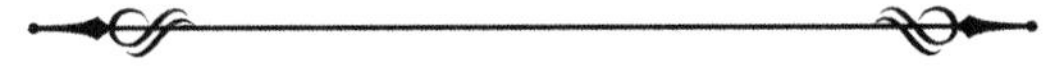

But now, it is time to reinforce your faith in the truth and to commit yourself wholeheartedly to helping others receive the profound gifts that Jesus secured for them through His sacrifice on the Cross. Do not allow setbacks to hinder your journey or that of your companions. Remember, the adversary would rejoice at your surrender, hoping you'd abandon your faith. Yet this is your cue to stand resolutely and commit to ushering others toward the blessings Jesus intended for them to claim. Embrace this opportunity to grab hold of God's promises for yourself and to help others grasp the inheritance bestowed through Christ's selfless redemptive act.

In the next, final chapter, I want to present you with a wide array of scriptures that we've explored throughout this book, but from a multitude of translations and interpretations. I trust that these verses, in their diverse translations, will become mighty tools in your defense against disease, illness, and sickness. So let's journey to the final chapter, where I want to load you with scriptural ammunition. With these, you'll be able to shoot down the enemy when he tries to threaten your physical or mental well-being or the well-being of those you know and love.

Scan the QR code to watch Rick teach more on this subject.

# QUESTIONS TO PONDER AND DISCUSS

1. Jesus paid a great price for us to walk in the benefits of our redemption — reconciliation to the Father and well-being in spirit, soul, and body, to name a few. What have you read in this book that has solidified your faith in God's eternal Word and His integrity and faithfulness? No matter what happens in the world around you, the just shall live by the faith that works by love and that pleases God, who rewards our faith — and our faith is the victory that overcomes the world (*see* Romans 3:17; Galatians 3:11; 5:6; Hebrews 10:38; 11:6; 1 John 5:4).

2. What is one of your favorite verses on healing that you rehearse over and over again that is really "in" you? What verse did you read in this chapter about Heaven and our departure to be with Christ that excites you about the life to come? It's important never to fear death, but to view it correctly, in light of the Word of God and eternity — so you can determine to run your race well here on Earth and look forward to Heaven's rewards.

3. Rather than throw in the towel and surrender to an early death — a premature departure — we should be determined to deal with every issue, visible or invisible, to make sure we're not hindered from receiving what Christ died for us to receive. And we should determine to help others do the same. Can you think of someone who needs to hear that God wants him to overcome his challenge and do the will of God, bringing glory to His name? How will you encourage that person after reading this book?

4. Do you know someone who lost his or her battle on Earth and left this life early to be with Christ in Heaven? If that person was saved, he didn't lose the battle ultimately, because for the believer, the Bible says, "O death, where is thy sting? O grave, where is thy victory?" (1 Corinthians 15:55). Does it comfort you to know that person is completely restored and full of life and light in the presence of the Lord — and that all the answers to any question

that can be asked are fully known and understood by him or her? How would you console someone else who has lost a loved one to death?

5. Of the New Testament verses listed in the first question about walking by faith, which one is most meaningful to you? In what areas are you expecting God to reward your faith?

# FIFTEEN

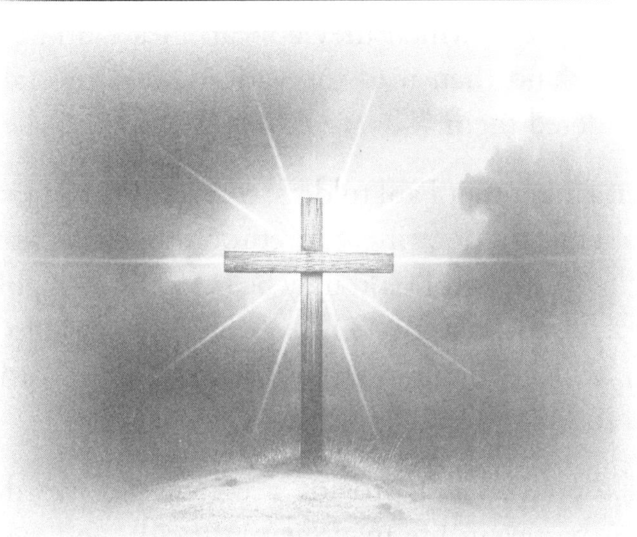

# SCRIPTURES ON DIVINE HEALING IN VARIOUS TRANSLATIONS

In the concluding chapter of this book, my aim is to present you with various interpretations of key verses that we have covered throughout the previous pages. Crafting such a chapter demands a significant investment of time and effort, and we have done our utmost to spare you any additional toil by compiling it for you. It is my hope that these passages reinforce the themes and insights I shared in previous chapters.

I want to express how profoundly grateful I am to Dr. Chip Beaulieu for his thoroughly researched work *Our Healing Covenant*.[1] His remarkable book has been a personal resource for me and one that I highly recommend to you. I am thankful to Dr. Beaulieu for generously permitting me to incorporate some of his compilation of healing scriptures in this chapter.

The following verses are listed according to the chronological appearance of the books of the Bible in which they appear. Please find the verse you wish to study more deeply and then read the various ways several interpreters and translators have rendered them.

As you read, remember that Paul told us, "All scripture is given by inspiration of God, and is profitable for doctrine, for reproof, for correction, for instruction in righteousness: that the man of God may be perfect, throughly furnished unto all good works" (2 Timothy 3:16-17). Let these verses help you renew your mind to the truth, which will allow the power of God's Word to wholly equip and empower you to valiantly wage the noble battle of faith.

At the end of the chapter, I provide a concluding word and a reminder that, although your battles in life may seem difficult, and even unwinnable at times, God's desire for you is unchanging — that you walk healed, healthy, and prosperous in life to His honor and glory. *And He is rooting for you!* He's on your side, and He is a present help when you call on Him in faith to meet your every need.

### Genesis 2:15

**[KJV]** And the Lord God took the man, and put him into the garden of Eden to dress it and to keep it.

**[AMPC]** And the Lord God took the man and put him in the Garden of Eden to tend and guard *and* keep it.

**[CEB]** The Lord God took the human and settled him in the garden of Eden to farm it and to take care of it.

**[CSB]** The Lord God took the man and placed him in the garden of Eden to work it and watch over it.

**[DARBY]** And Jehovah Elohim took Man, and put him into the garden of Eden, to till it and to guard it.

**[GNT]** Then the Lord God placed the man in the Garden of Eden to cultivate it and guard it.

**[NET]** The Lord God took the man and placed him in the orchard in Eden to care for it and to maintain it.

**[NIV]** The Lord God took the man and put him in the Garden of Eden to work it and take care of it.

### Genesis 3:17

**[KJV]** And unto Adam he said, Because thou hast hearkened unto the voice of thy wife, and hast eaten of the tree, of which I commanded thee, saying, Thou shalt not eat of it: cursed is the ground for thy sake; in sorrow shalt thou eat of it all the days of thy life.

**[CEB]** To the man he said, "Because you listened to your wife's voice and you ate from the tree that I commanded, 'Don't eat from it,' cursed is the fertile land because of you; in pain you will eat from it every day of your life."

**[CJB]** To Adam he said, "Because you listened to what your wife said and ate from the tree about which I gave you the order, 'You are not to eat from it,' the ground is cursed on your account; you will work hard to eat from it as long as you live."

**[CSB]** And he said to the man, "Because you listened to your wife and ate from the tree about which I commanded you, 'Do not eat from it': The ground is cursed because of you. You will eat from it by means of painful labor all the days of your life."

**[GNT]** And he said to the man, "You listened to your wife and ate the fruit which I told you not to eat. Because of what you have done, the ground will be under a curse. You will have to work hard all your life to make it produce enough food for you."

**[NIV]** To Adam he said, "Because you listened to your wife and ate fruit from the tree about which I commanded you, 'You must not eat from it,' Cursed is the ground because of you; through painful toil you will eat food from it all the days of your life."

## Exodus 20:7

**[KJV]** Thou shalt not take the name of the Lord thy God in vain; for the Lord will not hold him guiltless that taketh his name in vain.

**[AMPC]** You shall not use *or* repeat the name of the Lord your God in vain [that is, lightly or frivolously, in false affirmations or profanely]; for the Lord will not hold him guiltless who takes His name in vain.

**[CEB]** Do not use the Lord your God's name as if it were of no significance; the Lord won't forgive anyone who uses his name that way.

**[ERV]** You must not use the name of the Lord your God to make empty promises. If you do, the Lord will not let you go unpunished.

**[GNT]** Do not use my name for evil purposes, for I, the Lord your God, will punish anyone who misuses my name.

**[NLT]** You must not misuse the name of the Lord your God. The Lord will not let you go unpunished if you misuse his name.

**[WEB]** You shall not misuse the name of Yahweh your God, for Yahweh will not hold him guiltless who misuses his name.

## Exodus 20:12

**[KJV]** Honour thy father and thy mother: that thy days may be long upon the land which the Lord thy God giveth thee.

**[AMPC]** Regard (treat with honor, due obedience, and courtesy) your father and mother, that your days may be long in the land the Lord your God gives you.

**[CEB]** Honor your father and your mother so that your life will be long on the fertile land that the Lord your God is giving you.

**[ERV]** "You must honor and respect your father and your mother. Do this so that you will have a full life in the land that the Lord your God gives you."

**[GNT]** "Respect your father and your mother, so that you may live a long time in the land that I am giving you."

**[NLT]** "Honor your father and mother. Then you will live a long, full life in the land the Lord your God is giving you."

## Deuteronomy 4:40

**[KJV]** Thou shalt keep therefore his statutes, and his commandments, which I command thee this day, that it may go well with thee, and with thy children after thee, and that thou mayest prolong thy days upon the earth, which the Lord thy God giveth thee, for ever.

**[CEB]** Keep the Lord's regulations and his commandments. I'm commanding them to you today for your well-being and for the well-being of your children after you, so that you may extend your time on the fertile land that the Lord your God is giving you forever.

**[CEV]** Today I am explaining his laws and teachings. And if you always obey them, you and your descendants will live long and be successful in the land the Lord is giving you.

**[ERV]** "And you must obey his laws and commands that I give you today. Then everything will go well with you and your children who live after you. And you will live a long time in the land the Lord your God is giving you—it will be yours forever."

**[GNT]** "Obey all his laws that I have given you today, and all will go well with you and your descendants. You will continue to live in the land that the Lord your God is giving you to be yours forever."

**[NET]** "Keep his statutes and commandments that I am setting forth today so that it may go well with you and your descendants and that you may enjoy longevity in the land that the Lord your God is about to give you as a permanent possession."

**[NLT]** "If you obey all the decrees and commands I am giving you today, all will be well with you and your children. I am giving you these instructions so you will enjoy a long life in the land the Lord your God is giving you for all time."

## Deuteronomy 5:33

**[KJV]** Ye shall walk in all the ways which the Lord your God hath commanded you, that ye may live, and that it may be well with you, and that ye may prolong your days in the land which ye shall possess.

**[CEB]** You must walk the precise path that the Lord your God indicates for you so that you will live, and so that things will go well for you, and so you will extend your time on the land that you will possess.

**[CSB]** Follow the whole instruction the Lord your God has commanded you, so that you may live, prosper, and have a long life in the land you will possess.

**[ERV]** You must live the way the Lord your God commanded you. Then you will continue to live, and everything will be fine with you. You will live a long life in the land that will belong to you.

**[GNT]** Obey them all, so that everything will go well with you and so that you will continue to live in the land that you are going to occupy.

**[GW]** Follow all the directions the Lord your God has given you. Then you will continue to live, life will go well for you, and you will live for a long time in the land that you are going to possess.

**[NIV]** Walk in obedience to all that the Lord your God has commanded you, so that you may live and prosper and prolong your days in the land that you will possess.

**[NLT]** Stay on the path that the Lord your God has commanded you to follow. Then you will live long and prosperous lives in the land you are about to enter and occupy.

### Deuteronomy 6:1-2

**[KJV]** Now these are the commandments, the statutes, and the judgments, which the Lord your God commanded to teach you, that ye might do them in the land whither ye go to possess it: That thou mightest fear the Lord thy God, to keep all his statutes and his commandments, which I command thee, thou, and thy son, and thy son's son, all the days of thy life; and that thy days may be prolonged.

**[CEB]** Now these are the commandments, the regulations, and the case laws that the Lord your God commanded me to teach you to follow in the land you are entering to possess, so that you will fear the Lord your God by keeping all his regulations and his commandments that I am commanding you—both you and your sons and daughters—all the days of your life and so that you will lengthen your life.

**[CEV]** The Lord told me to give you these laws and teachings, so you can obey them in the land he is giving you. Soon you will cross the Jordan River and take that land. And if you and your descendants want to live a long time, you must always worship the Lord and obey his laws.

**[ERV]** "These are the commands, the laws, and the rules that the Lord your God told me to teach you. Obey these laws in the land that you are entering to live in. You and your descendants must respect the Lord your God as long as you live. You must obey all his laws and commands that I give you. If you do this, you will have a long life in that new land."

**[GNT]** "These are all the laws that the Lord your God commanded me to teach you. Obey them in the land that you are about to enter and occupy. As long as you live, you and your descendants are to honor the Lord your God and obey all his laws that I am giving you, so that you may live in that land a long time."

**[NLT]** "These are the commands, decrees, and regulations that the Lord your God commanded me to teach you. You must obey them in the land you are about to enter and occupy, and you and your children and grandchildren must fear the Lord your God as long as you live. If you obey all his decrees and commands, you will enjoy a long life."

### Deuteronomy 30:19-20

**[KJV]** I call heaven and earth to record this day against you, that I have set before you life and death, blessing and cursing: therefore choose life, that both thou and thy seed may live. That thou mayest love the Lord thy God, and that thou mayest obey his voice, and that thou mayest cleave unto him: for he is thy life, and the length of thy days: that thou mayest dwell in the land which the Lord sware unto thy fathers, to Abraham, to Isaac, and to Jacob, to give them.

**[ERV]** "Today I am giving you a choice of two ways. And I ask heaven and earth to be witnesses of your choice. You can choose life or death. The first choice will bring a blessing. The other choice will bring a curse. So choose life! Then you and your children will live. You must love the Lord your God and obey him. Never leave him, because he is your life. And he will give you a long life in the land that he, the Lord, promised to give to your ancestors—Abraham, Isaac, and Jacob."

**[GNT]** I am now giving you the choice between life and death, between God's blessing and God's curse, and I call heaven and earth to witness the choice you make. Choose life. Love the Lord your God, obey him and be faithful to him, and then you and your descendants will live long in the land that he promised to give your ancestors, Abraham, Isaac, and Jacob.

†**[Knox]** I call heaven and earth to witness this day that I have set such a choice before thee, life or death, a blessing or a curse. Wilt thou not choose life, long life for thyself and for those that come after thee? Wilt thou not learn to love the Lord thy God, and obey him, and keep close to his side? Thou hast no life, no hope of long continuance, but in him; shall not the land which he promised as a gift to thy fathers, Abraham, Isaac and Jacob, be thine to dwell in?

**[NLT]** "Today I have given you the choice between life and death, between blessings and curses. Now I call on heaven and earth to witness the choice you make. Oh, that you would choose life, so that you and your descendants might live! You can make this choice by loving the Lord your God, obeying him, and committing yourself firmly to him. This is the key to your life. And if you love and obey the Lord, you will live long in the land the Lord swore to give your ancestors Abraham, Isaac, and Jacob."

## 1 Kings 3:14

**[KJV]** And if thou wilt walk in my ways, to keep my statutes and my commandments, as thy father David did walk, then I will lengthen thy days.

**[CEB]** "And if you walk in my ways and obey my laws and commands, just as your father David did, then I will give you a very long life."

**[CEV]** If you obey me and follow my commands, as your father David did, I'll let you live a long time.

**[ERV]** "And I will give you a long life if you follow me and obey my laws and commands as your father David did."

**[ISV]** "If you will live life my way, keeping my statutes and my commands, just like your father David did, I'll also increase the length of your life."

**[NET]** "If you follow my instructions by obeying my rules and regulations, just as your father David did, then I will grant you long life."

**[NIV]** "And if you walk in obedience to me and keep my decrees and commands as David your father did, I will give you a long life."

## Job 5:26

**[KJV]** Thou shalt come to thy grave in a full age, like as a shock of corn cometh in in his season.

**[CEB]** You will come to your grave in old age as bundles of grain stacked up at harvesttime.

**[CEV]** You will live a very long life, and your body will be strong until the day you die.

**[CJB]** You will come to your grave at a ripe old age, like a pile of grain that arrives in season.

**[ERV]** You will be like the wheat that grows until harvest time. Yes, you will live to a ripe old age.

**[GNT]** Like wheat that ripens till harvest time, you will live to a ripe old age.

**[ISV]** You'll go to your grave at a ripe old age; like a stack of grain that's harvested at just the right time.

## Psalm 91:16

**[KJV]** With long life will I satisfy him, and shew him my salvation.

**[CEB]** "I'll fill you full with old age. I'll show you my salvation."

**[CEV]** "You will live a long life and see my saving power."

**[CJB]** "I will satisfy him with long life and show him my salvation."

†**[Douay-Rheims]** I will fill him with length of days; and I will shew him my salvation.

**[GW]** I will satisfy you with a long life. I will show you how I will save you.

**[ISV]** I will satisfy him with long life; I will show him my deliverance.

†**[JPS-OT 1985]** "I will let him live to a ripe old age, and show him My salvation."

†**[NAB]** With length of days I will satisfy them and show them my saving power.

**[NLV]** I will please him with a long life. And I will show him My saving power.

**[NLT]** "I will reward them with a long life and give them my salvation."

†**[TPT]** "You will be satisfied with a full life and with all that I do for you. For you will enjoy the fullness of my salvation!"

## Psalm 92:13-15

**[KJV]** Those that be planted in the house of the Lord shall flourish in the courts of our God. They shall still bring forth fruit in old age; they shall be fat and flourishing; To shew that the Lord is upright: he is my rock, and there is no unrighteousness in him.

**[AMPC]** Planted in the house of the Lord, they shall flourish in the courts of our God.

[Growing in grace] they shall still bring forth fruit in old age; they shall be full of sap [of spiritual vitality] and [rich in the] verdure [of trust, love, and contentment]. [They are living memorials] to show that the Lord is upright *and* faithful to His promises; He is my Rock, and there is no unrighteousness in Him.

**[CEB]** Those who have been replanted in the Lord's house will spring up in the courtyards of our God. They will bear fruit even when old and gray; they will remain lush and fresh in order to proclaim: "The Lord is righteous. He's my rock. There's nothing unrighteous in him."

**[CEV]** They will take root in your house, Lord God, and they will do well. They will be like trees that stay healthy and fruitful, even when they are old. And they will say about you, "The Lord always does right! God is our mighty rock."

**[ERV]** They are planted in the house of the Lord. They grow strong there in the courtyards of our God. Even when they are old, they will continue producing fruit like young, healthy trees. They are there to show everyone that the Lord is good. He is my Rock, and he does no wrong.

**[GNT]** They are like trees planted in the house of the Lord, that flourish in the Temple of our God, that still bear fruit in old age and are always green and strong. This shows that the Lord is just, that there is no wrong in my protector.

**[NLT]** For they are transplanted to the Lord's own house. They flourish in the courts of our God. Even in old age they will still produce fruit; they will remain vital and green. They will declare, "The Lord is just! He is my rock! There is no evil in him!"

### Psalm 103:2-5

**[KJV]** Bless the Lord, O my soul, and forget not all his benefits: Who forgiveth all thine iniquities; who healeth all thy diseases; Who redeemeth thy life from destruction; who crowneth thee with lovingkindness and tender mercies; Who satisfieth thy mouth with good things; so that thy youth is renewed like the eagle's.

**[AMPC]** Bless (affectionately, gratefully praise) the Lord, O my soul, and forget not [one of] all His benefits — Who forgives [every one of] all your iniquities, Who heals [each one of] all your diseases, Who redeems your life from the pit *and* corruption, Who beautifies, dignifies, *and* crowns you with loving-kindness and tender mercy; Who satisfies your mouth [your necessity and desire at your personal age and situation] with good so that your youth, renewed, is like the eagle's [strong, overcoming, soaring]!

**[CEB]** Let my whole being bless the Lord and never forget all his good deeds: how God forgives all your sins, heals all your sickness, saves your life from the pit, crowns you with faithful love and compassion, and satisfies you with plenty of good things so that your youth is made fresh like an eagle's.

**[CEV]** With all my heart I praise the Lord! I will never forget how kind he has been. The Lord forgives our sins, heals us when we are sick, and protects us from death. His kindness and love are a crown on our heads. Each day that we live, he provides for our needs and gives us the strength of a young eagle.

†**[NEB]** Bless the Lord, my soul, and forget none of his benefits. He pardons all my guilt and heals all my suffering. He rescues me from the pit of death and surrounds me with constant love, with tender affection; he contents me with all good in the prime of life, and my youth is ever new like an eagles.

**[NLV]** Praise the Lord, O my soul. And forget none of His acts of kindness. He forgives all my sins. He heals all my diseases. He saves my life from the grave. He crowns me with loving-kindness and pity. He fills my years with good things and I am made young again like the eagle.

†**[Parkhurst-Ps]** O my soul, bless Jehovah, and do not forget any of his rewards. He forgiveth all thy iniquities; and healeth all thy ulcerations. Who delivereth thy life from destruction; and whose abundant mercy encompasseth thee. Who moreover satisfieth even thee with good things; thy youth is renewed like an eagle's.

†**[Slavitt-Ps]** Let the soul of my soul praise His name, exalt, laud, and extol His kindness, remembering all the ways He has forgiven our sins and healed our sickness to save our lives. Wherever we look, there is revealed His generous bounty. His people thrives. We are weak, we stagger and fall, but He snatches us back from the pit. We rise to a new day's bounty, surprised to be sustained like the eagle that soars and flies on powerful updrafts of air, effortless, beautiful there.

**[YLT]** Bless, O my soul, Jehovah, And forget not all His benefits, Who is forgiving all thine iniquities, Who is healing all thy diseases, Who is redeeming from destruction thy life, Who is crowning thee — kindness and mercies, Who is satisfying with good thy desire, Renew itself as an eagle doth thy youth.

## Psalm 119:89

**[KJV]** For ever, O Lord, thy word is settled in heaven.

**[CEV]** Our Lord, you are eternal! Your word will last as long as the heavens.

**[CSB]** Lord, your word is forever; it is firmly fixed in heaven.

**[GNT]** Your word, O Lord, will last forever; it is eternal in heaven.

**[GW]** O Lord, your word is established in heaven forever.

**[NET]** O Lord, your instructions endure; they stand secure in heaven.

**[NIV]** Your word, Lord, is eternal; it stands firm in the heavens.

## Proverbs 3:1-2

**[KJV]** My son, forget not my law; but let thine heart keep my commandments: for length of days, and long life, and peace, shall they add to thee.

**[AMPC]** My son, forget not my law *or* teaching, but let your heart keep my commandments; for length of days and years of a life [worth living] and tranquility [inward and outward and continuing through old age till death], these shall they add to you.

**[CEB]** My son, don't forget my instruction. Let your heart guard my commands, because they will help you live a long time and provide you with well-being.

**[CEV]** My child, remember my teachings and instructions and obey them completely. They will help you live a long and prosperous life.

**[ERV]** My son, don't forget my teaching. Remember what I tell you to do. What I teach will give you a good, long life, and all will go well for you.

**[GNT]** My child, don't forget what I teach you. Always remember what I tell you to do. My teaching will give you a long and prosperous life.

**[NIV]** My son, do not forget my teaching, but keep my commands in your heart, for they will prolong your life many years and bring you peace and prosperity.

**[NLT]** My child, never forget the things I have taught you. Store my commands in your heart.

If you do this, you will live many years, and your life will be satisfying.

### Proverbs 3:16

**[KJV]** Length of days is in her right hand; and in her left hand riches and honour.

**[CEB]** In her right hand is a long life; in her left are wealth and honor.

**[CEV]** In her right hand Wisdom holds a long life, and in her left hand are wealth and honor.

**[ERV]** With her right hand, Wisdom offers long life — with the other hand, riches and honor.

**[GNT]** Wisdom offers you long life, as well as wealth and honor.

**[NCV]** With her right hand wisdom offers you a long life, and with her left hand she gives you riches and honor.

### Proverbs 4:10

**[KJV]** Hear, O my son, and receive my sayings; and the years of thy life shall be many.

**[CEB]** Listen, my son, and take in my speech, then the years of your life will be many.

**[CEV]** My child, if you listen and obey my teachings, you will live a long time.

**[ERV]** Son, listen to me. Do what I say, and you will live a long time.

**[GNT]** Listen to me, my child. Take seriously what I am telling you, and you will live a long life.

**[NET]** Listen, my child, and accept my words, so that the years of your life will be many.

**[NLT]** My child, listen to me and do as I say, and you will have a long, good life.

### Proverbs 4:23

**[KJV]** Keep thy heart with all diligence; for out of it are the issues of life.

**[CEB]** More than anything you guard, protect your mind, for life flows from it.

**[CEV]** Carefully guard your thoughts because they are the source of true life.

**[ERV]** Above all, be careful what you think because your thoughts control your life.

**[GNT]** Be careful how you think; your life is shaped by your thoughts.

**[NIV]** Above all else, guard your heart, for everything you do flows from it.

**[NLT]** Guard your heart above all else, for it determines the course of your life.

### Proverbs 9:11

**[KJV]** For by me thy days shall be multiplied, and the years of thy life shall be increased.

**[CEB]** Through me your days will be many; years will be added to your life.

**[CEV]** I am Wisdom. If you follow me, you will live a long time.

**[ERV]** Wisdom will help you live longer; she will add years to your life.

**[NIV]** For through wisdom your days will be many, and years will be added to your life.

**[NLT]** Wisdom will multiply your days and add years to your life.

### Proverbs 10:27

**[KJV]** The fear of the Lord prolongeth days: but the years of the wicked shall be shortened.

**[CEB]** The fear of the Lord increases one's life, but the years of the wicked will be cut short.

**[CEV]** If you respect the Lord, you will live longer; if you keep doing wrong, your life will be cut short.

**[ERV]** Respect for the Lord will add years to your life, but the wicked will have their lives cut short.

**[GNT]** Obey the Lord, and you will live longer. The wicked die before their time.

**[NIV]** The fear of the Lord adds length to life, but the years of the wicked are cut short.

### Proverbs 14:30

**[KJV]** A sound heart is the life of the flesh: but envy the rottenness of the bones.

**[AMPC]** A calm *and* undisturbed mind *and* heart are the life *and* health of the body, but envy, jealousy, *and* wrath are like rottenness of the bones.

**[CEB]** A peaceful mind gives life to the body, but jealousy rots the bones.

**[CEV]** It's healthy to be content, but envy can eat you up.

**[CJB]** A tranquil mind gives health to the body, but envy rots the bones.

**[GNT]** Peace of mind makes the body healthy, but jealousy is like a cancer.

**[NIV]** A heart at peace gives life to the body, but envy rots the bones.

**[NLT]** A peaceful heart leads to a healthy body; jealousy is like cancer in the bones.

**[NLV]** A heart that has peace is life to the body, but wrong desires are like the wasting away of the bones.

**[YLT]** A healed heart [is] life to the flesh, And rottenness to the bones [is] envy.

## Proverbs 17:22

**[KJV]** A merry heart doeth good like a medicine: but a broken spirit drieth the bones.

**[GNT]** Being cheerful keeps you healthy. It is slow death to be gloomy all the time.

†**[Jerusalem]** A glad heart is excellent medicine, a spirit depressed wastes the bones away.

†**[Knox]** A cheerful heart makes a quick recovery, it is crushed spirits that waste a man's frame.

†**[Moffatt]** A glad heart is a healing medicine; but a broken spirit dries up the bones.

†**[REB]** A glad heart makes for good health, but low spirits sap one's strength.

†**[Rotherham]** A joyful heart, worketh an excellent cure, — but, a stricken spirit, drieth up the bone.

†**[SAAS-OT]** A cheerful heart makes a man healthy, but the bones of a sorrowful man dry him up.

†**[T4T]** Being cheerful is like swallowing good medicine; being discouraged/gloomy all the time will drain away your energy/cause you to become weak.

†**[WSP-OT]** A joyful heart bringeth healing; but a wounded spirit drieth the bones.

## Isaiah 1:19

**[KJV]** If ye be willing and obedient, ye shall eat the good of the land.

**[CEB]** If you agree and obey, you will eat the best food of the land.

**[CEV]** If you willingly obey me, the best crops in the land will be yours.

**[ERV]** If you listen to what I say, you will get the good things from this land.

**[GNT]** If you will only obey me, you will eat the good things the land produces.

**[NET]** If you have a willing attitude and obey, then you will again eat the good crops of the land.

**[NLT]** If you will only obey me, you will have plenty to eat.

## Isaiah 53:3-5

**[KJV]** He is despised and rejected of men; a man of sorrows, and acquainted with grief: and we hid as it were our faces from him; he was despised, and we esteemed him not. Surely he hath borne our griefs, and carried our sorrows: yet we did esteem him stricken, smitten of God, and afflicted. But he was wounded for our transgressions, he was bruised for our iniquities: the chastisement of our peace was upon him; and with his stripes we are healed.

**[AMPC]** He was despised and rejected *and* forsaken by men, a Man of sorrows *and* pains, and acquainted with grief *and* sickness; and like One from Whom men hide their faces He was despised, and we did not appreciate His worth *or* have any esteem for Him. Surely He has borne our griefs (sicknesses, weaknesses, and distresses) and carried our sorrows *and* pains [of punishment], yet we [ignorantly] considered Him stricken, smitten, and afflicted by God [as if with leprosy]. But He was wounded for our transgressions, He was bruised for our guilt *and* iniquities; the chastisement [needful to obtain] peace *and* well-being for us was upon Him, and with the stripes [that wounded] Him we are healed *and* made whole.

†**[Anchor]** He was despised, the lowest of men: a man of pains, familiar with disease, one from whom men avert their gaze — despised, and we reckoned him as nothing. But it was our diseases that he bore, our pains that he carried, while we counted him as one stricken, touched by God with affliction. He was wounded for our rebellions, crushed for our transgressions; the chastisement that reconciled us fell upon him, and we were healed by his bruises.

†**[CT-OT]** Despised and rejected by men, a man of pains and accustomed to illness, and as one who hides his face from us, despised and we held him of no account. Indeed, he bore our illnesses, and our pains-he carried them, yet we accounted him as plagued, smitten by God and oppressed. But he was pained because of our transgressions, crushed because of our iniquities; the chastisement of our welfare was upon him, and with his wound we were healed.

**[GNT]** We despised him and rejected him; he endured suffering and pain. No one would even look at him — we ignored him as if he were nothing. But he endured the suffering that should have been ours, the pain that we should have borne. All the while we thought that his suffering was punishment sent by God. But because of our sins he was wounded, beaten because of the evil we did. We are healed by the punishment he suffered, made whole by the blows he received.

†**[Haupt]** Despised was he, and forsaken of men, a man of many pains, and familiar with sickness, yea, like one from whom men hide the face, Despised, and we esteemed him not. But our sickness, alone, he bore, and our pains — he carried them, whilst we esteemed him stricken, Smitten of God, and afflicted. But alone he was humiliated because of our rebellions, alone he was crushed because of our iniquities; a chastisement, all for our peace, was upon him, and to us came healing through his stripes.

†**[Moffatt]** He was despised and shunned by men, a man of pain, who knew what sickness was; like one from whom men turn with shuddering, he was despised, we took no heed of him. And yet ours was the pain he bore, the sorrow he endured! We thought him suffering from a stroke at God's own hand; yet he was wounded because we had sinned, 'twas our misdeeds that crushed

him; 'twas for our welfare that he chastised, the blows that fell to him have brought us healing.

**[NCV]** He was hated and rejected by people. He had much pain and suffering. People would not even look at him. He was hated, and we didn't even notice him. But he took our suffering on him and felt our pain for us. We saw his suffering and thought God was punishing him. But he was wounded for the wrong we did; he was crushed for the evil we did. The punishment, which made us well, was given to him, and we are healed because of his wounds.

†**[NEB]** He was despised, he shrank from the sight of men, tormented and humbled by suffering; we despised him, we held him of no account, a thing from which men turn away their eyes. Yet on himself he bore our sufferings, our torments he endured, which we counted him smitten by God, struck down by disease and misery; but he was pierced for our transgressions, tortured for our iniquities; the chastisement he bore is health for us and by his scourging we are healed.

†**[Ottley-Isa-Heb]** Despised and avoided of men; a man of pains, and one that knew sickness; and as one from whom faces are hid; despised, and we esteemed him not. Surely he bore our sicknesses; and our pains, he supported them; and we, (on our part,) did esteem him stricken, smitten of God, and afflicted. And he was pierced for our rebellions, bruised for our iniquities; the chastisement of our peace was upon him; and in his stripes was there healing for us.

## Hosea 4:6

**[KJV]** My people are destroyed for lack of knowledge: because thou hast rejected knowledge, I will also reject thee, that thou shalt be no priest to me: seeing thou hast forgotten the law of thy God, I will also forget thy children.

**[CEB]** My people are destroyed from lack of knowledge. Since you have rejected knowledge, so I will reject you from serving me as a priest. Since you have forgotten the Instruction of your God, so also I will forget your children.

**[CEV]** You priests have rejected me, and my people are destroyed by refusing to obey. Now I'll reject you and forget your children, because you have forgotten my Law.

**[ERV]** My people are destroyed because they have no knowledge. You priests have refused to learn, so I will refuse to let you be priests for me. You have forgotten the law of your God, so I will forget your children.

**[GNT]** My people are doomed because they do not acknowledge me. You priests have refused to acknowledge me and have rejected my teaching, and so I reject you and will not acknowledge your sons as my priests.

**[NET]** You have destroyed my people by failing to acknowledge me! Because you refuse to acknowledge me, I will reject you as my priests. Because you reject the law of your God, I will reject your descendants.

**[NLT]** My people are being destroyed because they don't know me. Since you priests refuse to know me, I refuse to recognize you as my priests. Since you have forgotten the laws of your God, I will forget to bless your children.

**[NLV]** My people are destroyed because they have not learned. You were not willing to learn. So I am not willing to have you be My religious leader. Since you have forgotten the Law of your God, I also will forget your children.

### Matthew 8:17

**[KJV]** That it might be fulfilled which was spoken by Esaias the prophet, saying, Himself took our infirmities, and bare our sicknesses.

**[AMPC]** And thus He fulfilled what was spoken by the prophet Isaiah, He Himself took [in order to carry away] our weaknesses *and* infirmities and bore away our diseases.

†**[Barclay-NT]** This happened that the statement made through the prophet Isaiah might come true: 'He took upon himself our weaknesses and carried the burden of our diseases.'

**[CEB]** This happened so that what Isaiah the prophet said would be fulfilled: *He is the one who took our illnesses and carried away our diseases.*

**[CEV]** So God's promise came true, just as the prophet Isaiah had said, "He healed our diseases and made us well."

†**[Madsen-NT]** So the word of the prophet Isaiah was fulfilled: He has taken our sickness from us, he has borne all our infirmities.

†**[Moffatt]** That the word spoken by the prophet Isaiah might be fulfilled, He took away our sicknesses and our diseases he removed.

†**[NEB]** To make good the prophecy of Isaiah: 'He took away our illnesses and lifted our diseases from us.'

**[NLV]** It happened as the early preacher Isaiah said it would happen. He said, "He took on Himself our sickness and carried away our diseases."

†**[TPT]** In doing this, Jesus fulfilled the prophecy of Isaiah: He put upon himself our weaknesses, and he carried away our diseases and made us well.

## Matthew 12:34

**[KJV]** O generation of vipers, how can ye, being evil, speak good things? for out of the abundance of the heart the mouth speaketh.

**[CEB]** Children of snakes! How can you speak good things while you are evil? What fills the heart comes out of the mouth.

**[CJB]** You snakes! How can you who are evil say anything good? For the mouth speaks what overflows from the heart.

**[EHV]** You offspring of vipers! How can you say anything good, since you are evil? For what the mouth speaks flows from the heart.

**[ERV]** You snakes! You are so evil. How can you say anything good? What people say with their mouths comes from what fills their hearts.

**[NIV]** You brood of vipers, how can you who are evil say anything good? For the mouth speaks what the heart is full of.

**[PHILLIPS]** "You serpent's brood, how can you say anything good out of your evil hearts? For a man's words depend on what fills his heart. A good man gives out good — from the goodness stored in his heart; a bad man gives out evil — from his store of evil. I tell you that men will have to answer at the day of judgment for every careless word they utter — for it is your words that will acquit you, and your words that will condemn you."

## Mark 11:23

**[KJV]** For verily I say unto you, That whosoever shall say unto this mountain, Be thou removed, and be thou cast into the sea; and shall not doubt in his heart, but shall believe that those things which he saith shall come to pass; he shall have whatsoever he saith.

†**[Authentic-NT]** 'I tell you positively, if anyone should say to this hill, "Go and hurl yourself into the sea," and should have not the slightest doubt, but fully believe that what he says will happen, he will bring it about.'

†**[Barclay-NT]** 'I tell you truly, if anyone were to say to this hill: "Be picked up and flung into the sea," if there are no doubts in his mind, but if he really believes that what he is saying will happen, what he asks will be done.'

†**[BrownKrueger]** For verily I say unto you, that whosoever shall say unto this mountain, Take thyself away, and cast thyself into the sea, and shall not waver in his heart, but shall believe that those things which he saith, shall come to pass, whatsoever he saith, shall be done to him.

†**[BV-KJV-NT]** You see, amen, I tell you that whoever might say to this mountain, 'Be picked up and thrown into the sea,' and in his heart does not consider it to be wrong, but trusts that what he speaks is happening, he will have whatever he said.

†**[Condon-Mk]** Truly I say to you, if anyone says to this mountain: "Be lifted and thrown into the sea", without hesitation in his heart but with faith that what he says will come true, it will be done for him.

**[GW]** I can guarantee this truth: This is what will be done for someone who doesn't doubt but believes what he says will happen: He can say to this mountain, 'Be uprooted and thrown into the sea,' and it will be done for him.

†**[HRB]** For truly I say to you, that he who says to this mountain, "Be lifted up and fall into the sea." And does not become divided in his heart but believes that it will happen. That thing which he said it will happen.

†**[Norlie-NT]** "I tell you," He continued, "if anyone would say to this mountain, 'Move! Throw yourself into the sea!' and have no doubt in his heart, but would be sure that what he said would come to pass, then it would so happen."

†**[TPT]** Listen to the truth I speak to you: If someone says to this mountain with great faith and having no doubt, 'Mountain, be lifted up and thrown into the midst of the sea,' and believes that what he says will happen, it will be done.

## Mark 16:17-18

**[KJV]** And these signs shall follow them that believe; In my name shall they cast out devils; they shall speak with new tongues; They shall take up serpents; and if they drink any deadly thing, it shall not hurt them; they shall lay hands on the sick, and they shall recover.

**[AMPC]** And these attesting signs will accompany those who believe: in My name they will drive out demons; they will speak in new languages; They will pick up serpents; and [even] if they drink anything deadly, it will not hurt them; they will lay their hands on the sick, and they will get well.

†**[Barclay-NT]** 'These are the visible demonstrations of the action of God which will accompany the life of those who believe. By using my name they will eject demons. They will speak in strange languages. They will lift snakes in their bare

hands. Even if they drink any deadly poison, it will not hurt them. They will place their hands on the sick and they will be cured.'

**[CJB]** And these signs will accompany those who do trust: in my name they will drive out demons, speak with new tongues, not be injured if they handle snakes or drink poison, and heal the sick by laying hands on them.

**[ERV]** And the people who believe will be able to do these things as proof: They will use my name to force demons out of people. They will speak in languages they never learned. If they pick up snakes or drink any poison, they will not be hurt. They will lay their hands on sick people, and they will get well.

**[GNT]** Believers will be given the power to perform miracles: they will drive out demons in my name; they will speak in strange tongues; if they pick up snakes or drink any poison, they will not be harmed; they will place their hands on sick people, and these will get well.

†**[Magiera-NT]** And these signs will follow those who believe, in my name they will cast out demons and they will speak with new tongues. And they will capture snakes, and if they should drink a deadly poison, it will harm not them and they will place their hands on the sick and they will be made whole.

†**[Original-NT]** And these signs shall attend those who have believed: they shall expel demons in my name; they shall speak in tongues; they shall take up snakes; if they drink anything poisonous it will not harm them; and they shall lay hands on the sick and cure them.

†**[TPT]** And these miracle signs will accompany those who believe: They will drive out demons in the power of my name. They will speak in tongues. They will be supernaturally protected from snakes and from drinking anything poisonous. And they will lay hands on the sick and heal them.

## Luke 10:19

**[KJV]** Behold, I give unto you power to tread on serpents and scorpions, and over all the power of the enemy: and nothing shall by any means hurt you.

**[AMPC]** Behold! I have given you authority *and* power to trample upon serpents and scorpions, and [physical and mental strength and ability] over all the power that the enemy [possesses]; and nothing shall in any way harm you.

†**[Harwood-NT]** Behold! I endow you with power to vanquish your most fell and implacable adversaries — and all their determined rage and rancor shall not be able to injure you or your cause.

†**[Norlie-NT]** Now listen! I have given you authority to trample on serpents and scorpions and all the might of the satanic foe, and nothing will harm you in any way.

**[PHILLIPS]** It is true that I have given you the power to tread on snakes and scorpions and to overcome all the enemy's power — there is nothing at all that can do you any harm.

†**[T4T]** Listen! I have given you authority so that if you oppose evil spirits they will not hurt you. I have given you authority to defeat our enemy, Satan. Nothing shall hurt you.

†**[TPT]** Now you understand that I have imparted to you all my authority to trample over his kingdom. You will trample upon every demon before you and overcome every power Satan possesses. Absolutely nothing will be able to harm you as you walk in this authority.

†**[Wade]** Listen! I have given to you the authority needed for trampling upon the agencies of evil, poisonous as serpents and scorpions — yes, authority over all the power of the Enemy; and nothing shall harm you.

## Luke 17:3

**[KJV]** Take heed to yourselves: If thy brother trespass against thee, rebuke him; and if he repent, forgive him.

**[CEB]** Watch yourselves! If your brother or sister sins, warn them to stop. If they change their hearts and lives, forgive them.

**[CEV]** So be careful what you do. Correct any followers of mine who sin, and forgive the ones who say they are sorry.

**[ESV]** Pay attention to yourselves! If your brother sins, rebuke him, and if he repents, forgive him.

**[NLT]** So watch yourselves! "If another believer sins, rebuke that person; then if there is repentance, forgive."

**[PHILLIPS]** Then Jesus said to his disciples, "It is inevitable that there should be pitfalls, but alas for the man who is responsible for them! It would be better for that man to have a mill-stone hung round his neck and be thrown into the sea, than that he should trip up one of these little ones. So be careful how you live. If your brother offends you, take him to task about it, and if he is sorry, forgive him. Yes, if he wrongs you seven times in one day and turns to you and says, 'I am sorry' seven times, you must forgive him."

**[YLT]** 'Take heed to yourselves, and, if thy brother may sin in regard to thee, rebuke him, and if he may reform, forgive him.'

## Luke 17:6

**[KJV]** And the Lord said, If ye had faith as a grain of mustard seed, ye might say unto this sycamine tree, Be thou plucked up by the root, and be thou planted in the sea; and it should obey you.

**[AMPC]** And the Lord answered, If you had faith (trust and confidence in God) even [so small] like a grain of mustard seed, you could say to this mulberry tree, Be pulled up by the roots, and be planted in the sea, and it would obey you.

**[ASV]** And the Lord said, If ye had faith as a grain of mustard seed, ye would say unto this sycamine tree, Be thou rooted up, and be thou planted in the sea; and it would obey you.

**[CJB]** The Lord replied, "If you had trust as tiny as a mustard seed, you could say to this fig tree, 'Be uprooted and replanted in the sea!' and it would obey you."

**[CSB]** "If you have faith the size of a mustard seed," the Lord said, "you can say to this mulberry tree, 'Be uprooted and planted in the sea,' and it will obey you."

**[ERV]** The Lord said, "If your faith is as big as a mustard seed, you can say to this mulberry tree, 'Dig yourself up and plant yourself in the ocean!' And the tree will obey you."

**[NIV]** He replied, "If you have faith as small as a mustard seed, you can say to this mulberry tree, 'Be uprooted and planted in the sea,' and it will obey you."

### Acts 1:8

**[KJV]** But ye shall receive power, after that the Holy Ghost is come upon you: and ye shall be witnesses unto me both in Jerusalem, and in all Judaea, and in Samaria, and unto the uttermost part of the earth.

**[AMPC]** But you shall receive power (ability, efficiency, and might) when the Holy Spirit has come upon you, and you shall be My witnesses in Jerusalem and all Judea and Samaria and to the ends (the very bounds) of the earth.

**[CEB]** "Rather, you will receive power when the Holy Spirit has come upon you, and you will be my witnesses in Jerusalem, in all Judea and Samaria, and to the end of the earth."

**[CEV]** "But the Holy Spirit will come upon you and give you power. Then you will tell everyone about me in Jerusalem, in all Judea, in Samaria, and everywhere in the world."

**[CSB]** "But you will receive power when the Holy Spirit has come on you, and you will be my witnesses in Jerusalem, in all Judea and Samaria, and to the ends of the earth."

**[ERV]** "But the Holy Spirit will come on you and give you power. You will be my witnesses. You will tell people everywhere about me — in Jerusalem, in the rest of Judea, in Samaria, and in every part of the world."

**[ESV]** "But you will receive power when the Holy Spirit has come upon you, and you will be my witnesses in Jerusalem and in all Judea and Samaria, and to the end of the earth."

**[PHILLIPS]** To this he replied, "You cannot know times and dates which have been fixed by the Father's sole authority. But you are to be given power when the Holy Spirit has come to you. You will be witnesses to me, not only in Jerusalem, not only throughout Judea, not only in Samaria, but to the very ends of the earth!"

**[YLT]** 'But ye shall receive power at the coming of the Holy Spirit upon you, and ye shall be witnesses to me both in Jerusalem, and in all Judea, and Samaria, and unto the end of the earth.'

## Acts 10:38

**[KJV]** How God anointed Jesus of Nazareth with the Holy Ghost and with power: who went about doing good, and healing all that were oppressed of the devil; for God was with him.

**[AMPC]** How God anointed *and* consecrated Jesus of Nazareth with the [Holy] Spirit and with strength *and* ability *and* power; how He went about doing good and, in particular, curing all who were harassed *and* oppressed by [the power of] the devil, for God was with Him.

†**[Barclay-NT]** You know about Jesus of Nazareth, and how God anointed him with the Holy Spirit and with power, and how he went about helping everyone, and curing all those who were under the tyranny of the devil, because God was with him.

†**[Doddridge-NT]** I mean the report [concerning] Jesus of Nazareth, how God anointed him with the Holy Spirit, and with a power of performing the most extraordinary miracles in attestation of his divine mission; who went about, and passed through the whole country, doing good wherever he came, and particularly healing all those who were oppressed by the tyranny of the devil,

dispossessing those malignant spirits of darkness with a most apparent and irresistible superiority to them; for God himself was with him, and wrought by him to produce those astonishing effects.

†**[Madsen-NT]** He was anointed by God with the Holy Spirit and with great power. You know how he went through the land, helping and bringing healing to all who had fallen into the power of the Adversary. The power of God was with him.

†**[Moffatt]** How God consecrated Jesus of Nazaret with the holy Spirit and power, and how he went about doing good and curing all who were harassed by the devil; for God was with him.

†**[Morgan-NT]** How God anointed Jesus, the Nazarene, with the holy spirit, and power, who traveled benefiting and healing all oppressed, by the devil, for God was with him.

†**[Original-NT]** Telling of Jesus of Nazareth, whom God anointed with holy Spirit and power, who went about doing good and curing all who were in the Devil's clutches; for God was with him.

**[PHILLIPS]** You must have heard how God anointed him with the power of the Holy Spirit, of how he went about doing good and healing all who suffered under the devil's power — because God was with him.

†**[Sawyer-7590]** How God anointed him with the Holy Spirit and power, who went about doing good and curing all that were subjugated by the devil, for God was with him.

†**[TPT]** "Jesus of Nazareth was anointed by God with the Holy Spirit and with great power. He did wonderful things for others and divinely healed all who were under the tyranny of the devil, for God had anointed him."

## Romans 3:24

**[KJV]** Being justified freely by his grace through the redemption that is in Christ Jesus.

**[CEB]** But all are treated as righteous freely by his grace because of a ransom that was paid by Christ Jesus.

**[CEV]** But God treats us much better than we deserve, and because of Christ Jesus, he freely accepts us and sets us free from our sins.

**[ERV]** They are made right with God by his grace. This is a free gift. They are made right with God by being made free from sin through Jesus Christ.

**[GNT]** But by the free gift of God's grace all are put right with him through Christ Jesus, who sets them free.

**[ISV]** By his grace they are justified freely through the redemption that is in the Messiah Jesus.

**[NLT]** Yet God, in his grace, freely makes us right in his sight. He did this through Christ Jesus when he freed us from the penalty for our sins.

## Romans 5:12

**[KJV]** Wherefore, as by one man sin entered into the world, and death by sin; and so death passed upon all men, for that all have sinned.

**[ASV]** Therefore, as through one man sin entered into the world, and death through sin; and so death passed unto all men, for that all sinned.

**[CEB]** Just as through one human being sin came into the world, and death came through sin, so death has come to everyone, since everyone has sinned.

**[ERV]** Sin came into the world because of what one man did. And with sin came death. So this is why all people must die — because all people have sinned.

**[ESV]** Therefore, just as sin came into the world through one man, and death through sin, and so death spread to all men because all sinned.

**[NIV]** Therefore, just as sin entered the world through one man, and death through sin, and in this way death came to all people, because all sinned.

**[NLT]** When Adam sinned, sin entered the world. Adam's sin brought death, so death spread to everyone, for everyone sinned.

## Romans 5:17

**[KJV]** For if by one man's offence death reigned by one; much more they which receive abundance of grace and of the gift of righteousness shall reign in life by one, Jesus Christ.

**[AMPC]** For if because of one man's trespass (lapse, offense) death reigned through that one, much more surely will those who receive [God's] overflowing grace (unmerited favor) and the free gift of righteousness [putting them into right standing with Himself] reign as kings in life through the one Man Jesus Christ (the Messiah, the Anointed One).

**[CEB]** If death ruled because of one person's failure, those who receive the multiplied grace and the gift of righteousness will even more certainly rule in life through the one person Jesus Christ.

**[CEV]** Death ruled like a king because Adam had sinned. But that cannot compare with what Jesus Christ has done. God has treated us with undeserved grace, and he has accepted us because of Jesus. And so we will live and rule like kings.

**[ERV]** One man sinned, and so death ruled all people because of that one man. But now some people accept God's full grace and his great gift of being made right. Surely they will have true life and rule through the one man, Jesus Christ.

**[NIV]** For if, by the trespass of the one man, death reigned through that one man, how much more will those who receive God's abundant provision of grace and of the gift of righteousness reign in life through the one man, Jesus Christ!

**[NLT]** For the sin of this one man, Adam, caused death to rule over many. But even greater is God's wonderful grace and his gift of righteousness, for all who receive it will live in triumph over sin and death through this one man, Jesus Christ.

**[PHILLIPS]** For if one man's offence meant that men should be slaves to death all their lives, it is a far greater thing that through another man, Jesus Christ, men by their acceptance of his more than sufficient grace and righteousness, should live all their lives like kings!

### Romans 5:21

**[KJV]** That as sin hath reigned unto death, even so might grace reign through righteousness unto eternal life by Jesus Christ our Lord.

**[AMPC]** So that, [just] as sin has reigned in death, [so] grace (His unearned and undeserved favor) might reign also through righteousness (right standing with God) which issues in eternal life through Jesus Christ (the Messiah, the Anointed One) our Lord.

**[CEB]** The result is that grace will rule through God's righteousness, leading to eternal life through Jesus Christ our Lord, just as sin ruled in death.

**[CEV]** Sin ruled by means of death. But God's gift of grace now rules, and God has accepted us because of Jesus Christ our Lord. This means that we will have eternal life.

**[GNT]** So then, just as sin ruled by means of death, so also God's grace rules by means of righteousness, leading us to eternal life through Jesus Christ our Lord.

**[NLT]** So just as sin ruled over all people and brought them to death, now God's wonderful grace rules instead, giving us right standing with God and resulting in eternal life through Jesus Christ our Lord.

**[PHILLIPS]** Now we find that the Law keeps slipping into the picture to point the vast extent of sin. Yet though sin is shown to be wide and deep, thank God his grace is wider and deeper still! The whole outlook changes — sin used to be the master of men and in the end handed them over to death: now grace is the ruling factor, with righteousness as its purpose and its end the bringing of men to the eternal life of God through Jesus Christ our Lord.

## Romans 6:17

**[KJV]** But God be thanked, that ye were the servants of sin, but ye have obeyed from the heart that form of doctrine which was delivered you.

**[CEB]** But thank God that although you used to be slaves of sin, you gave wholehearted obedience to the teaching that was handed down to you, which provides a pattern.

**[CEV]** You used to be slaves of sin. But I thank God that with all your heart you followed the example set forth in the teaching you received.

**[ERV]** In the past you were slaves to sin — sin controlled you. But thank God, you fully obeyed what you were taught.

**[GNT]** But thanks be to God! For though at one time you were slaves to sin, you have obeyed with all your heart the truths found in the teaching you received.

**[NIV]** But thanks be to God that, though you used to be slaves to sin, you have come to obey from your heart the pattern of teaching that has now claimed your allegiance.

**[PHILLIPS]** Thank God that you, who were at one time the servants of sin, honestly responded to the impact of Christ's teaching when you came under its influence. Then, released from the service of sin, you entered the service of righteousness.

## Romans 8:11

**[KJV]** But if the Spirit of him that raised up Jesus from the dead dwell in you, he that raised up Christ from the dead shall also quicken your mortal bodies by his Spirit that dwelleth in you.

**[AMPC]** And if the Spirit of Him Who raised up Jesus from the dead dwells in you, [then] He Who raised up Christ *Jesus* from the dead will also restore to life your mortal (short-lived, perishable) bodies through His Spirit Who dwells in you.

†**[Authentic-NT]** And if the Spirit that raised up Jesus from the dead resides in you, then he that raised Christ Jesus from the dead will also give life to your mortal bodies by very reason of his Spirit indwelling in you.

†**[BV-KJV-NT]** If the Spirit of the One who got Jesus up from the dead has a house in you, the One who got the Anointed King up from the dead will also give your dying bodies life through His Spirit that is housed in you.

**[ERV]** God raised Jesus from death. And if God's Spirit lives in you, he will also give life to your bodies that die. Yes, God is the one who raised Christ from death, and he will raise you to life through his Spirit living in you.

†**[Madsen-NT]** If the Spirit of HIM who awakened Jesus from the dead lives in you, then HE who raised Christ Jesus from the dead will create life for your death-riddled bodies also. He does that, because HIS Spirit dwells in you.

**[PHILLIPS]** Once the Spirit of him who raised Christ Jesus from the dead lives within you he will, by that same Spirit, bring to your whole being, yes even your mortal bodies, new strength and vitality. For he now lives in you.

†**[Rotherham]** If, moreover, the Spirit of him that raised Jesus from among the dead dwelleth in you, he that raised from among the dead Christ Jesus, shall make alive [even] your death-doomed bodies, through means of his indwelling Spirit within you.

†**[TPT]** Yes, God raised Jesus to life! And since God's Spirit of Resurrection lives in you, he will also raise your dying body to life by the same Spirit that breathes life into you!

## Romans 12:2

**[KJV]** And be not conformed to this world: but be ye transformed by the renewing of your mind, that ye may prove what is that good, and acceptable, and perfect, will of God.

**[CEB]** Don't be conformed to the patterns of this world, but be transformed by the renewing of your minds so that you can figure out what God's will is — what is good and pleasing and mature.

**[CEV]** Don't be like the people of this world, but let God change the way you think. Then you will know how to do everything that is good and pleasing to him.

**[ERV]** Don't change yourselves to be like the people of this world, but let God change you inside with a new way of thinking. Then you will be able to understand and accept what God wants for you. You will be able to know what is good and pleasing to him and what is perfect.

**[GNT]** Do not conform yourselves to the standards of this world, but let God transform you inwardly by a complete change of your mind. Then you will be able to know the will of God — what is good and is pleasing to him and is perfect.

**[PHILLIPS]** With eyes wide open to the mercies of God, I beg you, my brothers, as an act of intelligent worship, to give him your bodies, as a living sacrifice, consecrated to him and acceptable by him. Don't let the world around you squeeze you into its own mould, but let God re-mould your minds from within, so that you may prove in practice that the plan of God for you is good, meets all his demands and moves towards the goal of true maturity.

### 1 Corinthians 2:5

**[KJV]** That your faith should not stand in the wisdom of men, but in the power of God.

**[AMPC]** So that your faith might not rest in the wisdom of men (human philosophy), but in the power of God.

**[CEB]** I did this so that your faith might not depend on the wisdom of people but on the power of God.

**[CEV]** That way you would have faith because of God's power and not because of human wisdom.

**[GNT]** Your faith, then, does not rest on human wisdom but on God's power.

**[PHILLIPS]** Plainly God's purpose was that your faith should not rest upon man's cleverness but upon the power of God.

### 1 Corinthians 6:19-20

**[KJV]** What? know ye not that your body is the temple of the Holy Ghost which is in you, which ye have of God, and ye are not your own? For ye are bought with a price: therefore glorify God in your body, and in your spirit, which are God's.

**[AMPC]** Do you not know that your body is the temple (the very sanctuary) of the Holy Spirit Who lives within you, Whom you have received [as a Gift] from God? You are not your own. You were bought with a price [purchased with a preciousness and paid for, made His own]. So then, honor God *and* bring glory to Him in your body.

†**[Barclay-NT]** Are you not aware that your body is the temple of the Holy Spirit, who dwells within us, and whom we have received from God, and that you therefore do not belong to yourselves? He bought you for himself — and it did not cost him nothing. Therefore honour God with your body.

**[CEV]** You surely know that your body is a temple where the Holy Spirit lives. The Spirit is in you and is a gift from God. You are no longer your own. God paid a great price for you. So use your body to honor God.

†**[Madsen-NT]** Do you not know that your body is a temple of the indwelling Holy Spirit in you? You have received it from God: you do not belong to yourselves. Your freedom was bought for you for a high price. So now let your body become a revelation of God.

†**[TPT]** Have you forgotten that your body is now the sacred temple of the Spirit of Holiness, who lives in you? You don't belong to yourself any longer, for the gift of God, the Holy Spirit, lives inside your sanctuary. You were God's expensive purchase, paid for with tears of blood, so by all means, then, use your body to bring glory to God!

## 1 Corinthians 9:27

**[KJV]** But I keep under my body, and bring it into subjection: lest that by any means, when I have preached to others, I myself should be a castaway.

**[CEB]** Rather, I'm landing punches on my own body and subduing it like a slave. I do this to be sure that I myself won't be disqualified after preaching to others.

**[CEV]** I keep my body under control and make it my slave, so I won't lose out after telling the good news to others.

**[ERV]** It is my own body I fight to make it do what I want. I do this so that I won't miss getting the prize myself after telling others about it.

**[GNT]** I harden my body with blows and bring it under complete control, to keep myself from being disqualified after having called others to the contest.

**[NIV]** No, I strike a blow to my body and make it my slave so that after I have preached to others, I myself will not be disqualified for the prize.

**[PHILLIPS]** I run the race then with determination. I am no shadow-boxer, I really fight! I am my body's sternest master, for fear that when I have preached to others I should myself be disqualified.

## 1 Corinthians 10:31

**[KJV]** Whether therefore ye eat, or drink, or whatsoever ye do, do all to the glory of God.

**[AMPC]** So then, whether you eat or drink, or whatever you may do, do all for the honor *and* glory of God.

**[CEB]** So, whether you eat or drink or whatever you do, you should do it all for God's glory.

**[CEV]** When you eat or drink or do anything else, always do it to honor God.

**[ERV]** So if you eat, or if you drink, or if you do anything, do it for the glory of God.

**[NLV]** So if you eat or drink or whatever you do, do everything to honor God.

**[PHILLIPS]** Because, whatever you do, eating or drinking or anything else, everything should be done to bring glory to God.

### 1 Corinthians 11:27

**[KJV]** Wherefore whosoever shall eat this bread, and drink this cup of the Lord, unworthily, shall be guilty of the body and blood of the Lord.

**[AMPC]** So then whoever eats the bread or drinks the cup of the Lord in a way that is unworthy [of Him] will be guilty of [profaning and sinning against] the body and blood of the Lord.

**[CEB]** This is why those who eat the bread or drink the cup of the Lord inappropriately will be guilty of the Lord's body and blood.

**[CEV]** But if you eat the bread and drink the wine in a way that isn't worthy of the Lord, you sin against his body and blood.

**[CSB]** So, then, whoever eats the bread or drinks the cup of the Lord in an unworthy manner will be guilty of sin against the body and blood of the Lord.

**[ERV]** So if you eat the bread or drink the cup of the Lord in a way that does not fit its meaning, you are sinning against the body and the blood of the Lord.

## 1 Corinthians 11:29-30

**[KJV]** For he that eateth and drinketh unworthily, eateth and drinketh damnation to himself, not discerning the Lord's body. For this cause many are weak and sickly among you, and many sleep.

**[AMPC]** For anyone who eats and drinks without discriminating *and* recognizing with due appreciation that [it is Christ's] body, eats and drinks a sentence (a verdict of judgment) upon himself. That [careless and unworthy participation] is the reason many of you are weak and sickly, and quite enough of you have fallen into the sleep of death.

†**[Authentic-NT]** For he who eats and drinks is eating and drinking a judgment on himself, not discerning the body. That is why many of you are infirm and ailing, and a number have gone to their rest.

**[CEV]** If you fail to understand that you are the body of the Lord, you will condemn yourselves by the way you eat and drink. This is why many of you are sick and weak and why a lot of others have died.

**[NLT]** For if you eat the bread or drink the cup without honoring the body of Christ, you are eating and drinking God's judgment upon yourself. That is why many of you are weak and sick and some have even died.

**[NLV]** Anyone who eats the bread and drinks from the cup, if his spirit is not right with the Lord, will be guilty as he eats and drinks. He does not understand the meaning of the Lord's body. This is why some of you are sick and weak, and some have died.

†**[Norlie-NT]** For if one eats and drinks unworthily he eats and drinks judgment on himself, not recognizing the Lord's body. Because of this indifference, many of you are feeble and sickly, and some have died.

**[PHILLIPS]** He that eats and drinks carelessly is eating and drinking a judgment on himself, for he is blind to the presence of the Lord's body. It is this careless participation which is the reason for many feeble and sickly Christians in your church, and the explanation of the fact that many of you are spiritually asleep.

†**[Wand-NT]** He who partakes of this food without recognizing it as the Body eats and drinks to his own condemnation. For this reason many among you are weak and sickly and some are just spiritual corpses.

†**[Williams-NT]** For whoever eats and drinks without recognizing His body, eats and drinks a judgment on himself. This is why many of you are sick and feeble, and a considerable number are falling asleep.

## 1 Corinthians 12:9

**[KJV]** To another faith by the same Spirit; to another the gifts of healing by the same Spirit.

**[AMPC]** To another [wonder-working] faith by the same [Holy] Spirit, to another the extraordinary powers of healing by the one Spirit.

†**[Bowes-NT]** To another faith in the same Spirit; but to another gracious gifts of healings in the one Spirit.

†**[Erasmus-NT]** To another by the inspiration of the same Spirit has come the strength of faith that moves even mountains from their place, according to the promise of the Lord; to another through the same Spirit has come the power to heal disease.

†**[Goodspeed-NT]** Another, from his union with the same Spirit receives faith, another, by one and the same Spirit, the ability to cure the sick.

†**[Green-NT]** And to another faith, in the same Spirit; to another endowments of healings, in the one Spirit.

†**[Guyse-NT]** To another is given, by the same Holy Spirit, a full assent to the truth of the gospel, and boldness in preaching it, together with a firm trust in Christ for all divine assistance, that shall be needful in every dangerous and

difficult service, to which he may be called: To another is communicated the gift of healing all manner of bodily diseases, in an instant, without the use of ordinary means, for confirmation of the gospel, by the same good Spirit.

†**[Knox]** One, through the same Spirit, is given faith; another, through the same Spirit, powers of healing.

†**[MLV]** And miraculous faith to different one in the same Spirit; and gifts of healing to another in the same Spirit.

**[NLV]** One person receives the gift of faith. Another person receives the gifts of healing. These gifts are given by the same Holy Spirit.

†**[Shuttleworth-NT]** To another again is given a submiss and firm confidence in the doctrines of revelation; to another, the gift of healing diseases; but still again it is the same Spirit which manifests itself under these distinct appearances.

†**[TCNT]** To another faith by the same Spirit; to another power to cure diseases by the one Spirit; to another supernatural powers.

### 2 Corinthians 5:7

**[KJV]** (For we walk by faith, not by sight.)

**[AMPC]** For we walk by faith [we regulate our lives and conduct ourselves by our conviction or belief respecting man's relationship to God and divine things, with trust and holy fervor; thus we walk] not by sight *or* appearance.

**[CEB]** We live by faith and not by sight.

**[CJB]** For we live by trust, not by what we see.

**[ERV]** We live by what we believe will happen, not by what we can see.

**[GNT]** For our life is a matter of faith, not of sight.

**[GW]** Indeed, our lives are guided by faith, not by sight.

**[NLT]** For we live by believing and not by seeing.

**[NLV]** Our life is lived by faith. We do not live by what we see in front of us.

**[WE]** We do not see these things, but we believe them.

## 2 Corinthians 10:4-5

**[KJV]** (For the weapons of our warfare are not carnal, but mighty through God to the pulling down of strong holds;) Casting down imaginations, and every high thing that exalteth itself against the knowledge of God, and bringing into captivity every thought to the obedience of Christ.

**[CEB]** Our weapons that we fight with aren't human, but instead they are powered by God for the destruction of fortresses. They destroy arguments, and every defense that is raised up to oppose the knowledge of God. They capture every thought to make it obedient to Christ.

**[CEV]** Or fight our battles with the weapons of this world. Instead, we use God's power that can destroy fortresses. We destroy arguments and every bit of pride that keeps anyone from knowing God. We capture people's thoughts and make them obey Christ.

**[ERV]** The weapons we use are not human ones. Our weapons have power from God and can destroy the enemy's strong places. We destroy people's arguments, and we tear down every proud idea that raises itself against the knowledge of God. We also capture every thought and make it give up and obey Christ.

**[GNT]** The weapons we use in our fight are not the world's weapons but God's powerful weapons, which we use to destroy strongholds. We destroy false arguments; we pull down every proud obstacle that is raised against the knowledge of God; we take every thought captive and make it obey Christ.

**[NIV]** The weapons we fight with are not the weapons of the world. On the contrary, they have divine power to demolish strongholds. We demolish arguments and every pretension that sets itself up against the knowledge of God, and we take captive every thought to make it obedient to Christ.

**[NLT]** We use God's mighty weapons, not worldly weapons, to knock down the strongholds of human reasoning and to destroy false arguments. We destroy every proud obstacle that keeps people from knowing God. We capture their rebellious thoughts and teach them to obey Christ.

**[PHILLIPS]** The truth is that, although of course we lead normal human lives, the battle we are fighting is on the spiritual level. The very weapons we use are not those of human warfare but powerful in God's warfare for the destruction of the enemy's strongholds. Our battle is to bring down every deceptive fantasy and every imposing defence that men erect against the true knowledge of God. We even fight to capture every thought until it acknowledges the authority of Christ.

**[WE]** We do not use the things of this world in our fighting, but we use the power of God. This power can break down the walls where the enemy hides. We can break down what people think and every big idea that tries to stop people from knowing God. And we can make every thought a prisoner to obey Christ.

## 2 Corinthians 12:7

**[KJV]** And lest I should be exalted above measure through the abundance of the revelations, there was given to me a thorn in the flesh, the messenger of Satan to buffet me, lest I should be exalted above measure.

**[RIV]** Because of the phenomenal revelations I have received and on account of the vast number of these revelations that God has entrusted to me — and to hinder the highly visible progress I am making — a special messenger has been sent from Satan to harass me with constant distractions and headaches. There's no doubt about it! Satan wants my head on a stake! Satan is constantly trying to buffet and distract me in an attempt to keep me from reaching a higher level of visibility and recognition and to sidetrack me from preaching my revelations.

**[DARBY]** And that I might not be exalted by the exceeding greatness of the revelations, there was given to me a thorn for the flesh, a messenger of Satan that he might buffet me, that I might not be exalted.

## Galatians 3:13

**[KJV]** Christ hath redeemed us from the curse of the law, being made a curse for us: for it is written, Cursed is every one that hangeth on a tree:

**[AMPC]** Christ purchased our freedom [redeeming us] from the curse (doom) of the Law [and its condemnation] by [Himself] becoming a curse for us, for it is written [in the Scriptures], Cursed is everyone who hangs on a tree (is crucified).

†**[Doddridge-NT]** But ever adored be the riches of divine grace, Christ hath redeemed us who believe in his name from the terrible curse of the law, and bought us off from that servitude and misery to which it inexorably doomed us, by being himself made a curse for us, and enduring the penalty which our sins had deserved: for such was the death which he bore in our stead; not only when considered as a capital punishment, which universally implies something of this, but as thus stigmatized by the express declaration of the law against everyone in such a particular circumstance; for it is written, "Cursed is everyone that hangeth on a tree." Now Christ, as you well know, was hung upon a tree; he expired on the cross, and his dead body hung for some time upon it.

†**[EEBT]** As a result of the Jews' rules, God would have had to punish us. God would have had to make us separate from himself. But Christ bought us, to make us free, because God punished him on our behalf. It says in the Old Testament: 'When people hang someone on a tree to kill him, that person must be separate from God.'

†**[Erasmus-NT]** Christ alone of all was not subject to the curse, for he was wholly innocent and owed nothing to the law. We were guilty and for this reason accursed. But he freed the guilty from the curse, changing our guilt into

innocence and our curse into a blessing. He is very far from wanting you to be led into servitude to the law. How has he liberated you? Though innocent himself, he paid the penalty owed for our crimes, thus taking upon himself the curse which held us firmly in its grasp. He did this though otherwise free from the curse and a partner in the blessing. Did he not take our crimes upon himself when as a criminal among criminals he underwent the ignominious punishment of the cross to redeem us? For we read in Deuteronomy: 'Cursed is anyone who hangs on a tree.'

**[ERV]** The law says we are under a curse for not always obeying it. But Christ took away that curse. He changed places with us and put himself under that curse. The Scriptures say, "Anyone who is hung on a tree is under a curse."

†**[NEB]** Christ bought us freedom from the curse of the law by becoming for our sake an accursed thing; for Scripture says, 'Cursed is everyone who is hanged on a tree.'

**[NLV]** Christ bought us with His blood and made us free from the Law. In that way, the Law could not punish us. Christ did this by carrying the load and by being punished instead of us. It is written, "Anyone who hangs on a cross is hated and punished."

†**[TPT]** Yet Christ paid the full price to set us free from the curse of the law. He absorbed it completely as he became a curse in our place. For it is written: "Everyone who is hung upon a tree is doubly cursed."

†**[Wand-NT]** Now, Christ bought us off the curse of the Law at the cost of being accursed for our sakes, 'Cursed is everyone who suffers a criminal's death.'

## Galatians 6:7

**[KJV]** Be not deceived; God is not mocked: for whatsoever a man soweth, that shall he also reap.

**[AMPC]** Do not be deceived *and* deluded *and* misled; God will not allow Himself to be sneered at (scorned, disdained, or mocked by mere pretensions or professions, or by His precepts being set aside.) [He inevitably deludes himself who attempts to delude God.] For whatever a man sows, that *and* that only is what he will reap.

**[CEB]** Make no mistake, God is not mocked. A person will harvest what they plant.

**[ERV]** If you think you can fool God, you are only fooling yourselves. You will harvest what you plant.

**[GNT]** Do not deceive yourselves; no one makes a fool of God. You will reap exactly what you plant.

**[NIV]** Do not be deceived: God cannot be mocked. A man reaps what he sows.

**[NLT]** Don't be misled — you cannot mock the justice of God. You will always harvest what you plant.

**[PHILLIPS]** Don't be under any illusion: you cannot make a fool of God! A man's harvest in life will depend entirely on what he sows.

### Ephesians 1:7

**[KJV]** In whom we have redemption through his blood, the forgiveness of sins, according to the riches of his grace.

**[AMPC]** In Him we have redemption (deliverance and salvation) through His blood, the remission (forgiveness) of our offenses (shortcomings and trespasses), in accordance with the riches *and* the generosity of His gracious favor.

**[CEB]** We have been ransomed through his Son's blood, and we have forgiveness for our failures based on his overflowing grace.

**[CEV]** Christ sacrificed his life's blood to set us free, which means our sins are now forgiven. Christ did this because of God's gift of undeserved grace to us. God has great wisdom and understanding.

**[ERV]** In Christ we are made free by his blood sacrifice. We have forgiveness of sins because of God's rich grace.

**[GNT]** For by the blood of Christ we are set free, that is, our sins are forgiven. How great is the grace of God.

**[NLT]** He is so rich in kindness and grace that he purchased our freedom with the blood of his Son and forgave our sins.

**[PHILLIPS]** It is through the Son, at the cost of his own blood, that we are redeemed, freely forgiven through that full and generous grace which has overflowed into our lives and opened our eyes to the truth.

**[WE]** Jesus Christ has given his blood [died] to make us free. He has forgiven us for our wrong ways. We have been put right with God freely because of his great kindness.

## Ephesians 2:10

**[KJV]** For we are his workmanship, created in Christ Jesus unto good works, which God hath before ordained that we should walk in them.

**[AMPC]** For we are God's [own] handiwork (His workmanship), recreated in Christ Jesus, [born anew] that we may do those good works which God predestined (planned beforehand) for us [taking paths which He prepared ahead of time], that we should walk in them [living the good life which He prearranged and made ready for us to live].

**[CEB]** Instead, we are God's accomplishment, created in Christ Jesus to do good things. God planned for these good things to be the way that we live our lives.

**[CEV]** God planned for us to do good things and to live as he has always wanted us to live. This is why he sent Christ to make us what we are.

**[ERV]** God has made us what we are. In Christ Jesus, God made us new people so that we would spend our lives doing the good things he had already planned for us to do.

**[GNT]** God has made us what we are, and in our union with Christ Jesus he has created us for a life of good deeds, which he has already prepared for us to do.

**[ISV]** For we are God's masterpiece, created in the Messiah Jesus to perform good actions that God prepared long ago to be our way of life.

**[NET]** For we are his creative work, having been created in Christ Jesus for good works that God prepared beforehand so we can do them.

†**[TPT]** We have become his poetry, a re-created people that will fulfill the destiny he has given each of us, for we are joined to Jesus, the Anointed One. Even before we were born, God planned in advance our destiny and the good works we would do to fulfill it!

## Ephesians 4:23

**[KJV]** And be renewed in the spirit of your mind.

**[CEB]** Instead, renew the thinking in your mind by the Spirit.

**[CEV]** Let the Spirit change your way of thinking.

**[ERV]** You must be made new in your hearts and in your thinking.

**[GNT]** Your hearts and minds must be made completely new.

**[GW]** However, you were taught to have a new attitude.

**[ISV]** To be renewed in your mental attitude.

**[NIV]** To be made new in the attitude of your minds.

**[NLT]** Instead, let the Spirit renew your thoughts and attitudes.

**[PHILLIPS]** But you have learned nothing like that from Christ, if you have really heard his voice and understood the truth that he has taught you. No, what you learned was to fling off the dirty clothes of the old way of living, which were rotted through and through with lust's illusions, and, with yourselves mentally and spiritually re-made, to put on the clean fresh clothes of the new life which was made by God's design for righteousness and the holiness which is no illusion.

**[WE]** Have a new mind and heart.

## Ephesians 4:27

**[KJV]** Neither give place to the devil.

**[AMPC]** Leave no [such] room *or* foothold for the devil [give no opportunity to him].

†**[Beck]** Don't give the Devil a chance to work.

†**[Erasmus-NT]** Let harmony, by itself, make you safe against the scoffing of the devil; if it is torn apart by hatreds and mutual affronts, there will be laid open to the foe a fissure through which he may burst in, to your destruction. Against those who are of one mind he is feeble; against the divided, powerful. To him you will be giving a place if a place is given to hatred.

**[ERV]** Don't give the devil a way to defeat you.

†**[Heberden-NT]** Neither give place to the evil suggestions of the devil.

†**[Kneeland-NT]** And give no advantage to the impostor.

**[NLV]** Do not let the devil start working in your life.

†**[Norlie-NT]** Do not let the devil get that satisfaction.

†**[Williams-NT]** Stop giving the devil a chance.

†**[Worsley-NT]** And give not the devil room to ensnare you.

†**[Wuest-NT]** And stop giving an occasion for acting [opportunity] to the devil.

## Ephesians 6:12

**[KJV]** For we wrestle not against flesh and blood, but against principalities, against powers, against the rulers of the darkness of this world, against spiritual wickedness in high places.

**[AMPC]** For we are not wrestling with flesh and blood [contending only with physical opponents], but against the despotisms, against the powers, against [the master spirits who are] the world rulers of this present darkness, against the spirit forces of wickedness in the heavenly (supernatural) sphere.

†**[EEBT]** You need to be strong because we are not fighting against human enemies. No, but instead we are fighting against the rulers and the powerful spirits that have authority over this dark world. We are fighting against powerful bad spirits who live in the heavens.

†**[Macrae]** For our wrestling is not with flesh and blood alone, but with (diabolical) principalities and powers, who rule in the darkness (i.e. ignorance, error, and wickedness) of this world, with wicked spirits, with respect to heavenly things.

†**[Madsen-NT]** For our part is not to fight against powers of flesh and blood, but against spirit-beings, mighty in the stream of time, against spirit-beings, powerful in the moulding of earth's substance, against the cosmic powers whose darkness rules the present time, against beings who, in the spiritual worlds, are themselves the powers of evil.

**[NLV]** Our fight is not with people. It is against the leaders and the powers and the spirits of darkness in this world. It is against the demon world that works in the heavens.

†**[Norlie-NT]** For our struggle is not so much against wicked men, but rather against the forces, authorities and master-spirits that rule this world in its present darkness. Yes, our war is against the wicked spiritual forces of the underworld itself.

†**[Shuttleworth-NT]** For the Christian's warfare is not against flesh and blood, which is able to destroy the body, but against spiritual beings leagued for his eternal destruction, the various orders of evil angels who rule over the dark elements of this world, and who surround the earth, looking down upon us, and seeking whom they may devour.

†**[Way-NT]** For we have to close in grapple not with human flesh and blood alone, But with Principalities, with Powers, With the Lords of Darkness whose present sway is world-wide, With the spirit-host of Wicked Beings that haunt the upper air.

†**[Weymouth-NT]** For ours is not a conflict with mere flesh and blood, but with the despotisms, the empires, the forces that control and govern this dark world — the spiritual hosts of evil arrayed against us in the heavenly warfare.

## Philippians 4:6

**[KJV]** Be careful for nothing; but in every thing by prayer and supplication with thanksgiving let your requests be made known unto God.

†**[Beck]** Don't worry about anything, but in everything go to God, and pray to let Him know what you want, and give thanks.

†**[BV-KJV-NT]** Worry about nothing, but in everything by the prayer and the plea with thankfulness, your requests must be made known to God.

†**[Doddridge-NT]** In the mean time, whatever necessities or whatever oppressions may arise, be anxious about nothing, so as to disquiet or distress your minds; but in every thing that occurs, in every condition and on every occasion, let your petitions be made known, and breathed out before God, in humble prayer and fervent supplication, to be still mingled with thanksgiving, as there is always room for praise, and always occasion for it, even in circumstances of the greatest affliction and distress.

†**[Harwood-NT]** Suffer not your minds to be corroded with anxious cares about any thing: in every situation of life do you, with fervent prayer and devout gratitude, address your petitions to the Supreme.

†**[Jerusalem]** There is no need to worry; but if there is anything you need, pray for it, asking God for it with prayer and thanksgiving.

†**[Madsen-NT]** Let no anxiety take root in your hearts, but let your concerns in all things be known to God by sending your thankful thoughts upwards in supplication and prayer.

†**[Stevens-NT]** Be not distracted by anxious care, but in prayer and praise commit your wants and desires to God.

†**[TPT]** Don't be pulled in different directions or worried about a thing. Be saturated in prayer throughout each day, offering your faith-filled requests before God with overflowing gratitude. Tell him every detail of your life.

†**[Williams-NT]** Stop being worried about anything, but always, in prayer and entreaty, and with thanksgiving, keep on making your wants known to God.

†**[Wuest-NT]** Stop worrying about even one thing, but in everything by prayer whose essence is that of worship and devotion and by supplication which is a cry for your personal needs, with thanksgiving let your requests for the things asked for be made known in the presence of God.

## Colossians 1:13-14

**[KJV]** Who hath delivered us from the power of darkness, and hath translated us into the kingdom of his dear Son: In whom we have redemption through his blood, even the forgiveness of sins.

**[AMPC]** [The Father] has delivered *and* drawn us to Himself out of the control *and* the dominion of darkness and has transferred us into the kingdom of the Son of His love, In Whom we have our redemption through His blood, [which means] the forgiveness of our sins.

**[CEB]** He rescued us from the control of darkness and transferred us into the kingdom of the Son he loves. He set us free through the Son and forgave our sins.

**[CJB]** He has rescued us from the domain of darkness and transferred us into the Kingdom of his dear Son. It is through his Son that we have redemption — that is, our sins have been forgiven.

†**[Haweis-NT]** Who hath plucked us out from the dominion of darkness, and transferred us into the kingdom of the Son of his love: in whom we have redemption through his blood, and forgiveness of sins.

**[PHILLIPS]** For we must never forget that he rescued us from the power of darkness, and re-established us in the kingdom of his beloved Son, that is, in the kingdom of light. For it is by his Son alone that we have been redeemed and have had our sins forgiven.

†**[TCNT]** For God has rescued us from the tyranny of Darkness, and has removed us into the Kingdom of his Son, who is the embodiment of his love, and through whom we have found deliverance in the forgiveness of our sins.

## Colossians 3:10

**[KJV]** And have put on the new man, which is renewed in knowledge after the image of him that created him.

**[AMPC]** And have clothed yourselves with the new [spiritual self], which is [ever in the process of being] renewed *and* remolded into [fuller and more perfect knowledge upon] knowledge after the image (the likeness) of Him Who created it.

**[CEB]** And put on the new nature, which is renewed in knowledge by conforming to the image of the one who created it.

**[CEV]** Each of you is now a new person. You are becoming more and more like your Creator, and you will understand him better.

**[ERV]** Now you are wearing a new life, a life that is new every day. You are growing in your understanding of the one who made you. You are becoming more and more like him.

**[GNT]** And have put on the new self. This is the new being which God, its Creator, is constantly renewing in his own image, in order to bring you to a full knowledge of himself.

**[NLT]** Put on your new nature, and be renewed as you learn to know your Creator and become like him.

**[WE]** And now you have become a new person. That new person is always learning more and more until he becomes like God who made him.

### 1 Thessalonians 4:4

**[KJV]** That every one of you should know how to possess his vessel in sanctification and honour.

**[AMPC]** That each one of you should know how to possess (control, manage) his own body in consecration (purity, separated from things profane) and honor.

**[CEB]** And learn how to control your own body in a pure and respectable way.

**[ERV]** God wants each one of you to learn to control your own body. Use your body in a way that is holy and that gives honor to God.

**[EHV]** He wants each of you to learn to obtain a wife for yourself in a way that is holy and honorable.

**[NET]** That each of you know how to possess his own body in holiness and honor.

**[NLV]** God wants each of you to use his body in the right way by keeping it holy and by respecting it.

**[PHILLIPS]** Every one of you should learn to control his body, keeping it pure and treating it with respect, and never regarding it as an instrument for self-gratification, as do pagans with no knowledge of God.

## 1 Thessalonians 5:23

**[KJV]** And the very God of peace sanctify you wholly; and I pray God your whole spirit and soul and body be preserved blameless unto the coming of our Lord Jesus Christ.

**[AMPC]** And may the God of peace Himself sanctify you through and through [separate you from profane things, make you pure and wholly consecrated to God]; and may your spirit and soul and body be preserved sound *and* complete [and found] blameless at the coming of our Lord Jesus Christ (the Messiah).

**[CEB]** Now, may the God of peace himself cause you to be completely dedicated to him; and may your spirit, soul, and body be kept intact and blameless at our Lord Jesus Christ's coming.

**[CJB]** May the God of *shalom* make you completely holy — may your entire spirit, soul and body be kept blameless for the coming of our Lord Yeshua the Messiah.

**[ERV]** We pray that God himself, the God of peace, will make you pure — belonging only to him. We pray that your whole self — spirit, soul, and body — will be kept safe and be blameless when our Lord Jesus Christ comes.

†**[MCC-NT]** Then may the God of Peace Himself sanctify you quite perfectly; and may your whole Frame, Spirit, Soul and Body, be preserved unblameable, till our Lord Jesus Christ's Advent.

†**[Knox]** So may the God of peace sanctify you wholly, keep spirit and soul and body unimpaired, to greet the coming of our Lord Jesus Christ without reproach.

**[NLV]** May the God of peace set you apart for Himself. May every part of you be set apart for God. May your spirit and your soul and your body be kept complete. May you be without blame when our Lord Jesus Christ comes again.

**[PHILLIPS]** May the God of peace make you holy through and through. May you be kept in soul and mind and body in spotless integrity until the coming of our Lord Jesus Christ.

## 1 Timothy 4:8

**[KJV]** For bodily exercise profiteth little: but godliness is profitable unto all things, having promise of the life that now is, and of that which is to come.

**[CEB]** While physical training has some value, training in holy living is useful for everything. It has promise for this life now and the life to come.

**[ERV]** Training your body helps you in some ways. But devotion to God helps you in every way. It brings you blessings in this life and in the future life too.

**[GNT]** Physical exercise has some value, but spiritual exercise is valuable in every way, because it promises life both for the present and for the future.

**[NIV]** For physical training is of some value, but godliness has value for all things, holding promise for both the present life and the life to come.

**[PHILLIPS]** Bodily fitness has a certain value, but spiritual fitness is essential both for this present life and for the life to come. There is no doubt about this at all, and Christians should remember it.

## 1 Timothy 6:12

**[KJV]** Fight the good fight of faith, lay hold on eternal life, whereunto thou art also called, and hast professed a good profession before many witnesses.

†**[Barclay-NT]** Strain every nerve, as the noble athlete of faith, to win the prize of eternal life. It was to this you were called, when you nobly and publicly confessed your faith in the presence of many witnesses.

**[CEB]** Compete in the good fight of faith. Grab hold of eternal life — you were called to it, and you made a good confession of it in the presence of many witnesses.

**[CJB]** Fight the good fight of the faith, take hold of the eternal life to which you were called when you testified so well to your faith before many witnesses.

†**[Goodspeed-NT]** Enter the great contest of faith! Take hold of eternal life, to which God called you, when before many witnesses you made the great profession of faith.

†**[Haweis-NT]** Strain every nerve in the noble conflict of faith, lay fast hold on eternal life, unto which also thou hast been called, and hast confessed the good confession before many witnesses.

†**[Macknight-NT]** Combat the good combat of faith: Lay hold on eternal life, to which also thou wast called; and confess the good confession in the presence of many witnesses.

**[PHILLIPS]** Fight the worthwhile battle of the faith, keep your grip on that life eternal to which you have been called, and to which you boldly professed your loyalty before many witnesses.

†**[Spencer-NT]** Strive in the noble contest of the faith, seize hold of the life eternal to which thou wert called and of which thou madest that noble confession before many witnesses.

†**[TPT]** So fight with faith for the winner's prize! Lay your hands upon eternal life, for this is your calling — celebrating in faith before the multitude of witnesses!

†**[Weymouth-NT]** Exert all your strength in the honourable struggle for the faith; lay hold of the Life of the Ages, to which you were called, when you made your noble profession of faith before many witnesses.

## 2 Timothy 1:7

**[KJV]** For God hath not given us the spirit of fear; but of power, and of love, and of a sound mind.

**[AMPC]** For God did not give us a spirit of timidity (of cowardice, of craven and cringing and fawning fear), but [He has given us a spirit] of power and of love and of calm *and* well-balanced mind *and* discipline *and* self-control.

†**[BV-KJV-NT]** You see, God did not give us a spirit of cowardice, but of ability, of love, and of proper focus.

†**[GT]** God did not give us a cowardly attitude. No, God gave us one of power, of giving of self to others, for their good, expecting nothing in return, and good sense.

†**[Guyse-NT]** You ought by no means to be discouraged in the exercise of those gifts, on account of the opposition of your adversaries: For the temper and disposition, which God by his spirit has formed in us, whom he hath called and fitted for holy ministrations, is not a spirit of cowardice and dread of our enemies, whether men or devils; but is a spirit of holy fortitude and undaunted courage to encounter all difficulties and dangers; and of fervent love to Christ and his cause, and to immortal souls; and of sobriety and good judgment, in a due government of our passions, and in stedfastly adhering to, and patiently suffering for, the true gospel of Christ.

†**[Mace-NT]** For the spirit, which God has given us, is not a spirit of timidity, but of fortitude, of benevolence, and of moderation.

†**[Macknight-NTc]** For God hath not infused into us a spirit of cowardice which shrinks at danger, but of courage, such as becometh those who possess the gifts of inspiration and miracles, and of benevolence, which disposes us to communicate the gospel to all mankind, and of self-government, to behave with prudence on every occasion.

†**[MCC-NT]** For God has not given Us an Impulse of Dismay, but of Power, and of Love, and of Discretion.

†**[Shuttleworth-NT]** For the precious gift was not communicated that it might lie dormant through timidity, but that it might operate by miracles, and works of Christian charity, and well-regulated zeal.

†**[T4T]** Remember that God has put his Spirit within us. His Spirit does not cause us to be afraid. Instead, he causes us to be powerful to work for God, and he helps us to love others and to control what we say and do.

†**[Weymouth-NT]** For the Spirit which God has given us is not a spirit of cowardice, but one of power and of love and of sound judgement.

### Titus 2:14

**[KJV]** Who gave himself for us, that he might redeem us from all iniquity, and purify unto himself a peculiar people, zealous of good works.

**[AMPC]** Who gave Himself on our behalf that He might redeem us (purchase our freedom) from all iniquity and purify for Himself a people [to be peculiarly His own, people who are] eager *and* enthusiastic about [living a life that is good and filled with] beneficial deeds.

**[CEB]** He gave himself for us in order to rescue us from every kind of lawless behavior, and cleanse a special people for himself who are eager to do good actions.

**[CEV]** He gave himself to rescue us from everything evil and to make our hearts pure. He wanted us to be his own people and to be eager to do right.

**[CJB]** He gave himself up on our behalf in order to free us from all violation of Torah and purify for himself a people who would be his own, eager to do good.

**[ERV]** He gave himself for us. He died to free us from all evil. He died to make us pure — people who belong only to him and who always want to do good.

**[GNT]** He gave himself for us, to rescue us from all wickedness and to make us a pure people who belong to him alone and are eager to do good.

**[NLT]** He gave his life to free us from every kind of sin, to cleanse us, and to make us his very own people, totally committed to doing good deeds.

**[PHILLIPS]** For he gave himself for us all, that he might rescue us from all our evil ways and make for himself a people of his own, clean and pure, with our hearts set upon living a life that is good.

### Hebrews 2:1

**[KJV]** Therefore we ought to give the more earnest heed to the things which we have heard, lest at any time we should let them slip.

**[CEB]** This is why it's necessary for us to pay more attention to what we have heard, or else we may drift away from it.

**[ERV]** So we must be more careful to follow what we were taught. We must be careful so that we will not be pulled away from the true way.

**[GNT]** That is why we must hold on all the more firmly to the truths we have heard, so that we will not be carried away.

**[NET]** Therefore we must pay closer attention to what we have heard, so that we do not drift away.

**[NLT]** So we must listen very carefully to the truth we have heard, or we may drift away from it.

**[NLV]** That is why we must listen all the more to the truths we have been told. If we do not, we may slip away from them.

**[PHILLIPS]** We ought, therefore, to pay the greatest attention to the truth that we have heard and not allow ourselves to drift away from it.

## Hebrews 4:16

**[KJV]** Let us therefore come boldly unto the throne of grace, that we may obtain mercy, and find grace to help in time of need.

†**[Bowes-NT]** Let us therefore approach with freedom of speech the throne of grace, that we may receive mercy and find grace for seasonable support.

†**[BV-NT]** So we may come with openness to the throne of the generosity so that we might receive forgiving kindness and find generosity for well-timed help.

†**[Madsen-NT]** Let us then approach the throne of grace with confident freedom, that we may experience compassionate goodness and find a share in the grace which sends us help in the right hour.

**[NLV]** Let us go with complete trust to the throne of God. We will receive His loving-kindness and have His loving-favor to help us whenever we need it.

**[PHILLIPS]** Let us therefore approach the throne of grace with fullest confidence, that we may receive mercy for our failures and grace to help in the hour of need.

†**[SG]** So let us come with courage to God's throne of grace to receive his forgiveness and find him responsive when we need his help.

†**[Stevens-NT]** We may therefore fearlessly approach his heavenly seat in the assurance that he will receive us with favor and will strengthen us to resist and overcome the power of evil when we are tempted.

†**[Way-NT]** Let us, then, approach God's throne of grace with a fearlessly-outspoken plea, that we may gain God's mercy, and find His grace bestowed for our help just when it can best avail us.

## Hebrews 10:23

**[KJV]** Let us hold fast the profession of our faith without wavering; (for he is faithful that promised.)

**[AMPC]** So let us seize *and* hold fast *and* retain without wavering the hope we cherish *and* confess *and* our acknowledgement of it, for He Who promised is reliable (sure) *and* faithful to His word.

†**[Barclay-NT]** Let us hold inflexibly to the hope which we tell the world we possess, for we can rely on the word of him who promised it to us.

**[GW]** We must continue to hold firmly to our declaration of faith. The one who made the promise is faithful.

†**[Hammond-NT]** Let not all the afflictions and dangers that can approach us move us so much as to waver in our Christian profession, which, having the hope of eternal life joined with it, is fortification enough against all the terrors of this world, having God's fidelity engaged to make good the promise to us.

†**[Knox]** Do not let us waver in acknowledging the hope we cherish; we have a promise from one who is true to his word.

†**[NEB]** Let us be firm and unswerving in the confession of our hope, for the Giver of the promise may be trusted.

**[PHILLIPS]** In this confidence let us hold on to the hope that we profess without the slightest hesitation — for he is utterly dependable.

†**[Sacred-NT]** Let us hold fast the confession of the hope, unmoved; for he is faithful, who has promised.

†**[Stevens-NT]** And let us steadfastly adhere to the assurance of salvation given us in Christ, for this promise of God will not fail of its fulfilment.

†**[T4T]** We must unwaveringly keep professing what we believe. Since God faithfully does all he promised to do, we must confidently expect him to keep doing that.

†**[TCNT]** Let us maintain the confession of our hope unshaken, for he who has given us his promise will not fail us.

†**[Wand-NT]** Let us cling to the statement of our hope without any weakening, for He who gave us the promise is utterly trustworthy.

## Hebrews 13:8

**[KJV]** Jesus Christ the same yesterday, and to day, and for ever.

**[AMPC]** Jesus Christ (the Messiah) is [always] the same, yesterday, today, [yes] and forever (to the ages).

†**[EEBT]** Jesus Christ is the same today as he was yesterday. And he will be the same always.

†**[Goodspeed-NT]** Jesus Christ is the same today that he was yesterday, and he will be so forever.

†**[Rotherham]** Jesus Christ, yesterday, and today, is the same, — and unto the ages.

†**[T4T]** Jesus Christ is the same now as he was previously, and he will be the same forever.

†**[TCNT]** Jesus Christ is the same yesterday and to-day — yes, and for ever!

†**[TPT]** Jesus, the Anointed One, is always the same — yesterday, today, and forever.

†**[Wade]** Jesus Christ, the object of their faith, is, in the past, in the present, and for all time to come, ever the Same.

†**[Wand-NT]** Jesus Christ is for you just what He was for them, the same yesterday, to-day and for ever.

## James 1:3

**[KJV]** Knowing this, that the trying of your faith worketh patience.

**[RIV]** You need to know — really know, and never forget, that difficult situations come to see if you are serious about your stance of faith and if your faith is really all it claims to be or if it will break under pressure. But finally… when those tests let up, and your faith is still standing strong, it will have proven your faith to be real. When you push back to resist the tests that have been sent to break you — that pushback triggers a release of divine endurance that fills you from the top of your head clear to the bottom of your feet! It's a supernatural endurance that will enable you to bear up under any heavy load, and it will give you the ability to stay put, to keep your position, and to never surrender. I'm talking about a power that will enable you to hold on; hold out; never give up; neither bend nor break; outlast; persevere; and stick it out. This power will strengthen you to hold on to whatever promise or territory is under assault.

**[AMPC]** Be assured and understand that the trial *and* proving of your faith bring out endurance *and* steadfastness *and* patience.

**[CEB]** After all, you know that the testing of your faith produces endurance.

**[GNT]** For you know that when your faith succeeds in facing such trials, the result is the ability to endure.

**[NIV]** Because you know that the testing of your faith produces perseverance.

**[NLT]** For you know that when your faith is tested, your endurance has a chance to grow.

**[NLV]** You know these prove your faith. It helps you not to give up.

**[PHILLIPS]** Realise that they come to test your faith and to produce in you the quality of endurance.

**[WE]** You know this, that when you prove you believe, you become stronger to take troubles.

## James 1:4

**[KJV]** But let patience have her perfect work, that ye may be perfect and entire, wanting nothing.

**[RIV]** But you're the one who must make the choice to let this God-given endurance do its work. And if you'll let endurance run its full course, it will advance you into higher levels of spiritual maturity. Choosing to let endurance run its full course takes work — but if you'll stick with this process all the way to the end, you'll advance to high spiritual levels in your life. Not only that, but you'll have in your possession the quality necessary to possess your God-given inheritance — ending up with no deficits, shortages, or lack of any kind, and I mean none whatsoever.

**[AMPC]** But let endurance *and* steadfastness *and* patience have full play *and* do a thorough work, so that you may be [people] perfectly and fully developed [with no defects], lacking in nothing.

**[CJB]** But let perseverance do its complete work; so that you may be complete and whole, lacking in nothing.

**[ERV]** If you let that patience work in you, the end result will be good. You will be mature and complete. You will be all that God wants you to be.

**[GNT]** Make sure that your endurance carries you all the way without failing, so that you may be perfect and complete, lacking nothing.

**[NIV]** Let perseverance finish its work so that you may be mature and complete, not lacking anything.

**[NLT]** So let it grow, for when your endurance is fully developed, you will be perfect and complete, needing nothing.

**[NLV]** Learn well how to wait so you will be strong and complete and in need of nothing.

**[PHILLIPS]** But let the process go on until that endurance is fully developed, and you will find you have become men of mature character with the right sort of independence.

### James 1:5-6

**[KJV]** If any of you lack wisdom, let him ask of God, that giveth to all men liberally, and upbraideth not; and it shall be given him. But let him ask in faith, nothing wavering. For he that wavereth is like a wave of the sea driven with the wind and tossed.

**[RIV]** But if — as I'm sure is actually the case — there is anyone among you who lacks insight about why these principles aren't already working, my advice is that you draw near to the side of the giving God to ask your questions with the full expectation of an answer from the One who always generously responds with an open hand to every person who comes to Him. And when you come to Him with your questions, He will not berate, reprimand, or scold you for asking the questions you put before Him — for answers are always generously given to the person who draws near to God to find them. But this next point is important, so pay close attention. Whoever is asking must do it with an expectation that God will actually answer him. In other words, he must ask, being rooted in faith (with unwavering confidence). The one who doesn't stick with it, but who habitually changes his mind — who is up one day and down the next, flip-flopping and going back and forth "all over the place" in what he asks or believes — is a lot like the waves of the sea. Just as waves rise, fall, and tumble back into the sea over and over, a doubting person is one who keeps changing his mind again and again. He appears to be making progress, but then, suddenly, he changes his mind again and tumbles back into indecision. He is up and down, back and forth, indecisive, and unstable. And as the waves of the sea are endlessly tossed by ferocious winds, one who doubts is thrown here, there, and all around. A person who can't make up his mind about what he asks and believes doesn't realize the dangerous predicament he's in — for like a dangerous riptide, his doubt and wavering can pull him perpetually into a sea of indecision.

**[CEB]** But anyone who needs wisdom should ask God, whose very nature is to give to everyone without a second thought, without keeping score. Wisdom will certainly be given to those who ask. Whoever asks shouldn't hesitate. They should ask in faith, without doubting. Whoever doubts is like the surf of the sea, tossed and turned by the wind.

**[CEV]** If any of you need wisdom, you should ask God, and it will be given to you. God is generous and won't correct you for asking. But when you ask for something, you must have faith and not doubt. Anyone who doubts is like an ocean wave tossed around in a storm.

**[ERV]** Do any of you need wisdom? Ask God for it. He is generous and enjoys giving to everyone. So he will give you wisdom. But when you ask God, you must believe. Don't doubt him. Whoever doubts is like a wave in the sea that is blown up and down by the wind.

**[GNT]** But if any of you lack wisdom, you should pray to God, who will give it to you; because God gives generously and graciously to all. But when you pray, you must believe and not doubt at all. Whoever doubts is like a wave in the sea that is driven and blown about by the wind.

**[GW]** If any of you needs wisdom to know what you should do, you should ask God, and he will give it to you. God is generous to everyone and doesn't find fault with them. When you ask for something, don't have any doubts. A person who has doubts is like a wave that is blown by the wind and tossed by the sea.

**[NIV]** If any of you lacks wisdom, you should ask God, who gives generously to all without finding fault, and it will be given to you. But when you ask, you must believe and not doubt, because the one who doubts is like a wave of the sea, blown and tossed by the wind.

**[PHILLIPS]** And if, in the process, any of you does not know how to meet any particular problem he has only to ask God — who gives generously to all men without making them feel foolish or guilty — and he may be quite sure that the necessary wisdom will be given him. But he must ask in sincere faith without secret doubts as to whether he really wants God's help or not. The man who trusts God, but with inward reservations, is like a wave of the sea, carried forward by the wind one moment and driven back the next.

**[WE]** If any of you need to be wise, ask God to make you wise. He gives plenty of wisdom to all people. He is not angry because you ask him. He will make you wise. But when you ask, you must believe that God will do it. You must not doubt and think, 'Perhaps God will not do it.' A person who doubts is like a wave on the sea. The wind drives it this way and that way.

## James 3:16

**[KJV]** For where envying and strife is, there is confusion and every evil work.

**[RIV]** For it is a fact that whenever one is driven to see his view or agenda adopted at the expense of others, and he is irritated, irate, annoyed, provoked, fuming, or incensed at those who have other views — so filled with strife in his heart that he is blinded to the desires or needs of others — and jockeys for advantage or position even at the expense of others, there is anarchy, chaos, confusion, and insubordination. And that leads to instability, upheaval, unrest, and absolutely every kind of dead, decaying, foul, and stinking activity and business.

**[AMPC]** For wherever there is jealousy (envy) and contention (rivalry and selfish ambition), there will also be confusion (unrest, disharmony, rebellion) and all sorts of evil *and* vile practices.

**[ASV]** For where jealousy and faction are, there is confusion and every vile deed.

**[CSB]** For where there is envy and selfish ambition, there is disorder and every evil practice.

**[CEB]** Wherever there is jealousy and selfish ambition, there is disorder and everything that is evil.

**[CEV]** Whenever people are jealous or selfish, they cause trouble and do all sorts of cruel things.

**[DARBY]** For where emulation and strife [are], there [is] disorder and every evil thing.

**[ERV]** Where there is jealousy and selfishness, there will be confusion and every kind of evil.

**[GW]** Wherever there is jealousy and rivalry, there is disorder and every kind of evil.

**[WE]** If people are jealous of others, their lives are not right. They do every kind of wrong thing to get what they want. They confuse and upset people.

## James 4:7

**[KJV]** Submit yourselves therefore to God. Resist the devil, and he will flee from you.

**[RIV]** It is imperative that you make the decision to properly align yourselves under the authority of God — in a submitted position that actually provides you with protection. Being submitted to His authority gives you the ability to defy, oppose, stand steadfastly against, and withstand the accusing, slanderous, trap-setting behavior of the devil. In fact, he'll be so terrified of you that he'll move his feet as fast as he can to get away from you. Not only will he flee from you, he'll run like a criminal terrified of prosecution — so scared that he'll want to do all he can to put as much space between him and you as possible.

**[AMPC]** So be subject to God. Resist the devil [stand firm against him], and he will flee from you.

†**[Authentic-NT]** Submit yourselves to God therefore, but oppose the Devil and he will fly from you.

**[CEV]** Surrender to God! Resist the devil, and he will run from you.

†**[Doddridge-NT]** Subject yourselves therefore to God; and in being listed in his army, keep the rank which he has assigned you; resist the devil steadily and courageously, as the great enemy of your eternal salvation: and though he may for a while combat you with his varied temptations, he will at length flee from you, and your progress in religion, and your victory over your spiritual adversaries, will grow daily more easy.

**[NCV]** So give yourselves completely to God. Stand against the devil, and the devil will run from you.

†**[NEB]** Be submissive then to God. Stand up to the devil and he will turn and run.

**[NLT]** So humble yourselves before God. Resist the devil, and he will flee from you.

†**[Shuttleworth-NT]** Submit yourselves then to God's blessed protection, and under his support resist the devil, and he will flee from you.

†**[T4T]** So submit yourselves to God. Resist the devil/Refuse to do what the devil wants, and as a result he will run away from you.

†**[Wuest-NT]** Be subject with implicit obedience to God at once and once for all. Stand immovable against the onset of the devil and he will flee from you.

## James 5:14-16

**[KJV]** Is any sick among you? let him call for the elders of the church; and let them pray over him, anointing him with oil in the name of the Lord. And the prayer of faith shall save the sick, and the Lord shall raise him up; and if he have committed sins, they shall be forgiven him. Confess your faults one to another, and pray one for another, that ye may be healed. The effectual fervent prayer of a righteous man availeth much.

**[RIV]** Is anyone among you weak, sick, or incapacitated due to illness? Let that person personally call for the ordained leaders of the local assembly to come and passionately petition God on his behalf. Let the leaders hover over him in prayer, anointing the sick person with oil and operating in the stead of Jesus — that is, acting on His behalf and using the authority and reputation of the name of the Lord — the One who has authority in every seen and unseen realm [and that certainly includes authority and mastery over sickness and disease]. And the heartfelt prayer of rock-solid, steadfast, unwavering faith will deliver, heal, liberate, and physically save the person weakened from sickness — and as a result, the Lord — the One with supreme authority in every realm, seen and unseen — will raise him up. And if — as the case may be — he has carried out behaviors that have missed the mark of what is right and are sinful in nature, he will be forgiven and freed from them. Confess reciprocally to each other areas where you have sinned and missed the mark, and come to the altar of God together to earnestly pray on behalf of and for the betterment of one another so that you may be healed. Oh, how vast, mighty, effective, energizing, and powerful is the concrete and clearly stated petition of a righteous person.

**[AMPC]** Is anyone among you sick? He should call in the church elders (the spiritual guides). And they should pray over him, anointing him with oil in the Lord's name. And the prayer [that is] of faith will save him who is sick, and the Lord will restore him; and if he has committed sins, he will be forgiven. Confess to one another therefore your faults (your slips, your false steps, your offenses, your sins) and pray [also] for one another, that you may be healed *and* restored [to a spiritual tone of mind and heart]. The earnest (heartfelt, continued) prayer of a righteous man makes tremendous power available [dynamic in its working].

**[ERV]** Are you sick? Ask the elders of the church to come and rub oil on you in the name of the Lord and pray for you. If such a prayer is offered in faith, it will heal anyone who is sick. The Lord will heal them. And if they have sinned, he will forgive them. So always tell each other the wrong things you have done. Then pray for each other. Do this so that God can heal you. Anyone who lives the way God wants can pray, and great things will happen.

†**[Etheridge-NT]** And if he be sick, let him call for the presbyters of the church, and they will pray over him and anoint him with oil in the name of our Lord. And the prayer of faith shall make whole him who was sick, and our Lord shall raise him up; and if he have committed sins, they shall be forgiven him. But confess your faults one to another, and pray one for another, that you may be healed. For great is the power of that prayer which the righteous prayeth.

†**[MW-NT]** Is any among you sick? Let him call for the elders of the congregation, and let them pray over him, anointing him with oil in the name of the Lord. Then the prayer of faith will heal the one who is sick, and the Lord will raise him up. If he has committed sins, he will be forgiven. Confess your offenses to each other, and pray for each other, that you may be healed. The earnest entreaty of a righteous man is very powerful.

†**[NJB]** Any one of you who is ill should send for the elders of the church, and they must anoint the sick person with oil in the name of the Lord and pray over him. The prayer of faith will save the sick person and the Lord will raise him up again; and if he has committed any sins, he will be forgiven. So confess your sins to one another, and pray for one another to be cured; the heartfelt prayer of someone upright works very powerfully.

**[NLV]** Is anyone among you sick? He should send for the church leaders and they should pray for him. They should pour oil on him in the name of the Lord. The prayer given in faith will heal the sick man, and the Lord will raise him up. If he has sinned, he will be forgiven. Tell your sins to each other. And pray for each other so you may be healed. The prayer from the heart of a man right with God has much power.

**[PHILLIPS]** If anyone is ill he should send for the church elders. They should pray over him, anointing him with oil in the Lord's name. Believing prayer will save the sick man; the Lord will restore him and any sins that he has committed will be forgiven. You should get into the habit of admitting your sins to each other, and praying for each other, so that you may be healed. Tremendous power is made available through a good man's earnest prayer.

†**[T4T]** Whoever among you is sick should call the leaders of the congregation to come to pray for him. They should put olive oil on him and, with the Lord's authority (OR, calling on the Lord to heal him), pray. And if they truly trust in the Lord when they pray, the sick person will be healed. The Lord will heal him. And if that person has sinned in a way that caused him to be/and because of that he became sick, if he confesses what he did/says that he did what is wrong, he will be forgiven {the Lord will forgive him}. So, because the Lord is able to heal the sick and to forgive sins, tell each other the sinful things that you have done, and pray for each other in order that you may be healed {that God may heal you} physically and spiritually. If righteous people pray and ask fervently for God to do something, God will act powerfully and will certainly do it.

**[YLT]** Is any infirm among you? let him call for the elders of the assembly, and let them pray over him, having anointed him with oil, in the name of the Lord, and the prayer of the faith shall save the distressed one, and the Lord shall raise him up, and if sins he may have committed, they shall be forgiven to him. Be confessing to one another the trespasses, and be praying for one another, that ye may be healed; very strong is a working supplication of a righteous man.

## 1 Peter 1:13

**[KJV]** Wherefore gird up the loins of your mind, be sober, and hope to the end for the grace that is to be brought unto you at the revelation of Jesus Christ.

**[RIV]** On account of all this, you must gather up all the loose and dangling ends of your mind. Like a runner who gathers up all the dangling ends of his garment and tucks them under his belt to get them out of the way so he can run an unobstructed race, you must gather up the loins of your mind so that your spiritual productivity will be unobstructed. Be serious-minded and unaffected by urges, impulses, whims, and fluctuating emotions — and have a confident and expectant hope, reaching a level of maturity due to the grace that will be delivered to you in the day the curtains are pulled back and Jesus Christ is suddenly, fully revealed.

**[CEB]** Therefore, once you have your minds ready for action and you are thinking clearly, place your hope completely on the grace that will be brought to you when Jesus Christ is revealed.

**[CEV]** Be alert and think straight. Put all your hope in how God will treat you with undeserved grace when Jesus Christ appears.

**[ERV]** So prepare your minds for service. With complete self-control put all your hope in the grace that will be yours when Jesus Christ comes.

**[GNT]** So then, have your minds ready for action. Keep alert and set your hope completely on the blessing which will be given you when Jesus Christ is revealed.

**[GW]** Therefore, your minds must be clear and ready for action. Place your confidence completely in what God's kindness will bring you when Jesus Christ appears again.

**[NIV]** Therefore, with minds that are alert and fully sober, set your hope on the grace to be brought to you when Jesus Christ is revealed at his coming.

**[NLT]** So prepare your minds for action and exercise self-control. Put all your hope in the gracious salvation that will come to you when Jesus Christ is revealed to the world.

**[PHILLIPS]** So brace up your minds, and, as men who know what they are doing, rest the full weight of your hopes on the grace that will be yours when Jesus Christ reveals himself.

## 1 Peter 2:24

**[KJV]** Who his own self bare our sins in his own body on the tree, that we, being dead to sins, should live unto righteousness: by whose stripes ye were healed.

**[RIV]** Who Himself, like a priest serving at an altar, offered up each and every one of our sins in His very own body upon the Cross — which became the altar of sacrifice — in order that we, being dead to sin and wrongdoing, would be separated from them, emerge completely different and new, and henceforth live a life of righteousness. Furthermore, by the terrible lashing and stripes laid upon His body, you have been physically healed.

**[ERV]** Christ carried our sins in his body on the cross. He did this so that we would stop living for sin and live for what is right. By his wounds you were healed.

**[GW]** Christ carried our sins in his body on the cross so that freed from our sins, we could live a life that has God's approval. His wounds have healed you.

†**[Hanson-NT]** Who bore our sins himself, in his body, on the tree, that we, having died to sins, might live to righteousness; by whose hurt you were healed.

†**[Mace-NT]** He himself canceled our sins by the crucifixion of his body, that we being set free from sin, might live in the service of virtue. It is by his bruises that you were healed.

†**[Moffatt]** He bore our sins in his own body on the gibbet, that we might break with sin and live the good life; it is by his wounds that you have been healed.

**[PHILLIPS]** And he personally bore our sins in his own body on the cross, so that we might be dead to sin and be alive to all that is good. It was the suffering that he bore which has healed you.

**[WE]** Christ in his own body took the wrong things we have done to the cross. He did this so that we would stop our bad ways and live right. Because he was punished, you were healed.

†**[Weekes-NT]** He himself bore our sins in his own body upon the cross, in order that we, having become separated from our sins, should be alive to righteousness; for by his bruise ye have been healed.

†**[Wuest-NT]** Who himself carried up to the Cross our sins in His body and offered himself there as on an altar, doing this in order that we, having died with respect to our sins, might live with respect to righteousness, by means of whose bleeding stripe [the word "stripe" is in the singular here; a picture of our Lord's back after the scourging, one mass of raw, quivering flesh with no skin remaining, trickling with blood] you were healed.

### 1 Peter 3:10-11

**[KJV]** For he that will love life, and see good days, let him refrain his tongue from evil, and his lips that they speak no guile: Let him eschew evil, and do good; let him seek peace, and ensue it.

**[RIV]** For the person who fully intends to have a life that is full of gusto and zest — that is, a life really worth having and loving — and who wishes to see and personally experience really good and profitable days, times, and seasons in life, let him make sure his tongue refrains and ceases from speaking evil — [if a person wants to have a life filled with gusto and zest — a life really worth having and loving — that is, blessed] he must purposely put distance between himself and evil. And that includes watching what he says, no longer allowing his mouth to spue [reckless words] or to converse in such a way that baits others and drags them into negative conversations. For the person who really wants to have a good life must decide to permanently bow out of and forever put to bed such negative and rotten talk and to instead start producing speech that has beneficial, good, and profitable results. Let him wholeheartedly seek after peace — specifically the peace that causes cessation of conflict in relationships; a time of rebuilding and reconstruction with distractions removed; a time of relational prosperity; order in the place of relational chaos; and a calm, inner stability that results in one's ability to conduct himself peacefully even in circumstances that would normally be traumatic or upsetting. But to have this type of peace, one must mentally put on his "hunting gear" to pursue it like a hunter in pursuit of his prey. Because such peace tends to be elusive, it means one must determine that he will not stop his pursuit of it until he has finally apprehended it.

**[AMPC]** For let him who wants to enjoy life and see good days [good—whether apparent or not] keep his tongue free from evil and his lips from guile (treachery, deceit). Let him turn away from wickedness *and* shun it, and let him do right. Let him search for peace (harmony; undisturbedness from fears, agitating passions, and moral conflicts) and seek it eagerly. [Do not merely desire peaceful relations with God, with your fellowmen, and with yourself, but pursue, go after them!]

**[CEB]** For those who want to love life and see good days should keep their tongue from evil speaking and their lips from speaking lies. They should shun evil and do good; seek peace and chase after it.

**[CEV]** "Do you really love life? Do you want to be happy? Then stop saying cruel things and quit telling lies. Give up your evil ways and do right, as you find and follow the road to peace."

**[ERV]** The Scriptures say, "If you want to enjoy true life and have only good days, then avoid saying anything hurtful, and never let a lie come out of your mouth. Stop doing what is wrong, and do good. Look for peace, and do all you can to help people live peacefully."

**[GNT]** As the scripture says, "If you want to enjoy life and wish to see good times, you must keep from speaking evil and stop telling lies. You must turn away from evil and do good; you must strive for peace with all your heart."

**[NIV]** For, "Whoever would love life and see good days must keep their tongue from evil and their lips from deceitful speech. They must turn from evil and do good; they must seek peace and pursue it."

**[NLT]** For the Scriptures say, "If you want to enjoy life and see many happy days, keep your tongue from speaking evil and your lips from telling lies. Turn away from evil and do good. Search for peace, and work to maintain it."

**[WE]** The holy writings say, 'A man who wants to live and have good days must not say wrong things. He must not say anything that is not true. He must turn away from anything wrong and do what is good. He must try hard to find peace, and keep on looking for it.'

## 1 Peter 5:8-9

**[KJV]** Be sober, be vigilant; because your adversary the devil, as a roaring lion, walketh about, seeking whom he may devour: Whom resist stedfast in the faith, knowing that the same afflictions are accomplished in your brethren that are in the world.

**[RIV]** Think cautiously, clearly, coherently, level-headedly, and soberly — and keep your head on straight, staying free of the kind of hallucinatory thinking that is so indicative of drunks who can't think right because they are "under the influence." You need to be clear-headed, on high alert, watchful, wide awake, and determined to maintain your guard and protect what is yours. You need to know that the adversary is one who works like a prosecutor, looking for any tid-bit of information he can get his hands on to accuse you, prosecute you, and try to take you down. I'm talking about the devil — the one who is always hurling lies at people, verbally wrangling with them, and trying his best to ensnare and entrap them with accusations, lies, and slander. Exactly like a fierce, voracious lion who threatens and roars incessantly — nonstop — your adversary prowls around seriously searching and seeking for an exact prey or victim that he can devour to the point of slurping up everything that remains, until nothing is left of the victim at all. You must intentionally and strategically make a plan by which you can resist this enemy, and you must do everything you can to bolster and reinforce yourself in faith (and in really knowing what you believe). And you must continually know and never forget that the same identical kinds of physical distresses and mental and spiritual agonies are also coming against your brothers — the whole Christian family — who exist throughout the world.

**[AMPC]** Be well balanced (temperate, sober of mind), be vigilant *and* cautious at all times; for that enemy of yours, the devil, roams around like a lion roaring [in fierce hunger], seeking someone to seize upon *and* devour. Withstand him; be firm in faith [against his onset—rooted, established, strong, immovable, and determined], knowing that the same (identical) sufferings are appointed to your brotherhood (the whole body of Christians) throughout the world.

†**[HRB]** Be sensible, watch, because your adversary the Devil walks about as a roaring lion seeking someone he may devour; therefore resist him, being stead-fast in the faith: and know that the same sufferings befall your brethren that are in the world.

†**[NEB]** Awake! be on the alert! Your enemy the devil, like a roaring lion, prowls round looking for someone to devour. Stand up to him, firm in faith, and remember that your brother Christians are going through the same kinds of suffering while they are in the world.

**[NCV]** Control yourselves and be careful! The devil, your enemy, goes around like a roaring lion looking for someone to eat. Refuse to give in to him, by standing strong in your faith. You know that your Christian family all over the world is having the same kinds of suffering.

**[NLV]** Keep awake! Watch at all times. The devil is working against you. He is walking around like a hungry lion with his mouth open. He is looking for someone to eat. Stand against him and be strong in your faith. Remember, other Christians over all the world are suffering the same as you are.

**[PHILLIPS]** Be self-controlled and vigilant always, for your enemy the devil is always about, prowling like a lion roaring for its prey. Resist him, standing firm in your faith, remembering that the strain is the same for all your fellow-Christians in other parts of the world.

†**[TPT]** Be well balanced and always alert, because your enemy, the devil, roams around incessantly, like a roaring lion looking for its prey to devour. Take a decisive stand against him and resist his every attack with strong, vigorous faith. For you know that your believing brothers and sisters around the world are experiencing the same kinds of troubles you endure.

†**[Wand-NT]** Don't get excited but be continually on the watch, for the Devil like a roaring lion is continually on the prowl to see of whom he can make a meal. Against him stand steadfast in your faith, remembering that the same tribute of suffering is being paid by the rest of the brotherhood throughout the world.

**[WE]** Keep awake! Watch! Your enemy the devil is walking around like a growling lion. He is looking for someone to catch. Fight against the devil. Be strong because you believe. Remember that your brothers all over the world suffer the same kind of trouble as you.

†**[Wycliffe-Noble]** Be ye sober, and wake ye, for your adversary, the devil, as a roaring lion goeth about, seeking whom he shall devour. Whom against stand ye, strong in the faith, witting that the same passion is made to that brotherhood of you, that is in the world [witting the same passion to be done to that your brotherhood, that is in the world].

## 1 John 3:14-15

**[KJV]** We know that we have passed from death unto life, because we love the brethren. He that loveth not his brother abideth in death. Whosoever hateth his brother is a murderer: and ye know that no murderer hath eternal life abiding in him.

**[AMPC]** We know that we have passed over out of death into Life by the fact that we love the brethren (our fellow Christians). He who does not love abides (remains, is held and kept continually) in [spiritual] death. Anyone who hates (abominates, detests) his brother [in Christ] is [at heart] a murderer, and you know that no murderer has eternal life abiding (persevering) within him.

**[CEB]** We know that we have transferred from death to life, because we love the brothers and sisters. The person who does not love remains in death. Everyone who hates a brother or sister is a murderer, and you know that murderers don't have eternal life residing in them.

**[GNT]** We know that we have left death and come over into life; we know it because we love others. Those who do not love are still under the power of death. Those who hate others are murderers, and you know that murderers do not have eternal life in them.

**[ISV]** We know that we have passed from death to life, because we love one another. The person who does not love remains spiritually dead. Everyone who hates his brother is a murderer, and you know that no murderer has eternal life present in him.

**[NLT]** If we love our brothers and sisters who are believers, it proves that we have passed from death to life. But a person who has no love is still dead. Anyone who hates another brother or sister is really a murderer at heart. And you know that murderers don't have eternal life within them.

**[NLV]** We know we have passed from death into life. We know this because we love the Christians. The person who does not love has not passed from death into life. A man who hates his brother is a killer in his heart. You know that life which lasts forever is not in one who kills.

**[PHILLIPS]** We know that we have crossed the frontier from death to life because we do love our brothers. The man without love for his brothers is living in death already. The man who actively hates his brother is a potential murderer, and you will readily see that the eternal life of God cannot live in the heart of a murderer.

**[WE]** We know that we have gone from death to life. We know this because we love the Christian brothers. Anyone who does not love them has not gone from death to life. Everyone who hates his brother is like a man who kills a person. And you know that no one who kills a person has life that will live for ever.

## 1 John 4:18

**[KJV]** There is no fear in love; but perfect love casteth out fear: because fear hath torment. He that feareth is not made perfect in love.

**[AMPC]** There is no fear in love [dread does not exist], but full-grown (complete, perfect) love turns fear out of doors *and* expels every trace of terror! For fear brings with it the thought of punishment, and [so] he who is afraid has not reached the full maturity of love [is not yet grown into love's complete perfection].

**[CEB]** There is no fear in love, but perfect love drives out fear, because fear expects punishment. The person who is afraid has not been made perfect in love.

**[CJB]** There is no fear in love. On the contrary, love that has achieved its goal gets rid of fear, because fear has to do with punishment; the person who keeps fearing has not been brought to maturity in regard to love.

**[ERV]** Where God's love is, there is no fear, because God's perfect love takes away fear. It is his punishment that makes a person fear. So his love is not made perfect in the one who has fear.

**[NET]** There is no fear in love, but perfect love drives out fear, because fear has to do with punishment. The one who fears punishment has not been perfected in love.

**[NIV]** There is no fear in love. But perfect love drives out fear, because fear has to do with punishment. The one who fears is not made perfect in love.

**[NLV]** There is no fear in love. Perfect love puts fear out of our hearts. People have fear when they are afraid of being punished. The man who is afraid does not have perfect love.

## 1 John 5:4

**[KJV]** For whatsoever is born of God overcometh the world: and this is the victory that overcometh the world, even our faith.

**[ERV]** Because everyone who is a child of God has the power to win against the world. It is our faith that has won the victory against the world.

†**[Moffatt-NT 1917]** For whatever is born of God conquers the world. Our faith, that is the conquest which conquers the world.

**[NLT]** For every child of God defeats this evil world, and we achieve this victory through our faith.

**[PHILLIPS]** In fact, this faith of ours is the only way in which the world can be conquered.

**[WE]** Everyone who is God's child wins a victory over the world. We win because we believe God.

†**[Wuest-NT]** because everything that has been born of God is constantly coming off victorious over the world. And this is the victory that has come off victorious over the world, our faith.

## 3 John 2

**[KJV]** Beloved, I wish above all things that thou mayest prosper and be in health, even as thy soul prospereth.

**[AMPC]** Beloved, I pray that you may prosper in every way and [that your body] may keep well, even as [I know] your soul keeps well *and* prospers.

†**[Douay-Rheims]** Dearly beloved, concerning all things I make it my prayer that thou mayest proceed prosperously, and fare well as thy soul doth prosperously.

**[ERV]** My dear friend, I know that you are doing well spiritually. So I pray that everything else is going well with you and that you are enjoying good health.

**[ISV]** Dear friend, I pray that you are doing well in every way and that you are healthy, just as your soul is healthy.

**[NLT]** Dear friend, I hope all is well with you and that you are as healthy in body as you are strong in spirit.

**[NLV]** Dear friend, I pray that you are doing well in every way. I pray that your body is strong and well even as your soul is.

†**[T4T]** Dear friend, I ask God that things may go well for you in every way, specifically, that you will be physically healthy just like you are spiritually healthy.

†**[Wade]** Beloved friend, I pray that all may go well with you materially, and especially that you may keep in good health, just as it goes well with your soul spiritually.

## IN CONCLUSION

It is my prayer that as you journeyed through the pages of this book with me, you have found clarity on healing as your redemptive right and why some are healed and others are not. If you are among those who are awaiting a manifestation of healing, take courage from what you have read and continue to fight the good fight of faith (*see* 1 Timothy 6:12). My desire is that you have discovered what Christ's redemptive work has secured for you and that you have found practical steps to guide you from your current circumstances into the wholeness and wellness that Jesus secured through His sacrifice on the Cross.

One personal request: If this book has helped you, would you please share it with others who also need to understand what rightfully belongs to them due to the profound sacrifice of Jesus' death on the Cross and His triumphant resurrection? We are all called to be overcomers, and that blessing includes living above the curse of disease, illness, and sickness.

Lastly, let us never forget God's intentions for us clearly articulated in Third John 2. According to the *RIV* (*Renner Interpretive Version*), this verse reminds us:

> **My dearly loved brothers, it is my strongest desire that you prosper in every way that concerns you — and that you not only have enough money to pay your basic bills, but enough to really enjoy yourselves on every road of life you take, *and* that you be healthy, in good, physical working order, sound physically in every way — and that includes being blessed with good mental health.**

Scan the QR code to watch Rick teach more on this subject.

# ENDNOTES

## Chapter 1

[1] Don Chapman, "The Story Behind: Just As I Am," hymncharts.com, https://www.hymncharts.com/the-story-behind-just-as-i-am. Accessed October 6, 2025; "Just as I Am, Without One Plea," Hymnary.org, https://hymnary.org/text/just_as_i_am_without_one_plea. Accessed October 6, 2025.

[2] "How Great Thou Art," Hymnary.org, https://hymnary.org/text/o_lord_my_god_when_i_in_awesome_wonder. Accessed October 6, 2025.

## Chapter 2

[1] Rabbi Joseph Telushkin, *A Code of Jewish Ethics, Volume 1: You Shall Be Holy* (New York, NY: Bell Tower, 2006) p. 458.

## Chapter 3

[1] Richard Barker, "Ignorance is Bliss — Meaning, Origin & Usage," History of English, February 5, 2025, https://www.thehistoryofenglish.com/ignorance-is-bliss-meaning-origin-usage. Accessed November 4, 2025.

## Chapter 4

[1] Steven Teske, "Cuban Refugee Crisis," CALS: Encyclopedia of Arkansas, March 19, 2025, https://encyclopediaofarkansas.net/entries/cuban-refugee-crisis-4248/. Accessed September 23, 2025.

[2] Herodotus, "THE HISTORY OF HERODOTUS" [Note: Sardis account referenced in Book I, Section 84], Translated into English by G. C. Macaulay, Gutenberg.org, https://www.gutenberg.org/files/2707/2707-h/2707-h.htm#link2H_4_0004. Accessed September 24, 2025.

**Chapter 5**

[1] "Consequences of Obesity," CDC: U.S. Centers for Disease Control and Prevention, March 7, 2025, https://www.cdc.gov/obesity/php/about/consequences.html. Accessed December 5, 2025.

**Chapter 6**

[1] Cristian Vasile, "Mental health and immunity (Review)," National Library of Medicine, October 14, 2020, https://pmc.ncbi.nlm.nih.gov/articles/PMC7604758/. Accessed December 5, 2025; "PSYCHONEUROIMMUNOLOGY: THE STUDY OF MIND-BODY INTERACTIONS," Immunize Nevada, September 27, 2024, https://immunizenevada.org/psychoneuroimmunology-the-study-of-mind-body-interactions/. Accessed December 5, 2025.

[2] Nikki Seay and Allan Schwartz, Ph.D, "How Resentment Harms Mental Health," MentalHealth.com, May 25, 2025, https://www.mentalhealth.com/library/resentment-like-holding-onto-hot-coals. Accessed October 2, 2025; "How does holding a grudge affect your health?" Piedmont.org, https://www.piedmont.org/living-real-change/how-does-holding-a-grudge-affect-your-health. Accessed October 2, 2025.

[3] "Forgiveness: Letting go of grudges and bitterness," Mayo Clinic, November 22, 2022, https://www.mayoclinic.org/healthy-lifestyle/adult-health/in-depth/forgiveness/art-20047692. Accessed October 1, 2025; Nikki Seay and Allan Schwartz, Ph.D, "How Resentment Harms Mental Health," MentalHealth.com, May 25, 2025, https://www.mentalhealth.com/library/resentment-like-holding-onto-hot-coals. Accessed October 2, 2025; "How does holding a grudge affect your health?" Piedmont.org, https://www.piedmont.org/living-real-change/how-does-holding-a-grudge-affect-your-health. Accessed October 2, 2025.

[4] "Why Jesus compared unforgiveness to the Sycamine Tree," Aledo Times Record, April4, 2013, https://www.aledotimesrecord.com/story/news/columns/2013/04/04/why-jesus-compared-unforgiveness-to/48983392007/. Accessed October 2, 2025.

[5] Ibid.

[6] Ibid.

[7] Ibid.

**Chapter 7**

[1] Rick Renner, *No Room for Compromise: Christ's Message to Today's Church*, (Shippensburg, PA: Harrison House, 2022) pp. 278-290.

[2] "Anxiety disorders," Mayo Clinic, July 29, 2025, https://www.mayoclinic.org/diseases-conditions/anxiety/symptoms-causes/syc-20350961. Accessed October 24, 2025; Alyssa, "Short Term and Long Term Effects of Anxiety," Banyan Treatment Center, https://mentalhealth.banyantreatmentcenter.com/blog/short-and-long-term-effects-of-anxiety-on-the-body. Accessed October 24, 2025; Kristeen Cherney, "Effects of Anxiety on the Body," healthline.com, November 13, 2023, https://www.healthline.com/health/anxiety/effects-on-body. Accessed October 24, 2025.

[3] "Stress & Autoimmune Disease: Navigating the Complex Relationship," Global Autoimmune Institute, https://www.autoimmuneinstitute.org/articles/stress-autoimmune-disease-navigating-the-complex-relationship/. Accessed October 24, 2025; "How Chronic Stress Impacts the Immune System," Supportive Care, April 25, 2025, https://www.thesupportivecare.com/blog/how-chronic-stress-impacts-the-immune-system. Accessed November 4, 2025.

**Chapter 8**

[1] Yohanan Petrovsky-Shtern, "Demons," The YIVO Encyclopedia of Jews in Eastern Europe, https://encyclopedia.yivo.org/article/2093. Accessed October 31, 2025.

[2] Ibid.

[3] "The Octavius 26 — The Ante-Nicene Fathers Volume IV: The Fathers of the Third Century by Philip Schaff," Church Writings, https://churchwritings.com/reader/minucius-felix-the-octavius?lang=en&ver=0&pos=26-1-1. Accessed October 31, 2025.

[4] "The Octavius 27 — The Ante-Nicene Fathers Volume IV: The Fathers of the Third Century by Philip Schaff," Church Writings, https://churchwritings.com/reader/minucius-felix-the-octavius?lang=en&ver=0&pos=27-1-1. Accessed October 31, 2025.

[5] "On the Opposing Powers.," Origen De Principiis — Origen, Bible Hub, https://biblehub.com/library/origen/origen_de_principiis/chapter_ii_on_the_opposing_powers.htm. Accessed October 31, 2025.
[6] "Origen. Contra Celsus: BOOK VII. CHAP. LXX.," Early Christian Writings, https://www.earlychristianwritings.com/text/origen167.html. Accessed October 31, 2025.
[7] "Contra Celsum, Book IV: Chapter 92," Translated by Frederick Crombie, NewAdvent.org, https://www.newadvent.org/fathers/04164.htm. Accessed October 31, 2025.
[8] "Divine Institutes, Book II (Of the Origin of Error): Chapter 15," Translated by William Fletcher, NewAdvent.org, https://www.newadvent.org/fathers/07012.htm. Accessed October 31, 2025.
[9] "Divine Institutes, Book II (Of the Origin of Error): Chapter 16," Translated by William Fletcher, NewAdvent.org, https://www.newadvent.org/fathers/07012.htm. Accessed October 31, 2025.
[10] "Origen. Contra Celsus: BOOK VIII. CHAP. XXXIV.," Early Christian Writings, https://www.earlychristianwritings.com/text/origen168.html. Accessed November 3, 2025.
[11] "Contra Celsum, Book III: Chapter 36," Translated by Frederick Crombie, NewAdvent.org, https://www.newadvent.org/fathers/04163.htm. Accessed November 3, 2025.
[12] "On the Mission of the Seventy Disciples, and Christ's Charge to them Precedents Drawn from the Old Testament. Absurdity of Supposing that Marcion's Christ could Have," The Five Books Against Marcion — Tertullian, Bible Hub, https://biblehub.com/library/tertullian/the_five_books_against_marcion/chapter_xxiv_on_the_mission_of.htm. Accessed November 4, 2025.
[13] Mike Greenberg, PhD, "Selene: The Goddess of the Moon," Mythology Source, July 15, 2020, https://mythologysource.com/selene-greek-goddess/. Accessed November 4, 2025; Liana Miate, "Selene," World History Encyclopedia, January 23, 2023, https://www.worldhistory.org/Selene/. Accessed December 5, 2025.
[14] Ibid.

## Chapter 9

[1] "Redeemed, How I Love to Proclaim It!" Hymnary.org, https://hymnary.org/text/redeemed_how_i_love_to_proclaim_it. Accessed November 4, 2025.
[2] "PRICE OF SLAVES IN ANCIENT ROME," Imperium Romanum, October 31, 2021, https://imperiumromanum.pl/en/curiosities/price-of-slaves-in-ancient-rome/. Accessed November 5, 2025.
[3] James McPherson, "A Brief Overview of the American Civil War," American Battlefield Trust, November 29, 2023, https://www.battlefields.org/learn/articles/brief-overview-american-civil-war. Accessed November 5, 2025.
[4] "Transcript of the Proclamation," National Archives, https://www.archives.gov/exhibits/featured-documents/emancipation-proclamation/transcript.html. Accessed November 5, 2025.
[5] Ibid.
[6] "13th Amendment to the U.S. Constitution: Abolition of Slavery (1865)," National Archives, https://www.archives.gov/milestone-documents/13th-amendment. Accessed November 5, 2025.

## Chapter 10

[1] "Church History (Book IV), Chapter 15. Under Verus, Polycarp with Others suffered Martyrdom at Smyrna.," Translated by Arthur Cushman McGiffert, NewAdvent.org, https://www.newadvent.org/fathers/250104.htm. Accessed October 17, 2024.

## Chapter 12

[1] Palanikumar Balasundaram and Prathipa Santhanam, "Eating Disorders," National Library of Medicine, June 26, 2023, https://www.ncbi.nlm.nih.gov/books/NBK567717/. Accessed November 25, 2025.
[2] "What are Eating Disorders?" American Psychiatric Association, https://www.psychiatry.org/patients-families/eating-disorders/what-are-eating-disorders. Accessed November 25, 2025.

[3] "Exercise: 7 benefits of regular physical activity," Mayo Clinic, August 26, 2023, https://www.mayoclinic.org/healthy-lifestyle/fitness/in-depth/exercise/art-20048389. Accessed November 26, 2025.
[4] "Iatrophobia (Fear of Doctors)," Cleveland Clinic, https://my.clevelandclinic.org/health/diseases/22191-iatrophobia-fear-of-doctors. Accessed December 1, 2025.

**Chapter 13**

[1] "Trends in health care spending," American Medical Association, April 17, 2025, https://www.ama-assn.org/about/ama-research/trends-health-care-spending. Accessed December 2, 2025.
[2] Erin Woulfe, "Federal Health Care Spending Hits $1.9 Trillion in FY 2024," National Insurance Services, March 20, 2025, https://blog.nisbenefits.com/federal-health-care-spending-fy-2024. Accessed December 2, 2025.
[3] "A surprising key to healthy aging: Strong social connections," Mayo Clinic, March 15, 2024, https://mcpress.mayoclinic.org/healthy-aging/a-surprising-key-to-healthy-aging-strong-social-connections/. Accessed December 2, 2025; "Social connection linked to improved health and reduced risk of early death," World Health Organization, June 30, 2025, https://www.who.int/news/item/30-06-2025-social-connection-linked-to-improved-heath-and-reduced-risk-of-early-death. Accessed December 2, 2025.
[4] Nina Avramova, "Friends and family may help Italians live healthier and longer," CNN, May 9, 2019, https://www.cnn.com/2019/05/09/health/social-connections-health-benefits-intl/index.html. Accessed December 2, 2025.
[5] "Social isolation, loneliness in older people pose health risks," Alzheimers.gov, https://www.alzheimers.gov/news/social-isolation-loneliness-older-people-pose-health-risks#. Accessed December 2, 2025.
[6] "What Happens When We Sleep?" BetterNight, August 23, 2022, https://betternight.com/news/what-happens-when-we-sleep. Accessed December 2, 2025; Kirsten Nunez, Karen Lamoreux, "What Is the Purpose of Sleep?" Healthline, August 9, 2024, https://www.healthline.com/health/why-do-we-sleep. Accessed December 2, 2025.

[7] Tae Won Kim, Jong-Hyun Jeong, Seung-Chul Hong, "The Impact of Sleep and Circadian Disturbance on Hormones and Metabolism," National Library of Medicine, International Journal of Endocrinology, March 11, 2015, https://pmc.ncbi.nlm.nih.gov/articles/PMC4377487/. Accessed December 2, 2025; "New study helps explain links between sleep loss and diabetes," UChicago Medicine, February 19, 2015, https://www.uchicagomedicine.org/forefront/news/new-study-helps-explain-links-between-sleep-loss-and-diabetes. Accessed December 2, 2025.

[8] ALZRA, "What You Should Know About Alzheimer's And Type 3 Diabetes?" Alzheimer's Research Association, August 15, 2022, https://www.alzra.org/blog/what-you-should-know-about-alzheimers-and-type-3-diabetes/. Accessed December 2, 2025.

[9] Ibid.

[10] Ibid.

[11] Stephanie Booth, "Type 3 Diabetes and Alzheimer's: What to Know," WebMD.com, November 14, 2024, https://www.webmd.com/diabetes/alzheimers-diabetes-link. Accessed December 2, 2025.

[12] Zoe Caplan, "U.S. Older Population Grew From 2010 to 2020 at Fastest Rate Since 1880 to 1890," United States Census Bureau, May 25, 2023, https://www.census.gov/library/stories/2023/05/2020-census-united-states-older-population-grew.html. Accessed December 2, 2025.

[13] Jean-Marie Robine, Sarah Cubaynes, "Worldwide demography of centenarians," National Library of Medicine, March 16, 2017, https://pubmed.ncbi.nlm.nih.gov/28315698/. Accessed December 2, 2025.

[14] Bill Gifford, "How Old Can Humans Get?", ScientificAmerican.com, July 31, 2023, https://www.scientificamerican.com/article/how-old-can-humans-get/. Accessed December 3, 2025; Victoria Burrows, "Can we live to be 1,000 years old? How science is on a mission to slow ageing and extend the human lifespan", South China Morning Post, March 15, 2020, https://www.scmp.com/magazines/style/well-being/article/3075102/can-we-live-be-1000-years-old-how-science-mission-slow. Accessed December 3, 2025.

[15] Marika Price Spitulski, "Never Too Old to Succeed: Inspiring People Who Achieved Great Things Later in Life," Nice News, May 20, 2023, https://nicenews.com/culture/people-achieved-great-things-later-life/. Accessed December 4, 2025; List25 Team, "25 Oldest People To Accomplish Amazing Feats," List25.com, July 19, 2024, https://list25.com/25-oldest-people-to-accomplish-amazing-feats/. Accessed December 4, 2025; "Oldest person to begin primary school," Guinness World Records, January 12, 2004, https://www.guinnessworldrecords.com/world-records/oldest-person-to-begin-primary-school. Accessed December 4, 2025.

[16] List25 Team, "25 Oldest People To Accomplish Amazing Feats," List25.com, July 19, 2024, https://list25.com/25-oldest-people-to-accomplish-amazing-feats/. Accessed December 4, 2025; "Oldest person to obtain a pilot's licence," Guinness World Records, September 1, 2010, https://www.guinnessworldrecords.com/world-records/oldest-person-to-obtain-a-pilots-licence. Accessed December 4, 2025.

[17] List25 Team, "25 Oldest People To Accomplish Amazing Feats," List25.com, July 19, 2024, https://list25.com/25-oldest-people-to-accomplish-amazing-feats/. Accessed December 4, 2025; "Dr. Leila Alice Daughtry Denmark," NIH: U.S. National Library of Medicine, June 3, 2015, https://cfmedicine.nlm.nih.gov/physicians/biography_78.html. Accessed December 4, 2025; Martin Childs, "Leila Denmark: Doctor whose work led to the whooping cough vaccine and who worked till 103," The-Independent.com, April 13, 2012, https://www.the-independent.com/news/obituaries/leila-denmark-doctor-whose-work-led-to-the-whooping-cough-vaccine-and-who-worked-till-103-7643878.html. Accessed December 4, 2025.

**Chapter 14**

[1] "CLEMENT OF ROME, First Epistle," Translated by J.B. Lightfoot, Early Christian Writings, https://www.earlychristianwritings.com/text/1clement-lightfoot.html. Accessed December 5, 2025.

[2] "De Viris Illustribus (On Illustrious Men)," Translated by Ernest Cushing Richardson, New Advent, https://www.newadvent.org/fathers/2708.htm. Accessed December 5, 2025.

[3] Rick Renner, *No Room for Compromise: Christ's Message to Today's Church*, (Shippensburg, PA: Harrison House, 2022) p. 180; "New Discoveries Relating to the Apostle Paul," Associates for Biblical Research, https://www.biblearchaeology.org/research/new-testament-era/4117-New-Discoveries-Relating-to-the-Apostle-Paul. Accessed December 5, 2025; David Farley, "Visiting St. Paul Outside the Walls: Rome's Hidden Basilica," WalksofItaly.com, February 5, 2025, https://www.walksofitaly.com/blog/travel-tips/st-paul-outside-the-walls. Accessed December 5, 2025.

**Chapter 15**

[1]References marked with this symbol † were taken from Dr. Chip Beaulieu, *Our Healing Covenant* (Charlestown, IN, Rock House Publishing, 2021). Used by permission.

# BIBLIOGRAPHY

**[RIV]** Scriptures quoted from the Renner Interpretive Version ® (RIV) copyrighted © 2020, 2024 by Teaching You Can Trust, LLC, and published by Harrison House Publishers. Used by permission. Renner.org. Harrisonhouse.com.

**[AMPC]** Scripture quotations marked (AMPC) are taken from the Amplified® Bible, Classic Edition. Copyright © 1954, 1958, 1962, 1964, 1965, 1987 by The Lockman Foundation. Used by permission. www.Lockman.org.

† **[Anchor]** McKenzie, John L. *The Anchor Bible – Second Isaiah*. Copyright © 1969 by Doubleday & Company, Inc. All Rights Reserved. 1st edition volume 20. Garden City New York: Doubleday & Company, Inc.

**[ASV]** American Standard Version, © 1901. Public Domain.

† **[Authentic-NT]** – Schonfield, Hugh J. *The Authentic New Testament*. Copyright © 1956 by Hugh J. Schonfield. London: Dennis Dobson Ltd.

† **[Barclay-NT]** – Barclay, Williams. *The New Testament, A New Translation*. London, New York: Collins, © 1968.

† **[Beck]** – Beck, William Fred *The Holy Bible – An American Translation* Copyright © 1976 by Mrs. William F. Beck. Used by permission.

† **[Bowes-NT]** – Bowes, John. *The New Testament Translated from the Purest Greek*. Copyright © 1870. Dundee.

† **[BrownKrueger]** – Brown, David L.; Krueger, James. *Geneva Bible - The Pilgrim's Bible*. Copyright © 2001 & 2005.

† **[BV-KJV-NT]** – Geide, Ray. *Breakthrough Version*. BREAKTHROUGH VERSION™, BV™ Copyright © 2018 by Ray Geide. Used by permission. All rights reserved worldwide. breakthroughversion.com. version 3.3.3. Breakthrough Version Publishing.

† **[BV-NT]** – Geide, Ray. *Breakthrough Version.* BREAKTHROUGH VERSION™, BV™ Copyright © 2018 by Ray Geide. Used by permission. All rights reserved worldwide. breakthroughversion.com. version 3.3.3. Breakthrough Version Publishing.

**[CEB]** *Scripture quotations from the COMMON ENGLISH BIBLE. © Copyright 2011. COMMON ENGLISH BIBLE. All rights reserved. Used by permission.*
**[CEV]** Scripture quotations marked (CEV) are from the Contemporary English Version Copyright © 1991, 1992, 1995 by American Bible Society. Used by Permission.

**[CJB]** Taken from the Complete Jewish Bible by David H. Stern. Copyright © 1998. All rights reserved. Used by permission of Messianic Jewish Publishers, 6120 Day Long Lane, Clarksville, MD 21029. www.messianicjewish.net.

† **[Condon-Mk]** – Schmid, Josef; Condon, Kevin. *The Gospel According to Mark.* Copyright © 1968. Cork: The Mercier Press.

**[CSB]** Scripture quotations marked CSB have been taken from the Christian Standard Bible®, Copyright © 2017 by Holman Bible Publishers. Used by permission. Christian Standard Bible® and CSB® are federally registered trademarks of Holman Bible Publishers.

† **[CT-OT]** – Rosenberg, A. J. *Judaica Press Prophets and Writings.* English Translation Copyright © Judaica Press. All rights reserved. Chabad.org. Judaica Press.

**[DARBY]** Darby Translation © 1890. Public Domain.

† **[Doddridge-NT]** – Doddridge, Philip. *Family Expositor.* Copyright © 1831. London: Frederick Westley and A. H. Davis.

† **[Douay-Rheims]** – *Douay Rheims Version of the Holy Bible*, Douay Bible House, New York, New York, 1942.

† **[EEBT]** – *EasyEnglish Bible.* Copyright © MissionAssist 2018 – Charitable Incorporated Organisation 1162807 easyenglish.bible. Wycliffe Associates.

**[EHV]** Scripture quotations are from the Holy Bible, Evangelical Heritage Version ® (EHV ®) © 2017 Wartburg Project, Inc. All rights reserved. Used by permission.

† **[Erasmus-NT]** – Erasmus. *Collected Works of Erasmus volume 42. Paraphrases on Romans and Galatians*. Copyright © 1984. University of Toronto Press.

**[ERV]** Scripture quotations are taken from the Holy Bible, Easy-to-Read Version, Copyright © 2006 by Bible League International. All rights reserved.

**[ESV]** Scripture quotations marked (ESV) are from The Holy Bible, English Standard Version. ESV® Text Edition: 2016. Copyright © 2001 by Crossway Bibles, a publishing ministry of Good News Publishers.

† **[Etheridge-NT]** – Etheridge, John Wesley. *New Testament - Acts, Epistles, and Revelation*. Copyright © 1849. London: Longman, Green, Brown, and Longmans.

**[GNT]** Scriptures marked as (GNT) are taken from the Good News Translation - Second Edition © 1992 by American Bible Society. Used by permission.

† **[Goodspeed-NT]** – Goodspeed, Edgar J. *The New Testament: An American Translation*. Copyright © 1923 by The University of Chicago. Used by permission.

† **[Green-NT]** – Green, Thomas Sheldon. *The Twofold New Testament: Being a New Translation Accompanying a Newly Formed Text. In Parallel Columns*. Copyright © 1865. London: Samuel Bagster and Sons.

† **[GT]** – *Galilee Translation*. Public Domain by the Galilee Translation Project.

† **[Guyse-NT]** – Guyse, John. *Exposition of the New Testament in the Form of a Paraphrase*. Copyright © 1739. Edinburg: Ross & Sons.

**[GW]** All Scripture marked with the designation (GW) is taken from GOD'S WORD®. © 1995, 2003, 2013, 2014, 2019, 2020 by God's Word to the Nations Mission Society. Used by permission.

† **[Hammond-NT]** – Hammond, Henry. *Paraphrase and Annotations Upon All Books of the New Testament*. Copyright © 1845. New edition. Oxford: University Press.

† **[Hanson-NT]** – Hanson, John Wesley. *The New Covenant*. Copyright © 1884 (vol. 1), 1885 (vol. 2). Boston and Chicago: The Universalist Publishing House.

† **[Harwood-NT]** – Harwood, Edward. *A Liberal Translation of the New Testament Being an Attempt to translate the Sacred Writings with the Same Freedom, Spirit, and Elegance, with which other English Translations of the Greek Classics have lately been executed: The Design and Scope of each Author being strictly and impartially explored, the True Signification and Force of the Original critically observed, and, as much as possible, transfused into our Language, and the Whole elucidated and explained upon a new and rational Plan: With Select Notes, Critical and Explanatory.* Copyright © 1768. London: Printed for T. Becket and P. A. De Hondt; and J. Johnson, in Paternoster Row; T. Cadell, at Bristol, J. Gore and J. Sibbald, at Liverpool; and T. Bancks, at Warrington.

† **[Haupt]** – Haupt, Paul *The Sacred Books of the Old and New Testament* © 1899 Dodd, Mead, and Company, New York.

† **[Haweis-NT]** – Haweis, Thomas. *A Translation of the New Testament from the Original Greek.* Copyright © 1795. London: T. Chapman.

† **[Heberden-NT]** – Heberden, William. *A Literal Translation of the Apostolic Epistles and Revelation with a Concurrent Commentary.* Copyright © 1839. London: Printed for J. G. & F. Rivington.

† **[HRB]** – Esposito, Don. *Hebraic Roots Bible - A Literal Translation.* © Copyright Word of Truth Publications, 2009, 2012, 2015. 3rd edition.

**[ISV]** Scripture taken from the Holy Bible: International Standard Version®. Copyright © 1996-forever by The ISV Foundation. ALL RIGHTS RESERVED INTERNATIONALLY. Used by permission.

† **[Jerusalem]** – *The Jerusalem Bible* © 1966 by Darton Longman & Todd Ltd and Doubleday and Company Ltd.

† **[JPS-OT 1985]** – JPS. *The Old Testament - JPS 1985.* Copyright © 1985 Jewish Publication Society. All rights reserved. Jps.org. Philadelphia: Jewish Publication Society of America.

† **[JUB]** – *The Jubilee Bible* (from the Scriptures of the Reformation) edited by Russell M. Stendal Copyright © 2000, 2001, 2010.

**[KJV]** *King James Version*, © 1987. Public Domain.

† **[Kneeland-NT]** – Kneeland, Abner. *The New Testament Being the English Only of the Greek and English Testament; Translated from the Original Greek according to Griesbach; upon the basis of the fourth London edition of the Improved Version, with an attempt to further improvements from the translations of Campbell, Wakefield, Scarlett, Macknight, and Thomson.* Copyright © 1823. Philadelphia: Published by the Editor.

† **[Knox]** – Knox, Monsignor Ronald. *The Holy Bible: A Translation from the Latin Vulgate in the Light of the Hebrew and Greek Originals.* Copyright © 1944, 1948, 1950 by Sheed & Ward, Inc., New York. Used by permission.

† **[Mace-NT]** – Mace, Daniel. *New Testament in Greek and English.* Copyright © 1739. London: J. Roberts.

† **[Macknight-NT]** – Macknight, James. *A New Literal Translation, from the Original Greek, of All the Apostolical Epistles.* Copyright © 1835. New Edition. Philadelphia: Desilver, Thomas, and Co. Note: [Macknight-NT] denotes a verse from the translation column while **[Macknight-NTc]** is from the commentary / paraphrase column.

† **[Macrae]** – Macrae, David. *A Revised Translation and Interpretation of the Sacred Scriptures.* Copyright © 1815. Glasgow: R. Hutchinson & Co.

† **[Madsen-NT]** – Madsen, Jon. *The New Testament: A Rendering.* Copyright © 1994 Floris Books. Floris Books.

† **[Magiera-NT]** – Magiera, Janet M. *Aramaic Peshitta New Testament Translation.* Copyright © 2009. Messianic Edition.

† **[MCC-NT]** – Williams, William. *A Modern, Correct, and Close, Translation of the New Testament; with Occasional Observations, and Arranged in Order of Time. With a Special Explanation of the Apocalypse.* Copyright © 1812. London: Printed for John Stockdale, Piccadilly.

† **[MLV]** – Walker, G. Allen. *Holy Bible Modern Literal Version.* Copyright © 2015, G. Allen Walker, co-editor of the MLV. mlvbible.com. CreateSpace Independent Publishing Platform.

† **[Moffatt]** – Moffatt, James A. R. *The Bible, A New Translation.* Copyright © 1922, 1924,1925,1926, 1935 by Harper Collins, San Francisco; copyright © 1950, 1952, 1953, 1954; and copyright © 1994 by Kregel Publications, Grand Rapids, Michigan. Used by permission.

† **[Moffatt-NT 1917]** – Moffatt, James. *The New Testament - A New Translation in Modern Speech.* Copyright © 1917. New Edition Revised. New York: Hodder & Stoughton, George H. Doran Company.

† **[Morgan-NT]** – Morgan, Jonathan. *The New Testament of Our Lord and Saviour Jesus Christ. Translated from the Greek, into Pure English; with Explanatory Notes, on Certain Passages, wherein the Author differs from other translators.* Copyright © 1848. Portland: S. H. Colesworthy; Boston: B. B. Mussey, New-York: P. Price; Philadelphia: J. Gibon, Cincinnati: A. T. Ames; Louisville: Noble and Dean.

† **[MW-NT]** – Gruber, Daniel. *The Messianic Writings.* Copyright © 2011. Daniel Gruber. All Rights reserved under International and Pan-American Copyright Conventions. Elijah Publishing.

**[NCV]** Scripture taken from the New Century Version®. Copyright © 2005 by Thomas Nelson. Used by permission. All rights reserved.

† **[NEB]** – *The New English Bible*, copyright © 1961, 1970 by The Delegates of the Oxford University Press and The Syndics of the Cambridge University Press. Used by permission.

**[NET]** NET Bible® copyright © 1996-2017 by Biblical Studies Press, L.L.C. http://netbible.com. All rights reserved.

**[NIV]** Scripture quotations marked (NIV) are taken from the Holy Bible, New International Version®, NIV® Copyright © 1973, 1978, 1984, 2011 by Biblica, Inc.® Used by permission. All rights reserved worldwide.

† **[NJB]** – *The New Jerusalem Bible.* Copyright © 1985 All Rights Reserved. Doubleday & Company.

**[NLT]** Scripture quotations marked (NLT) are taken from the Holy Bible, New Living Translation, copyright © 1996, 2004, 2015 by Tyndale House

Foundation. Used by permission of Tyndale House Publishers, Inc., Carol Stream, Illinois 60188. All rights reserved.

**[NLV]** Scripture quotations marked NLV are taken from the *New Life Version*, copyright © 1969 and 2003. Used by permission of Barbour Publishing, Inc., Uhrichsville, Ohio 44683. All rights reserved.

† **[Norlie-NT]** – Norlie, Olaf Morgan; Harrison, R. K. *Norlie's Simplified New Testament In Plain English - for Today's Reader. A New Translation from the Greek with The Psalms for Today A New Translation in Current English*, Toronto: Wycliffe College, University of Toronto. Copyright © 1961. Grand Rapids: Zondervan Publishing House.

† **[Original-NT]** – Schonfield, Hugh J. *The Original New Testament*. Copyright © 1985 by Hugh J. Schonfield. All rights reserved. 1st US edition. San Francisco: Harper & Row.

† **[Ottley-Isa]** – Ottley, Richard Rusden. *The Book of Isaiah According to the Septuagint (Codex Alexandrinus)*. Copyright © 1909. Cambridge: at the University Press. -Heb is translation from Hebrew.

† **[Parkhurst-Ps]** – Parkhurst, John. *Literal Translation of the Psalms of David*. Copyright © 1830. London: Samuel Bagster and Sons.

**[PHILLIPS]** Scripture references marked (J.B. Phillips) are taken from The New Testament in Modern English by J.B. Phillips copyright © 1960, 1972 J. B. Phillips. Administered by The Archbishops' Council of the Church of England. Used by Permission.

† **[REB]** – *The Revised English Bible with the Apocrypha*. Copyright © Oxford University Press and Cambridge University Press 1989. Oxford University Press, Cambridge University Press.

† **[Rotherham]** – Rotherham, Joseph Bryant. *Rotherham's Emphasized Bible* (EBR), 1902 – Public Domain.

† **[SAAS-OT]** – *The Orthodox Study Bible*. Scripture taken from the St. Athanasius Academy Septuagint™. Copyright © 2008 by St. Athanasius Academy of

Orthodox Theology. Used by permission. All rights reserved. Thomas Nelson, Inc.

† **[Sacred-NT]** – Campbell, George; Macknight, James; Doddridge, Philip. *The Sacred Writings of the Apostles and Evangelists of Jesus Christ. Commonly Styled the New Testament. Translated from the Original Greek*. Copyright © 1914. St. Louis 16th edition. St. Louis MO: Christian Board of Publication.

† **[Sawyer-7590]** – Sawyer, Leicester Ambrose. *The New Testament, Translated from the Original Greek, with Chronological Arrangement of the Sacred Books, and Improved Divisions of Chapters and Verses*. Copyright © 1861. Revised and Improved, 12th thousand. Boston: Walker, Wise and Company
† **[Sawyer-7590]** – Sawyer, Leicester Ambrose. *The Holy Bible, Containing the Old and New Testaments. Translated and Arranged, with Notes*; Copyright © 1861. vol 2. Boston: Walker, Wise and Company.

† **[SG]** – Smith, J. M. Powis; Goodspeed, Edgar J. *The Complete Bible - An American Translation. The Old Testament translated by J. M. Powis Smith and a Group of Scholars. The Apocrypha and the New Testament translated by Edgar J. Goodspeed* © 1945 University of Chicago Press.

† **[Shuttleworth-NT]** – Shuttleworth, Philip Nicholas. *A Paraphrasic Translation of the Apostolic Epistles, with Notes*. Copyright © 1854. 5th edition. London: Rivingtons.

† **[Slavitt-Ps]** – Slavitt, David R. *Sixty-One Psalms of David*. Copyright © 1996. New York: Oxford University Press.

† **[Spencer-NT]** – Spencer, Francis Aloysius. *The New Testament of Our Lord and Saviour Jesus Christ Translated into English from the Original Greek*. Copyright © 1951. New York: The Macmillan Company.

† **[Stevens-NT]** – Stevens, George Barker. *The Epistles of Paul in Modern English*. Copyright © 1898. New York: Charles Scribner's Sons.

† **[T4T]** – Deibler, Ellis W.; Jr. *A Translation for Translators*. Copyright © 2008-2017 Ellis W. Deibler, Jr. This translation is made available to you under the terms of the Creative Commons Attribution Share-Alike license 4.0.

† **[TCNT]** – *The Twentieth Century New Testament - A Translation into Modern English Made from the Original Greek (Westcott & Hort's Text).* Copyright © 1900, 1901, 1902, 1903, 1904 by Fleming H. Revell Company. Used by permission.

† **[TPT]** – Simmons, Brian. *The Passion Translation.* Scripture quotations marked TPT are from The Passion Translation®. Copyright © 2017 by BroadStreet Publishing® Group, LLC. Used by permission. All rights reserved. ThePassionTranslation.com.

† **[Wade]** – Wade, George Woosung. *Documents of the New Testament.* Copyright © 1934. London: Thomas Murby & Co.

† **[Wand-NT]** – Wand, J. W. C. *The New Testament Letters Prefaced and Paraphrased.* Copyright © 1950 Oxford University Press. 3rd impression. London, New York, Toronto: Oxford University Press (The Epistles).

† **[Way-NT]** – Way, Author Sanders. *The Letters of St. Paul to the Seven Churches and Three Friends with the Letter to the Hebrews.* Copyright © 1906. 2nd edition, revised. London: Macmillan and Co., Limited; New York: The Macmillan Co.

**[WE]** Taken from THE JESUS BOOK - The Bible in Worldwide English. Copyright © 1969, 1971, 1996, 1998 by SOON Educational Publications, Derby DE65 6BN, UK. Used by permission.

**[WEB]** *World English Bible,* ©1901. Public Domain.

† **[Weekes-NT]** – Weekes, Robert Dodd. *The New Dispensation - The New Testament Translated from the Greek.* Copyright © 1897. New York and London: Funk and Wagnalls.

† **[Weymouth-NT]** – Weymouth, Richard Francis. *The New Testament in Modern Speech.* Copyright © 1978 by Kregel Publications. Used by permission.

† **[Williams-NT]** – Williams, Charles Bray. *The New Testament - A Translation in the Language of the People.* Copyright © 1960. Boston: Bruce Humphries, Inc.

† **[Worsley-NT]** – Worsley, John. *New Testament or New Covenant.* Copyright © 1770. London: R. Hett.

† **[WSP-OT]** – Porter, John Scott; Smith, George Vance; Wellbeloved, Charles. *The Holy Scriptures of the Old Covenant in a Revised Translation.* Copyright © 1859. vol 1, © 1861 vol 2, © 1862 vol 3, London: Longman, Brown, Longmans, and Roberts.

† **[Wuest-NT]** – Wuest, Kenneth Samuel. *The New Testament: An Expanded Translation.* Copyright © 1961 by William B. Eerdmans Publishing Co., Grand Rapids, Michigan. Used by permission.

† **[Wycliffe-Noble]** – Noble, Terence P., *Wycliff's NT - Modern Spelling Edition.* Copyright © 2001 All rights reserved. For permission to reproduce significant portions of this book, please contact the publisher.

**[YLT]** – Young, Robert. *Young's Literal Translation of the Holy Bible,* © 1898. Public Domain.

Dear Friend,

If you enjoyed this book and believe others would benefit from reading it, please leave a review on Amazon and recommend it to others — or *consider sharing a copy with a friend or loved one!*

There is a great need for *"teaching you can trust"* among God's people.

Your friend in Christ and for His Gospel,

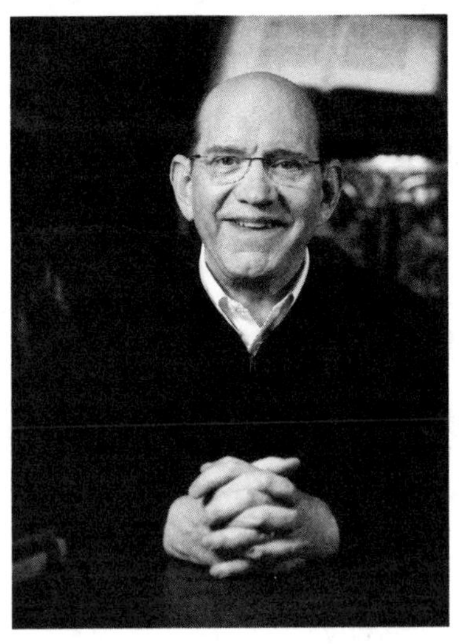

Rick Renner **(renner.org)** holds an earned ThD (Doctor of Theology) from a prominent Russian university and is a respected Bible teacher and leader in the international Christian community. He is the author of an extensive list of books, including best-sellers *Sparkling Gems From the Greek 1* and *2*, and his accumulated titles have sold millions of copies worldwide. Rick's understanding of the Greek language and biblical history opens up the Scriptures in a unique way that enables his audience to gain wisdom and insight while learning something brand new from the Word of God.

Today Rick is the overseer of the Good News Association of Churches, founder of the Moscow Good News Church, pastor of the Internet Good News Church, founder of Media Mir, and president of the Good News Channel — the largest Russian-speaking Christian satellite network in the world, which broadcasts the Gospel 24/7 to countless viewers in more than 83 nations. He is also founder of TBV, a national channel that broadcasts to all of Russia.

Rick is the founder of RENNER Ministries in Broken Arrow, Oklahoma, and host to his TV program, also seen around the world in multiple languages via television, Internet, and satellite. He leads this amazing work with Denise — his wife and life-long ministry partner — along with their sons and committed leadership team.

# CONTACT RENNER MINISTRIES

For further information about RENNER Ministries or to reach out for prayer, please contact the office nearest you or visit the ministry website at:
www.renner.org

**ALL USA CORRESPONDENCE:**
RENNER Ministries
1814 W. Tacoma St.
Broken Arrow, OK 74012
(918) 496-3213
Or 1-800-RICK-593
Email: renner@renner.org
Website: www.renner.org

**CANADA OFFICE:**
P. O. Box 275
Abbotsford, BC V2T 6Z6
Phone: 877-498-3427
Email: information@rickrenner.ca

**MOSCOW OFFICE:**
RENNER Ministries
P. O. Box 789
101000, Moscow, Russia
+7 (495) 727-1467
Email: blagayavestonline@ignc.org
Website: www.ignc.org

**OXFORD OFFICE:**
RENNER Ministries
Box 7, 266 Banbury Road
Oxford OX2 7DL, United Kingdom
+44 1865 521024
Email: europe@renner.org

**RIGA OFFICE:**
RENNER Ministries
Unijas 99
Riga LV-1084, Latvia
+371 67802150
Email: church@goodnews.lv
Website: www.goodnews.lv

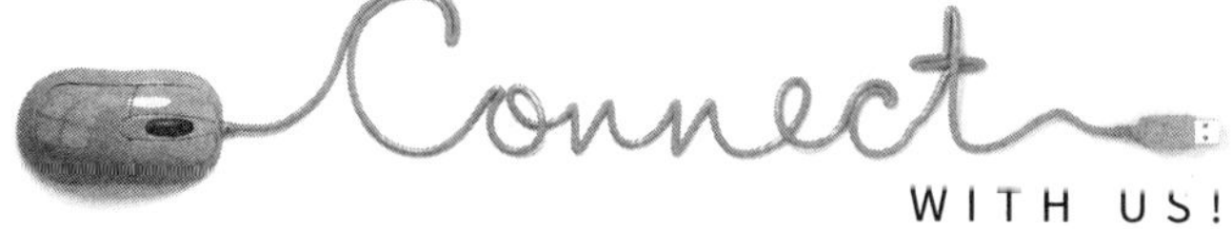


facebook.com/rickrenner • facebook.com/rennerdenise

youtube.com/rennerministries • youtube.com/deniserenner

instagram.com/rickrrenner • instagram.com/rennerministries_
instagram.com/rennerdenise

# BOOKS BY RICK RENNER

Apostles and Prophets
Build Your Foundation*
Chosen by God*
Christmas — The Rest of the Story
Dream Thieves*
Dressed To Kill*
Easter — The Rest of the Story
Fallen Angels, Giants, Monsters, and the World Before the Flood
The Holy Spirit and You*
How To Keep Your Head on Straight in a World Gone Crazy*
How To Receive Answers From Heaven!*
Igniting a Powerful Prayer Life
Insights on Successful Leadership*
Last-Days Survival Guide*
A Life Ablaze*
Life in the Combat Zone*
A Light in Darkness, Volume One,
*Seven Messages to the Seven Churches* series
The Love Test*
My Peace-Filled Day
My Spirit-Empowered Day
My Victory-Filled Day
No Room for Compromise, Volume Two,
*Seven Messages to the Seven Churches* series
Paid in Full*
The Point of No Return*
The Rapture, the Antichrist, and the Tribulation —
An End-Times Countdown and What Happens Next
The Rapture, the Antichrist, and the Tribulation —
An End-Times Countdown and What Happens Next — COMPANION WORKBOOK
Renner A to Z
Comments and Quotes by Rick Renner on 400 Bible Topics A to Z!
Renner Interpretive Version of James and Jude (RIV)
Renner Interpretive Version of First and Second Peter (RIV)
Repentance*
Signs You'll See Just Before Jesus Comes*
Sparkling Gems From the Greek Daily Devotional 1*
Sparkling Gems From the Greek Daily Devotional 2*
Spiritual Weapons To Defeat the Enemy*
Ten Guidelines To Help You Achieve Your Long-Awaited Promotion!*
Testing the Supernatural
365 Days of Increase
365 Days of Power
Turn Your God-Given Dreams Into Reality*
Unlikely — Our Faith-Filled Journey to the Ends of the Earth*
Why We Need the Gifts of the Holy Spirit*
The Will of God — The Key to Your Success*
You Can Get Over It*

*Digital version available for Kindle, Nook, and iBook.
**Note:** Books by Rick Renner are available for purchase at:
**www.renner.org**

# FALLEN ANGELS, GIANTS, MONSTERS, AND THE WORLD BEFORE THE FLOOD

## How the Events of Noah's Ark and the Flood Are Relevant to the End of the Age

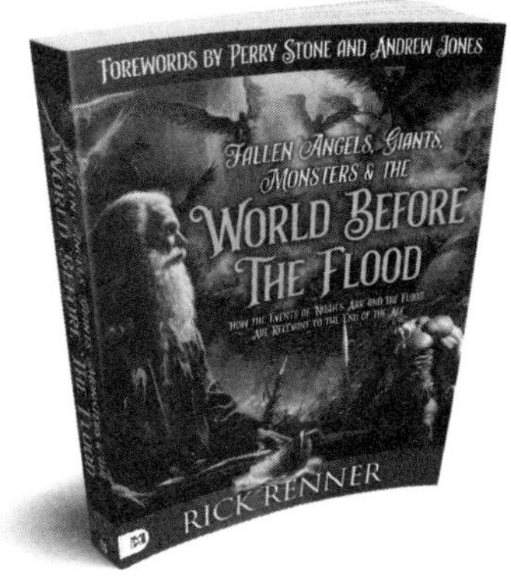


512 pages
(Paperback)

In his book *Fallen Angels, Giants, Monsters, and the World Before the Flood — How the Events of Noah's Ark and the Flood Are Relevant to the End of the Age* — which includes more than 300 photos and illustrations — Rick Renner answers long-held questions about the fascinating story of Noah's Ark.

Presenting Scripture as well as the recordings of early writers, such as Irenaeus, Josephus, Origen, Tertullian, and many others, Rick explains such details as the population explosion on the earth just before the Flood; the likely reason the writings of Enoch survived the Flood; who "the sons of God" and "the daughters of men" in Genesis were; why God ultimately saved only Noah and his family of eight; what happened when they finally exited the Ark; Jesus' own prophecy that certain elements of Noah's day would happen again; *and much, much more!*

Using findings from his own expedition of the remains of Noah's Ark in the Ararat mountains — along with other empirical evidence of the Ark's present location — Rick fascinates readers in this book and helps the Bible *come alive* concerning this favorite childhood story from the Bible!

God has had a plan from the beginning concerning Jesus as "the Seed born of a woman" who would destroy the works Satan wrought in the Fall of man. And just as God has faithfully executed that plan in the past, He will continue to carry it out until Christ's rapture of His Church *and beyond.*

To order, visit us online at: **www.renner.org**

Book resellers: Contact Harrison House at 800-722-6774
or visit **www.HarrisonHouse.com** for quantity discounts.

# SPARKLING GEMS FROM THE GREEK 1

## 365 Greek Word Studies for Every Day of the Year To Sharpen Your Understanding of God's Word

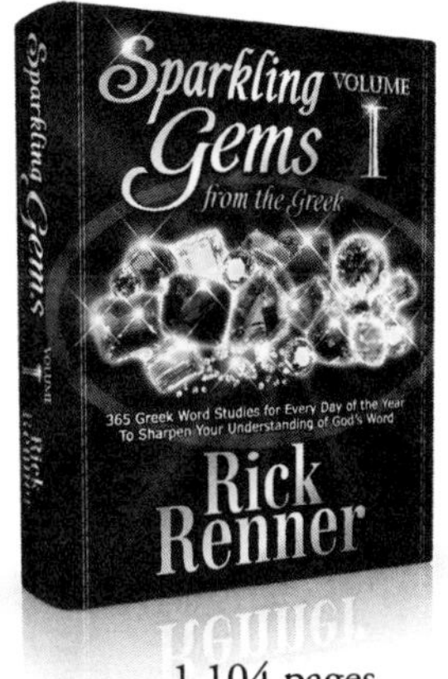


1,104 pages
(Hardback)

Rick Renner's *Sparkling Gems From the Greek 1* has gained widespread recognition for its unique illumination of the New Testament through more than 1,000 Greek word studies in a 365-day devotional format. *Sparkling Gems 1* remains a beloved resource that has spiritually strengthened believers worldwide. As many have testified, the wealth of truths within its pages never grows old. Year after year, *Sparkling Gems 1* continues to deepen readers' understanding of the Bible.

# SPARKLING GEMS FROM THE GREEK 2

## 365 New Gems To Equip and Empower You for Victory Every Day of the Year

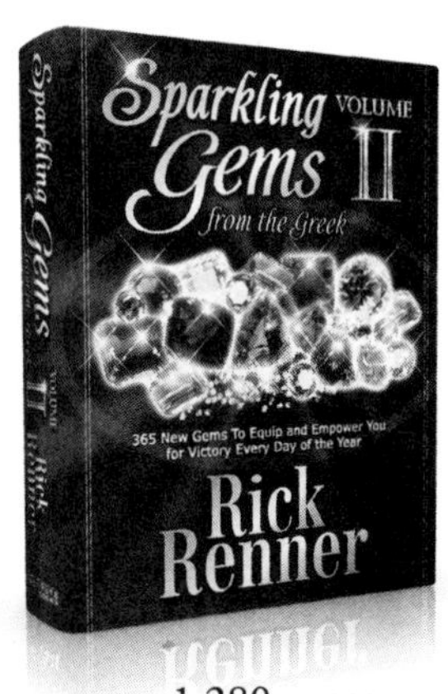


1,280 pages
(Hardback)

Rick infuses into *Sparkling Gems From the Greek 2* the added strength and richness of many more years of his own personal study and growth in God — expanding this devotional series to impact the reader's heart on a deeper level than ever before. This remarkable study tool helps unlock new hidden treasures from God's Word that will draw readers into an ever more passionate pursuit of Him.

To order, visit us online at: **www.renner.org**

Book Resellers: Contact Harrison House at 800-722-6774
or visit **www.HarrisonHouse.com** for quantity discounts.

# DRESSED TO KILL

## A Biblical Approach to Spiritual Warfare and Armor

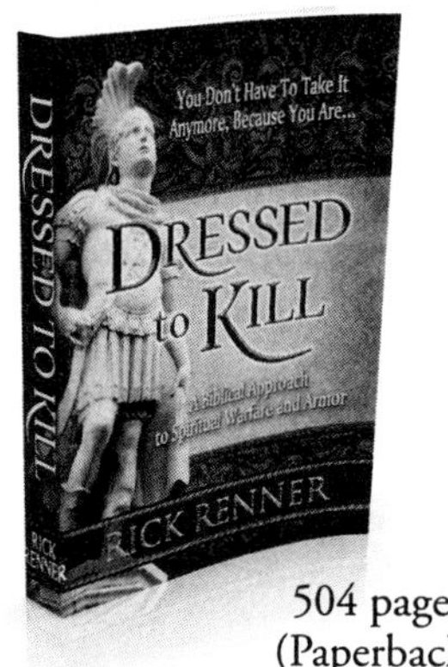


504 pages
(Paperback)

Rick Renner's book *Dressed To Kill* is considered by many to be a true classic on the subject of spiritual warfare. The original version, which sold more than 400,000 copies, is a curriculum staple in Bible schools worldwide. In this beautiful volume, you will find:

- 504 pages of reedited text in paperback
- 16 pages of full-color illustrations
- Questions at the end of each chapter to guide you into deeper study

In *Dressed To Kill*, Rick explains with exacting detail the purpose and function of each piece of Roman armor. In the process, he describes the significance of our *spiritual* armor not only to withstand the onslaughts of the enemy, but also to overturn the tendencies of the carnal mind. Furthermore, Rick delivers a clear, scriptural presentation on the biblical definition of spiritual warfare — what it is and what it is not.

When you walk with God in deliberate, continual fellowship, He will enrobe you with Himself. Armed with the knowledge of who you are in Him, you will be dressed and dangerous to the works of darkness, unflinching in the face of conflict, and fully equipped to take the offensive and gain mastery over any opposition from your spiritual foe. You don't have to accept defeat anymore once you are *dressed to kill*!

To order, visit us online at: **www.renner.org**

Book Resellers: Contact Harrison House at 800-722-6774
or visit **www.HarrisonHouse.com** for quantity discounts.

# CHRISTMAS

## THE REST OF THE STORY

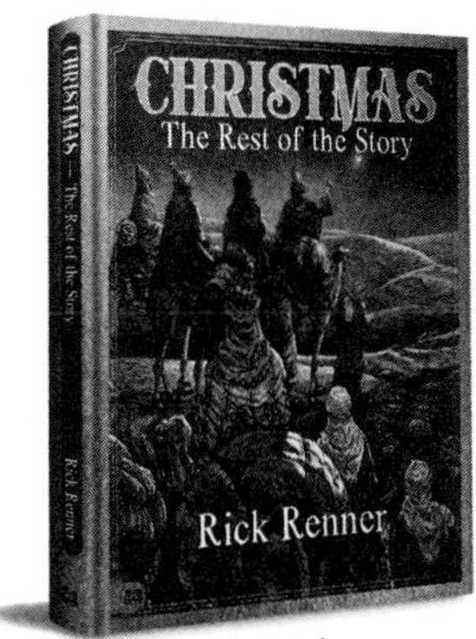


304 pages
(Hardback)

In this storybook of biblical history, Rick takes you on the "magical" journey of Christ's coming to Earth in a way you've probably never heard it before. Featuring full-color, original illustrations, *Christmas — The Rest of the Story* gives the spell-binding account of God's masterful plan to redeem mankind, and vividly portrays the wonder of the Savior's birth and His "ordinary" life marked by God's *extraordinary* plan.

If you want to be taken back in your imagination to this earth-shaking course of events that changed the history of the whole world, this book is a *must-have* not just for the Christmas season, but for all time. *Topics include:*

- Why God chose Mary and Joseph.
- The significance of the *manger* and *swaddling clothes*.
- Why angels viewed *God in the flesh* with such wonderment.
- Why King Herod was so troubled by this historical birth.
- How we can prepare for Christ's *next* coming.

*Christmas — The Rest of the Story* is sure to be a favorite in your family for generations to come! Jesus' birth is truly *the greatest story on earth* — perhaps never more uniquely told than in the pages of this book.

To order, visit us online at: **www.renner.org**
Book Resellers: Contact Harrison House at 800-722-6774
or visit **www.HarrisonHouse.com** for quantity discounts.

# EASTER

## The Rest of the Story

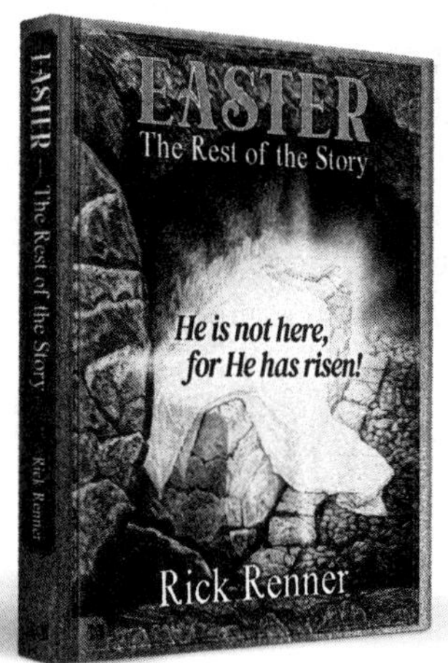


304 pages
(Hardback)

At the moment of Christ's death on the Cross, the day darkened and the earth shook — but what about the days and hours leading up to His crucifixion? What happened in those critical moments, and why did it happen?

In this *must-have* Easter classic, Rick Renner walks you through the pages of history, diving deep into the world's most famous story to reveal the riveting truths and harrowing details of Jesus' last moments on Earth. In this vivid storybook equipped with full-color, original illustrations, you'll learn:

- Why hundreds of soldiers — not just a few — met Jesus to arrest Him.
- The physical and mental abuse Jesus endured before the Crucifixion.
- What Jesus meant when He said, "It is finished!"
- What Jesus has been doing for the last 2,000 years.

Whether you've heard this story before or this is your first time reading it, Jesus' death and resurrection will come alive as you draw face to face with the brutality Jesus endured and the unflinching love He displayed on the Cross.

To order, visit us online at: **www.renner.org**
Book Resellers: Contact Harrison House at 800-722-6774
or visit **www.HarrisonHouse.com** for quantity discounts.

# THE RENNER INTERPRETIVE VERSION (RIV) OF JAMES AND JUDE

## A Parallel Study Bible for People of Faith

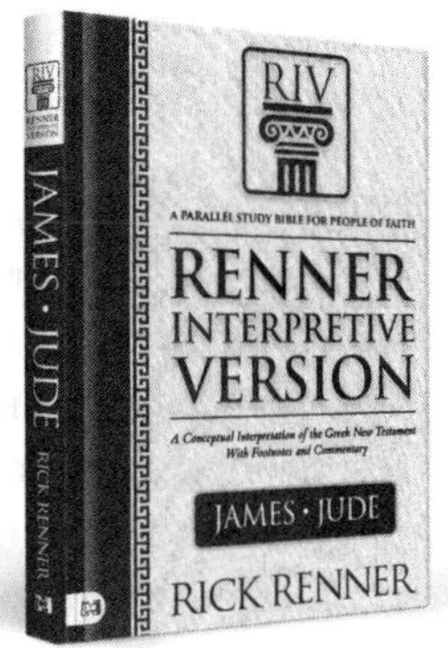


288 pages
(Hardback)

Do you long for deeper insight into your personal study of the Word of God? If so, the *RIV* is for you!

Equipped with footnotes and commentary, the *RIV* will open up the world of the New Testament in a whole new way. While it is not a word-for-word translation — the *RIV* is a conceptual interpretation that draws upon concepts in the Greek language and expresses them in a way that supplies a broader comprehension of Scripture. By bringing out imagery presented in the Greek language and conveying it to readers using contemporary speech, Rick helps draw lovers of the Bible into a deeper study of God's message to people for all time.

This first installment of the *RIV* is taken from the books written by James and Jude. James and Jude were Jesus' half-brothers, younger sons of Joseph and Mary, and in this representation, their Spirit-inspired words will thrill your heart, challenge your thinking, and open the eyes of your spirit in greater ways to see the unchanging nature of God — His wisdom, goodness, power, and love.

To order, visit us online at: **www.renner.org**

Book resellers: Contact Harrison House at 800-722-6774
or visit **www.HarrisonHouse.com** for quantity discounts.

# THE RENNER INTERPRETIVE VERSION (RIV) OF FIRST AND SECOND PETER

## A Parallel Study Bible for People of Faith

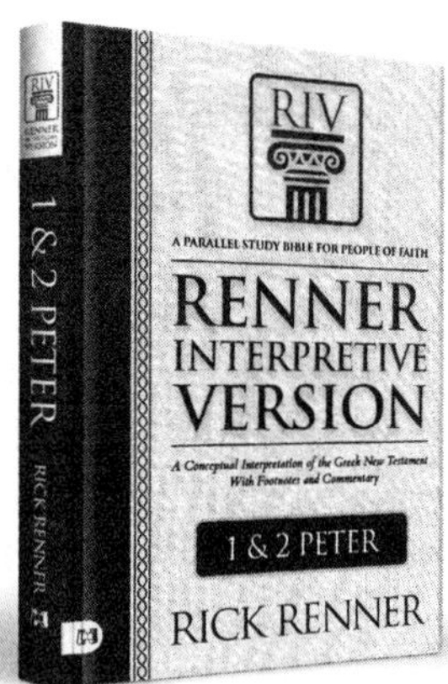


384 pages
(Hardback)

Dive deep into the Greek New Testament with Rick Renner in this brand-new volume of the *RIV*!

In these two power-packed epistles, Peter, an apostle and disciple of Jesus, wrote to the Church imploring believers to live holy lives and endure the persecution and suffering they were facing as a result of their faith, even warning them to remain steadfast as the time for Jesus' return draws near. As Rick expounds upon the original language of the Greek in contemporary speech that is easy to understand, you will learn that Peter's encouragement and warning was not only timely for the Early Church, but offers wisdom for believers facing hardship and deception in today's world as well.

Using the comprehensive footnotes and commentary found on each page, you can study the meaning behind the powerful words Peter wrote. The *RIV* will open the Scriptures like you've never seen them before, encouraging your faith, prompting your obedience, and preparing you for the soon return of our Lord Jesus. This is a volume you do not want to miss!

To order, visit us online at: **www.renner.org**

Book resellers: Contact Harrison House at 800-722-6774
or visit **www.HarrisonHouse.com** for quantity discounts.

# THE RAPTURE, THE ANTICHRIST, AND THE TRIBULATION —

## An End-Times Countdown and What Happens Next

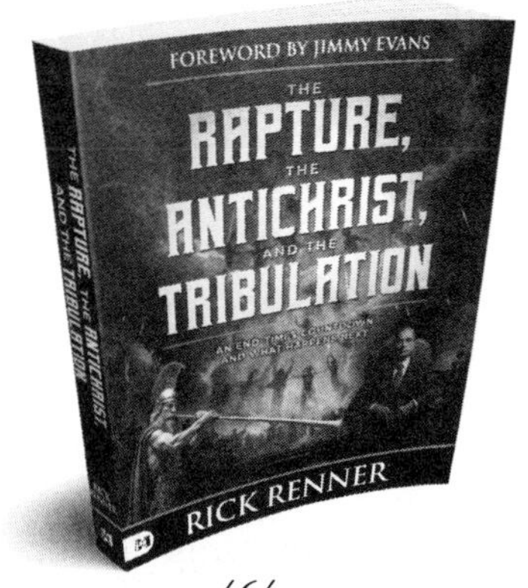


464 pages
(Paperback)

You've likely heard of the Rapture, but have you thought about what happens next? In this book, Rick Renner takes you deep into Scripture to show you that *Christ's rapture of His Church* is the domino-event that will set in motion the next phase of God's prophetic timeline.

The Rapture is the event God's people should desirously anticipate as they prepare to meet Him face to face. But the Rapture, Heaven, and the Marriage Supper of the Lamb are not the end for true believers in Christ, as Rick vividly explains.

In this book, you'll learn:

- The origin of the word "rapture" and every Greek instance of this word in the New Testament.
- How to be prepared for the Rapture in the dark, last hours of time.
- Attributes of the Antichrist and how to avoid contamination by the spirit of the Antichrist that is already in the world.
- Five important differences between *the Rapture* and *the Second Coming*.
- *And much more!*

This *may* be the most comprehensive look at all three topics — the Rapture, the Antichrist, and the Tribulation — you've ever read in just one book!

To order, visit us online at: **www.renner.org**

Book resellers: Contact Harrison House at 800-722-6774
or visit **www.HarrisonHouse.com** for quantity discounts.

# LAST-DAYS SURVIVAL GUIDE

## A Scriptural Handbook To Prepare You for These Perilous Times

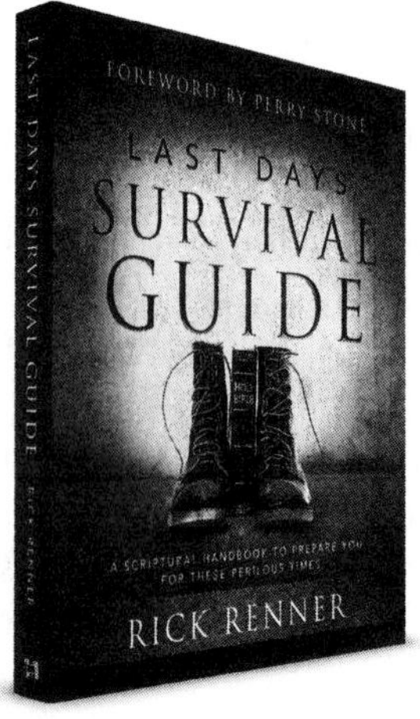


496 pages
(Paperback)

In his book *Last-Days Survival Guide*, Rick Renner masterfully expands on Second Timothy 3 to clearly reveal the last-days signs to expect in society as one age draws to a close before another age begins.

Rick also thoroughly explains how not to just *survive* the times, but to *thrive* in the midst of them. God wants you as a believer to be equipped — *outfitted* — to withstand end-time storms, to navigate wind-tossed seas, and to sail with His grace and power to fulfill your divine destiny on earth!

If you're concerned about what you're witnessing in society today — and even in certain sectors of the Church — the answers you need in order to keep your gaze focused on Christ and maintain your victory are in this book!

To order, visit us online at: **www.renner.org**

Book Resellers: Contact Harrison House at 800-722-6774
or visit **www.HarrisonHouse.com** for quantity discounts.

# PAID IN FULL

## An In-Depth Look at the Defining Moments of Christ's Passion

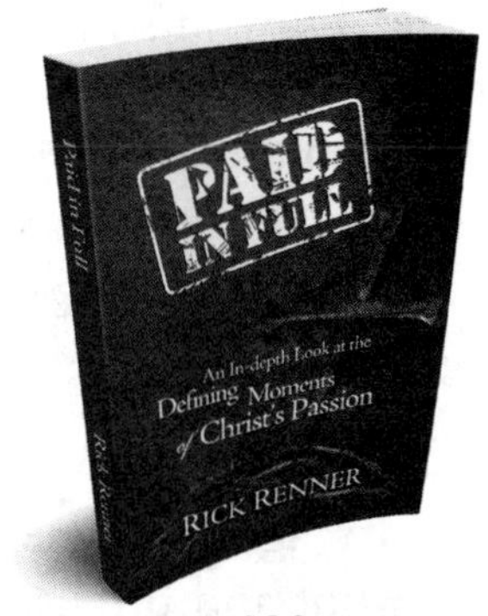


320 pages
(Paperback)

In *Paid in Full: An In-Depth Look at the Defining Moments of Christ's Passion*, Rick Renner offers unforgettable insights into the heart, emotions, and humanity of Jesus in His final days on the earth. Providing a brilliant historical backdrop from his studies of New Testament Greek, Rick guides you on an uncommon journey through each of Christ's encounters along His way from Gethsemane to Golgotha.

Jesus' responses to betrayal and suffering reveal rich, practical applications for our own lives when we're faced with disappointment and pain. As you gain a more intimate glimpse into Jesus' final hours and the great love He displayed, you will be moved in a way you will never forget and will gain more confidence than ever that God's plan for your life will stand!

Your redemption had a price. Discover just how completely that price was *paid in full*!

To order, visit us online at: **www.renner.org**

Book Resellers: Contact Harrison House at 800-722-6774 or visit **www.HarrisonHouse.com** for quantity discounts.

# A LIFE ABLAZE

## Ten Simple Keys to Living on Fire for God

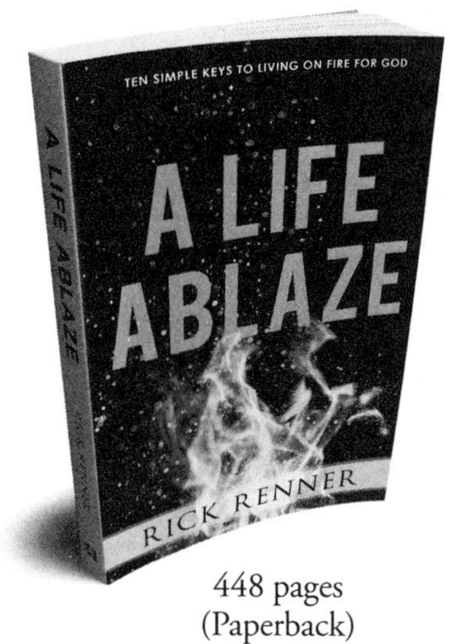


448 pages
(Paperback)

Do you struggle to keep the fire of the Holy Spirit burning in your heart as it may have burned earlier in your life? Do you sometimes feel like all that's left are a few small glowing embers — and that perhaps even those embers are starting to die out and become cold?

How do you stoke the embers of the fire within you so that those flames begin to burn red-hot in your heart again? Once you have that fire burning hot and bright, how do you sustain and grow the intensity of that inner fire for the rest of your time on this earth?

In *A Life Ablaze,* Rick teaches you about the ten different kinds of fuel you need to stay spiritually ablaze for years to come. As you learn about these fuels, you will discover how to throw them into the fire in your heart so you can keep burning spiritually.

Topics include:

- What is the real condition of your spiritual fire right now?
- What to do if your spiritual embers are about to go out.
- What to do to help others whose flames are burning low.

To order, visit us online at: **www.renner.org**

Book Resellers: Contact Harrison House at 800-722-6774
or visit **www.HarrisonHouse.com** for quantity discounts.

# SIGNS YOU'LL SEE JUST BEFORE JESUS COMES

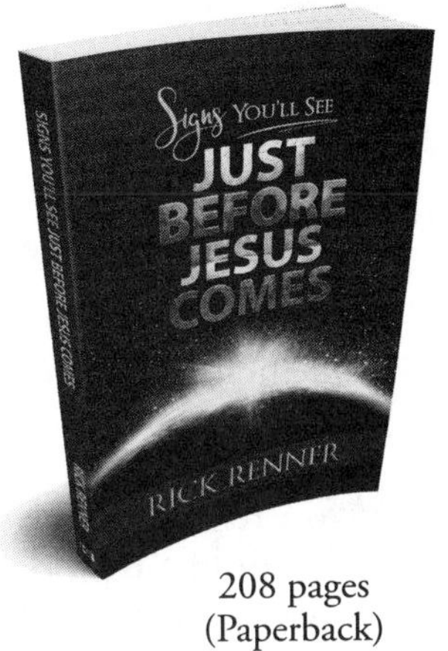


208 pages
(Paperback)

As we advance toward the golden moment of Christ's return for His Church, there are signs on the road we're traveling to let us know where we are in time. Jesus Himself foretold the types of events that will surely take place as we watch for His return.

In his book *Signs You'll See Just Before Jesus Comes*, Rick Renner explores the signs in Matthew 24:3-12, expounding on each one from the Greek text with his unique style of teaching. Each chapter is written to *prepare* and *embolden* a last-days generation of believers — not send them running for the hills!

The signs on the road are appearing closer together. We are on the precipice of something new. Soon we'll see the final sign at the edge of our destination as we enter the territory of the last days, hours, and minutes *just before Jesus comes*.

To order, visit us online at: **www.renner.org**

Book Resellers: Contact Harrison House at 800-722-6774
or visit **www.HarrisonHouse.com** for quantity discounts.

# WHO STOLE CINDERELLA?

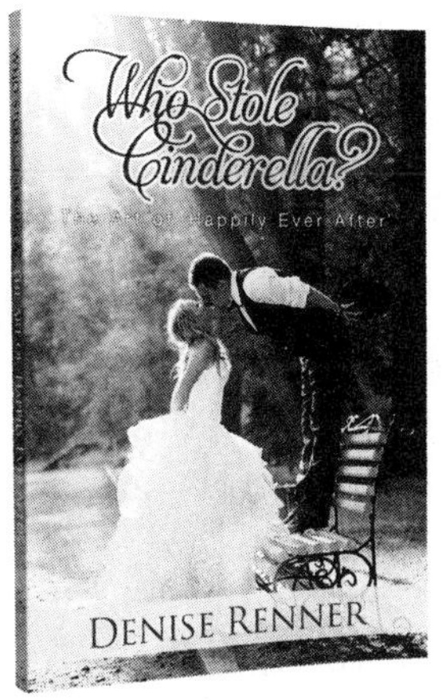


192 pages
(Paperback)

In ***Who Stole Cinderella?***, Denise Renner shows why "happily ever after" is not a gift for a selected few, but rather an art that anyone can master who is willing to learn. With genuine warmth and candor, Denise recounts the journey of her own struggles in marriage and the unique insights she learned along the way to attaining emotional health and happiness. Your life will be enriched by the biblical wisdom Denise imparts and the originality with which she sheds light on your path to *happily ever after* and shows you right where to begin again if you've lost your way.

Even if the clock shows "past midnight" in your marriage, don't give up on your dream of experiencing a happy ending. Cinderella and Prince Charming are not lost — they just need to be rediscovered *God's way*!

"This teaching, like precious pearls, has been obtained by diving into the deep to learn of God and His ways over the course of many years. It is yours for the reading — but believe me when I tell you that it has cost Denise extravagantly."

— Rick Renner

To order, visit us online at: **www.renner.org**

Book Resellers: Contact Harrison House at 800-722-6774 or visit **www.HarrisonHouse.com** for quantity discounts.

# UNSTOPPABLE

## Pressing Through Fear, Offense, and Negative Opinions To Fulfill God's Purpose

### By Denise Renner

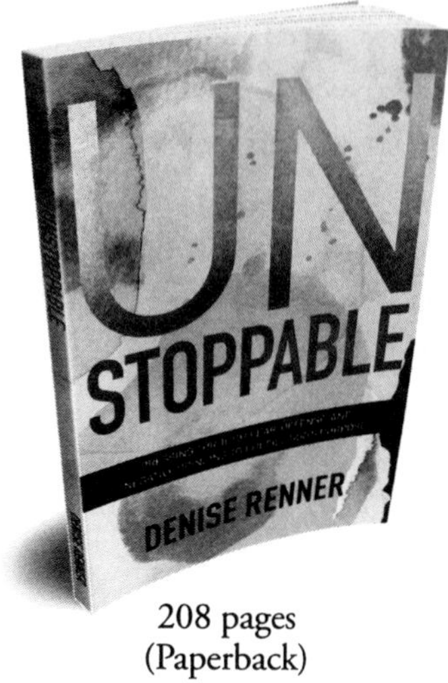


208 pages
(Paperback)

God has given every one of us a unique supply of His Spirit — with individual gifts and callings — that we are to contribute to the Body of Christ and to the plans and purposes of God on earth.

But what stops so many from entering this place of blessing and falling short of fulfilling their God-given destiny? The obstacles are plenteous because the enemy is most threatened when a believer takes his or her place in the perfect will of God. Some of these hindrances include fear, offense, and the negative opinions of others. But the good news is, God has given us power through His Word and His Spirit to overcome every obstacle and to *gloriously* manifest our supply for the blessing and benefit of others.

In her book *Unstoppable,* Denise Renner brings fresh insight from God's Word on how we can overcome key hindrances — whether it's fear of man, rejection, unforgiveness, other people's negative opinions, or even our own poor opinion of ourselves — that the enemy exploits to try to prevent our God-given gifts and talents from being used to bless others.

No one else can take your place; your part is absolutely crucial to God's plan. So don't let anyone or anything stop you from doing what Jesus wants you to do or from receiving what He wants you to receive. This book will help you be *unstoppable* as you push past every obstacle you are facing and keep pressing toward the glorious prize that awaits you in Christ Jesus!

To order, visit us online at: **www.renner.org**

Book Resellers: Contact Harrison House at 800-722-6774
or visit **www.HarrisonHouse.com** for quantity discounts.

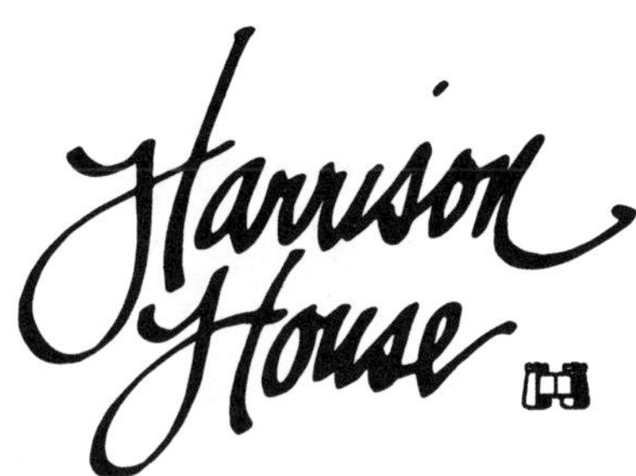

*Equipping Believers to Walk in the Abundant Life*

John 10:10b